DIRECTING AT DISNEY

The Original Directors of Walt's Animated Films

Don Peri
Pete Docter

Foreword by George Lucas

For information address Disney Editions, 77 West 66th Street, New York, New York 10023.

Editorial Director: **Wendy Lefkon**
Senior Editor: **Jennifer Eastwood**
Senior Design Manager: **Winnie Ho**
Senior Designer: **Lindsay Broderick**
Compositor: **Susan Gerber**
Managing Editor: **Monica Vasquez**
Production: **Marybeth Tregarthen**

Cover Image: Walt Disney and director Wilfred Jackson at work on *Alice in Wonderland* in March 1951.

ISBN 978-1-4847-5574-7

FAC-025383-24109

Printed in China

First Hardcover Edition, September 2024

10 9 8 7 6 5 4 3 2 1

Visit www.disneybooks.com

DIRECTING AT DISNEY

The Original Directors of Walt's Animated Films

Don Peri
Pete Docter

Foreword by **George Lucas**

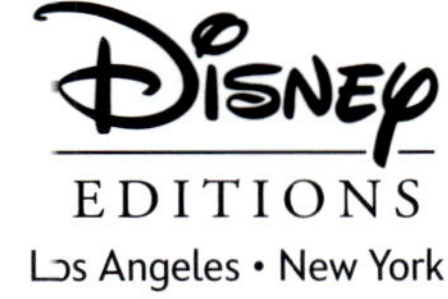

EDITIONS
Los Angeles • New York

This book is dedicated to the many people who worked alongside Walt Disney to make the films we love—and to the people who helped preserve their stories.

And to a man who loved Disney history but could also create art that belonged alongside the best of them, we dedicate this book to Ralph Eggleston.

—D.P. & P.D.

CONTENTS

The Animator's Prayer ix

Foreword by George Lucas x

Introduction xii

PART 1 / 1920–1931 xviii
"There Were No Directors at First"

Chapter 1 6
The Birth of the Disney Director

PART 2 / 1932–1935 18
"Extensions of Walt's Arms"

Chapter 2 22
Burt Gillett—The Man Who Directed *Three Little Pigs*

PART 3 / 1936–1948 42
"We Couldn't Have Done It Without Organization"

Chapter 3 46
Dave Hand—A Man Trapped, the Water Rising

Chapter 4 84
Ben Sharpsteen—The Organization Man

PART 4 / 1949–1961 116
"All of a Sudden, We Had to Grow Up"

Chapter 5 120
Wilfred Jackson—The Musical Man

Chapter 6 148
Ham Luske—A Team Player

Chapter 7 170
Gerry Geronimi—The Fight for Quality

PART 5 / 1936–1957 196
"You Pretty Much Had Full Autonomy"

Chapter 8 200
The Shorts Department—King, Hannah, Nichols, and Kinney

PART 6 / 1962–1973 226
"No Replacement for Walt"

Chapter 9 230
Woolie Reitherman—In the Director's Cockpit

Chapter 10 258
Legacy

Appendix A 269
Listing of All Sequence Directors and Production Supervisors

Appendix B 279
Disney Animated Films by Year and Director

Appendix C 293
Sequences by Director

Appendix D 307
Animation Directors Time Line

Appendix E 315
Dave Hand's 1938 Organization Diagram

Acknowledgments 318

Endnotes 324

Index 340

Selected Bibliography 346

Image Credits 348

THE ANIMATOR'S PRAYER

Our Director, who art above us,
Q! XX! QX! *** ! Q*! X! be Thy name!
Thy pictures Come
They will be done! In color as in black and white.
Give us this day our daily razz
And forgive us our animation,
As we forgive the stories that are written for us.
Lead us not into chase, but deliver us from
The Lay-Out Men.

AYE BEN.

"The Animator's Prayer," author unknown. Printed in the *Mickey Mouse Melodeon: House Organ of the Disney Studios*, Volume 1, Number 4, February 1933, page 5. Edited by Carolyn Shafer (later Churchill).

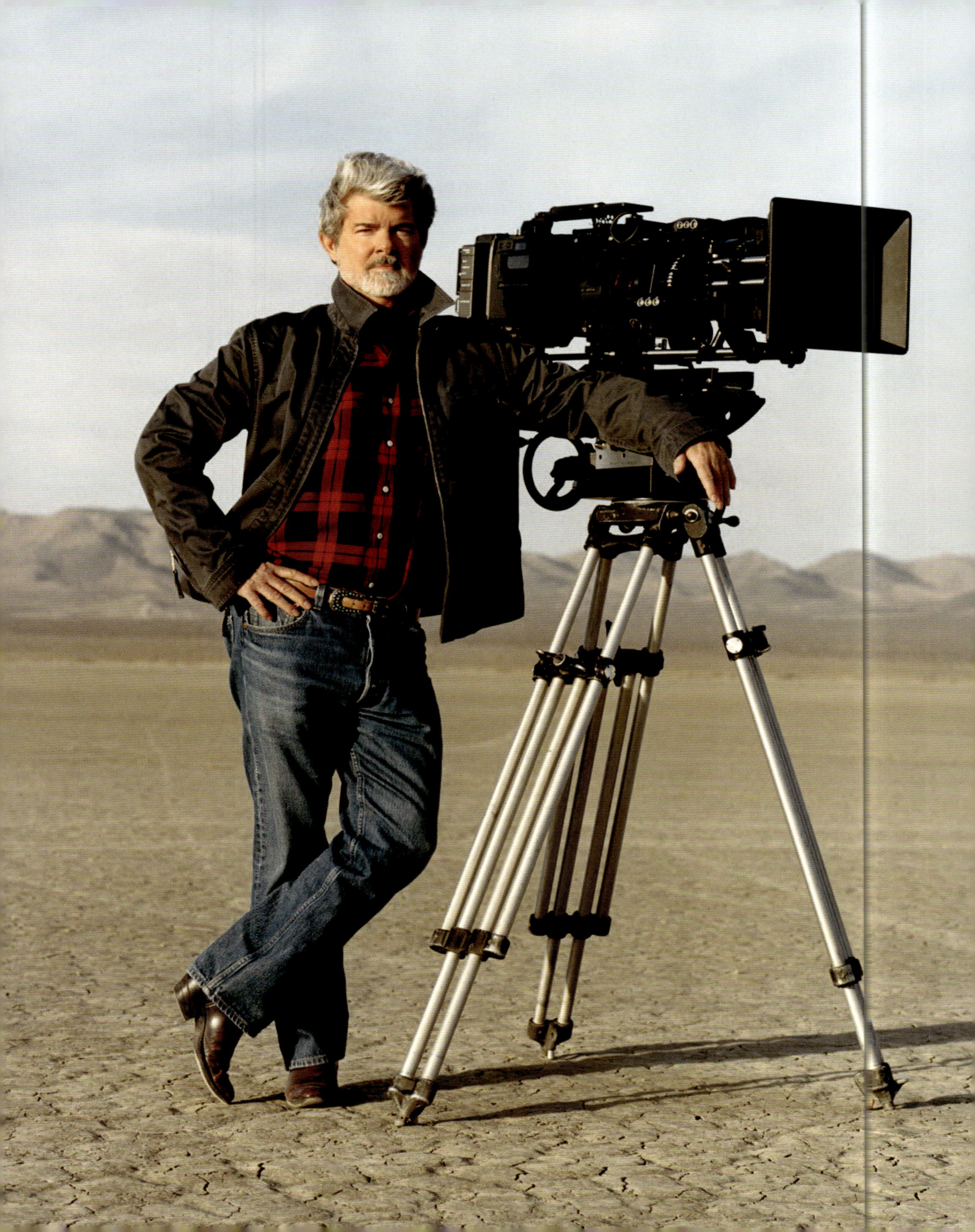

FOREWORD

I never had the opportunity to meet Walt Disney, but he was a hero of mine growing up. I loved his films and was among the first in line to visit Disneyland on the second day of its opening week. That experience filled my eleven-year-old mind with wonder. Walt Disney was the type of innovator and dreamer who comes along once in a lifetime. But as a creative producer, Mr. Disney faced challenges that few people stop to think about.

When I became a film director, it was my job to guide the talented cast and crew of *THX 1138*, *American Graffiti*, and *Star Wars*, focusing our collective creative skills to give form to the outside-the-box concepts of my imagination that would eventually appear on-screen. All my waking hours (and even some of my nonwaking ones) were dedicated to shaping the script, designing, casting, and thousands of other details.

Then, for *The Empire Strikes Back*, I asked Irvin Kershner to direct the film. A strong director, he would take on supervision of many aspects of the production as I had done for *Star Wars*. Yet the storyteller in me still had very specific ideas of what I wanted to see and feel. This presented an interesting challenge: How could I convey the mood, approach, innovation, and intention across every element of a universe I had created . . . for someone else to oversee?

As Lucasfilm grew, I produced films helmed by some of the most talented of directors with strong visions of their own, like Steven Spielberg (the Indiana Jones series), Francis Ford Coppola (*Tucker: The Man and His Dream*), and Ron Howard (*Willow*). Producing multiple projects, I found I still encountered the challenge of finding artistic balance, whether on set, in the editing room, or in making daily production decisions. I like to think that, in partnership with the directors and production teams on these films, I was able to combine our creative strengths to make these projects better.

Reading this book, I recognized the challenges Walt Disney faced on *Snow White and the Seven Dwarfs* and *Pinocchio*—films he didn't direct but clearly led creatively. I empathized as his creative appetite grew and he oversaw multiple projects. Without drawing, writing, or directing the actors and animators, how did Walt Disney manage to get what he wanted on the silver screen?

That is the challenge of the creative producer. And one of the keys to success is finding strong collaborators, like the directors you'll read about in this book.

Finding creative partners with whom you really click is one of the great joys of making movies. I always felt that Steven Spielberg and I had the ability to think along the same narrative lines, to connect through a shared vision of what we were after. When this happens, the trust is there and ideas flow. Everyone contributes within their area of expertise and the movie gets better at every turn.

Though Walt Disney was indeed a singular genius, he obviously recognized this crucial need for trusted associates—people who would not just execute but improve his ideas.

It is through these kinds of partnerships that the very best movies are made.

—George Lucas

INTRODUCTION

PETE Some years ago, I was watching *Peter Pan* with my kids. As Peter, Wendy, Michael, and John leapt off Big Ben and flew over the clouds of London, I thought, *Wow, what a great shot! I wonder who came up with that. Was it the director? Come to think of it, who was the director?* As a huge fan of Disney films and history, I was embarrassed to admit I didn't know.

At the time, I was directing *Up* at Pixar Animation Studios. As with all my directorial efforts, I had come up with the core idea and worked with a small group to craft the story and characters. I worked with writers, guided designers, directed actors, and steered and approved every shot in the film through camera, editorial, animation, effects, lighting, and final sound.

Was this true of directors who had worked with Walt Disney?

My embarrassingly large shelf of Disney books revealed precious few facts—and even scant mention—of directors or their job. Why was this key position so unsung? I knew one person who might know more: my friend and Disney historian Don Peri.

DON I have always been a "who" person, meaning that my interest in Disney has always centered on Walt Disney and the people who worked with and for him. Sure, I have loved the movies, the theme parks, some of the television shows, but I am not an artistic person, so the "how" of making films has been less a focus for me than who made them and their working relationships.

My odyssey through Disney history really took flight fifty years ago when the cover art for a college magazine led to a meeting with Ben Sharpsteen, a retired Disney animator, director, and producer. Ben and I both lived in Northern California, so we easily developed a working relationship: I helped him record his memoirs and he helped me expand my knowledge of Disney history in general and particularly his history and the history of those in his orbit. We worked together for three years, and then I ventured out to conduct many more interviews and to teach courses on Disney history, all the while honing my skills and knowledge. One of my interviews, with director Wilfred Jackson, led to a meeting with director Pete Docter. We shared a love of Disney history, and Pete not only knew the "how" of animation, but also yearned to know more about the "who." This was the beginning of a beautiful friendship.

PETE As Don and I researched and interviewed, we found Disney directors to be a bundle of contradictions. All artists they worked with saw directors as a central and powerful figure in the making of Disney films. But many directors were hated. Several were seen as having "failed up" into their position.

Even the job description was confusing. Some spoke of the role as glorified assistant to Walt, the real director; others spoke of directors being completely in charge, coming up with the concepts and dictating creative choices. We eventually found both to be true; the role changed over time and from project to project.

Ultimately we discovered the directors to be a fascinating insight into Walt himself. As he expanded from personally drawing a handful of short films and advertisements in the early twenties to overseeing shorts, features, television shows, and theme parks in the fifties, Walt developed people and processes that still allowed him to achieve his vision. In many ways, the evolution of the role of the director reflected Disney's own growth as a creative leader.

DON Walt Disney has always fascinated us, inspiring childhood wonder at the stories and worlds he introduced and then the more mature appreciation of the challenges he faced and the innovations in storytelling, animation, filmmaking, and technology he created with his dedicated team. It all came full circle when we watched Disney films or enjoyed his theme parks with our young families and relived his world through their lives.

The dilemma we faced with this book is that while we have the greatest respect and admiration for Walt, he was a taskmaster, and he would be the first to admit it. So in telling the stories of his band of animation directors, we see how his drive and ambition both inspired them and stressed them.

PETE One quote that stuck with me was from a February 10, 1941, speech that Walt gave to his animation staff: "Those men who have worked closely with me in trying to organize and keep the studio rolling, and keep its chin above the water, should not be envied. Frankly, those fellows catch plenty of hell, and a lot of you can feel lucky that you don't have too much contact with me."[1]

DON But I think they would all say—were they still alive—that they would gladly do it again, because they believed strongly in his vision, were in awe of him personally, and readily attached themselves to his star for as long as they could hang on. His hold on their hearts and minds stayed long after his passing. I can remember interviewing many of them at the studio years later, and as we talked, they gradually shifted from the past tense to the present tense when speaking of him, and Walt was still alive for them. Swept up in their memories, I almost expected to hear his cough and see him come around the corner to join us.

Walt was a different person to each of his directors, depending on his needs at the time and their skills at delivering what he needed. Over the years, as his world expanded beyond animated films, his attention divided, and he expected his directors to take up the slack.

He often had an uneasy relationship with the role of director, which he virtually created within animation, and the men who filled that role. He was constantly changing the organization and studio process to fit his vision, and woe to the director who could not go with the flow.

For this book, we have simplified the evolution of the director into six periods or stages. These designations were certainly not anything discussed during their time, but they seemed the best way to explain the changes in this complex and sometimes technical role. Each section begins with a simple explanation of the job at that time and place.

But most of this book is devoted to the careers of the often unknown, unsung directors. Rising from the animation ranks, these men were a wide and varied group of characters. Capable of incredibly demanding precision, some delegated willingly, while others demanded meticulous control. They were boisterous, quiet, exacting, and creative. Some smoked and drank heavily. Some were hated, others revered. They all worked long hours. It was a highly stressful position, likely contributing to declining health for some in their later years.

As generals of the small armies it took to make these animated films, directors had an unequalled view of the art, craft, and organization it took to make them. And as Walt's closest creative partners, they saw a side of Walt seen by very few.

We're excited to introduce you to the talented but unknown people who directed some of the world's favorite films.

—Don Peri and Pete Docter
February 2023

P.S. Within these pages, you will not see a lot of diversity. While today this is slowly changing, the films and the processes discussed in this book are products of their time. With hope of a more diverse group of directors in the future, we feel these stories have plenty of lessons to offer all filmmakers and historians today.

—D.P. & P.D.

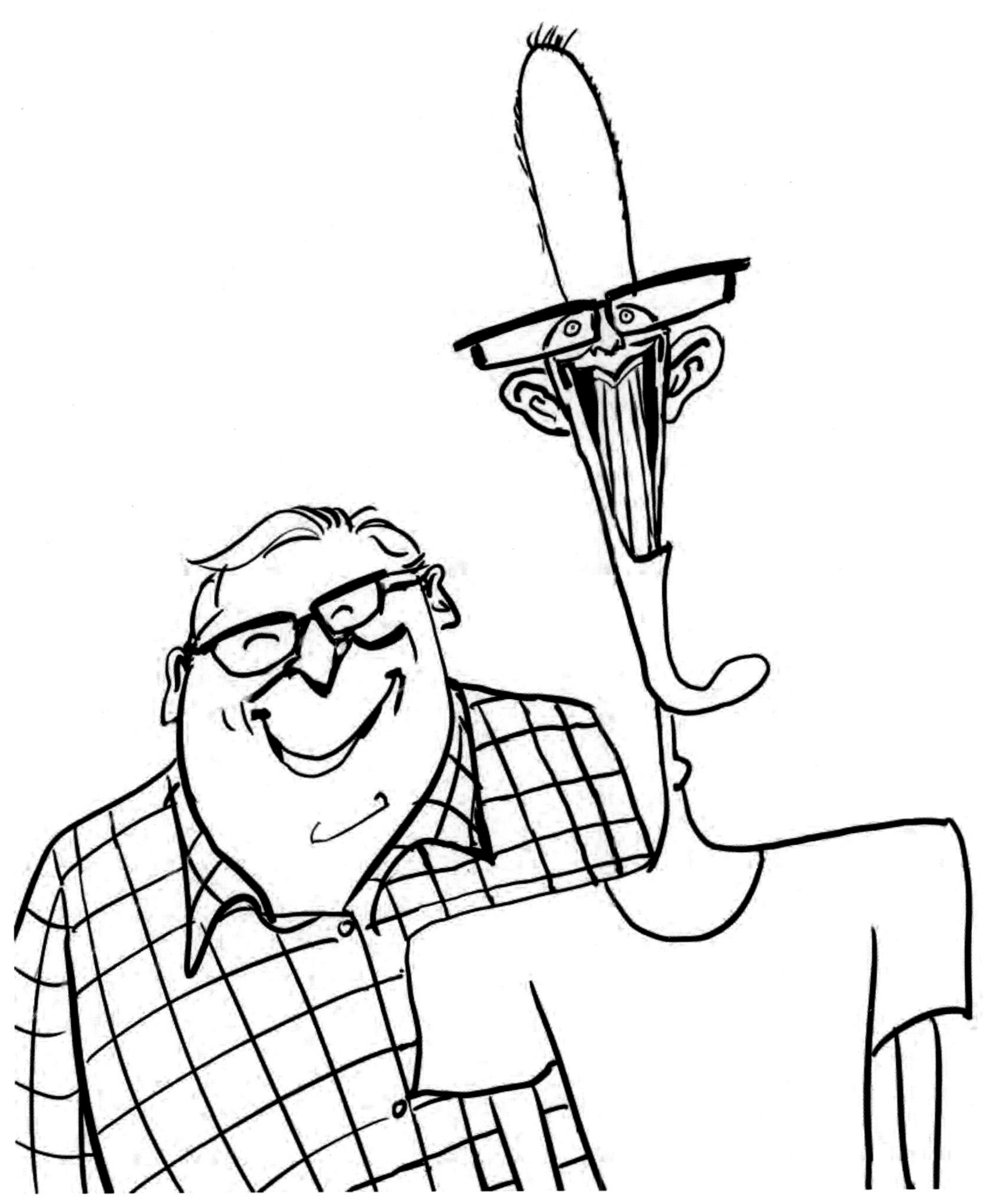

Caricature by John Musker.

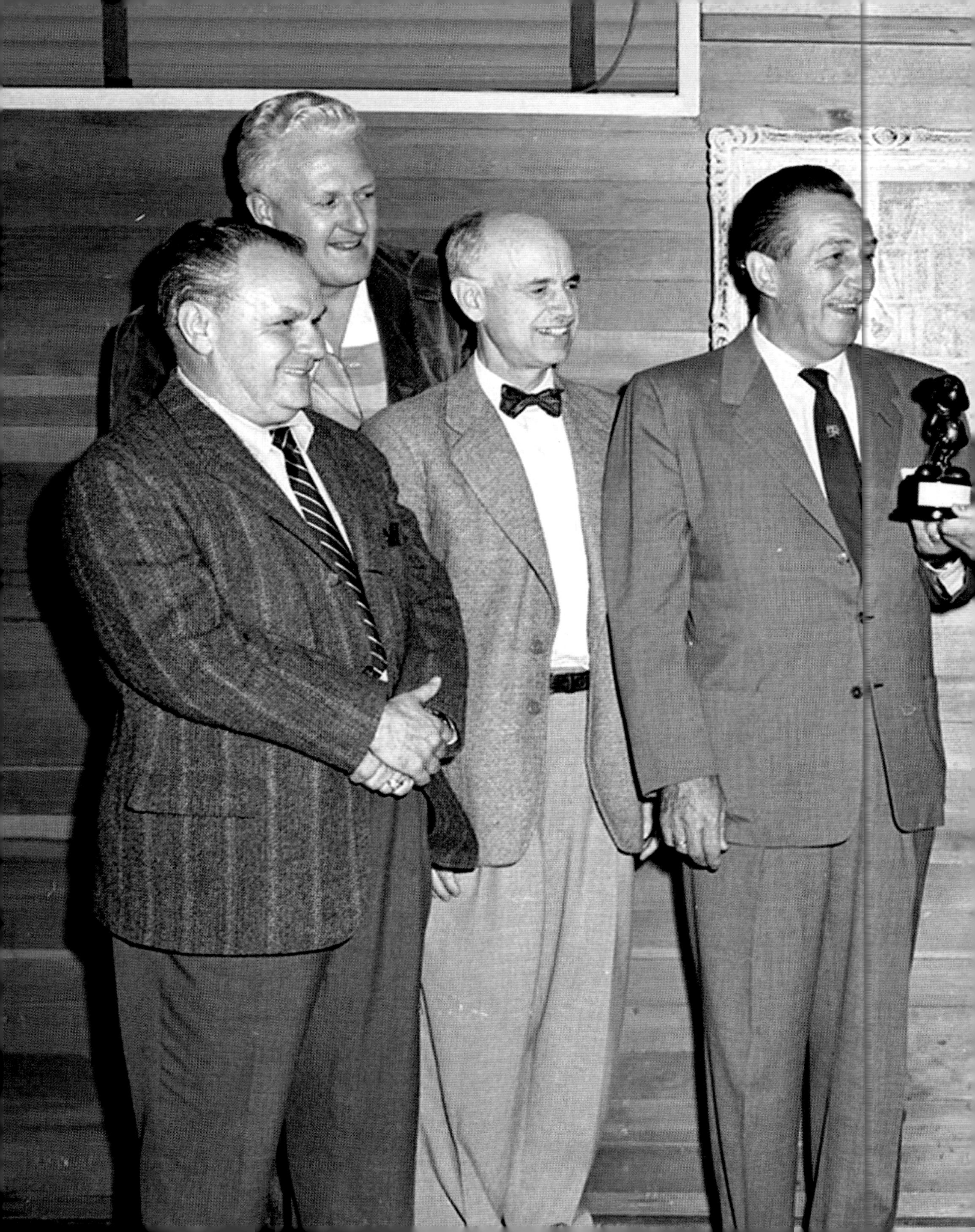

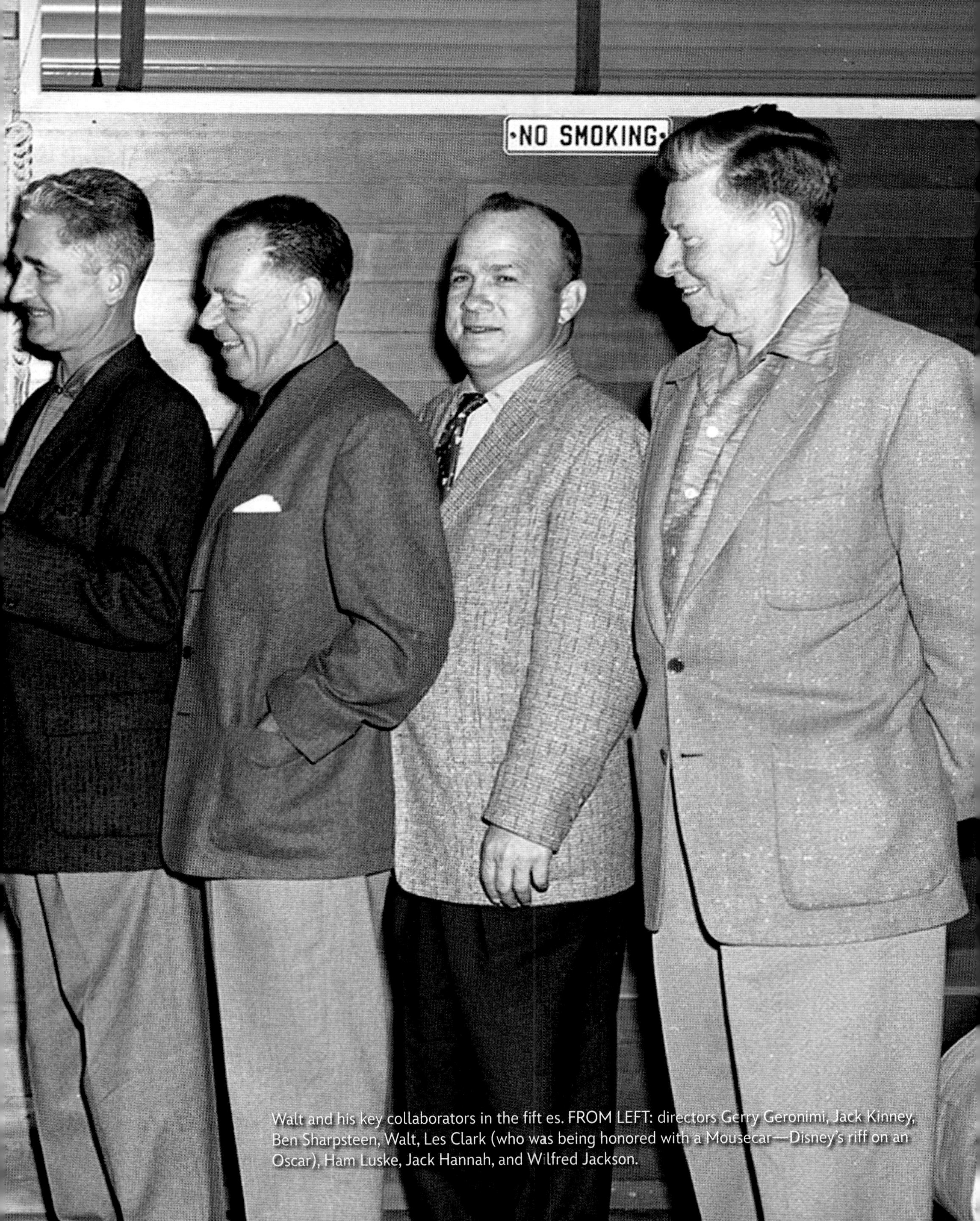

Walt and his key collaborators in the fift es. FROM LEFT: directors Gerry Geronimi, Jack Kinney, Ben Sharpsteen, Walt, Les Clark (who was being honored with a Mousecar—Disney's riff on an Oscar), Ham Luske, Jack Hannah, and Wilfred Jackson.

PART 1

“THERE WERE NO DIRECTORS AT FIRST”

1920–1931

Throughout time, the job of the director changed. In an attempt to show this, we have created a series of simplified flowcharts, based largely on graphs prepared in the late 1970s by Frank Thomas and Ollie Johnston for use in their book *The Illusion of Life*. Ultimately unused, they still provided a firsthand account of the evolving system. Please note these charts are simplified, especially as time goes on, and are focused on the director's duties and jurisdiction rather than on details of the production process.

1920s

NEW YORK STUDIOS

No directors; animators do everything in making the film.

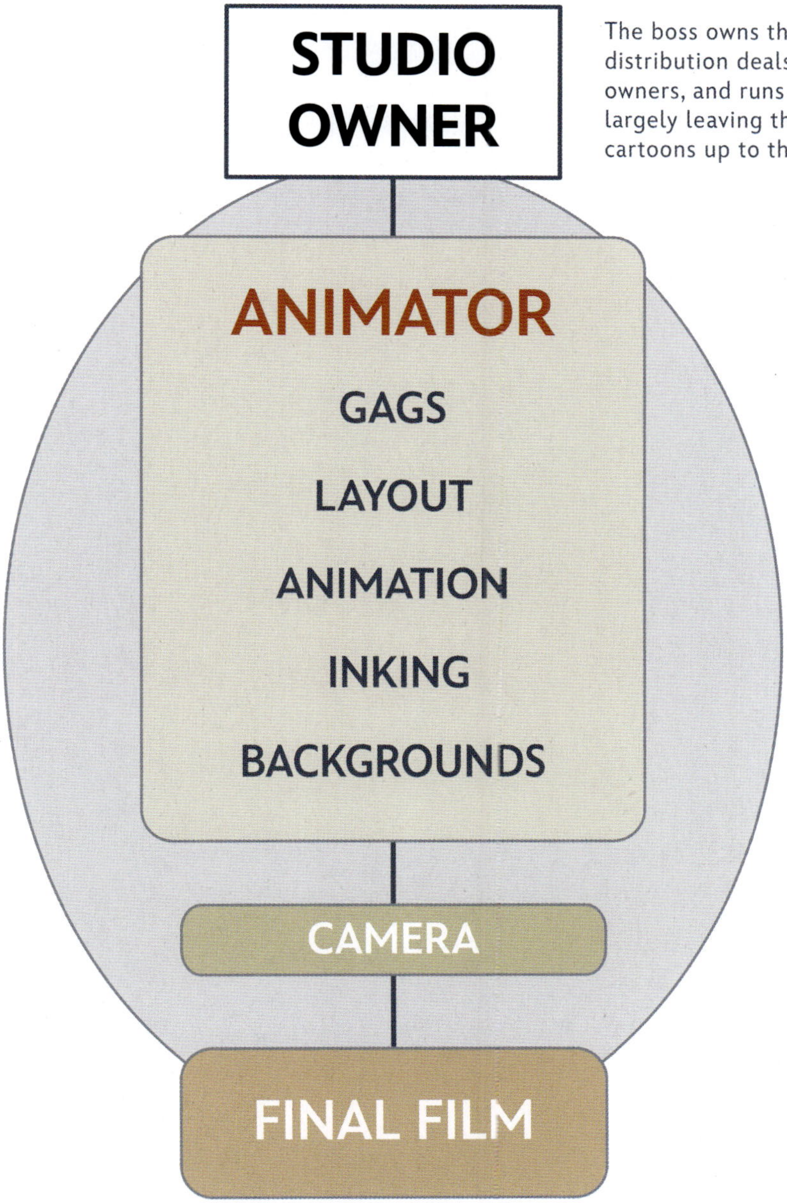

STUDIO OWNER

The boss owns the studio, makes distribution deals with theater owners, and runs the business, largely leaving the making of cartoons up to the animator.

ANIMATOR

GAGS

LAYOUT

ANIMATION

INKING

BACKGROUNDS

Each short is divided among two to four animators. Each thinks up gags for their own section, stages them, makes the animation drawings, inks them, and inks a background on a cel to lay over the paper drawings of the character. With luck, the cameraman can draw, in case something doesn't work or has been left out.

CAMERA

FINAL FILM

Output: one short a week

1920–1928

THE EARLY DAYS AT DISNEY'S

No directors; Walt determines what will end up on the screen, as well as the timing.

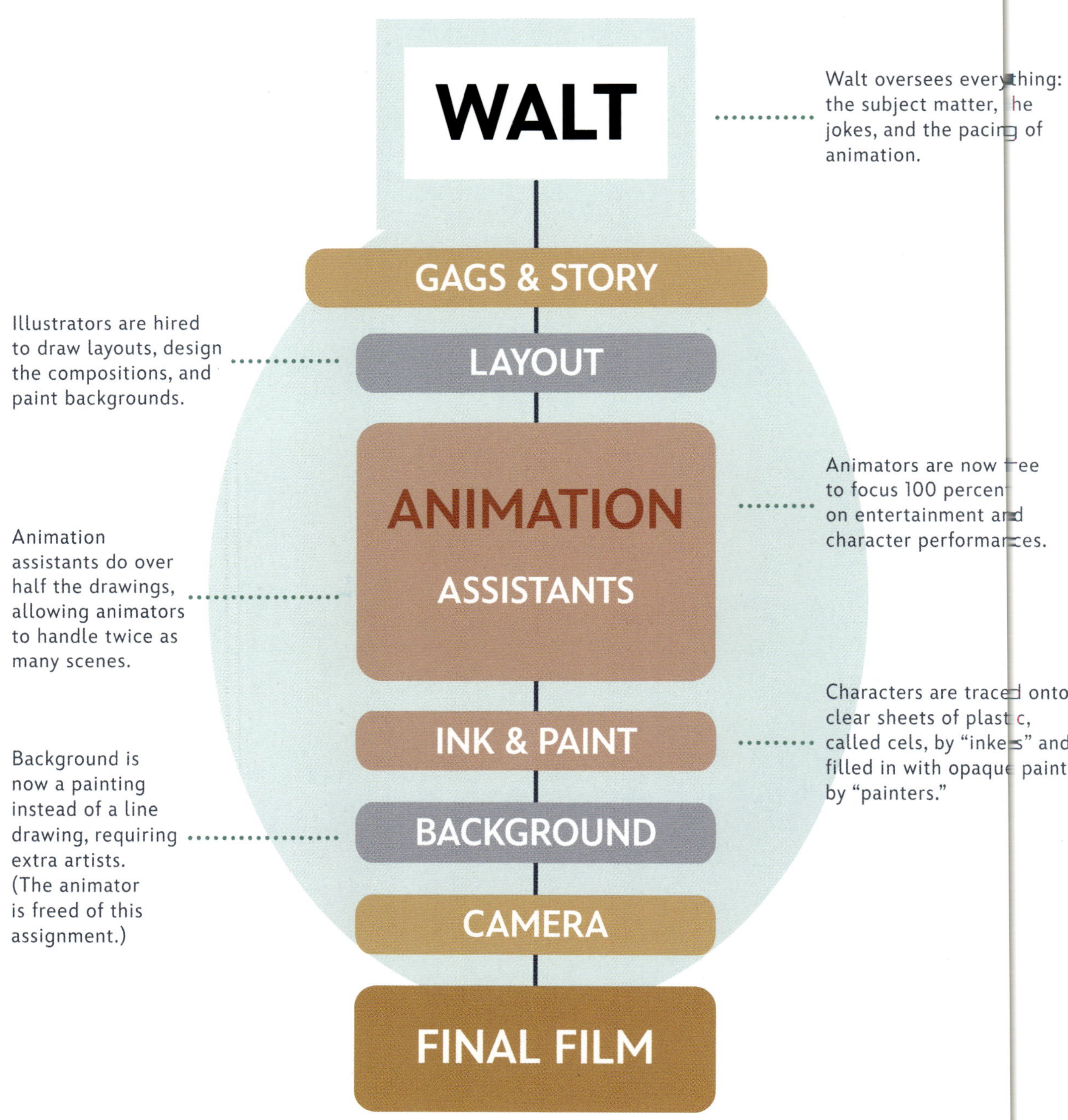

Output: one short every two weeks

1929–1931

THE PROTO-DIRECTOR

The role of the Director (called the "Story Man" at this point) is created to make sure the gags come off as discussed in prior meetings, and alleviate Walt's time spent on details.

The Story Man's job:
- Hand out shots to animators with spoken description of what is expected
- Review rough and cleaned-up animation
- Time out drawings, often removing or revising instructions to camera how many frames each should be seen on-screen

The Director's job includes the planning and recording of sound, usually done at the end of the picture.

The inclusion of sound calls for a cutter (editor) to keep everything in sync.

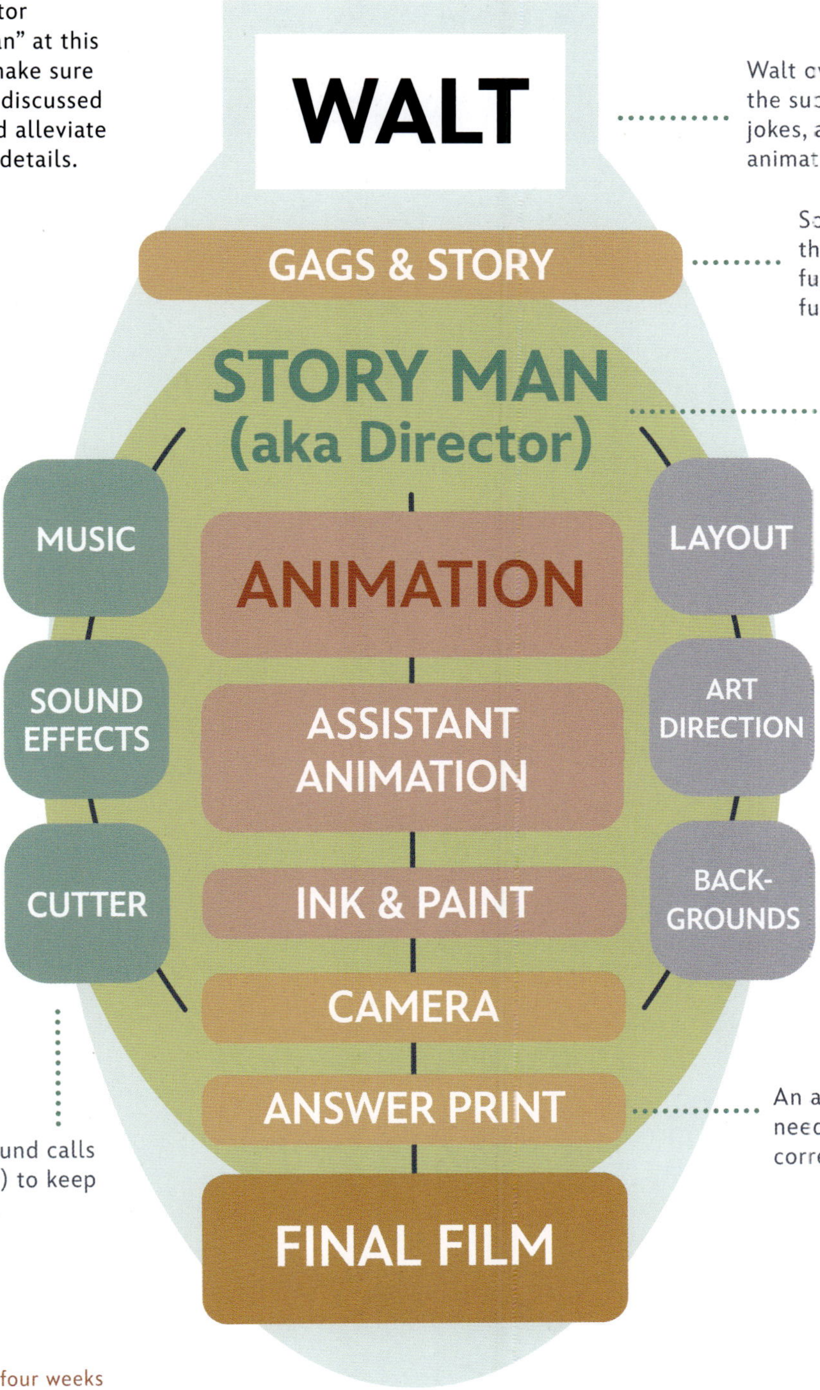

WALT

GAGS & STORY

STORY MAN (aka Director)

MUSIC

SOUND EFFECTS

CUTTER

ANIMATION

ASSISTANT ANIMATION

INK & PAINT

CAMERA

ANSWER PRINT

FINAL FILM

LAYOUT

ART DIRECTION

BACK-GROUNDS

Walt oversees everything: the subject matter, the jokes, and the pacing of animation.

Someone better at gags than animation gets a full-time job thinking up funny business.

The Story Man oversees the largely organizational issues complicated by sound while Walt makes most creative decisions.

Layout and background artists have the added responsibility of selecting colors.

An answer print is now needed to check color corrections.

Output: one short every four weeks

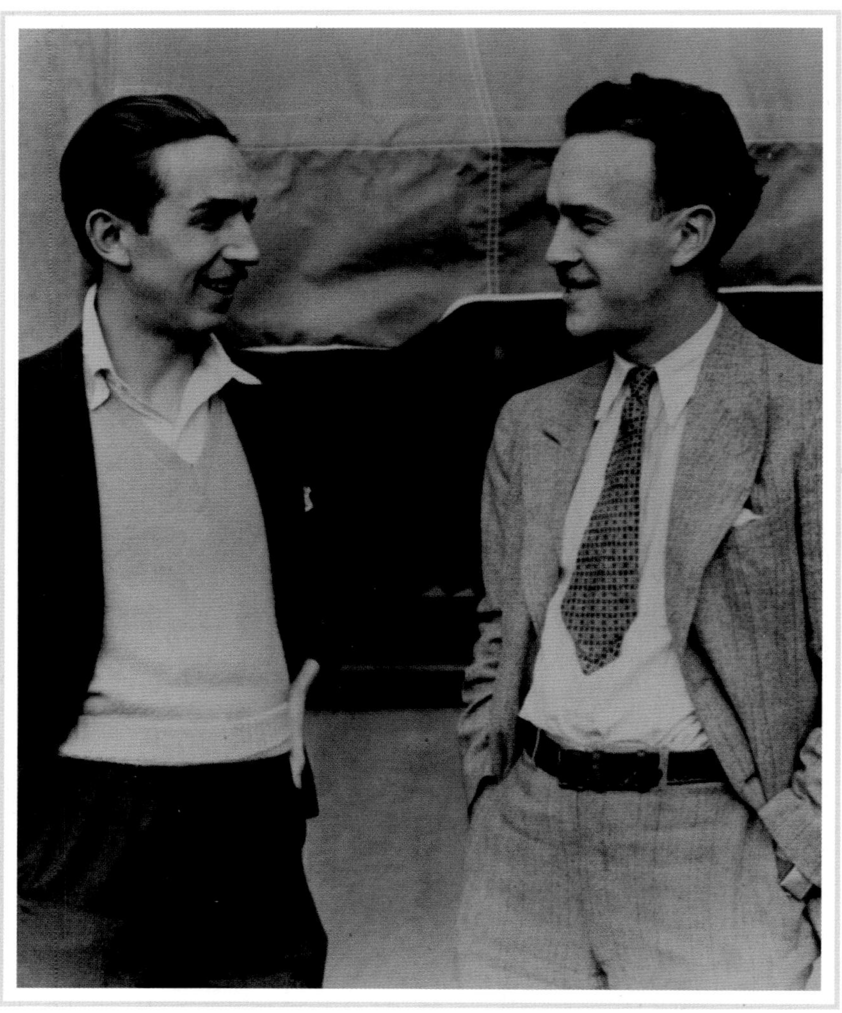

Walt Disney and Ub Iwerks circa 1928, as sound revolutionized the movie industry.

CHAPTER 1

THE BIRTH OF THE DISNEY DIRECTOR

"There were no directors at first. Disney produced directors—or rather, created them."[1]

—Animator/Director Dick Huemer

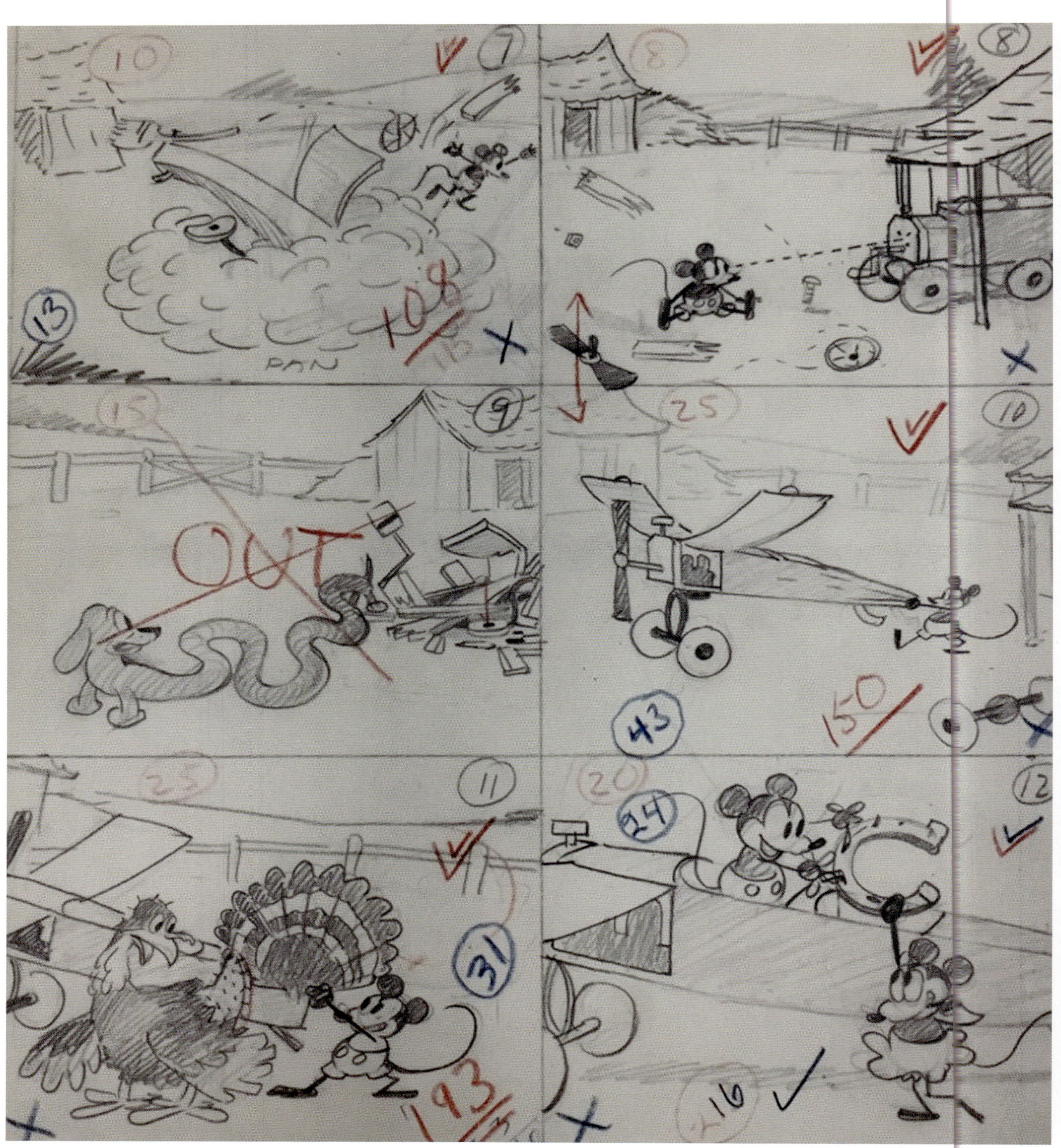

One of several pages of proto-storyboard drawings by Ub Iwerks for *Plane Crazy*, initially planned as a silent.

LIGHTS! CAMERA! ACTION! *SOUND!*

When Al Jolson tells a cabaret crowd in *The Jazz Singer*, "You ain't heard nothin' yet," he meant more than he could possibly know. The movie studios were initially dismissive of this film from the upstart Warner Bros. Studio, but the public enthusiastically embraced it. And what the industry hoped was a fad in fact changed movies forever.

Sound meant big things for Walt Disney as well, establishing both him and Mickey Mouse as household names. It also ushered in a new position in the production of animated films: that of director.

BEFORE DIRECTORS

When the very first animated films appeared around the turn of the twentieth century, there were no directors. The position would have been superfluous; with no actors, sets, costumes, or sound, what appeared on-screen was simply decided and drawn by the animator. Since early films were usually made by one or two artists, there was very little need for planning.

Even as small studios grew to churn out a more regular diet of cartoons, organization was loose. As then-animator Clyde "Gerry" Geronimi said of his work in New York around 1920, "There were no storyboards [visual scripts] in those days. We had just a typewritten sheet, with an outline of what we were going to do."[2] Animator Dick Huemer's reference to his work at the Mintz Studio (Screen Gems) reflected a similar improvisational approach: "Sid [Marcus], Art [Davis], and myself each took a third of the picture, animated and amplified it on our own, with hardly any consultation with each other. We each considered our section our own private affair—gags, interpretation, and all."[3]

When he started in Kansas City, Walt Disney followed the same process. Along with fellow artist and friend Ub Iwerks, he animated on shorts and advertising products.

The failure of Walt's first two studios precipitated a move to California, where he and brother Roy again hired Iwerks, recognizing his amazing ability to animate fast and with high quality. At the same time, Walt found that his strength was in story and character. "I am in no sense of the word a great artist, not even a great animator; I have always had men working for me whose skills were greater than my own. I am an idea man."[4] "It wasn't that Walt couldn't do it [animate], he could," recalled Ub years later. "But since I had joined him in 1924, he found he could do more for his pictures with gags and doing writing than by sitting over a drawing board. I don't think Walt made any drawings after 1924."[5]

Walt wanted stories that were cohesive, unlike the loose themes pieced together at other studios. He began writing outlines, describing what would appear scene by scene. Soon the text was accompanied by a sketch previsualizing the layout, giving all animators working on the film a clear vision of how their parts fit into the whole.

Instead of just letting animators draw whatever they wanted, Walt and Ub now had a plan for their films, much like architectural blueprints for a building. While this planning took more time, it added immeasurably to the quality of the films, which seemed to be Walt's single-minded goal.

Walt shepherded the stories from their inception through every revision and gag. He approved every camera angle. He dictated what happened in every shot, sometimes every frame, obsessing over every detail. While not credited as such on-screen, Walt was the first Disney director.

But it was sound that would really bring the position into focus.

"MICKEY'S NIGHTMARE"

1- Iris opens on M.L.S. of Mickey's bed room-----------Candle on night-stand lights the room------------moon in sky seen through window----------alarm clock and Minnie's picture on night-stand---other pictures of Minnie all over the walls. Mickey is dressed in over-sized pajamas and is kneeling beside his bed with hands crossed and head bowed-------Pluto is in same position beside him---------Mickey says in whisper---------"GOD BLESS MINNIE, GOD BLESS PLUTO, GOD BLESS EVERYBODY,"---------then he says in loud voice,-------"A-MEN!!!! "-----------after this he hops up quickly and jumps into bed----------Pluto prances and barks and hops into bed with him.

2- M.C.U. of Mickey and Pluto in bed----------Mickey sees Pluto beside him-----------looks surprised---------Pluto smiles at him in manner begging Mickey to let him sleep with him-------Mickey gives him an exasperated look and sternly points off scene to Pluto's bed---------------Pluto's happy expression wilts and he looks off scene in direction of bed with a very disheartened expression.

3- C.U. of Pluto's bed-----------small miniature of Mickey's bed.

4- Cut back to M.C.U. of Mickey pointing to Pluto's bed in stern manner------Pluto looks to Mickey in pleading manner and whines-------Mickey points again and says sternly------"GO ON"-------Pluto wilts------turns-------and hops down and walks dejectedly over to own bed----------(Pan over to bed and exclude Mickey)---------Pluto stops by bed-------looks back to Mickey with pleading expression----------(off stage voice)-------------"GO ON"----------Pluto jumps when Mickey speaks-------turns looks at bed---------sniffs at it-----------hops into bed--------goes around and around in circles in manner od dog preparing to lie down-----------finally he settles down------crosses his paws-------lays chin on paws and snorts in disgusted manner. closes both eyes - opens 1 eye - peats

5- M.C.U. of Mickey in bed watching Pluto-------(alarm clock, Minnie's picture-----statue of cupid and candle on night-stand) Mickey smiles when he sees Pluto obeying him---------then he lays back in bed with hands behind his head----------he looks over at Minnie's picture on the night-stand-----------then Mickey leans over in bed and looks at picture in love-sick manner--------throws her a kiss-------sighs-------sees cupid statue---------picks it up---------looks at it with goofy smile---------winks at it and sets it down on night-standin position by Minnie's picture-------throws another kiss---------sighs again---------and lays back in bed----------blinks eyes in goofy love-sick manner.

6- M.C.U. Pluto in his bed---------he raises up and looks at Mickey in an inquisitive manner.

Hold that Line

Scene 1 - Coach of football players working out on field - Show action of football players tackling dummy, running and kicking football - Peg Leg Pete as coach and Mickey as quarterback - Coach tells them to go to the showers and players follow orders

Scene ② Night - Room where players sleep -
Mickey gets off of bed and tries to sneak out looks out window. and sees Minnie in garden -

Scene ③ Garden and Moonlight showing -
Minnie waves that she's waiting - Mickey's in window in silhouette -

Scene ④ - Same as ②
Mickey tries to open window but hears noise He jumps up and lands on a fat pig's stomach and sneaks to bed - Pig wakes up and wonders what it's all about - Coach enters and pig goes to bed right away -
Coach is satisfied and leaves -
Mickey gets up and goes through window -

Scene ⑤ Show him going down sliding in pipe -
As he reaches down a mob kidnaps him + take him in car.
Minnie follows them -

ABOVE AND RIGHT: Examples of early written outlines, for *Mickey's Nightmare* and *Hold that Line* (released as *Hold that Pose*), courtesy Hans Perk.

THE COST OF SOUND

Recovering from a loss of most of their animators as well as their star Oswald the Lucky Rabbit to a rival, Walt started a new series with a newly created character, Mickey Mouse. The first two Mickey cartoons created, *The Gallopin' Gaucho* and *Plane Crazy*, were silent. These two films did not attract distributors, so Walt decided to add sound—synchronized sound—to the third Mickey, *Steamboat Willie*. One historic evening, Walt and his animation crew, including top animator Ub Iwerks and animators Les Clark, Johnny Cannon, and Wilfred Jackson, tested sound on a scene from what would become *Steamboat Willie*, with a makeshift microphone, a few musical instruments, and Walt's vocals, before a captive audience of wives and girlfriends. Each performer took a turn to see the effect of sound synchronized with action, and they concluded that it worked. Mild-mannered and taciturn Ub Iwerks recalled, "It was wonderful; there was no precedent of any kind. I've never been so thrilled in my life. Nothing since has ever equaled it. That evening proved that an idea could be made to work."[6] Now all Walt had to do was find a sound system, an orchestra to synchronize the score to the completed cartoon, *and* a distributor to release his films. Walt traveled to New York City in the fall of 1928 to do just that.

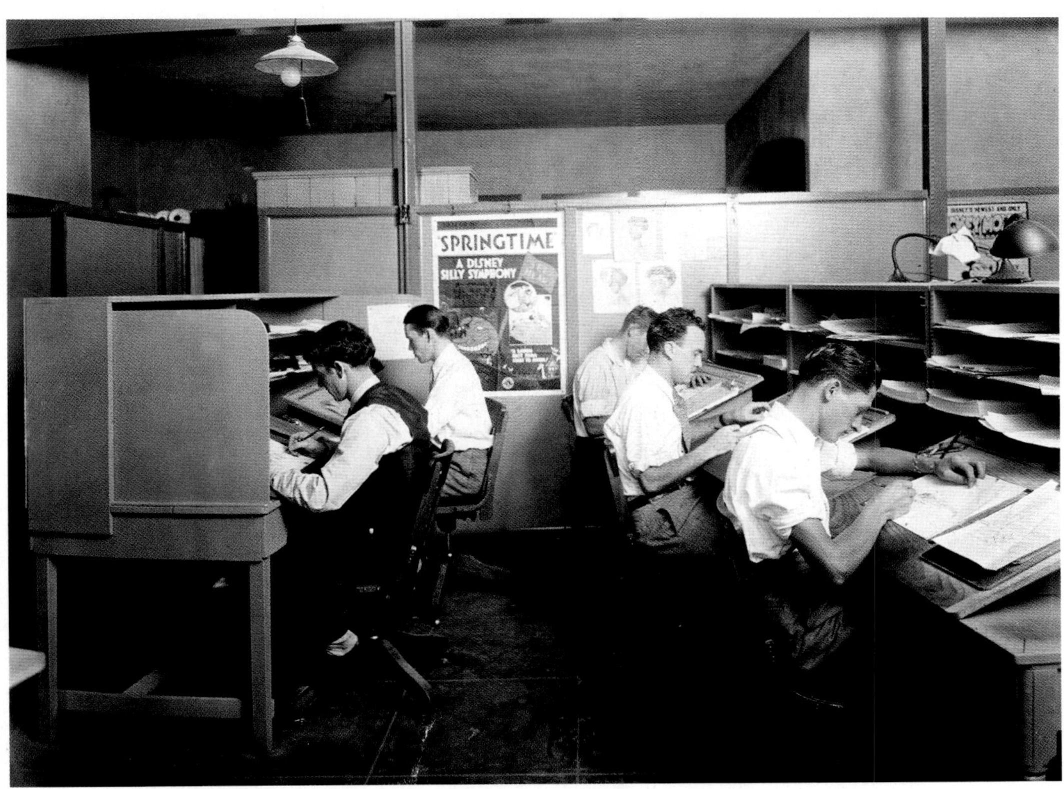

The Disney animation staff in December 1929. CLOCKWISE (FROM LEFT): Johnny Cannon, Jack Cutting, Wilfred Jackson, Ub Iwerks, and Les Clark (who is drawing a scene from *Summer*, released January 16, 1930).

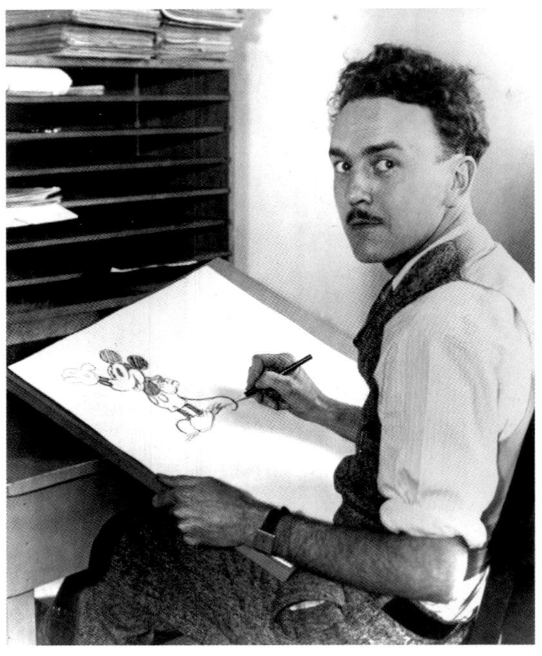

Ub Iwerks at the drawing board.

Steamboat Willie premiered on November 18, 1928, at the Colony Theatre in New York City, and it set the world on fire. It brought Walt to the attention of the animation industry and movie fans everywhere, who were captivated with its synchronized sound. Beyond more Mickey shorts (sound was added to *Plane Crazy* and *Gallopin' Gaucho* prior to their release), Walt put a new series, the Silly Symphonies, into production, doubling the studio's output[7]. In the Mickey series, the story's action took precedence over the music. In the Silly Symphonies, it was just the opposite, but in both cases, synchronization is what gave the Disney cartoons a magical quality that put them above their competitors with moviegoing audiences.

The success of sound in Disney's cartoons was undeniable, but with it came a tax. Stories had to be carefully planned to synchronize with the music, dialogue, and sound effects across multiple animators working on any given film. With Walt's focus spent on crafting the stories, not to mention his role as the studio's leader, someone else would need to do this planning.

Walt gradually let Ub take over some of the duties that Walt had performed, and around the same time hired animator Burt Gillett to assist Ub (see Chapter 2). Ub preplanned the film, drawing backgrounds rather than letting animators draw their own, which at that point in time was often the practice. Ub guided the animators—usually three to five other artists—making sure that their work reflected what he and Walt had planned and that different artists' scenes matched up.

THE STORY MAN

Walt was evolving the role of the director (which he initially called the story man). Whether he had planned to do that or simply needed more help, Burt and Ub were the pioneers on that trail.

Wilfred Jackson recalled the general process for creating a story in the late twenties and early thirties:

- Decide on a concept—usually from Walt, but now becoming the director's responsibility and frequently coming from him
- Hold a preliminary gag meeting, pulling ideas from all the crew (sometimes even brainstorming for a concept if none was brought in by Walt or the director)
- Develop the rough story line and musical treatment, done by the director and musician, with the help of the gag men and Walt
- Refine the ideas into the final continuity, done by the director and musician as they

The Production Staff of
MICKEY MOUSE and
SILLY SYMPHONY
CARTOONS
EXTEND THEIR CONGRATULATIONS
to WALT DISNEY
TED SEARS
· Gags ·
BURT GILLETT
· Story ·
WILFRED JACKSON
· Story ·
FLOYD GOTTFREDSON
· Artist ·
TOM PALMER
· Artist ·
BEN SHARPSTEEN
· Artist ·
BILL COTTRELL
· Cameraman ·
DAVE HAND
· Artist ·
WALT DISNEY
JOHNNY CANNON
· Artist ·
EMIL FLOHRI
· Scenic ·
FRENCHY DE TREMAUDAN
· Artist ·
NORMAN FERGUSON
· Artist ·
RUDY ZAMORA
· Artist ·
HAZEL SEWELL
· Inking ·
LES CLARK
· Artist ·
JACK CUTTING
· Artist ·
BILL GARITY
· Recording Engineer ·
DICK LUNDY
· Artist ·
FRANK CHURCHILL
· Musician ·
BERT LEWIS
· Musician ·
EARL DUVALL
· Gags ·
CARICATURES by JACK KING
· Artist ·

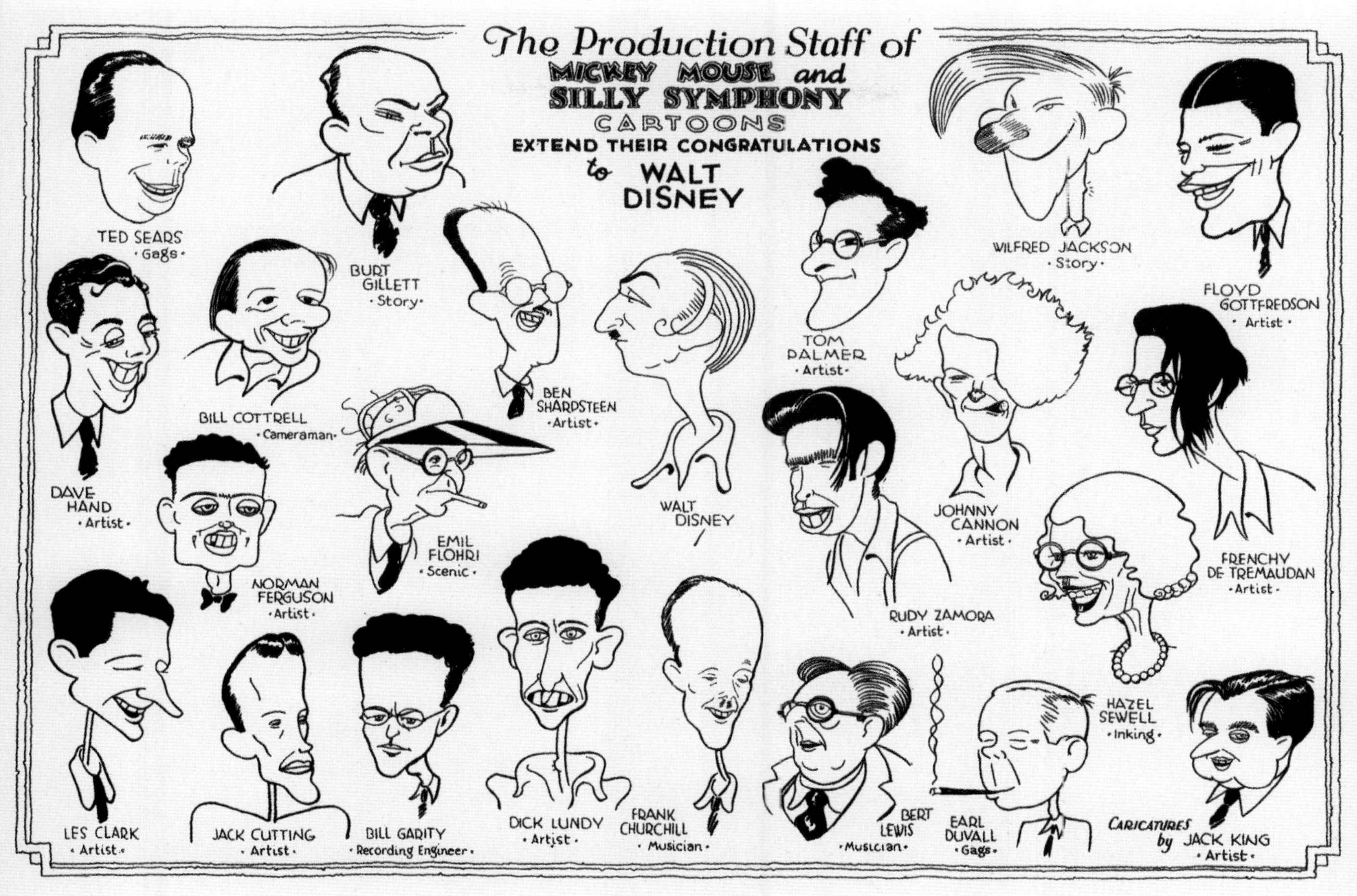

Jack King's caricatures of the Disney staff appeared in the June 20, 1931, edition of *Motion Picture Daily*. Even after the departure of Ub, directors Burt Gillett and Wilfred Jackson were still called "story men" or, in this case, just "Story."

pre-timed the action, with Walt's supervision. By this phase, the gag men were helping another director with his early story work on another story.

- Build and improve details of the business during animation (by Walt, the director, and the animators)[8]

And the story men weren't the only ones being pushed by Walt. Ben Sharpsteen, a recent hire from the New York studios, recognized that Walt Disney could visualize things beyond what was being done at other studios, which called for better, but more difficult, animation. "Walt knew how to take an animator's work, he knew how to feed the animator ideas, and he knew how to put them together and produce a picture. Just that alone was a terrific talent that nobody else in the producing end of the animated cartoon business had. In other words,

Walt's ideas were oftentimes more difficult to portray than we would have selected at another studio. We would think up something that could be portrayed before we started to animate it, so we naturally lapsed into a tail end way of doing something. We wouldn't try something that we didn't think we could get away with. Therefore, the animation possibilities were extremely limited."[9]

The role of the director would expand and change over the years, reflecting the amount of trust Walt had in the men he worked with, his interest in a specific project, and other projects he had on his plate. Given Walt's exacting standards, the job would not be easy. Walt expected them to follow instructions—which were occasionally vague and indefinite—but also to improve the work at every turn. When results didn't meet his high expectations, Walt didn't mince words.

By now the written outlines and quick sketches had been replaced with a new innovation called a storyboard. To a portable 4x8-foot panel, artists pinned consecutive drawings representing the action and continuity. Ideas could be added, discarded, or reordered easily, allowing everyone a view of what the film would look like before they made it. Once again, this innovation took more time up front, but would prove a valuable tool to ensure quality. Storyboards were used throughout Walt's life and continue to be used today. Dick Huemer said:

> Would you like to know the name of the genius who invented the concept of the storyboard? Most think that it was Walt Disney's idea and there are those who claim the honor for Webb Smith. But take it from me, an unimpeachable source; it was Ted Sears who first thought of it and submitted it to the [Fleischer Studios] back in New York when he was working for them in the twenties. According to how I heard it, they didn't go for it. So later when Ted made the switch to Disney and again unveiled the idea to that perfectionist, his nibs, seeing in the concept still another way to improve his product, promptly ordered it done. The rest, to uncoin a phrase, is no mystery.[10]

THE TEAM SPLITS

The storyboard also became a way for Walt to plan and lock down a version of the film, which he could then hand off to directors. If a picture is worth a thousand words, a board with sixty or so drawings pinned to it was a way for Walt to ensure that his directors wouldn't stray too far from the specific desires he had for the film.

Burt supervised production of the Mickey cartoons, and Ub took on the Silly Symphonies while animating as well. Ub directed a handful of Disney cartoons, including *Springtime*, *Hell's Bells*, *Summer*, and *Autumn*.[11]

Ub seemed to be a natural for the position. He was the top animator, a minority partner in the studio, and, as mentioned, a longtime friend and associate of Walt and Roy's. He was also mechanically minded, responsible, and good with new employees.

But Walt and Ub began to clash, mostly over Ub's animation practices. Ub preferred to animate "straight ahead"—that is, animating the action in a linear fashion, one frame following the other, by himself. Walt wanted Ub to animate "pose to pose," capturing the key extreme poses, leaving others to draw the drawings in between that would create smooth movement. Leaving all these inbetweens to others was a better use of Ub's valuable time, reasoned Walt. But Ub strongly disagreed and felt it would handicap his process.

Timing the action was another sore spot between Walt and Ub. Walt would often return late at night to change how long each drawing should appear on-screen. For instance, if a character shoots his arm into the air, should it move in one frame or two? The difference is $\frac{1}{24}$ of a second—a miniscule detail—yet the difference could determine whether the scene gets a laugh.

Ub was a quiet man, unwilling to battle Walt directly, and he began to foster some resentment. He'd worked as long and hard toward the success of the studio as Walt, and in the end, Ub's drawings were what the public saw on-screen. But their partnership was not an equal one. As Dave Hand said later, "They were partners, but Walt was the boss!"[12] Ub felt that it was time for him to leave.

Walt and Roy were shocked when Ub came to Roy while Walt was in New York on business and told him that he was resigning. Ub shared a minimum amount of information about his motivations until Roy, in Walt's absence, pressed him: "For pity's sake, say something, and at least try to keep us from having such a nasty mean opinion of you as circumstances and conditions are forcing us to have as long as you keep your mouth shut!"[13] Roy sent a letter to Walt saying Ub had "wilted" and had told him about an offer he'd received for a studio of his own and a considerably higher salary. He did not know until two days before he received his contract that the offer had come through an intermediary for Pat Powers, the Disney distributor (and a deceitful character to boot, as all would unfortunately learn in time). Ub did not want to hurt the studio but objected to Walt's

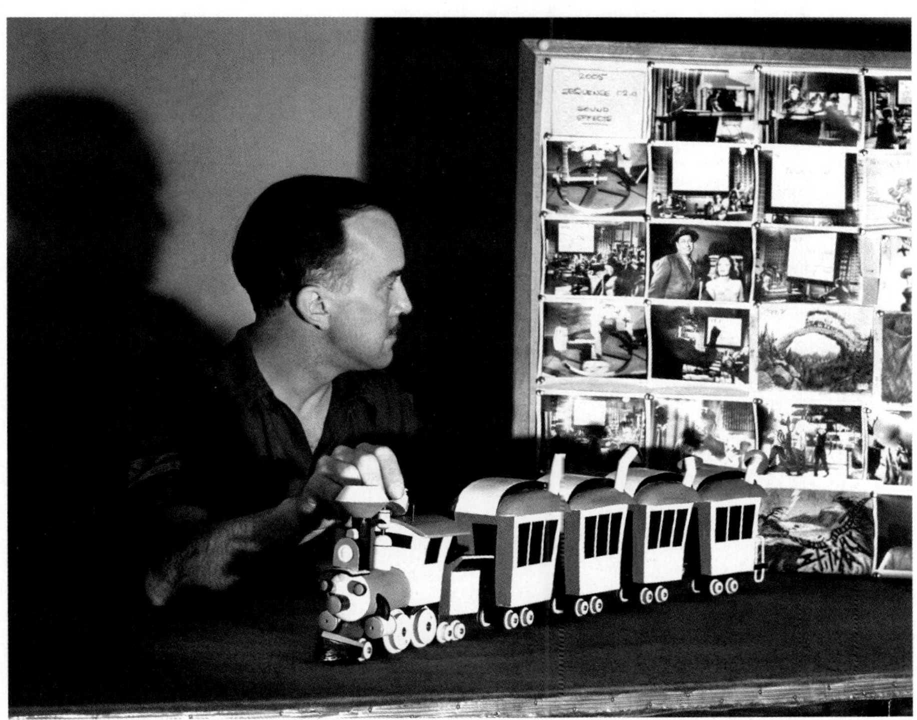

Ub back at the Disney Studios working with a model of the Casey Jr. train from *Dumbo*, as seen in *The Reluctant Dragon* (1941).

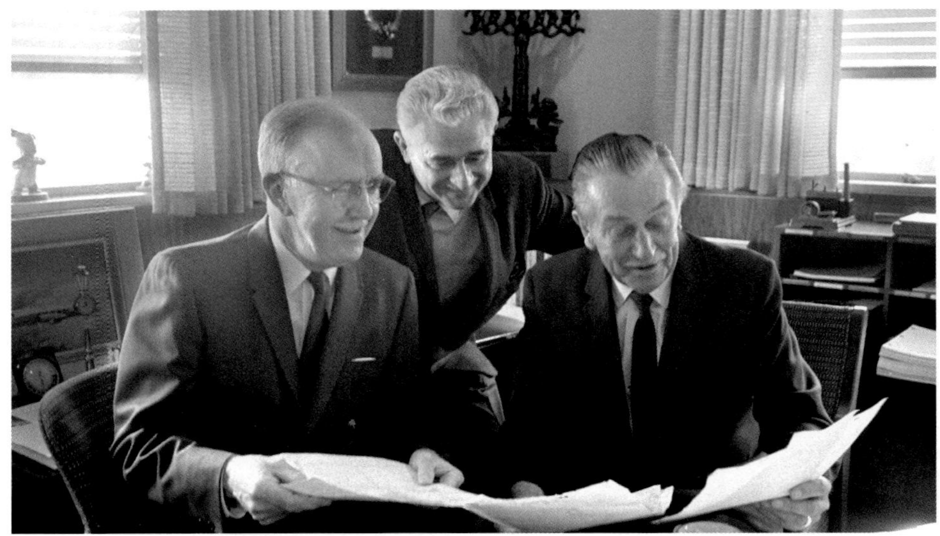

LEFT TO RIGHT: Ub, pioneering animator Les Clark, and Walt in 1966, reminiscing about the early days at the studio, and the early days of Mickey Mouse, specifically.

push for efficiency and continued "correcting" of his timing.

Disney Legend Bob Broughton, veteran Disney effects camera artist, had an interesting observation about Ub's position at Disney. "Well, he became one of two when Wilfred Jackson or Les Clark or one of them came in. And pretty soon he was one of ten. But up to that point, he was the only one. And he was asked less and less, and that was what drove him out or why he accepted the opportunity that came to him. He just became less significant than he had been."[14]

Although still feeling betrayed by Ub, Roy wrote to Walt that he'd told Ub how his leaving benefitted the company in a business sense:

> I had quite a talk with Ub . . . and I told him frankly that the worst feature of this whole affair was the fact that a fellow as close to us as he had been should turn on us at a time like this. I told him also that if we had deliberately planned to use him and Carl [Stalling, who also chose to leave] over the period of time which we really needed them, and when they were essential to the success of the pictures, and had planned and plotted to throw them over at the first opportunity for selfish motives, that the whole affair could not have worked out prettier. Also, I told him that from a financial angle we would benefit greatly by his withdrawal, but that we were deeply shocked and hurt at being treated as we have been by two fellows in whom we heretofore had every confidence and trust.[15]

Ub left in early 1930 and for a decade ran his own studio with, at best, mixed results. Though he was a talented animator and had an amazing technical mind, Ub soon discovered that Walt's creative focus was an essential part of their success, and that producing and directing were not Ub's strong suits. Ben Sharpsteen felt that "Ub Iwerks was a one hundred percent nice fellow, he was a wonderful man, but he was attempting to do something for which he was not qualified."[16]

Not finding success on his own, Ub returned to Disney in 1940 through the initial efforts of his friend Ben Sharpsteen. In a memo to Walt, the usually restrained Ben expressed his support in an upbeat way that might have surprised some at the studio, given his usual all-business attitude:

> . . . I feel, as you do, that he is almost a genius at things of an effects nature. Also I have

LIMERICKS ABOUT IWERKS

As Dick Huemer—a legendary pioneer in the animation industry both in New York and at The Walt Disney Studios as an animator, director, and story man—received a Lifetime Achievement Award from the International Animated Film Society (ASIFA) in 1978, he chose to humorously honor Ub Iwerks (who also received a Lifetime Achievement Award, posthumously) during his acceptance speech. Dick created a couple of limericks about Ub Iwerks.

ELECTRONICS! MATH-A-MATICS! AND HOW PI WORKS.
WAS SO MUCH DUCK SOUP FOR UB IWERKS!
HE'D EXPLAIN OFF THE CUFF,
FIFTH DIMENSION AND STUFF!
AND EVEN! HOW THE ZIPPER! ON YOUR FLY WORKS!

YOUNG UB! WAS THE BEST IN THE NATION!
A WIZ-Z-Z-ARD AT CARTOON CREATION!
ONE DAY, (THEY RECORD)
HE DOZED AT HIS BOARD,
AND INVENTED, SUSPENDED ANIMATION![18]

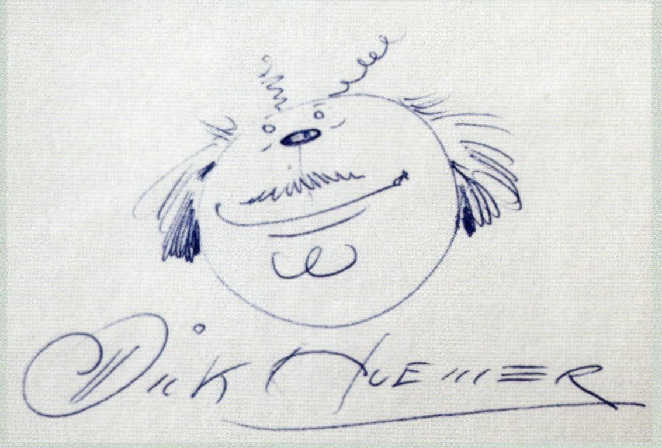

Huemer's self-caricature, at the end of a letter to Don Peri.

> always felt that Ub, outside of the fact that he is one hell of a swell fellow, that he made a definite contribution to this organization at one time, and . . . I, personally, like him very much and should be very happy to see him utilized in some way.[17]

Walt agreed and authorized Ben to hire him back. Ub directed at least one World War II training film and even did some animation at the studio, but made his lasting mark in the film industry through his technical innovations, primarily special visual effects, earning Academy Awards and other honors. Ub passed away in 1971 and received the Winsor McCay Award in 1978 and the Disney Legends Award in 1989.

Walt had learned that to produce his desired quantity of animated films and still get what he wanted on-screen, he could dictate through careful planning up front and delegate the actual production to others, supervised by a director. But this was more difficult than it had seemed. Artists—and directors—had egos. They had opinions about how things should be done, and sometimes their opinions clashed with his. Ub's tenure as a director was very short. Burt Gillett was still in the director's chair. Perhaps things would work better with him.

Ub Iwerks—Disney Director Filmography

Shorts:
- *Springtime* (1929)
- *Hell's Bells* (1929)
- *Summer* (1930)
- *Autumn* (1930)

Training Film:
- *Stop That Tank!* (1942)

PART 2

“EXTENSIONS OF WALT’S ARMS”

1932–1935

1932–1935

THE DIRECTOR EVOLVES

The Director's job, once Walt approves the story, is to previsualize and plan the film, essentially editing it before it is made. The Director is tasked with these responsibilities:

- Time out the action and cutting
- Collaborate with the composer to make sure the action and music work in synchrony
- Prepare work with the layout artist
- Hand out shots to animators with detailed expectations (exposure sheets, or "X-sheets") as to actions, reactions, and dialogue
- Review rough and cleaned-up animation before Walt sees it
- Supervise the cutting of picture and sound

The many specialized roles in making an animated cartoon are explained here by Frank Thomas and Ollie Johnston from an unused page of their book *The Illusion of Life*. Some of the information listed here goes beyond the scope of what we cover in this book.

PRODUCER
Determines what kind of picture this will be. Decides where, when, and how to make it. Makes all major decisions, hires crew, gets money, pays salaries, settles disputes, arranges for distribution of complete film.

WRITER
Many stories too subtle or too complicated for animation medium. Writer must adapt material to most effective use of this visual form. May submit script, but story will eventually have to be presented in drawings.

RECORDING
Highly creative process of capturing sounds on film that will make picture sparkle. This is responsibility of director with soundman. Must be alert to new ideas that might arise.

ASSISTANT DIRECTOR
Is troubleshooter and record-keeper. Must keep things in order at all times maintaining accurate records as scenes get shifted and shuffled during production.

VOICES
They determine the precise personalities of the characters . . . very important that just the right ones be found to suggest appropriate expressions and attitudes. Should stimulate animator.

SOUND EFFECTS
Ordinary sounds make a dull picture. Search for the unexpected, the exciting, the provocative. Good sounds will fortify actions making them stronger, funnier, more interesting.

MUSIC
Emphasizes moods of picture, accents, strengthens, pulls it together, works on feelings of audience, giving style and integrity to whole film.

CUTTER
Struggles to keep tracks in sync as reels are built, new sound added, footage changed, scenes shifted . . . prepares all reels for dubbing.

DUBBING
Combines all tracks, voices, sound effects, music onto one track, with best balance of all parts.

CAMERA
Photographs completed cels over finished background. Makes camera and peg moves as specified to give mobility within scenes.

ANSWER PRINT
Corrected and balance print for best color reproduction. Shows you what you are going to get instead of what you painted.

CHECKING
Everyone makes mistakes. Production time is saved if they are caught before they go too far. The checkers review all drawings and cels, catching errors in mechanics and missing details.

INBETWEENER
Does the drawings that are left to be finished by either animator or assistant. These drawings will be in between the key drawings they have done.

ASSISTANT ANIMATOR
Does whatever necessary to prepare the animator's work for duplicating and functions that follow . . . sees that all drawings match approval model.

ANIMATOR
He is the actor. Brings the story business to life in most interesting and entertaining way . . . makes the fantasy world real. Responsible for appearance of characters, and the efficient working of his unit.

BACKGROUND
Must be a strong painter with sense of dramatic, knowledge of color, ability to make the figure stage clearly in action without losing mood or scene. Should know current film processing problems.

COLOR MODEL
Establishes which specific colors give the best effect on the figures . . . balances color for hues or other characters, changes of light and moods of various sequences.

LAYOUT MAN
Adapts story sketches to needs of actual production. Controls appearance of film, staging, cutting, style, background, relative sizes, color . . . suggests patterns for animator.

INK & PAINT
Inkers trace the pencil drawings onto cels. Painters fill in the color areas, matching the color model.

STORY SKETCH
Works with writer to keep basic entertainment of story. His sketches must be concise, dramatic, appealing, provocative . . . he suggests the style, the characters, the mood, the staging. His drawings influence all who follow.

WALT
Walt still oversees every facet of production, with most of his focus on story. He has final approval on all important matters.

WRITERS & STORY SKETCH
DIRECTOR
Assistants track the increasing number of details in production.
MUSIC
ASSISTANT DIRECTOR
VOICES
CUTTER
SOUND EFFECTS
DUBBING
ANIMATION
ASSISTANTS
INBETWEENERS
Lead animators supervise small units of less experienced animators and assistants.
LAYOUT
ART DIRECTION
BACK-GROUNDS
INK & PAINT
CHECKING & STORY SKETCH
BACK-GROUNDS
Color necessitates Art Directors supervise color for each character and background.
CAMERA
ANSWER PRINT
FINAL FILM
Prerecorded sound elements can now be mixed together at the end of production.
Though the Director supervises the production, Walt has the final word and can call for fixes or adjustments at his discretion.

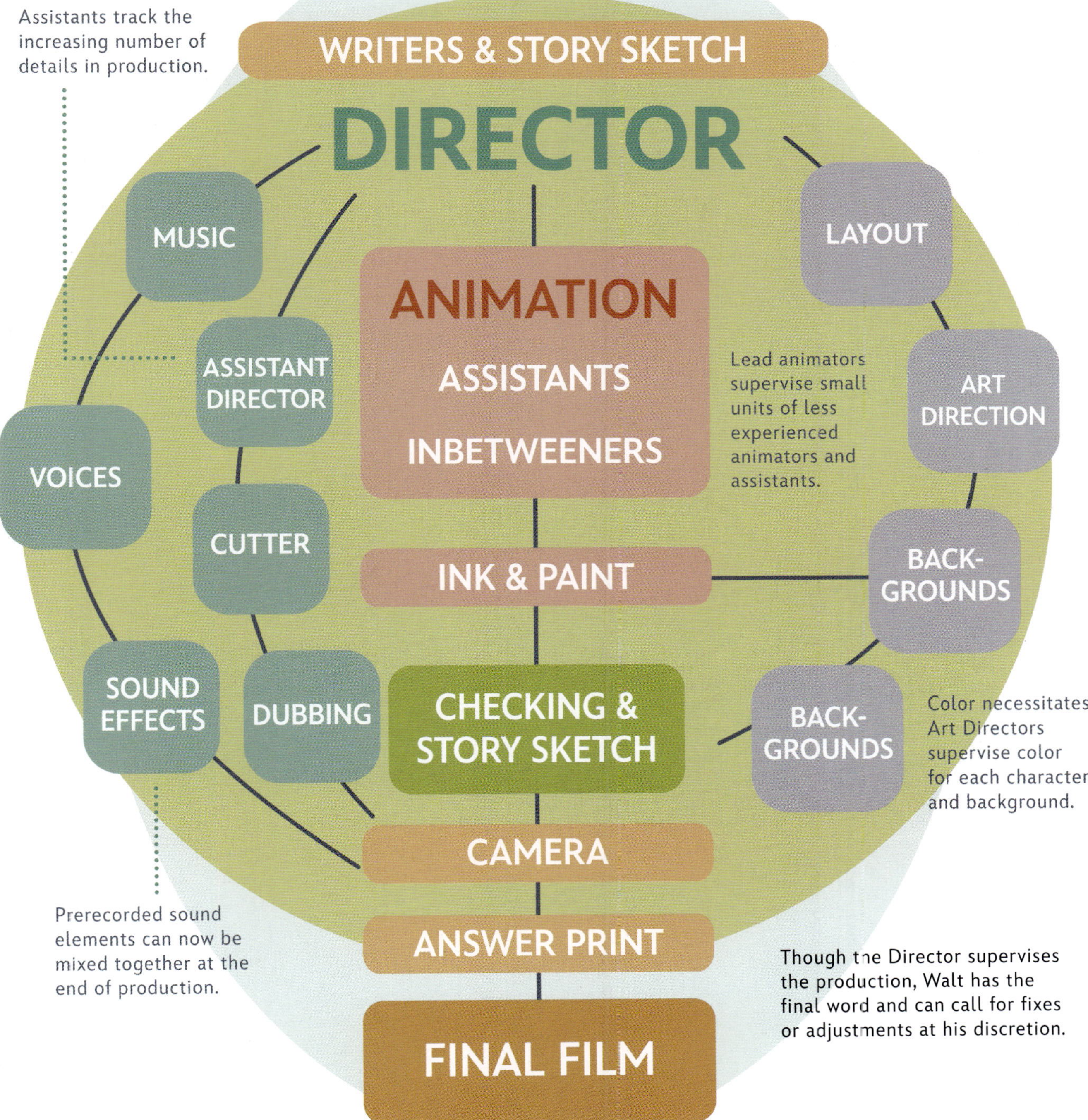

Output: one short every four weeks

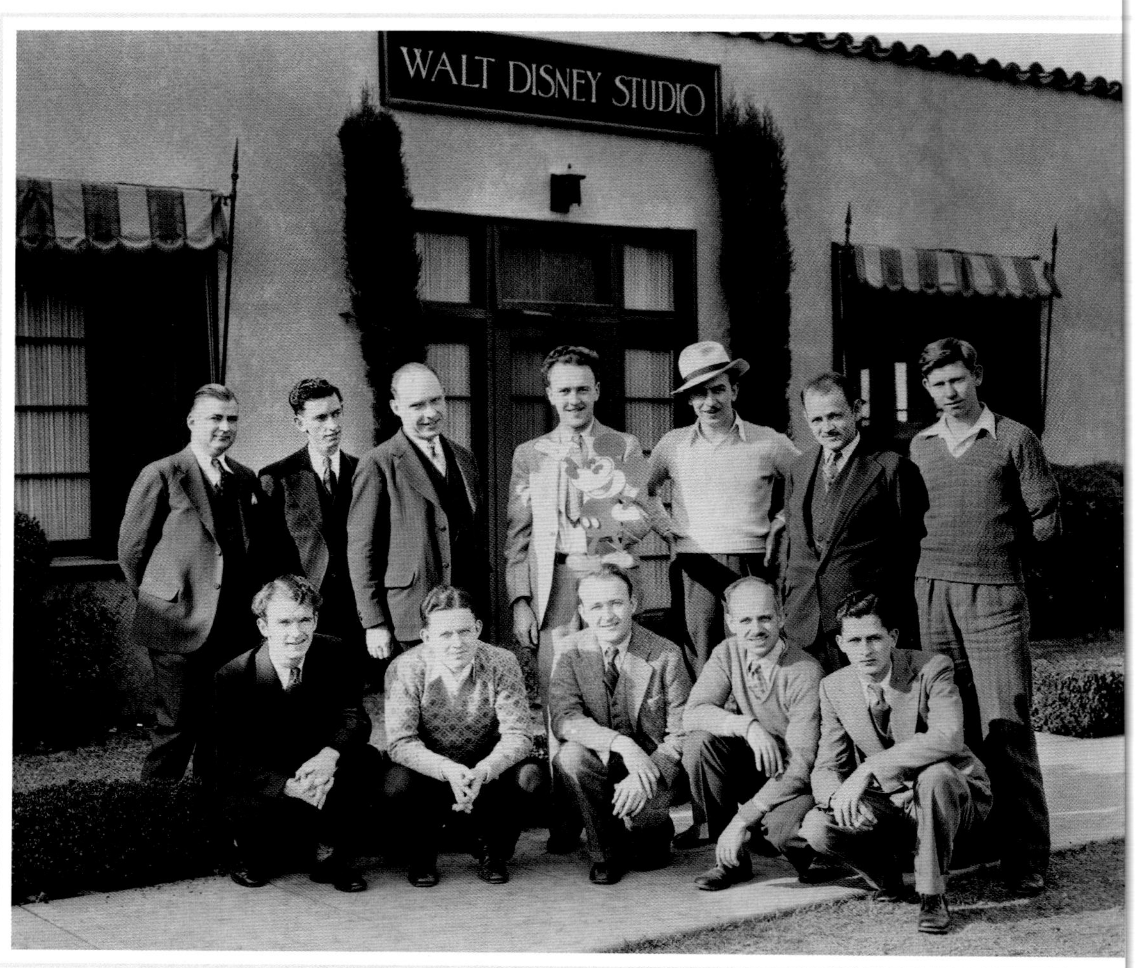

BACK ROW: Jack King, Dick Lundy, Burt Gillett, Ub Iwerks, Walt Disney, Carl Stalling, and Wilfred Jackson.
SQUATTING: Johnny Cannon, Norm Ferguson, Merle Gilson, Ben Sharpsteen, and Les Clark.

CHAPTER 2

BURT GILLETT—THE MAN WHO DIRECTED *THREE LITTLE PIGS*

"You could hear Gillett in there, putting his heart into it—and the fellow at the piano would be playing right along with him, just like the old silent-movie days, where they'd catch all the action on the screen. Gillett would roar, he'd holler, he'd scream, he'd jump on the desk, and onto the floor. And he'd say, 'Now, let's do it again.'"[1]

—Animator Eric Larson

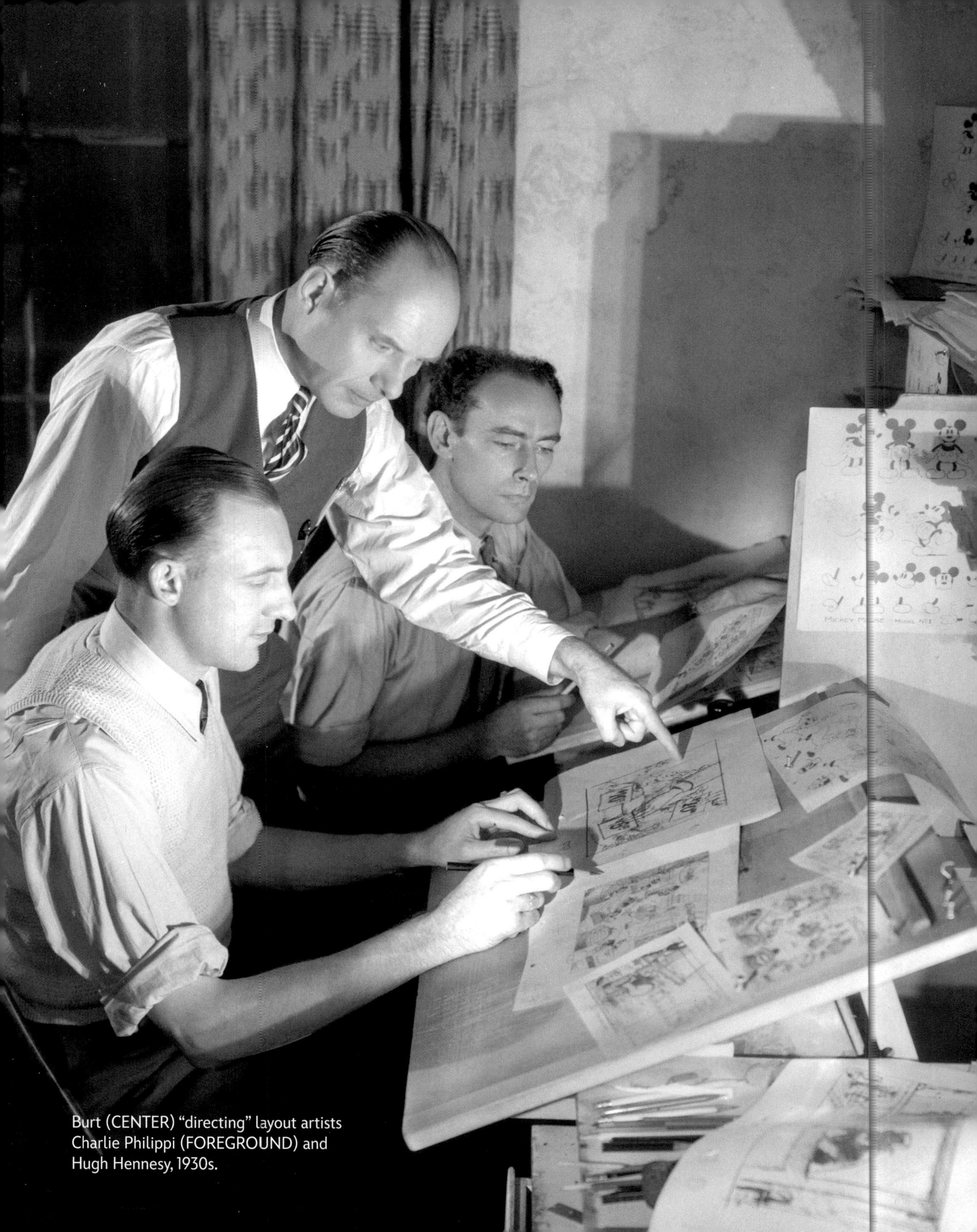

Burt (CENTER) “directing” layout artists Charlie Philippi (FOREGROUND) and Hugh Hennesy, 1930s.

"A VIVID IMPRESSION OF THE FEELING"

Ub Iwerks and Burt Gillett could not have been more different. While Ub was described as quiet, mild-mannered, non-demonstrative, and very likeable, Burt was intense, shameless, a wild man, full of excessive energy, and one who evoked strong positive and negative reactions from those who worked with him. Animator Shamus Culhane said, "He had a speech pattern that was unusual in that his words would come out with a machine-gun rapidity; then there would be a sudden stoppage, not always where one expected a natural pause. Then it would suddenly resume at breakneck speed. He never seemed to finish a thought, but skipped from one subject to the next, as a more compelling thought struck him."[2] Burt from all accounts was a force of nature at Disney and everywhere he worked before and after.

Burton Fred "Burt" Gillett was born in 1891 in Elmira, New York. He studied at the Art Students League in New York and worked as a cartoonist and reporter on local newspapers before entering the animation industry in 1916 at the Charles Bowers Studio. Over the next thirteen years, he worked at virtually all the New York studios, including Hearst International Film Service, Jefferson Film Company, Barre-Bowers Studio, Max Fleischer Studio, Bray Productions, and Pat Sullivan's studio, each with increasing responsibility. He was part of a cooperative, Associated Animators, with Dick Huemer, Ben Harrison, and Manny Gould, to revive production of *Mutt and Jeff* cartoons among others, but internal strife contributed to its early demise.

Walt, in a letter to Roy and Ub from New York on February 9, 1929, described his recruiting of animators from the New York studios and mentioned meeting Burt: "I have a fellow by the name of Gillette [sic]—he is now working at [Pat] Sullivan's studio on the new Felixes which he says are not so hot—he is the guy that made the last series of *Mutt and Jeff* . . . and was recommended to me by Jack King—He is a damn clever fellow—and a good gag man and animator. He made some good *Mutt and Jeff* stuff and had [Ben] Harrison and [Manny] Gould working for him—He is coming out as soon as he can get away—I am paying him $125—"[3] While talking with Walt in New York, Burt recommended that Walt contact Ben Sharpsteen, with whom Burt had worked at various New York studios over the years and who was now located on the West Coast. Walt did, and Ben joined the Disney Studios just ahead of Burt. (Ben has his own chapter. Stay tuned.) He was followed by New York veterans Jack King and Norman Ferguson over the next few months.

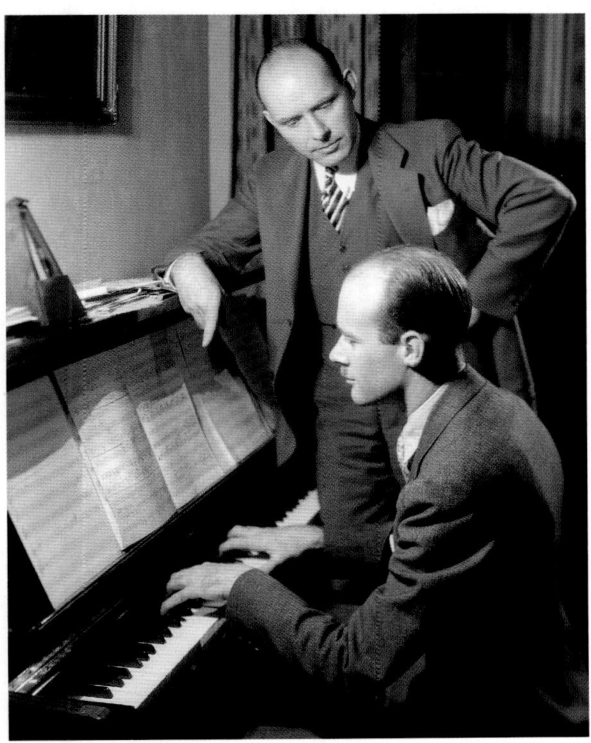

Burt Gillett watches as Frank Churchill plays.

FROM ANIMATOR TO DIRECTOR

Burt brought to the studio as much experience in the animation field as anyone currently on the roster, if not more. So it is not surprising that after a short stint as an animator, Burt began assisting Walt by handing out scenes to animators. Soon he moved into Walt's Music Room (the planning center of each Disney short) and took a bigger role in preparing the animation shorts for production.

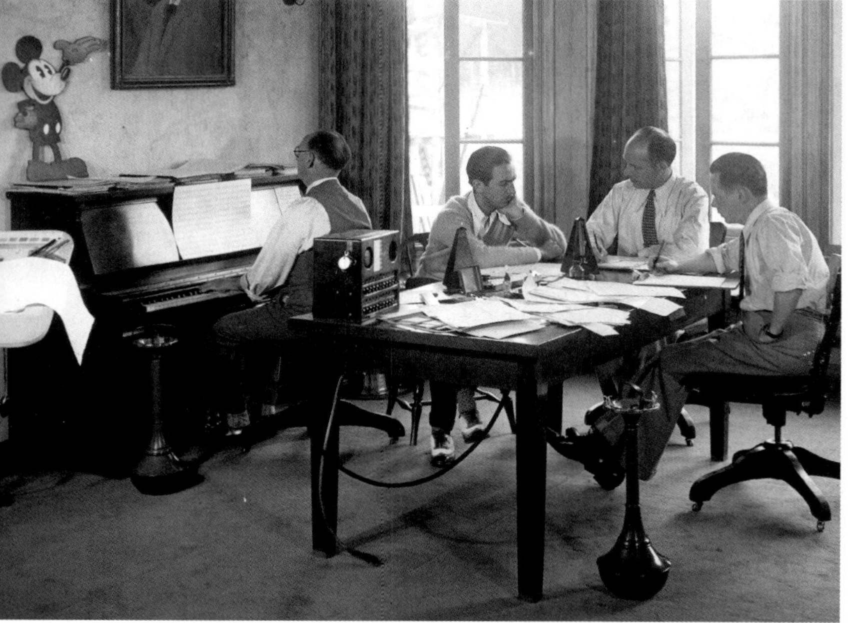

The Music Room, where the piano resided, home to the director, musician, layout artist, and occasional story writer. The fact it wasn't named the Director's Room perhaps gives an indication of what Disney felt was the important work being done here. This is Music Room 1, on the second floor of the Hyperion Avenue Studio. FROM LEFT TO RIGHT: Bert Lewis (musician), Walt, Burt Gillett, and Ted Sears (the first story writer). Next to Mickey hangs a painting of composer Victor Herbert by background artist Emil Flohri. This room was generally home to the Mickey and/or jazz-based cartoons.

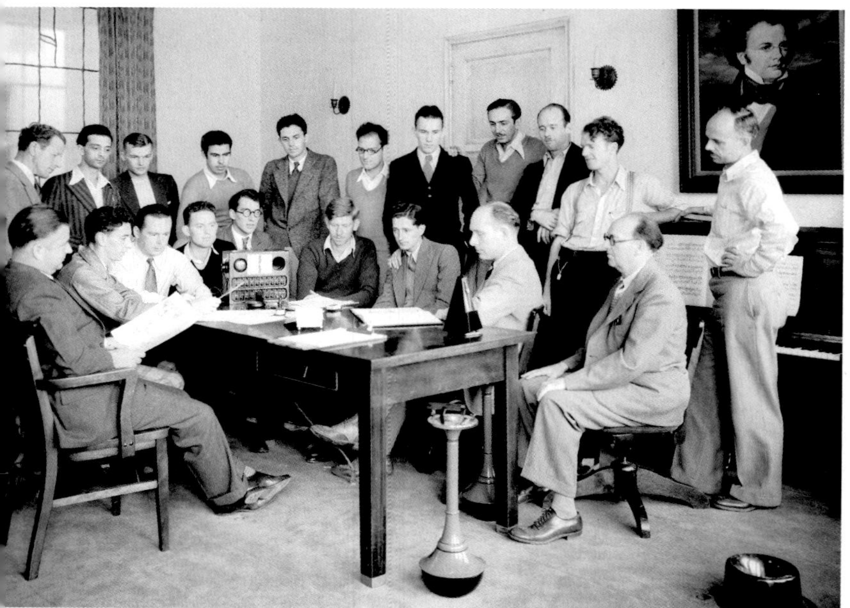

Music Room 2, downstairs, where classical Silly Symphony cartoons were helmed. A painting of Franz Schubert (by Flohri) hangs over that piano. STANDING LEFT TO RIGHT: Webb Smith, Otto Englander, Edmund Seward, Rudy Zamora, Dave Hand, Tom Palmer, Jack Cutting, Walt Disney, Frank Churchill, Johnny Cannon, Ben Sharpsteen. SITTING LEFT TO RIGHT: Jack King, Dick Lundy, Ted Sears, Norm Ferguson, Gilles Armand "Frenchy" de Trémaudan, Wilfred "Jaxon" Jackson, Les Clark, Burt Gillett, Bert Lewis.

TITLE "ARCTIC ANTICS" PROD. NO.- S-11

FOOTAGE	SCENE	ARTIST	STARTED	FINISHED		DESCRIPTION
59-8	1	TOM	5-22 A-M-	6-9 P-M	PAN	LITTLE BEAR ON MOTHER'S BACK.
28	2	JAXON	5-23 A.M	6-2 A-M-	PAN	L.S. BEARS AND SEALS on ICE CAKES
27-2	3	DAVE	5-24 A-M	6-2 A.M.	PAN	LITTLE BEAR ON ICE CAKE— USES TAIL AS PROPELLOR
30-4	4	LES-	5-26 P.M-	6-4 P-M-	PAN	BIG POLAR BEAR DANCING ON ICE CAKE —REAR VIEW—
30-3	5	FERGY	5-26 A-M	6-3 A.M.	PAN	WALRUS TRYING TO CATCH LITTLE FISH —
175-1 44-3	6	BEN	5-28 NOON	6-2 P.M.	PAN	4 SEALS DANCING ALONG - THEY DIVE AND BARK -
35-7	7	DICK	5-29 A.M.	6-9 P.M.		GIRL SEAL DOES HOOCH DANCE ——
41-9	8	JOHNNY	5-29 A.M.	6-9 P.M.		LITTLE SEAL PLAYS ON WALRUS'S NOSE, WHISKERS, TEETH
30-3	9	FERGY	6-3 NOON	6-5 P-M-		WALRUS SINGS —
7—	10	BEN	6-3 AM	6-7 P.M.		SEALS APPLAUD REPEAT FROM "WILD WAVES"
7 —	11	BEN	"	"		L.S. — SEAL TOSSES FISH TO WALRUS —
15-12	12	BEN	"	"	PAN	C.U. - WALRUS APPLAUDS. LITTLE FISH PEEKS OUT OF MOUTH
OUT						
72-9	14	JACK	6-2 NOON	6-12 NOON	PAN	START OF PENGUIN MARCH TO VERSE MUSIC
14-11	15	JAXON	6-2 P-M-	6-4 NOON		CLOSEUP OF GENERAL MARCHING AND GIVING COMMANDS
48-6 493-11	16	DAVE	6-2 P-M-	6-12 NOON	PAN	DRILL AND FORMATION MARCHING OF PENGUINS-ENTIRE ACTION REPEATS
51-14	17	JAXON	6-4 NOON	6-11 NOON	PAN	LITTLE PENGUIN FALLS IN WATER — THEN FALLS IN ICE-HOLE —COMES OUT 2ND HOLE.
19-4	18	LES-	6-5 A-M-	6-10 NOON	PAN	BIG PENGUIN MARCHES + DANCES TO DRUMMING
25-8	19	FERGY	6-6 A-M-	6-7 P.M.	PAN	L.S. PENGUINS MARCH + WHISTLE TO VERSE — CAMERA MOVES BACK—FINIS
590-5	TOTAL					

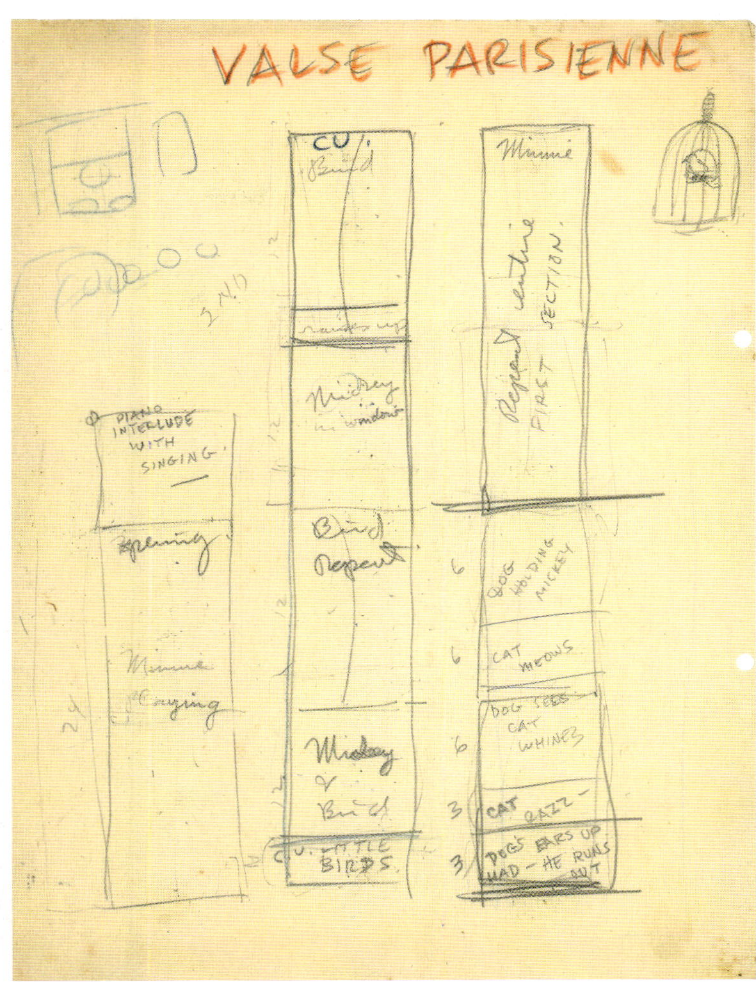

Examples of Gillett's planning, which would go on to become standard practice: (LEFT) an early version of what would become known as a draft, listing animators, scene numbers, and descriptions; (RIGHT) a vertical version of what would later be called a bar sheet. This was part of *Mickey Steps Out*, directed by Gillett and released July 7, 1931. Both courtesy Hans Perk.

Although not called directors, both Burt and Ub were functioning as such. Walt thought of them as story men, because their primary responsibility was to further story development (until artists like Ted Sears joined the staff and devoted their efforts purely to story development—always working under Walt—and a story department was born). But Ben Sharpsteen said, "There wasn't anything formal in the division there, and Walt wouldn't hesitate to criticize Gillett in front of one of us . . . Nothing was sacred to anybody then."[4] As Ben saw Burt: "Gillett was quite talkative, and a pretty good salesman . . . he'd act things out. It was pretty horrible, but that was what Walt wanted—it was stimulation. It comes right back to Walt again; who knew but Walt what the value of a man was?"[5] Both Burt and Ub were making layout drawings to guide the animators in staging, and they worked with Carl Stalling in preparing the blueprints for animation: bar sheets and exposure sheets.

BAR SHEETS

Imagine you are a Disney director. In front of you is a board with a hundred-plus drawings pinned to it, which describe a cartoon that does not yet exist. Your job is to figure out what actions happen when, and then communicate this to the dozens of people who will animate, write music, and make backgrounds for the cartoon.

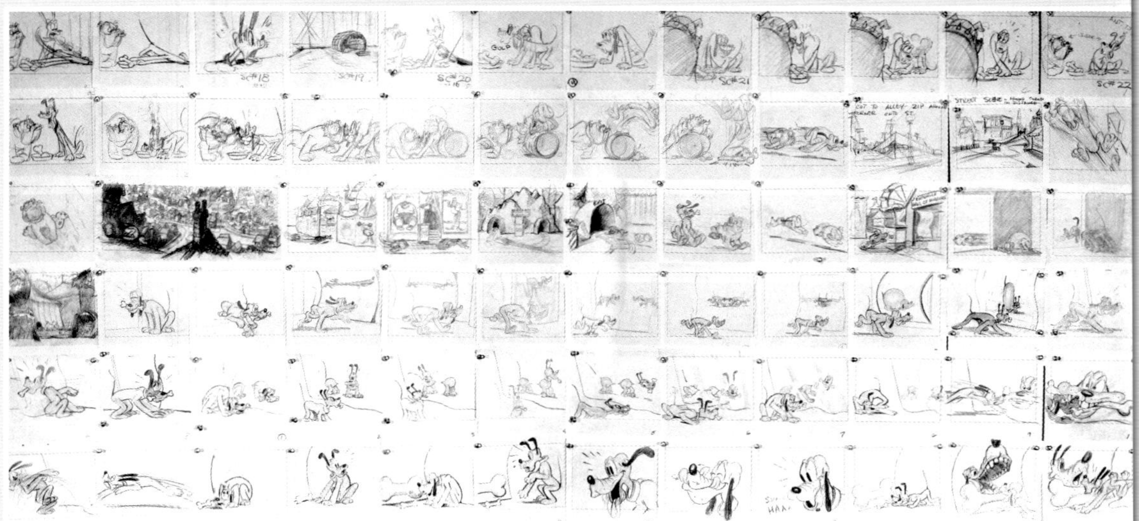

Storyboards from *Bone Trouble* (1940) dir. Jack Kinney.

How would you do it? You might start by making a list:

:00	Start cartoon. Begin iris open
:01	Iris full open
	Mickey walking down street, one footstep every eight frames. This goes on for 21 seconds, so footsteps fall on frames 24, 32, 40, 48, etc.
	at the same time:
:02:5	(Two and a half seconds in) Mickey begins whistling a jaunty tune, in rhythm to the footsteps
	This goes on for 12 seconds until:
:15.5	Pluto runs up, barking. Barks happen every 16 frames
:17.25	Mickey: "Down boy! Ha ha, down!" (Dialogue takes 3 seconds and 7 frames) etc.

This is mathematically clear, but not especially visual, and it's difficult to understand what sounds or actions overlap each other.

So what if we were to turn this into a timeline? You could make blocks that each represent a second (24 frames of film), with half seconds (12 frames) indicated as well.

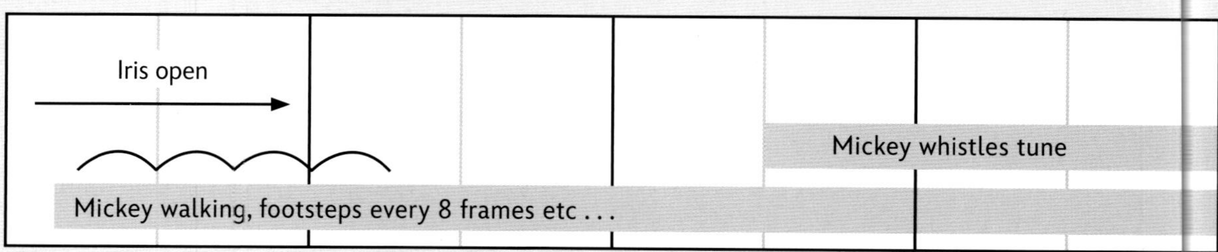

This is much easier to understand. And it's visual. Guess what? You've just invented a bar sheet! (Actually, it was invented by director Wilfred Jackson, who you'll read more about in chapter 5.)

Here's a bar sheet from *The Pointer* (1939), prepared and kept by assistant director Jack Cutting, following the timing by director Gerry Geronimi. As with the example on the lower left, each dark line marks off one second, showing four seconds every horizontal bar. The four blocks showing on this page add up to sixteen seconds, so a seven-minute cartoon would be planned out over twenty-seven pages.

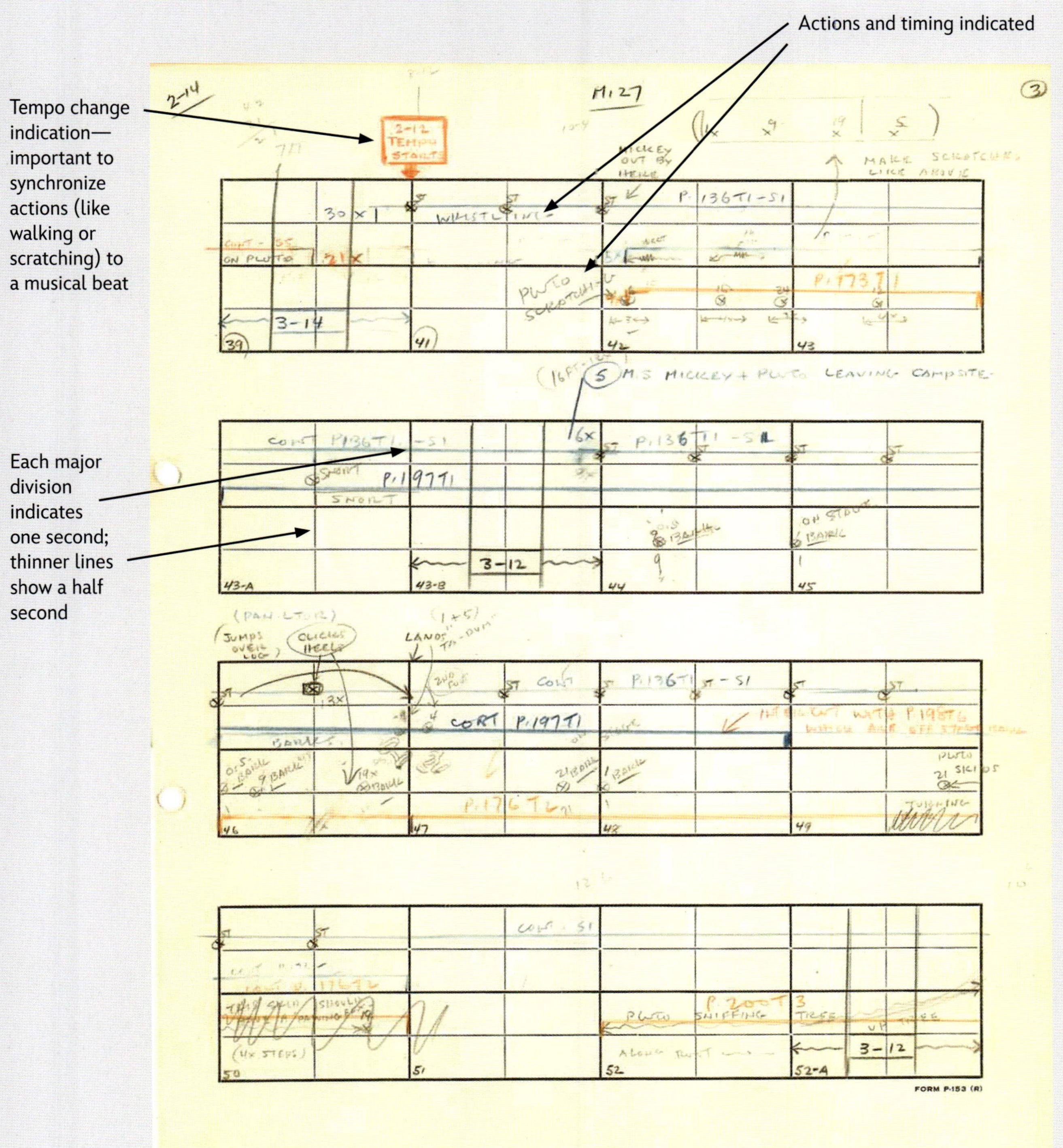

The director's bar sheets would then be transferred to a "main bar sheet" by the assistant director, to be used by the composer. Music was written to match the desired action on-screen.

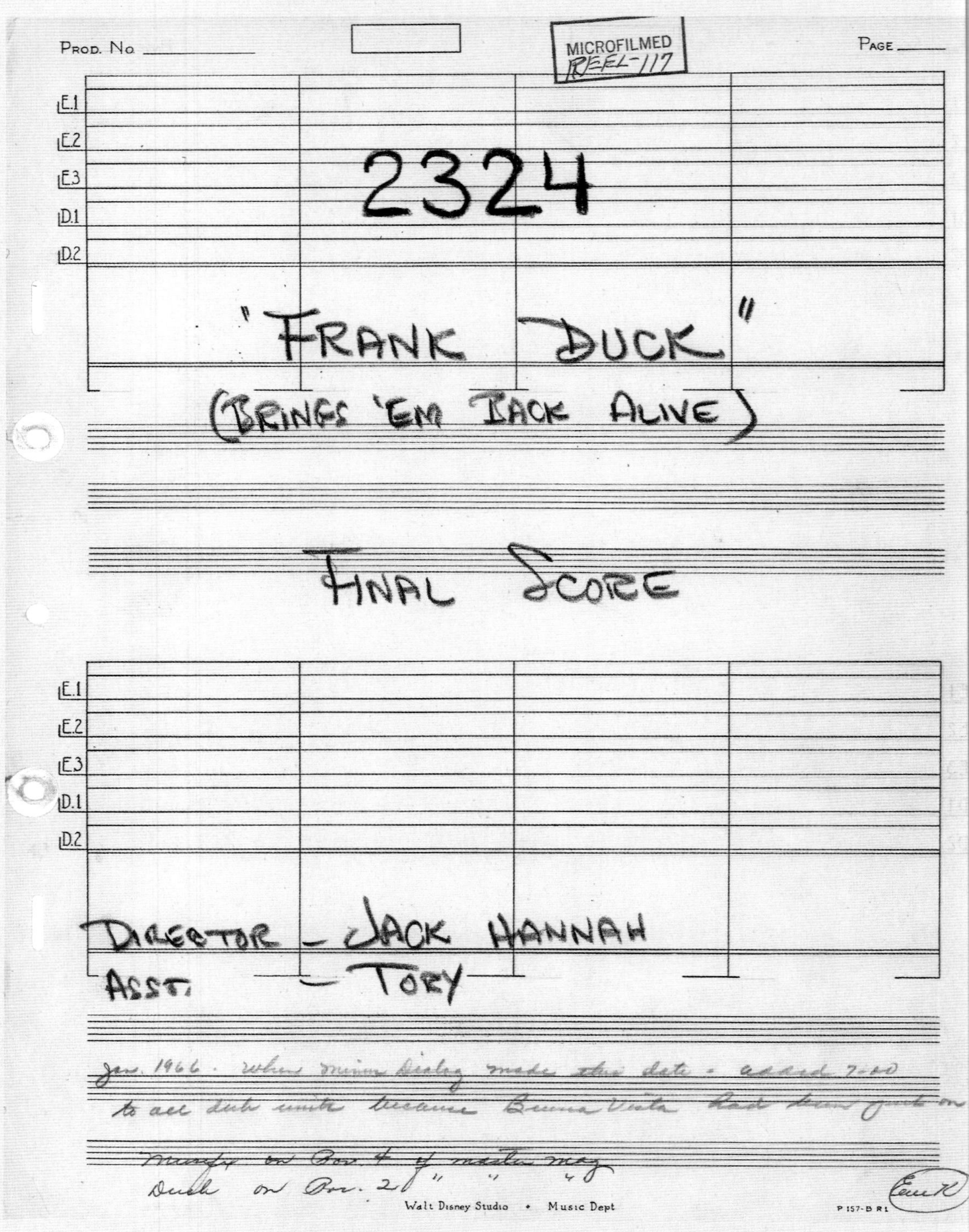

A 2-12 beat makes each measure equal to a second of screen time.

E1, E2, and E3 show sound effects tracks; D1 and D2 indicate dialogue.

Character's actions and timing are noted here.

Measure numbers (for music) are here.

A musical "sketch" (the basic melody) to be orchestrated later is here.

PROD. No 2324 2/12's PAGE 23

E1
E2 CRASH
E3
D.1 DUCK LAUGHTER
D.2

11 12 13 14

E.1
E.2
E3 RATTLING BARS RATTLING BARS
D.1 I GOT HIM – I GOT HIM – I GOT HIM – HEH-HEH BOY-OH-BOY – I –
D.2

15 16 17 18

Walt Disney Studio • Music Dept

From Prod. 2324, *Frank Duck Brings 'em Back Alive*, directed by Jack Hannah, released November 1, 1946.

X-SHEETS

X-sheets (short for exposure sheets) provided several functions. First, they communicated from director to animator what was meant to happen when on-screen. These timings were often adjusted as the animator worked—much to the director's frustration, as this would necessitate changes to the music and overall pacing of the film. Here is a page from prod. M-37, *Mickey's Grand Opera* (1936), assigned to animator Les Clark.

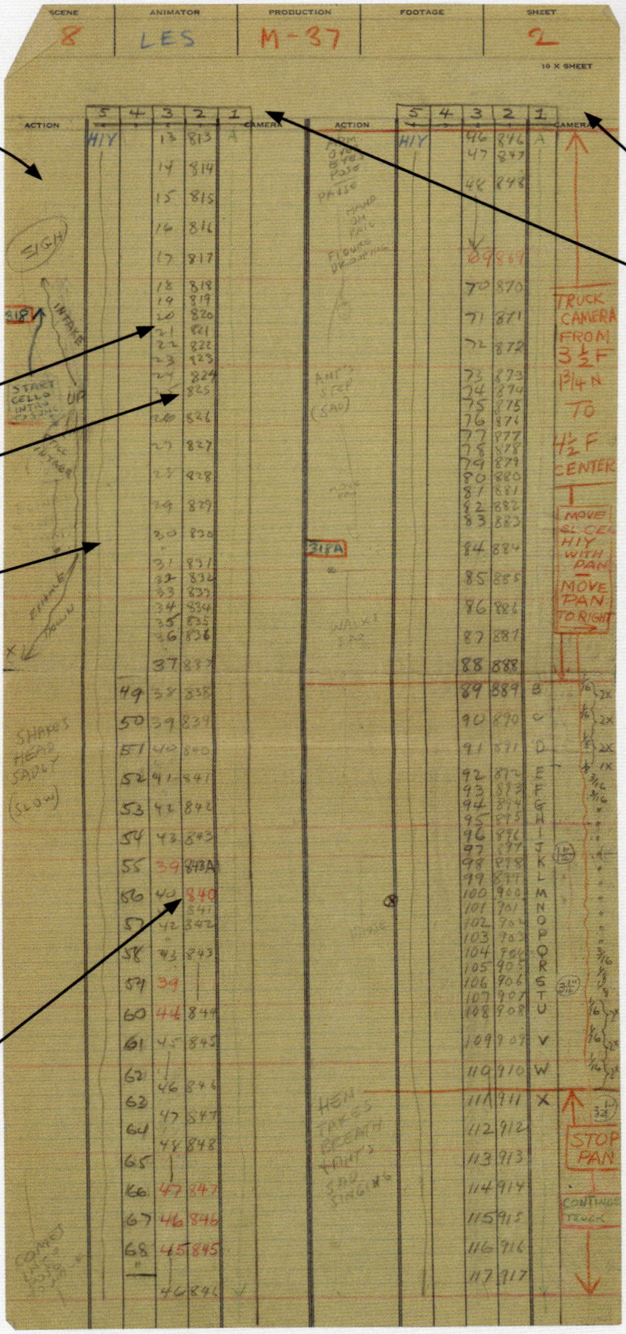

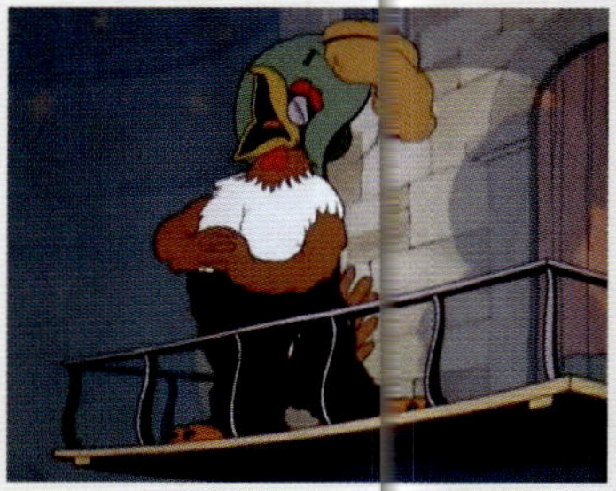

Each row across indicates one frame of film (there are 24 frames in one second).

Each column is a different layer of drawings. In this scene there are 5 levels, though that differs per scene. For example, here the hen is on level 3, her shadow on level 2, and the railing in front of her on level 5.

Character actions and other important info is indicated in left columns, initially by the director and added to by the animator.

Each number refers to a different animation drawing, each one different than the last, sometimes repeating or held across multiple frames of film.

This sheet has two columns per page; the left side ends at bottom, and continues on upper right.

Camera moves, such as pans, zooms, or tilts, are indicated here.

The X-sheet is vital to the cameraman, who would otherwise be receiving a confusing stack of drawings. This sheet gave precise instructions as to what should be shot on each frame of film.

The format of X-sheets changed over time, and several versions were usually prepared for each shot.

EXPERIENCE COUNTS

Burt focused mostly on the Mickey Mouse series and Ub on the Silly Symphonies, although Burt directed *Flowers and Trees*, the first Silly in color (and the first Academy Award winner in the new Best Animated Short category) a couple of years later. *Wild Waves* (1930) marked Burt's directorial debut, which was followed by a prolific career as a shorts director during his first stay at the studio: forty-four shorts between 1929 and 1934 with several outstanding entries, including *Mickey's Good Deed* (1932), *Mickey's Gala Premier* (1933), *Playful Pluto* (1934), and, of course, *Three Little Pigs* (1933). Animator and director Jack Kinney said, "Bert [sic] was the first 'tink-tink-tink' director. Every time Mickey took a step, there was a metallic 'tink.' . . . Everything moved to a rhythm and, by God, the animator better follow that beat . . . Gillett was very energetic and so were his Mickey Mouse pictures—loud and fast."[6]

Wilfred Jackson (who preferred to be called by his own creation: Jaxon), soon to join Burt as a director upon Ub's departure, valued the experience Burt brought to his position and felt that it put Burt on a much higher plane, at least from him. In a series of letters to animation historian Michael Barrier, Jackson stressed that Burt could draw on his experiences directing at New York studios to help guide him to successful directing ventures at Disney and that "he had already made a lot of the mistakes some of the rest of us still had to make in learning how to direct our cartoons, and he wouldn't have to make them again."[7] (The next two animators to become directors—Dave Hand and Ben Sharpsteen—also had extensive experience at the New York studios.)

Burt started at Disney at a time when, as Jaxon put it, "Walt wasn't yet so far ahead of the rest of us in knowing how to make our animation look life-like,"[8] giving Burt "a much broader background of experience with animation than any of the rest of us—maybe even including Walt."[9] Burt introduced several innovations from New York when he started that made quite an impression at the studio. One was the sliding cell. For anything to appear to move on-screen, each image must be different from the last. But instead of dozens of drawings of a car driving across the frame, for instance, the sliding cel allows one drawing to be used simply by positioning it in progressively different places. Or with a character walking, the animator could create a cycle of sixteen drawings for the walk, and then the camera operator could reposition those repeated drawings across the background, creating the sensation of movement and saving both time and labor.

Jaxon described Burt as older and more mature but as retaining a boyish enthusiasm for fun and excitement, demonstrated by things like his running out to follow a bell-clanging fire truck to observe how they put out a fire. Jaxon pointed out that as a director, Burt was thorough and "a stickler for detail." But what distinguished him from other Disney directors in Jaxon's mind was Burt's focus on the *feeling* of an action—the emotional content. Jaxon said that all the directors visualized the story's action in their minds but Burt did so with his whole body. This made him a noisy neighbor. His music room was above Jaxon's music room, and Jaxon was frequently subjected to jumping and pounding as Burt physically manifested the story plot moment to moment. Once, responding to "a sudden outburst of furious scuffling and thumping from above," Jaxon rushed upstairs "to discover that Burt had little Freddy Moore cornered against the wall and was throwing punches at him." While disagreements between animator and director were not uncommon, Jaxon was surprised to see it go this far. "But, as it turned out, Burt was only handing out some animation to Fred"[10] and was acting out the part to make sure Fred understood. Eric

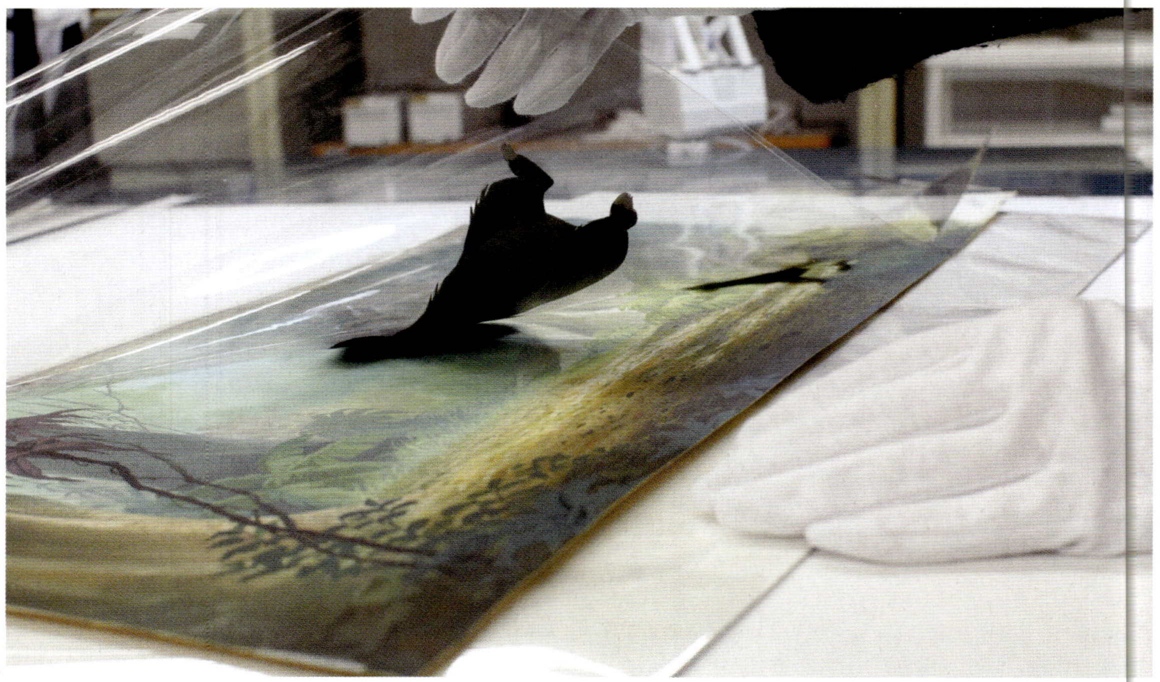

A cel (short for celluloid) placed over a background. Dozens, sometimes hundreds, of cels would create the illusion of movement while allowing the background to remain stationary.

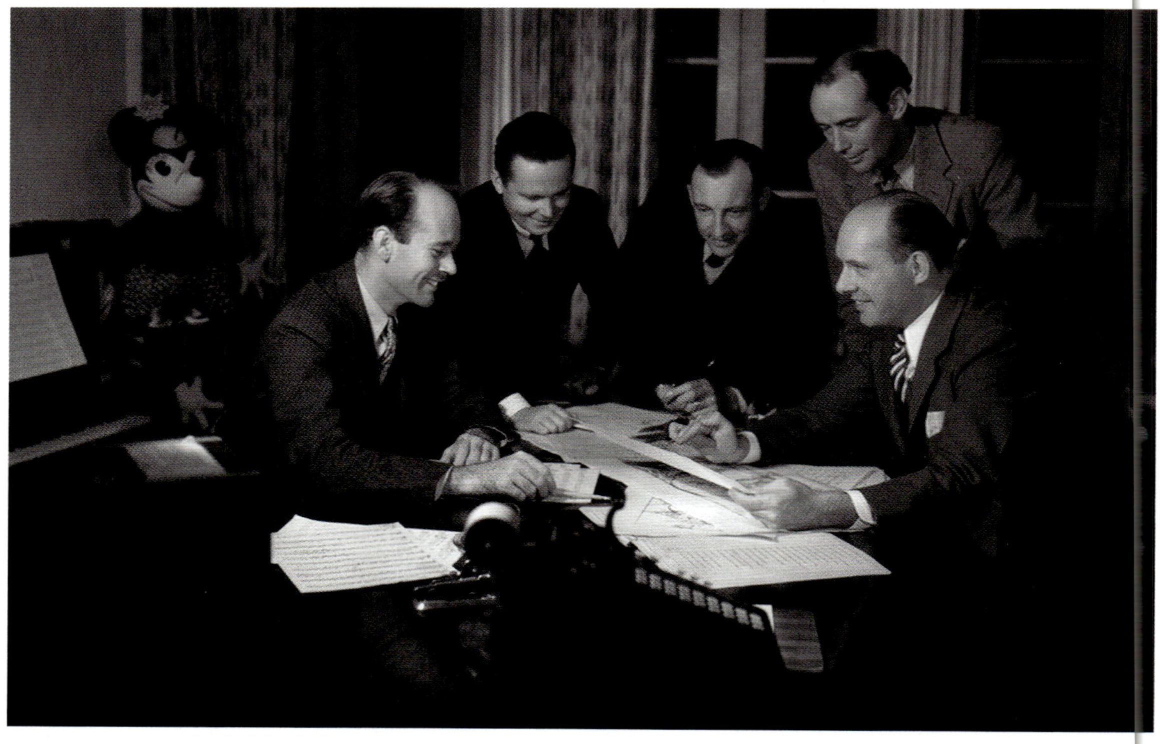

LEFT TO RIGHT: Frank Churchill, Ted Sears, Charlie Philippi, Hugh Hennesy, and Burt Gillett confer under the watchful eye of Minnie Mouse.

Larson, one of the more mild-mannered members of Walt Disney's "Nine Old Men" (a nickname Walt gave to his top animators), recalled witnessing the same phenomenon when he was an assistant to animator Ham Luske: "When he went over a scene with an animator . . . he ran around the room, jumping from floor to chair to table to floor, just as he wanted the character in the scene to do. He acted out tantrums and he pounded his fists on his desk for emphasis. As the villain in the scene, he growled ferociously, and as the little victim, he cried and cried." Eric concluded, "It was fun to listen in, but all the time I was hoping that should I ever become an animator, I would not have to work with Gillett. A great one, I told myself, but he would drive me up the wall."[11] Jaxon concluded, "The point I wanted to make is that when an animator picked up work from Burt, he went back to his room with a vivid impression of the *feeling* of the action he was to animate."[12]

Along with Burt's extensive experience animating and supervising at the New York studios, he brought an attitude of stubbornness beyond that evinced by any of the other directors in this early period. When he and Walt disagreed, if he couldn't win an argument with Walt outright, he would sometimes employ devious methods to achieve what he wanted, undoubtedly confident that he knew best. Stories circulated about Burt taking animation home to undo changes Walt had ordered over his objection. Walt would not see it until the preview, and then he would blame the animator for not making the change he had ordered.[13] But Jaxon, finding himself unwittingly thrown into the director's seat, turned to Burt as his role model. He reasoned: "Burt had already been doing a good job of directing pictures for Walt for some time. I had a tremendous respect for the result Burt was getting with his pictures and tried to find out what I could about how he went about it."[14]

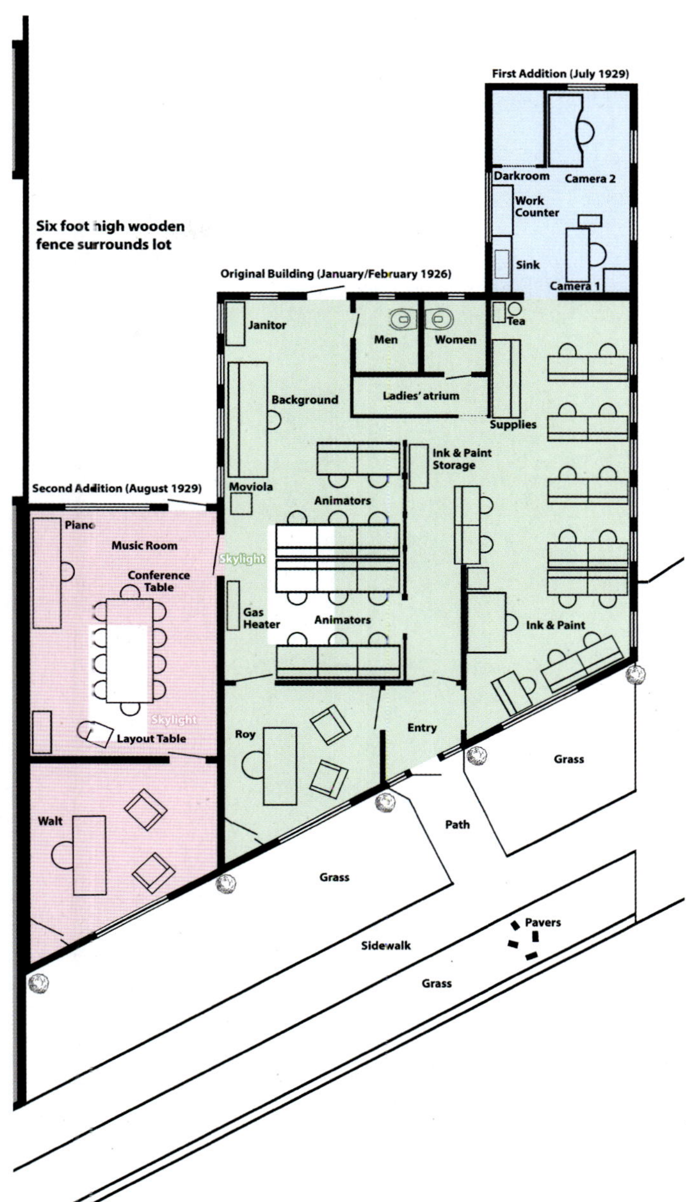

Walt and Roy moved into the Walt Disney Studio at 2719 Hyperion Avenue in January 1926. Until they moved to Burbank in 1940, the studio became a sort of Winchester Mystery House as it expanded to accommodate the growing staff. The above map by Hans Perk was pieced together from diagrams by Floyd Gottfredson and Wilfred Jackson, various photos, and verbal descriptions preserved in the Walt Disney Archives.

SUCCESS WITH PIGS

Walt perhaps shrewdly selected the team of Gillett and Frank Churchill to helm the Silly Symphony short *Three Little Pigs*. Walt knew that Burt would not be as exacting with the animators as Jaxon would have been, and consequently Fred Moore and Norm Ferguson were allowed to be more creative in developing each of the four characters with individual personalities. Frank Churchill, who went on to write much of Disney's most memorable music, struck gold with "Who's Afraid of the Big Bad Wolf?," which became almost an anthem for audiences struggling with the Great Depression. Some argue that *Three Little Pigs* is the best short cartoon ever made at the Disney Studios or anywhere else.

Animator Dick Huemer remembered Gillett as "difficult to work with, because he was never satisfied."[15] While he shared this trait with Walt, even Disney had a limit. In a letter to archivist Dave Smith, Burt's son, Fredric, recounted a story that captured some of the characteristics that ultimately led to Burt's downfall: "My father was the director on *Three Little Pigs*. In those days, Silly Symphonies were budgeted at $30,000. Near the end of the picture, Walt spent about a month in Cuba. My father did not like some of the animation so had them done over in Walt's absence. When Walt returned and ran the cost of the 'Pigs' it was running around $60,000. He took my father to task about it . . ."[16] In contrast to Fredric's account, Ben recalled: "Perhaps the high point in the animating of shorts, the greatest single factor

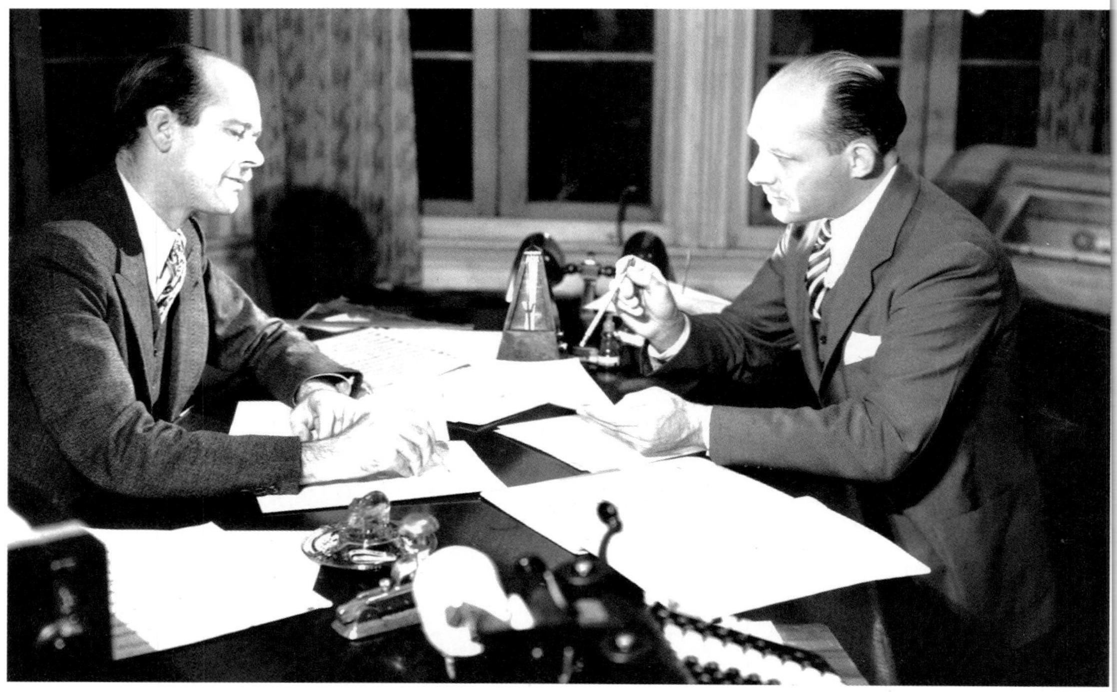

Composer Frank Churchill (LEFT) and Burt Gillett were a team on the production of *Three Little Pigs*.

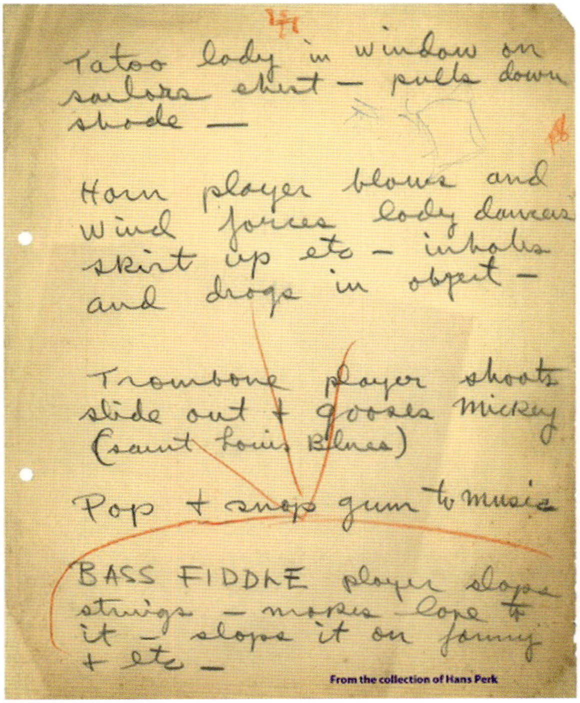

While Gillett was rightly praised for his work, these 1931 memos from Walt on *Blue Rhythm* reveal Disney's beat-by-beat involvement in every cartoon of that time. Courtesy Hans Perk.

that made Disney's name so popular with the moviegoing public was the *Three Little Pigs*. This was a picture where Walt practically lived in the Music Room while the director was working on it. . . . He visualized the entire picture, and he spent much more of his time on it than he had on any other picture up to that time. In spite of that, the picture was identified with the director."[17] In any event, within the industry, Burt Gillett was known as the director of the most successful short. His fame would have an unpredictable effect on his career and on Walt's attitude toward his directors.

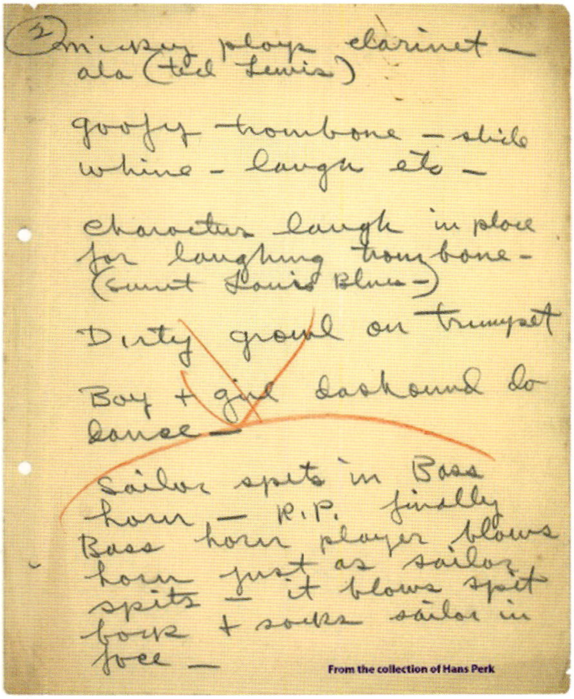

Amedee J. Van Beuren acquired Fables Pictures, which was known for its Aesop's Fables cartoons, in 1928. Paul Terry was in charge of animation; Van Beuren, headed the business operations. After Terry left in 1929, the studio carried on, but not as one of the top studios. Van Beuren wanted to improve his studio's output and saw Burt Gillett as the answer. After all, he had directed *Three Little Pigs*! In his autobiography, Joe Barbera said, "After some years in the cartoon business, I would learn that *everyone* who had been associated with Walt Disney either created the *Three Little Pigs* or *Snow White*. Burt Gillette [sic] claimed to have been responsible for both. But that was after we got to know one another."[18] Burt left Disney and joined Van Beuren as chief director and general manager. (It is ironic that Burt would go to this studio, because Disney successfully sued Van Beuren in 1931 over copyright infringements on Mickey Mouse.) Burt came in hoping to be the second coming of Walt, by hiring and firing at will, attempting to upgrade procedures by introducing pencil tests and the use of the Moviola—both standard practices at Disney—thwarting a movement to form a union, and doing whatever he could by threat or persuasion to elevate the quality of the studio's cartoons. He did make some improvements, but not quickly enough, and in 1936, RKO—the studio's distributor—dropped the studio when it signed a contract to distribute Disney pictures.

Frank Thomas quoted animator Bill Peet as saying about Walt: "I don't see how that guy ever got everybody to peak, to do their best work there at the studio. Everybody brought in, no matter how good they were before or after, did their top work while they were here."[19] Burt was just one of many who would prove Peet's point.

Meanwhile, back at the Disney Studios, Walt was not happy with the attention focused on Burt or any director, and wanted to organize the studio so that no one was indispensable. He tried two experiments without much success. The first was with *Mickey's Amateurs* (1937). The short was made by a group of animators with no assigned director; Walt would play a supervisory part. Ben Sharpsteen recalled, "The picture, however, turned out to be an extremely weak one. Walt complained that he himself had not had the time to put in on it, and that one of the animators, during the making of the picture, had dominated not only the story men, but also the other animators. He had monopolized the situation, and it was his poor judgment that was to blame. Walt never tried that experiment again, and I think he learned a lesson from it."[20] Next Walt decided that he *would* direct again, and he would use his top two animators—Freddy Moore and Norm Ferguson—to make a short. Again, Ben Sharpsteen: "Walt bragged to his directors about the merits of his animators. It was a backhanded way of telling you that if you wanted to get on the bandwagon, why, improve your work. In talking about this picture, he said he would make it, direct it himself. It was also because people in the studio were too inclined to associate the success of a particular picture with the director who was on it. I know that Walt resented this. I know that he wanted to prove that many other people could direct, even people who did not know the business."[21] The short, *The Golden Touch* (1935), was considered by the staff and the public to be a weak cartoon. It was another disappointing lesson for Walt.

Burt came back to Disney in September of 1936, despite the circumstances under which he had left and the fact that he had burned some bridges with the staff at Disney before his departure. During his slightly more than a year back at the studio, he directed *Lonesome Ghosts*, a very successful short—but resorted to some of his old ways of going over the maximum footage allowance and undercutting Walt's directives on story points. His eventual dismissal from Disney listed several reasons, including absence without cause or notification, not performing to the best of his ability (months behind schedule, cost run-ups, etc.), not attending art classes, and showing interest in business other than the studio's business.[22] He began direction on two more shorts—*Moth and the Flame* and *Brave Little Tailor*—but departed before they were finished.

After Disney, Burt worked at MGM under Fred Quimby for a short period and then for Walter Lantz, where he directed *A Haunting We Will Go* (1939) and a few other cartoons (and wrote his stories under the pen name Gil Burton). Lantz terminated his employment. Then his history becomes murky. He is listed in a 1942 Burbank directory as a writer[23] but then disappears from credits on any films that have come to light. Ben Sharpsteen did visit with him in San Francisco in the 1960s, describing it as a sad meeting of two old friends, with Burt not in the best of circumstances. He passed away at the age of eighty in 1971 in Panorama City, a neighborhood in Los Angeles. Burt had a major impact on animation history, but sadly, like the mythical Icarus, he flew too close to the sun and paid dearly for it.

Burt Gillett—Disney Director Filmography[24]

Shorts:

Wild Waves (1929)
Arctic Antics (1930)
Cannibal Capers (1930)
Frolicking Fish (1930)
The Fire Fighters (1930)
The Shindig (1930)
The Chain Gang (1930)
Monkey Melodies (1930)
The Gorilla Mystery (1930)
The Picnic (1930)
Winter (1930)
Pioneer Days (1930)
Playful Pan (1930)
The Birthday Party (1931)
Birds of a Feather (1931)
Traffic Troubles (1931)
Mother Goose Melodies (1931)
The Moose Hunt (1931)
The Delivery Boy (1931)
The Busy Beavers (1931)
Mickey Steps Out (1931)
Blue Rhythm (1931)
Fishin' Around (1931)
The Barnyard Broadcast (1931)
The Beach Party (1931)
Mickey Cuts Up (1931)
Mickey's Orphans (1931)
The Duck Hunt (1932)
The Mad Dog (1932)
Just Dogs (1932)
Flowers and Trees (1932) (Academy Award winner)
Mickey's Nightmare (1932)
King Neptune (1932)
Bugs in Love (1932)
The Wayward Canary (1932)
Babes in the Woods (1932)
Mickey's Good Deed (1932)
Mickey's Pal Pluto (1933)
Ye Olden Days (1933)
Three Little Pigs (1933) (Academy Award winner)
Mickey's Gala Premiere (1933)
The Steeple-Chase (1933)
Giantland (1933)
Shanghaied (1934)
Playful Pluto (1934)
The Big Bad Wolf (1934)
Gulliver Mickey (1934)
Orphan's Benefit (1934)
Mickey Plays Papa (1934)
Lonesome Ghosts (1937)
Moth and the Flame (1937)

By its second decade, the process of making animated films at the Disney Studios had become more or less standardized. The visual evolution of an animated film is depicted in this 1977 recruitment brochure, *Disney is Looking for some Colorful New Characters* (RIGHT), and the process itself was illustrated in these images created for *National Geographic* in the early 1960s (BELOW). It remained largely unchanged from the late twenties until computer ink and paint and digital editing arrived in the early 1990s.

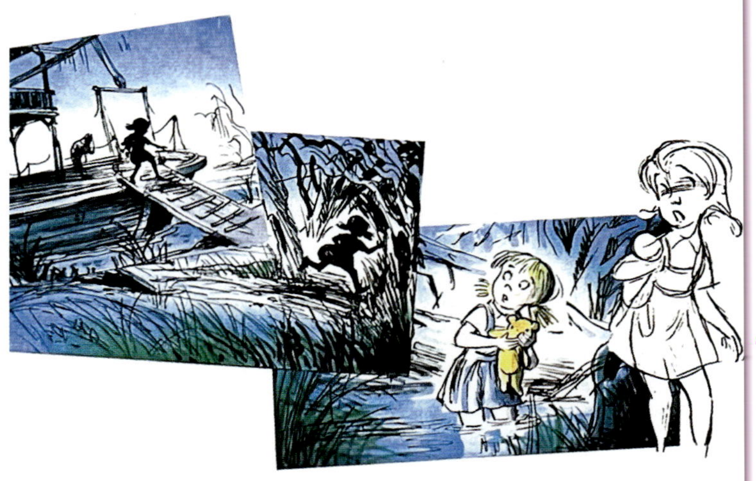

STORY / STORY SKETCH

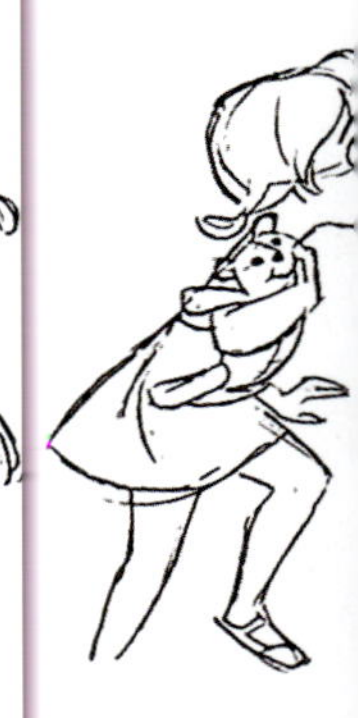

ANIMATION

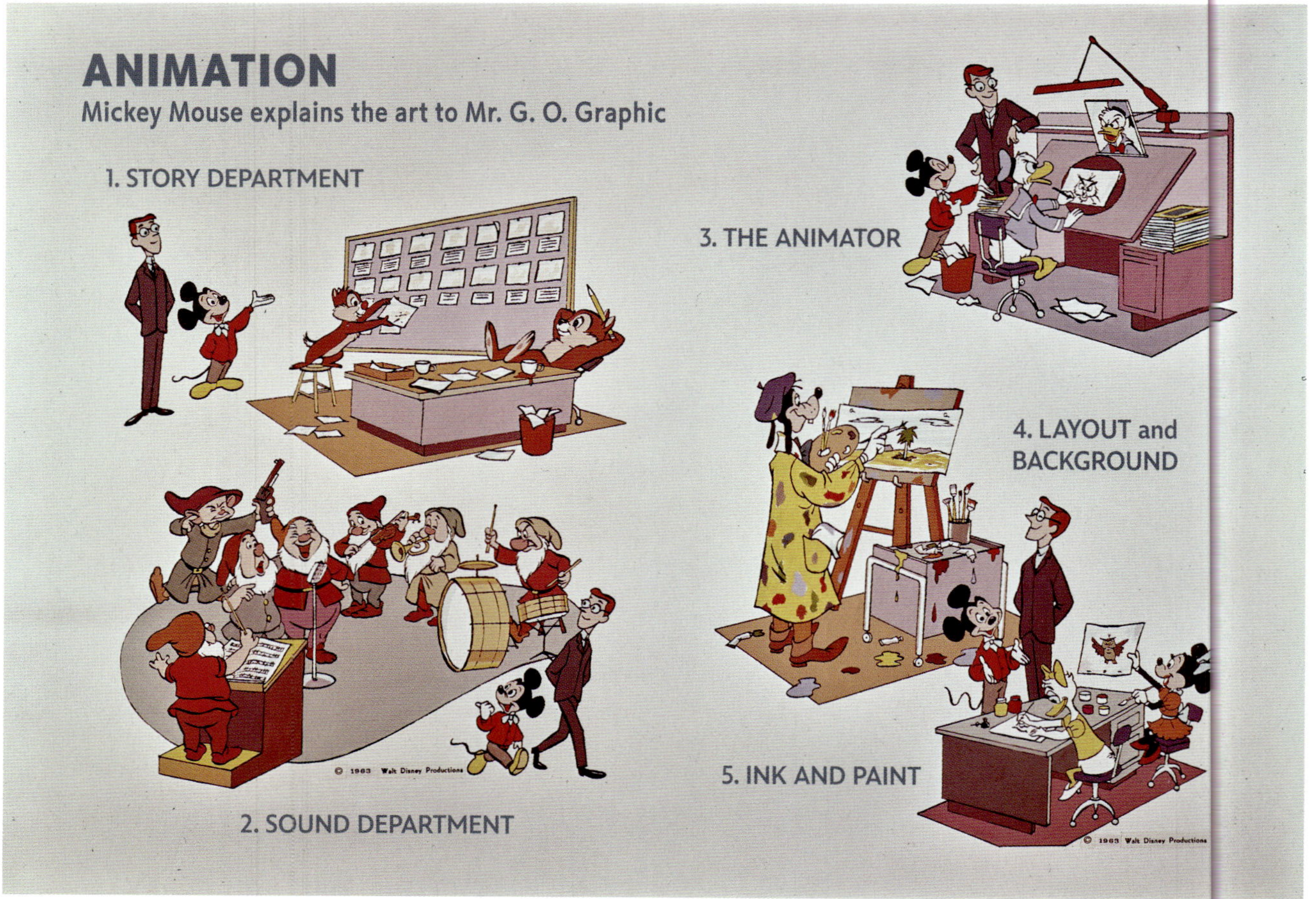

ANIMATION

Mickey Mouse explains the art to Mr. G. O. Graphic

1. STORY DEPARTMENT

2. SOUND DEPARTMENT

3. THE ANIMATOR

4. LAYOUT and BACKGROUND

5. INK AND PAINT

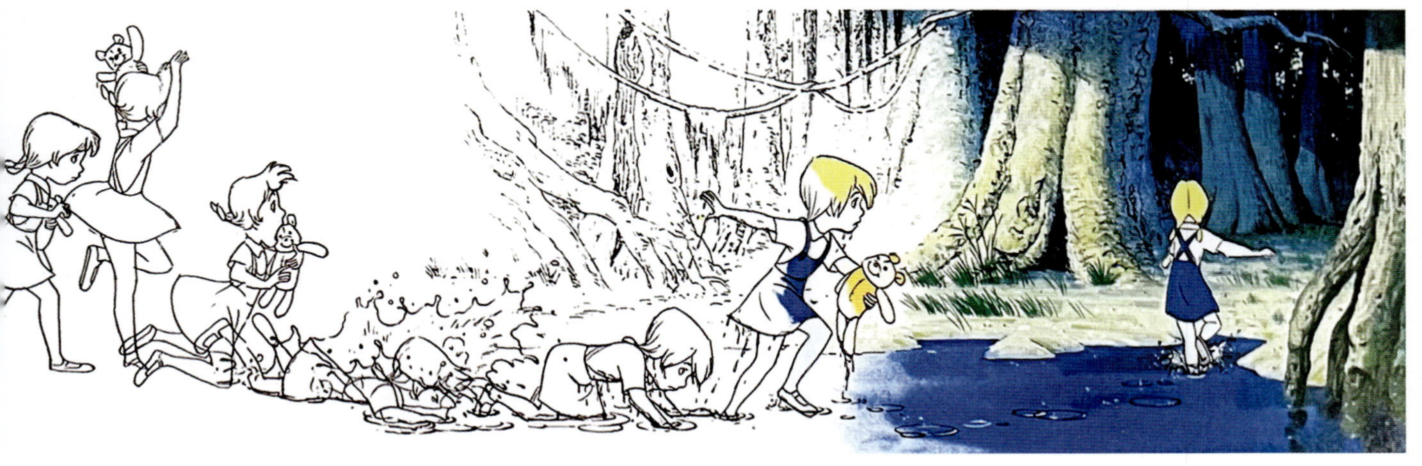

CLEAN-UP EFFECTS ANIMATION LAYOUT / BACKGROUND FINISHED PRODUCTION

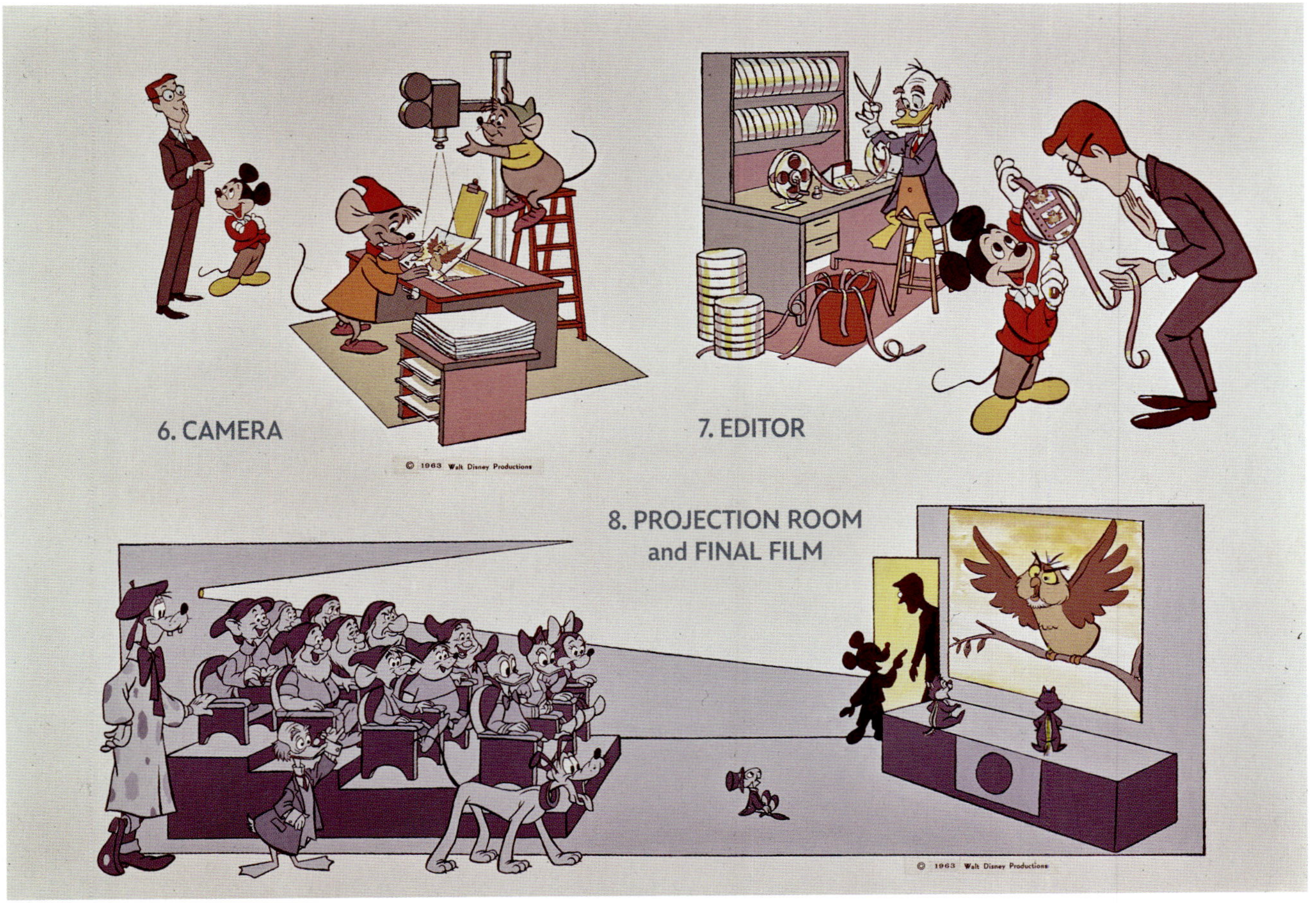

6. CAMERA

7. EDITOR

8. PROJECTION ROOM and FINAL FILM

PART 3

“WE COULDN’T HAVE DONE IT WITHOUT ORGANIZATION”

1936–1948

1936–1948

DIRECTING FEATURES

Under Walt's Creative Leadership

Story artists direct voice talent. Fixes or changes are handled by the Sequence Directors.

Each Sequence Director's job is to previsualize and plan their section(s) of the film:
- Time out the action and cutting
- Collaborate with the composer
- Prepare work with the layout artist
- Hand out and supervise animation
- Review animation
- Supervise cutting

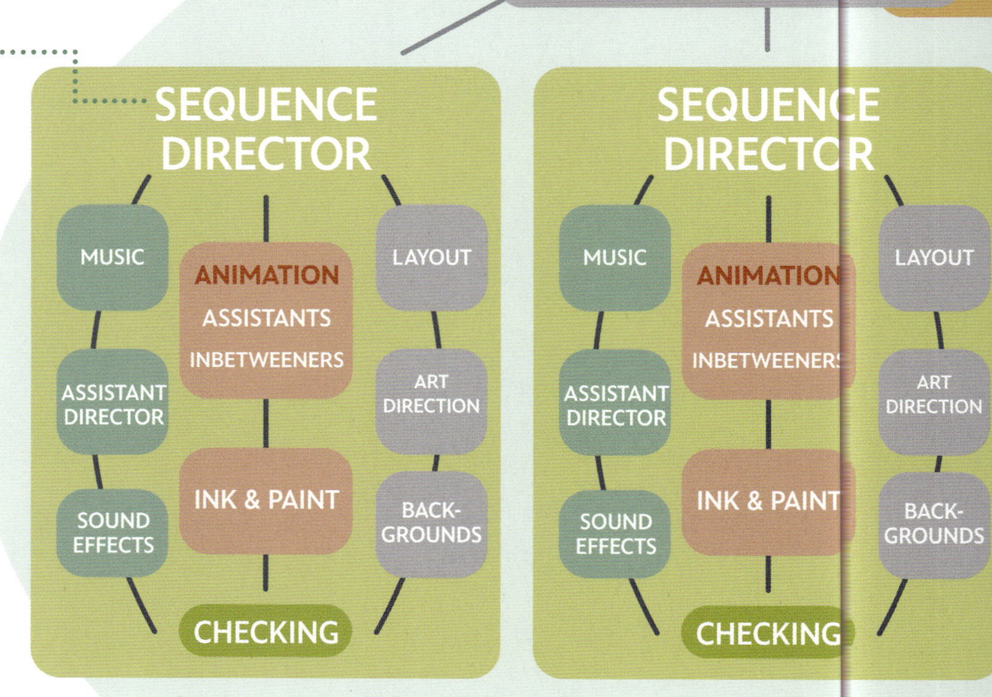

The "Package Films" made between 1946 and 1948 utilized a hybrid of the work process for features and shorts and introduced a Production Supervisor rather than a Supervising Director. That role would continue into the early features of the 1950s.

Later known as Final Sound Mix

Output: one feature every one to two years

The production process is simplified here; see Appendix E for more detail.

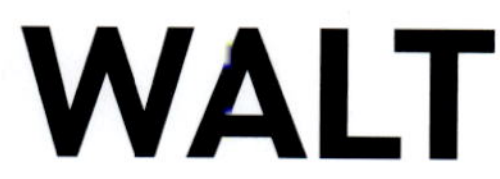

Walt is intimately involved in all aspects of production on the first two features. He delegates more to the Supervising Director for later films but still controls story.

The Supervising Director works under Walt and oversees eight to ten Sequence Directors to coordinate their efforts. The Supervising Director does not time out sequences or work directly with animators but is responsible for keeping the film faithful to Walt's vision.

DIRECTOR

WRITERS & STORY SKETCH

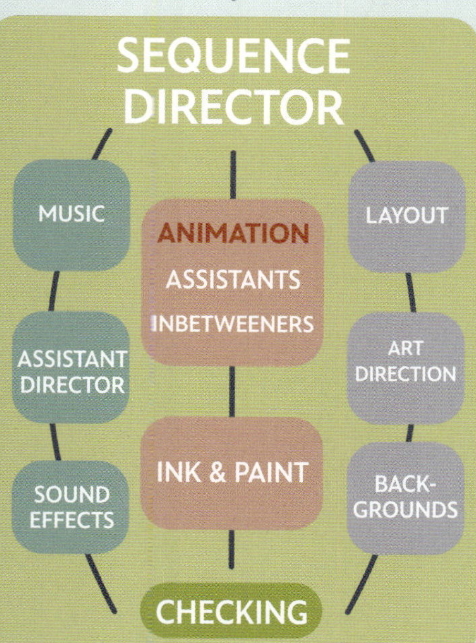

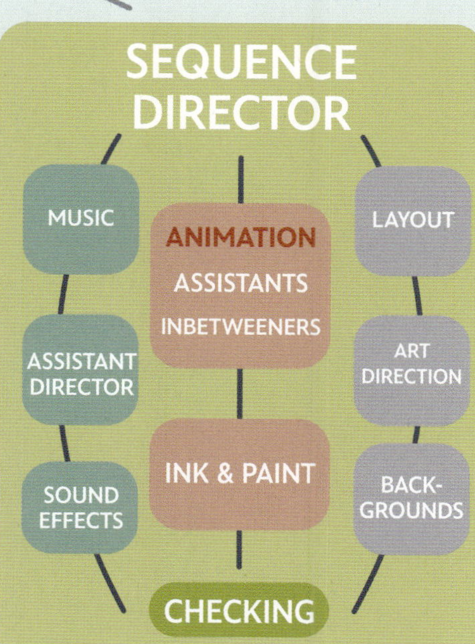

. . . ETC.

Each feature has six to ten Sequence Directors and associated teams who handle around thirty-five sequences for each movie.

CAMERA

ANSWER PRINT

RE-RECORDING

FINAL FILM

This diagram represents a single film; when more than one movie is in production, the above organization is duplicated for each film. Occasionally Sequence Directors work on multiple features simultaneously. Walt always has the final word.

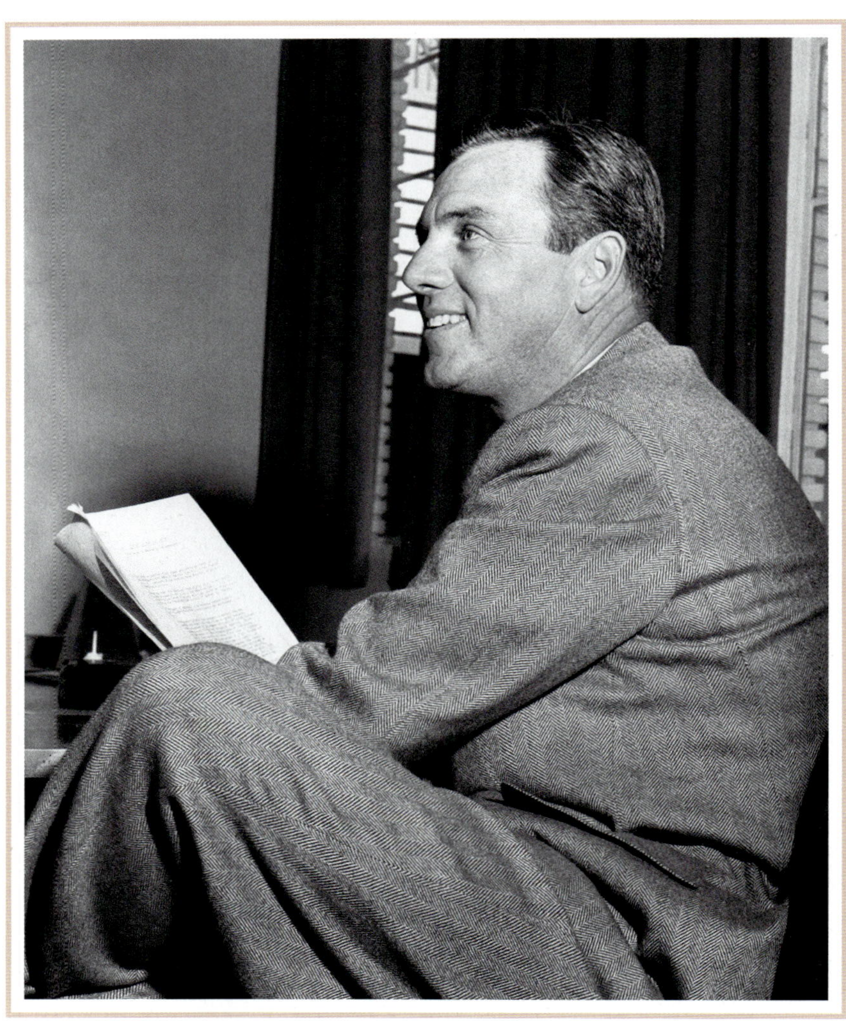

Dave Hand at the Disney Studios, May 1942.

CHAPTER 3

DAVE HAND—A MAN TRAPPED, THE WATER RISING

"What I am going to try to do is give you a bit of vision. By 'vision' I mean a realization that when you get in Dave Hand's position, you will just be starting. When you get up where I am, if I'm able, you'll see nothing but my smoke, because I'm going to be way ahead of you. Don't stop where Dave Hand, or Walt, is. Try to keep on going. Six years ago when I came here, Walt wasn't even where I am (that is, relatively speaking). Walt is a smart man—he has had the vision, he's going on and on. I can't catch him and you won't be able to catch me."

—Dave Hand[1]

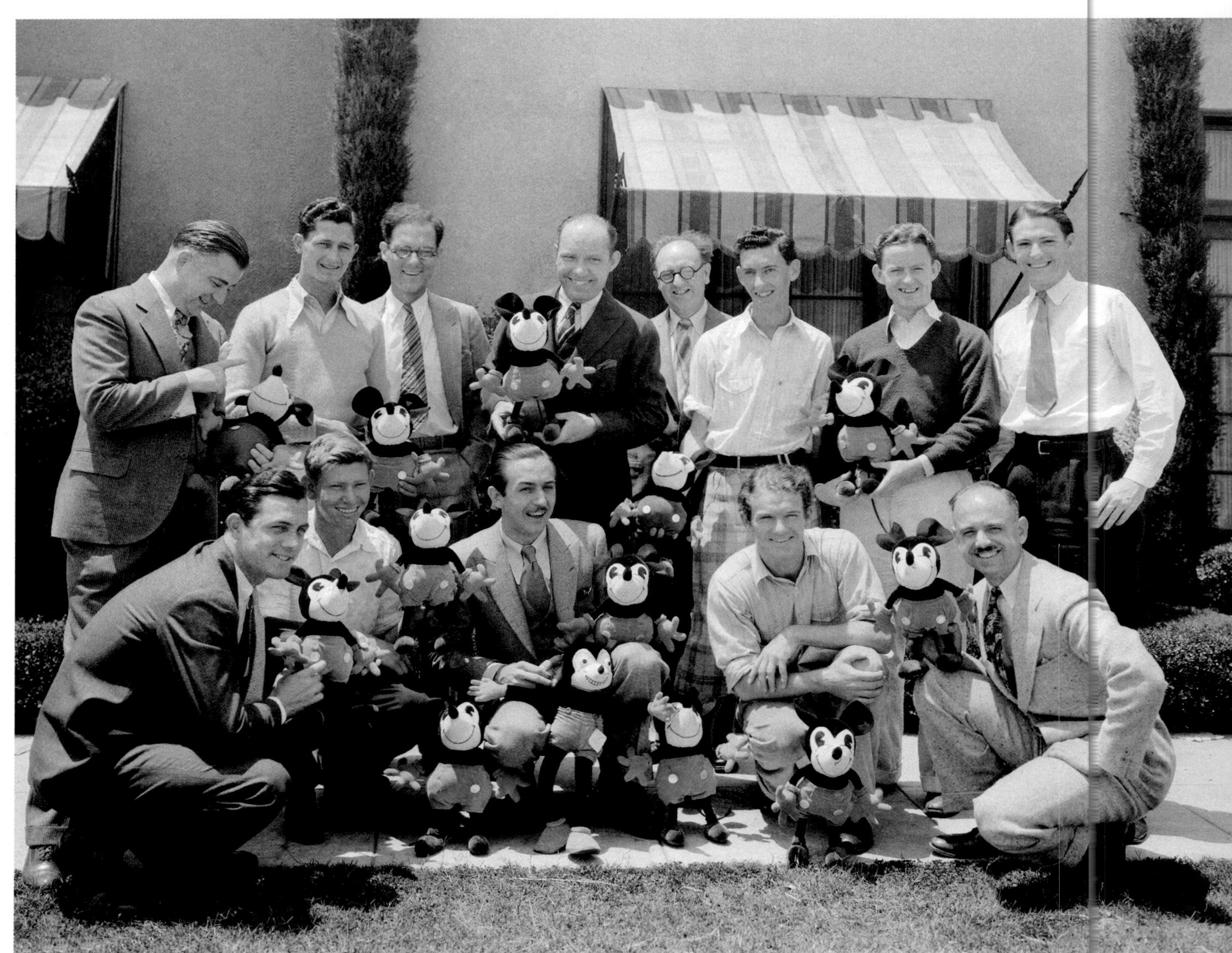

A group photo at the Disney Studios from 1930, the year Hand joined the staff. KNEELING, FROM LEFT: animator Dave Hand, director Wilfred Jackson, Walt Disney, animators Johnny Cannon and Ben Sharpsteen. STANDING, FROM LEFT: animators Jack King, Les Clark, and Tom Palmer; director Burt Gillett; composer Bert Lewis; animators Dick Lundy and Norm Ferguson; comic strip artist Floyd Gottfredson.

When the ambitious thirty-year-old Dave Hand showed up at the Disney Studios in January 1930 looking for a job, Ben Sharpsteen, who'd worked with Hand in New York, was reluctant to vouch for him.

Whether Sharpsteen was defending his own position or didn't think Hand was a fit, Dave turned out to be just the person Disney needed for his expanding and ambitious studio. Opinionated and decisive, Hand learned fast and looked to share his discoveries and creative responsibilities. His philosophy, as he counseled up-and-coming director Dick Lundy: "You've got to make decisions, and you've got to make them fast. If you're right fifty-one percent of the time, you're *right*."[2]

Hand became the supervising director of the studio's first feature, *Snow White*, and *Bambi*. At one point Walt told assistant director Paul Satterfield, "Dave Hand is the best director I've ever had." He was the first in the role of production supervisor, helping grow and give structure to Walt's rapidly expanding studio. He grew close to Walt socially, dining, playing polo, and even camping with him.

But as successful as he was, there was "some sort of friction between Hand and Walt," observed story man Joe Grant.[3] Hand left the studio in 1944, his relationship with Disney laced with unspoken tension, jealousy, and resentment.

BEFORE DISNEY

David Dodd Hand was born January 23, 1900, in Plainfield, New Jersey, and spent his youth working in his father's brickyard with his brother, Ernest. Hand's childhood love of cartoons led him to the Chicago Academy of Art and brief employment at Wallace Carlson's Chicago-based studio, where he animated Andy Gump, the popular comic strip character. After a salary dispute, Dave's colorful early life saw him as a lumberjack in Michigan, a railroad tie tamper in Montana, a western-bound hobo riding the rails, a Hollywood advertising cartoonist, and a shoe salesman back in Plainfield. He returned to animation at J.R. Bray Studios in New York, working on the *Dinky Doodle* series under Walter Lantz, and later at the Fleischer Studios, working on the *Out of the Inkwell* series. Living a Prohibition-era life of speakeasies and late-night parties in New York, Hand married fellow Chicago art student Jo Hale Marks and became a director at Fleischer Studios, the start of a promising career.

But Hand, like Disney, was compelled by the idea of becoming a live-action director. Dave and Jo drove across the country in their Model A to seek his fortune in Hollywood. And like Walt, after three months of finding no work, he fell back on his skills as an animator.

Dave had been impressed with the Disney Studios' ability to synchronize sound to picture, a problem that puzzled many New York competitors. With fortuitous timing, Hand applied and was hired on his birthday, January 23, 1930, just days after Ub Iwerks's departure. Though Hand's nine years of experience as an animator was seen as "nothing outstanding"[4] and "too mechanical"[5] by some coworkers, Hand won admiration for his logical approach and eye for speed—an approach he'd learned in New York, where "you were given so much money, and you got the picture out for that amount, or you got out."[6] But at Disney's[7], Dave soon learned that "if Walt didn't get what he wanted, you had to go back and do it over. And it didn't matter how often you did it over, you had to get what he wanted."[8]

Dave animated on some forty Mickey Mouse and Silly Symphony shorts, showing an aptitude

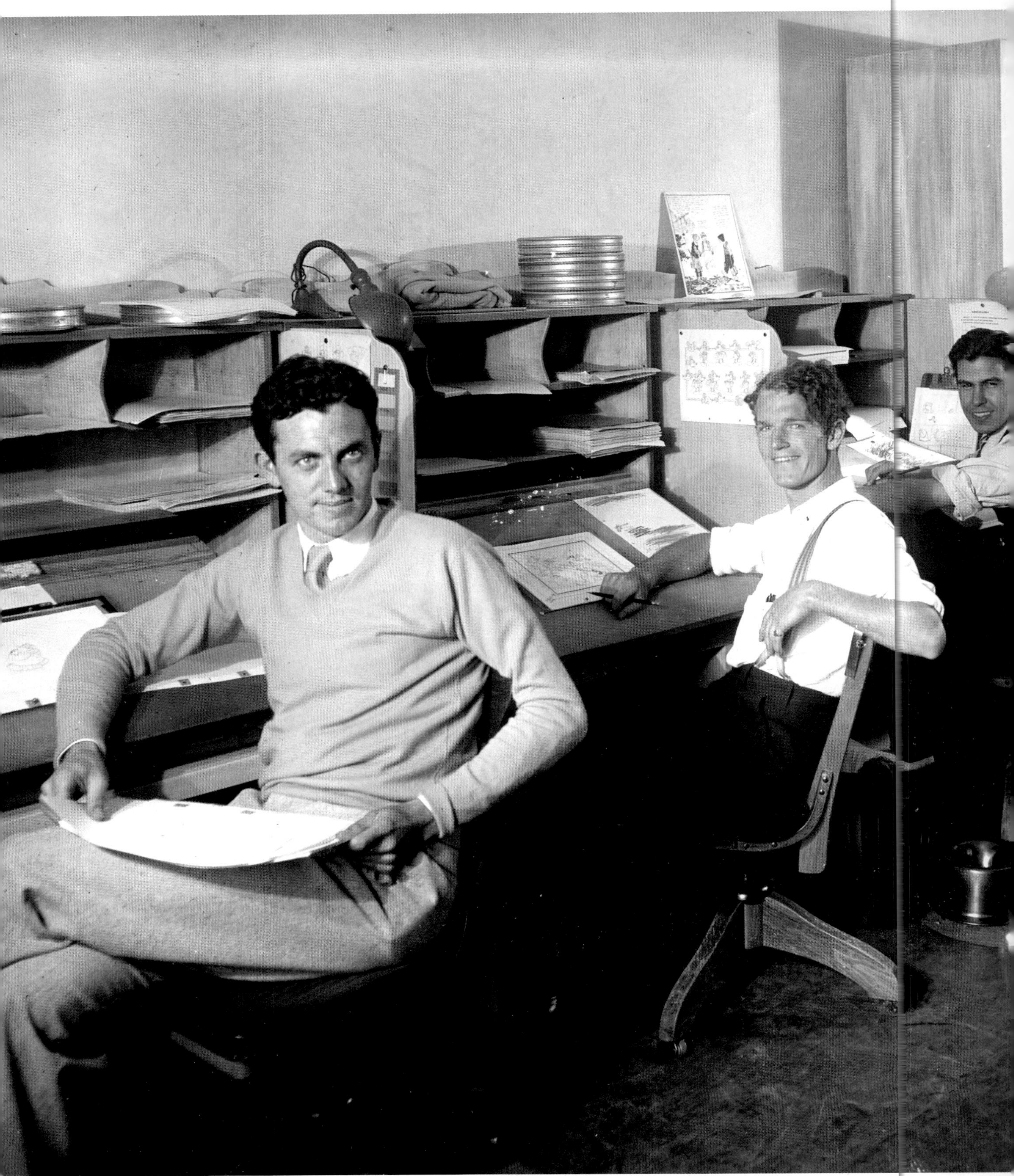

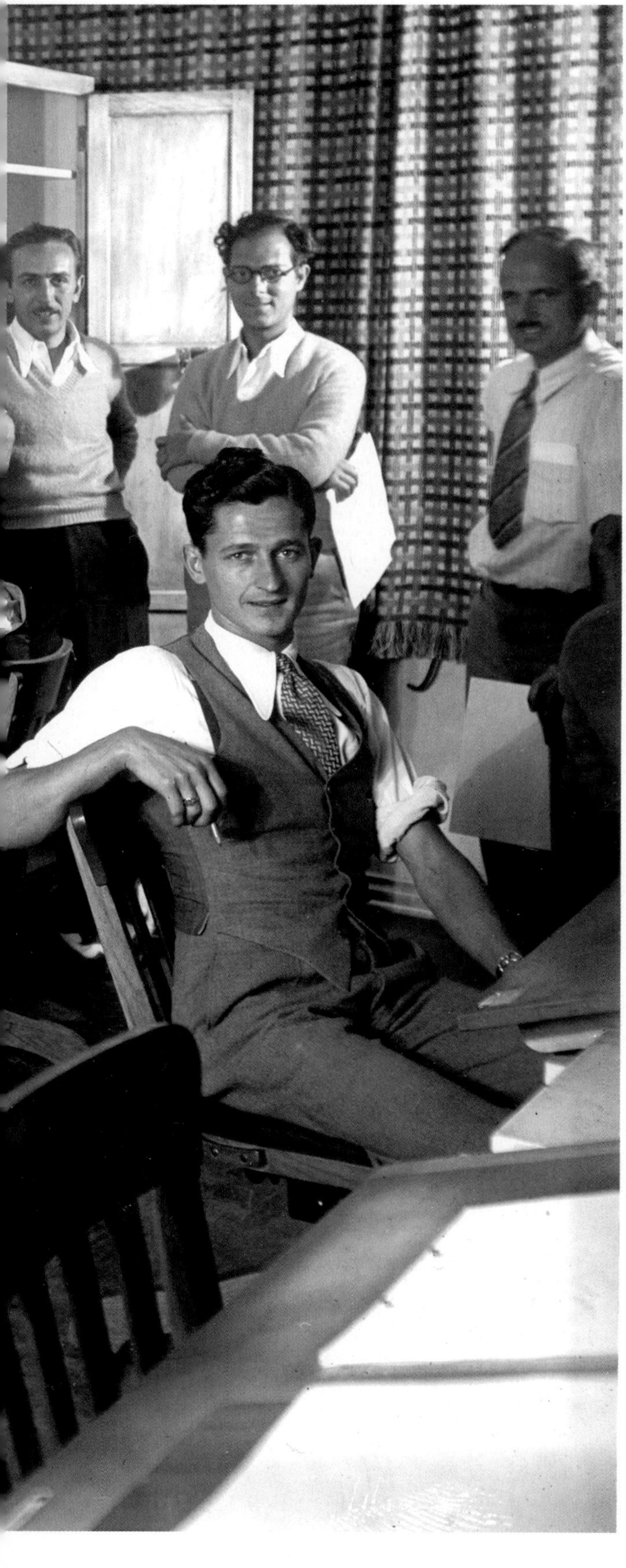

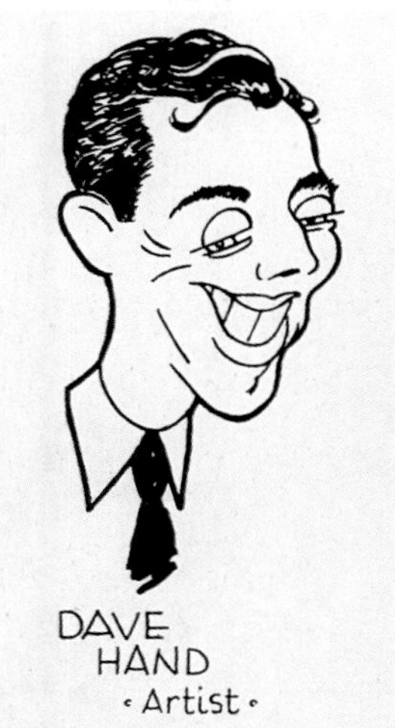

Hand as caricatured by animator Jack King in *Motion Picture Daily* magazine, June 20, 1931.

Hand as a young animator at Disney's in March or April of 1931, working on *The China Plate*, released May 23, 1931. SITTING FROM LEFT: Dave Hand, Johnny Cannon (seen here animating on *The Delivery Boy*), Rudy Zamora, Les Clark; STANDING (LEFT TO RIGHT): Walt Disney, Tom Palmer, Ben Sharpsteen.

for training and leading new artists. Like fellow New York animator Ben Sharpsteen, Hand took on large sections of the films, farming out scenes to juniors while animating important scenes himself. Initially wary, Ben later admitted that "Dave was an extremely positive person who had very positive ideas on how things should be done. I am sure that his attitude attracted the attention of Walt and, as a result, Walt made Dave a director."[9]

DAVE THE DIRECTOR

Hand's first break directing at Disney's was the 1933 short *Building a Building*, making him the fourth director after Ub Iwerks, Burt Gillett, and Wilfred Jackson. Although animator Ward Kimball suggested Dave was "kicked upstairs" because he was unable to keep up with advancements made by other artists,[10] story man Dick Huemer felt that Hand "was very effective and directed one of the best shorts of that time. When Walt really wanted a good picture and he had a real good story, I think he gave it to Dave, because Dave really put the stuff in it."[11]

Hand told of his first assignment on a story rejected by the other two directors and a brand-new crew of rookie animators; but Hand either misremembered or is exaggerating for a good story, as records show the film's animators to be the same who worked on many of the Mickeys of that era: Ben Sharpsteen, Johnny Cannon, Les Clark, Tom Palmer, Dick Lundy, Gerry Geronimi, and Frenchy de Trémaudan.[12] Regardless, the short was soon finished and, like all Disney shorts, screened for an advance test audience. Despite the film being enthusiastically received by the audience, Dave recalled Walt was not pleased, taking "about an hour and a half" to "knock me down until I was lower than a snake's belly."

Was Walt sincere in his opinion of Hand's ineptitude? Interestingly, this isn't the only account of Walt combining a promotion with a verbal smackdown;[13] perhaps it was Disney's way of keeping the power structure clear. Or maybe despite what he was bringing to the studio Walt already intuited Hand as something of a threat.

For his part, Hand claimed that he "never tried to do anything that wasn't Disney. We all said 'What does Walt want?' That was our loyalty to the man; we left our individualism behind someplace."[14] But Dave was also proud of his independence and fearlessness. "I always did say if I liked something or didn't like it, and say it openly and honestly and let the chips fall where they may. And I did that with Walt. And I think he liked that in me. I think he liked my not being a yes-man."[15]

Regardless of Disney's initial tirade, Hand must have balanced things right, because he went on to direct twenty-seven Mickey Mouse shorts and Silly Symphonies, including "some of the best Disney shorts," in the opinion of animation historian Michael Barrier.[16]

What did it mean to direct shorts at Disney's in the early thirties? "Walt was always in charge," said animator Eric Larson, "but Dave was a good wrangler. He could get stuff out. I have a great deal of respect for Dave."[17] Then-animator Dick Huemer offered that "direction really didn't mean that much to Walt at the time, because of the fact that he was really the producer-director, and the men who called themselves directors were, you might say, glorified assistant directors. They did a lot of the routine work, like timing and handing it out, and rough criticism, those technical tasks that had to be done. If something was obviously very bad, the director would see to fixing before Walt noticed it,

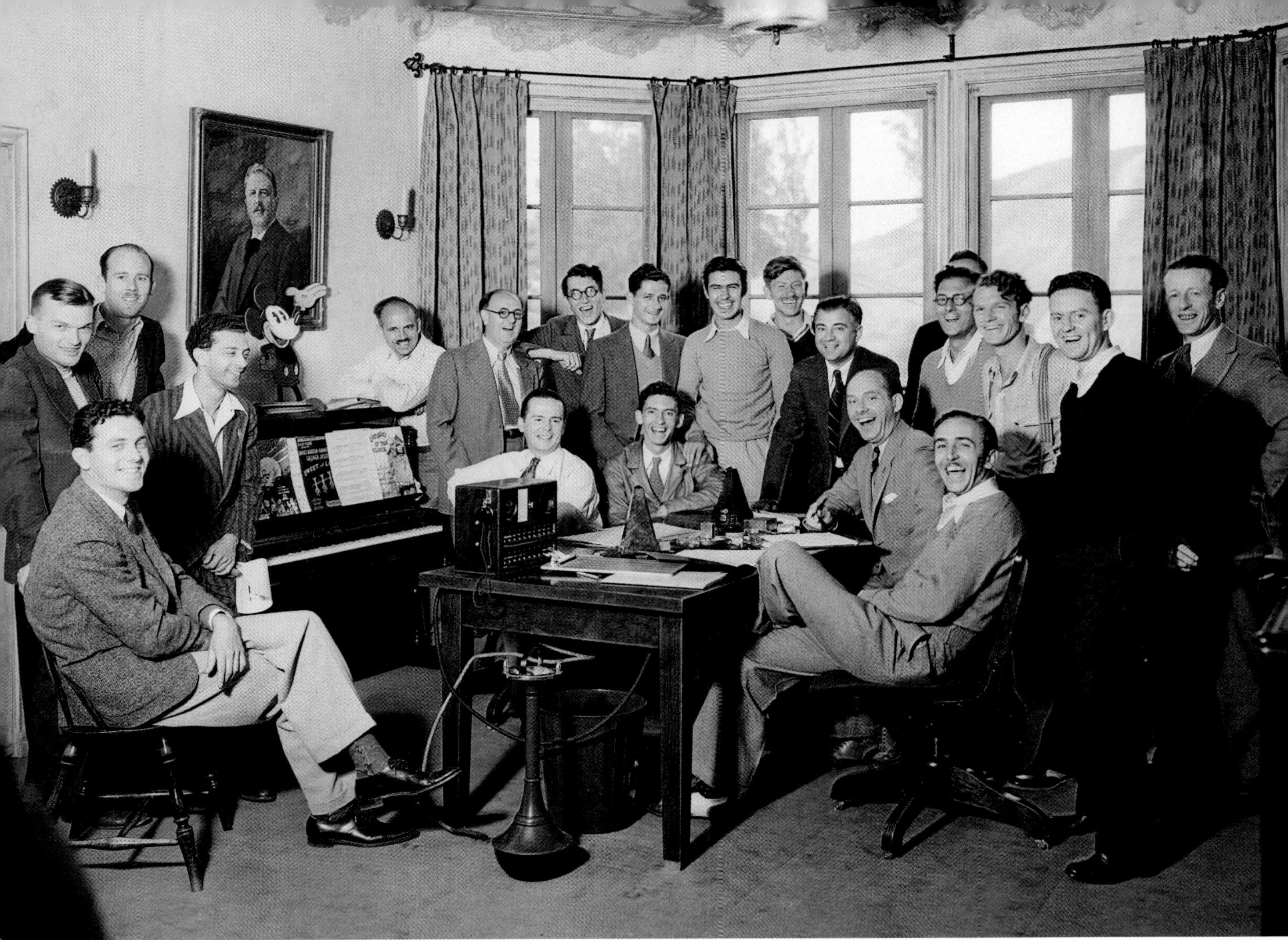

Dave Hand (SEATED AT LEFT) and others in Music Room 1 at the Hyperion Studio in mid-1933.

but when it came to making the decisions as to what to leave out or what to do next, the director per se didn't do it. Walt did it. But Walt needed this assistance, this guy to pick up the loose ends behind him and oversee the working out of a feature cartoon. Of course," remembered Huemer, "they also put in their own touches."[18]

Hand summed up his opinion of his own job in a 1936 studio lecture, "The Director's Relationship to the Picture and to the Animator": "To me, direction consists more or less of supervision and an ability to hold the picture together . . . His job is to see the picture as a whole at a distance." Dave's ability to do so was skillful and crisp. Animator and story man Chuck Couch remembered Hand as a "very practical guy" and said that "if Dave liked something, he'd tell you it was goddamn good. If it was bad, he'd say it stinks. You always knew where you stood."[19]

Assistant Jack Cutting said that Dave was a "colorful, interesting personality" who "just roared right on past everybody and his brother." Cutting recalled that "when Dave Hand was made a director, and he was very ambitious

PROPOSED PRODUCTION ROUTINE TO BE FOLLOWED IN THE FUTURE

Three directors: Gillett, Jackson and Hand. Musical director to each crew. At the present time three layout men. Philippi, Hennesy and Hurter. Horvath and Wood acting as assistants, will work where they are needed. Philippi and Hennesy are capable of handling everything themselves. Plan to have Ted Sears and the directors work more closely with Albert Hurter. When possible we will use Philippi and Hennesy on all the Mickey stories, and try to arrange to have Hurter do the layouts on the Symphonies or the greater part of them. The layout men will be assigned to each music room according to the type of story.

The layout man will come in when the director is ready to make the thumb-nail sketches of his story. The layout man and the director will sit down and work out together all the thumbnail sketches for the picture. It is not necessary that these thumbnail sketches be worked out to any extent where they are used for blow-ups, they are merely to figure out story angles, plan close-ups and long shots and arrange continuity.

It will be absolutely necessary that the director sit down with the layout man and plan his story. He is not merely to tell the layout man to make this kind of a sketch or to play around with something to see what he can get, he is to sit down with the layout man and work it out. In this manner the layout man will be able to get a better idea of what the director is driving for, and the same time the director will get a clearer idea of what he wants himself. On a six week schedule it is possible for the director to do this.

The main thing to be given to the layout man, is the director's angles; what he wants to put over, so that whenthe layout man makes the layouts he doesn't have to re-make them three or four times. The only way to accomplish this is for the director to sit down and actually work with the layout man in the making of the thumb-nail sketches and at this time definitely plan the way he is going to put over his gags and story. This will compel the director to thoroughly understand the story and gags that he intends to put over.

The layout man will work with the director until the thumbnail sketches are finished, then he will pick up from the thumbnail sketches and start making the layouts. He and the director will still work in close contact on the layouts, on account of various little changes which may come up, andwhich would not be anticipated in the thumb-nail sketches.

It is not necessary that the layout man go to great detail in his backgrounds. He can show by suggestions what he wants the background department to do. We should work out a code between the layouts and the background department which will eliminate unnecessary detail in background sketches.

All the background sketches and scenes layouts should be made first in the rough, (in the same manner as the animators make all their action in the rough) then the necessary detail should be added after the layouts have been OK'ed by the director. In this way, if after the rough layout is made, the director sees that a change is necessary, we are not wasting all the time and efforts of the layout men in making a detailed sketch. This gives the director two chances to catch anything that may be wrong; the first one is in the thumb-nail sketch and the second is the rough layout sketch.

The layout man will devote most of his time to planning the layouts and drawing them in the rough, then the assistants will put in the detail necessary, <u>but not any more than is necessary</u>.

This four-page internal memo from 1934 outlines the specific jobs of the director. Author is unknown; likely they are transcribed thoughts from Walt.

This same layout man who has made the thumb-nail sketches, and the original sketches for the animators to start work on, will then see that everything is carried out the way he and the director intended, when the sketches go to the background department to be finished. It will not be necessary for the director to have any contact with the background department, all of his contact will be with his layout man. The layout man will supervise the execution of the backgrounds in that department. The background department gets from the inking department celluloids depicting the action to take place on the scene, and with these cells it is very easy to see what is to be done. However, in the event the background department and the layout man come to something they do not understand or something on which they need advice, then they will call in the director and get his decision.

This entire plan is based on the angle that each man should do his own work and have his own responsibilities. In this way the director will have more time to concentrate on his present and future stories, and to see that the gags and action is being carried out as it should be by the animators., while the layout man will be able to see to the proper execution of the backgrounds.

The musicians will take more responsibility in fitting the music to the action. It will be up to the musicians to see that the music fits, and to relieve the director of the responsibility and worry of his music. The director's time must be spent constructing his story, directing the animation and putting over the gags.

All of the music will be in charge of Frank Churchill. He will be in charge of the other two musicians. Frank will have a crew of his own with which to work, but he will also be available to come in for suggestions and help on the other two crews. I want Frank Churchill to go over every score that is made here, and give his suggestions and ideas. He and the other musical directors will share the responsibility of the music in the pictures. Churchill should, of possible, be brought in when the music is being selected and fitted to the picture, and again when the score is ready for arranging. The directors will find that Churchill is very willing and very capable, and the other musical directors should fall right in line and work with Frank hand and glove.

With all the backing the director gets from the various departments, the gag department, the gags that come in from the fellows, the story outlines which are prepared ahead of time, and the various people who are available to help with the making of these stories, the director whould have no trouble in completing his picture in good clean shape within scheduled time. (approximately six weeks).

In order for the director to properly direct the story, it is necessary that he understand it thoroughly before he ever attempts to make a picture of it. In order to do this the director should be thinking on his future stories months ahead. This is possible I know because I have done it myself. I find that it works to better advantage when a man is thinkin of more than one thing at a time. He has the one story on which he is concentrating, but at times he lets him mind wander off to think of what the future story is going to be, and how he can work it out. This helps greatly, in that it keeps the director's mind fresh and keeps him from getting too stale on the story on which he is working.

The director should consider that the story on which he is going to work is his story and he should be throughly familiar with it before it is started. Conferences will be held far enough ahead in order that the Director will be able to determine at that time what his story should be, and whether he wants it and whether the story will mean a lot to him. If he doesn't think so, he should say so then, for there may be a director who is anxious for that story.

The director should be alert to any possible chances for saving the time of the animators; he should keep his mind open for ways in which he may get his gags over in a clearer and more simple manner, without going to a lot of unnecessary details. This plant is operated in such a manner that everyone is given a wonderful chance to bring out their talent. The amount of time we spend on our stories, compared to the other studios, is terrific. Some of the results that we have been getting with our efforts have been far below what the other studios are getting with half the cost. The main fault in our system is thatthere is too much time and thought given to unnecessary details which, in the long run, have nothing to do with puttin over the gags. We could take more simple and easier handling ofthe stories and get much better results.

The director should be able to make up his mind what he wants to do after we have finished talking the story over and building it up. He should take advantage of the advice of the various ones who are working with him, they may be more capable than he. The director should be thinking of his story plenty of time ahead. If he thinks of it far enough ahead, by the time he gets ready to start on it, he will find that he has the story practically worked out in his mind. He can't expect to sit down in a few days and out of a clear sky throw a story together. Good stories do not come that way; they come gradually.

Another plan that we are going to try to work out, is to try and avoid cutting the picture up into too many sequences; in other words, from allotting it to too many different animators. This plan is, that the animators will be spotted more on sequences, or on types of action, and that they will carry through this sequence. This may carry them over two or three pictures. Instead of giving an animator just a couple of scenes in each picture, give them longer sequences in one picture. This plan will enable the animator to give more concentrated thought to his work, more chance to see that the stuff carries through andthat the gags are put over.

The animators will be classed as to their types of work, such as dramatic, personality, action, etc. If the director will lay out his picture roughly as to types of action it contains, he can then look on his chart and see the various animators who are available and who can do that type of work, and in this way we will try to cast the animators for work in which they are best suited.

The director should not regulate his schedule according to how the animators are going in their production. He should see that his story is completed, his music in shape, his exposure sheets ready, and that his layouts are ready regardless of whether animators are waiting for them or not. If we keep waiting, one on another, we will never get the plant on schedule. Each department must put <u>itself</u> on schedule. If they do not, it will tie up the entire plant. If the animators find the layouts are not ready they slow up their work, take a longer time than is necessary, and more or less wait forthe layouts to be ready for them.

It is possible for the director to be starting on the next story even if he has only half of his other story handed out. I am not asking anything impossible, because after the story is once laid out, planned and put down, there is no further necessity for creative efforts on the part of the director, it is merely a routine to see that it is handed out and carried out.

The story men will be with the director only for the period allotted them. They cannot stay longer, and while he has them the director must make as much use of the story men as possible. If the director holds the story men beyond their allotted time it holds the next director up. We must keep the ball rolling.

DON'T BE RESPONSIBLE FOR THROWING THE OTHER FELLOW OFF SCHEDULE !

Another thing we musst put over is that we must get our gags over and make them to the point without a lot of ginger bread and unnecessary trimmings. It is up to the director to see that the gag is clear; it is up to him in the first place to know and understand the point of the gag, and then drive for it and see that the animators drive for it and put it over. Not to be fooling around with a lot of unnecessary details which in the long run do not show up or add to the picture enough to warrant or make it worth while.

We must improve the quality of our pictures all around. For the amount of effort, money, time and experience that everyone here has had, the pictures as not near what they should be. I have a wonderful vacation plan laid out for this organization, but it will be impossible for me ever to put it into effect until I get the full cooperation of all the departments, and until we operate on schedule. This plan is one that is far ahead of its time. I realize that creative work is nerve wracking, and it is necessary that men have relaxation. My whole plan is based on that fact. To get our plant on schedule I have equipped it with enough help, enough equipment that we should be able to turn out good pictures and have anough time left in a year for vacations. These vacations will not be possible until I get the full co-operation of everyone concerned, and get everyone driving for that one thing; to put the story over, without a lot of unnecessary details, which may seem of great importance but add nothing to the quality of the picture. Let's drive for the gags; for good stories, and make our pictures interesting, funny and full of personality.

Another important thing in my estimation, and one that will save a lot of time is this: The director must hand his scenes out to the enimator in such a manner that it is clear, to the point, and then follows it through to see that the animator thoroughly understands, and gets it correct. In this way we will save a lot of time, as I find the animators spend twice the amount of time they should on account of not having the idea correct in the first place, or because the director could not visualize what he wanted himself. The animators go to a lot of work making something and later the director find he has to have him change it. The time for the director to do his changing is when he is giving the scene to the animator. He has a second check-up in this, by looking at the rough tests of the animators drawing, not at the finished tests.

I would like to again impress the fact that the directors must give thought ahead of time to the stories coming up in the future. They must be thinking on future stories while they are laying out their present story; give them some thought outside of their regular time here. That is part of the director's job.

Copies of this proposed production routine have gone to the Directors, Musicians, Ben, the main animators, layout men and to the story men.

taking on multiple pictures, I said, 'Dave, couldn't you use an assistant because you've got all this work to do?' Lo and behold, a short time later he got in touch with me. He said he had spoken to Walt about it and Walt said why not try it. So I became his assistant."[20] Hand was the first to delegate work to assistants, which would soon become standard. "The more Hand found you could do, he would unload it on you," recalled Cutting. But Hand wasn't being lazy; Cutting found Dave to be "ambitious, doing a lot of work" and "a hard driver."[21] Mirroring Disney's own actions, handing work to others allowed Hand to take on even more.

Dave had strong opinions, sometimes resulting in heated arguments, even with Walt. But if later found to be wrong, he made a point to apologize. Said assistant Jack Cutting, "He was always very fair."[22] Hand could also be surprisingly sensitive. He opposed Walt's common use of "hurt gags" in the films and worried about potentially offensive gags, like the blind rabbits in *Funny Little Bunnies*. He worked well with animators. Animator Frank Thomas recalled, "When I worked with Dave he was most helpful, seeing that I had every help I needed without getting in the way of any fresh ideas I might have had."[23]

HOME LIFE

By the mid-1930s Dave's success enabled him to own two homes in Alhambra, a town just east of Los Angeles—with him and Jo in one, and Jo's parents in the other—and an empty lot between with a barn and fruit trees. In 1932 the Hands adopted two children, David Hale and Judy. The family had a cook and a full-time nurse for the kids, who later took piano, violin, ballet, and life drawing with Rico Lebrun, the master draftsman who taught the Disney artists on *Bambi*.[24]

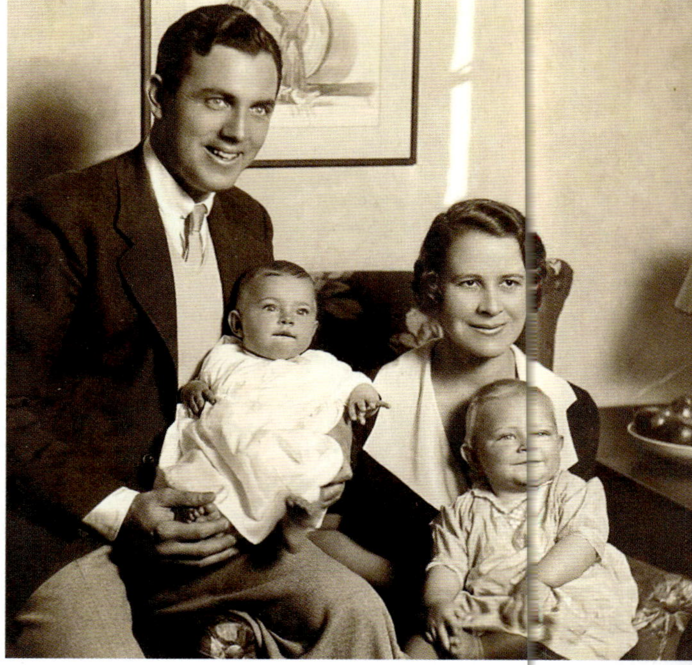

Dave, Jo, and children, David Hale and Judy, 1933.

Despite (or perhaps because of) his authoritative role at work, Dave was not a disciplinarian at home—that was Jo's job. "My father could always see the funny side of everything," remembered Judy.[25] Though half-day working Saturdays were standard at that time at the studio, son David Hale recalled his father kept horses at Will Rogers's ranch, where they would "go riding almost every Saturday afternoon. He was a great shot with both rifle and pistol. I mean, he wasn't a fast draw, but he could sure shoot. He'd put a beer can on a string and tie it to a tree, and then he would swing the can and he'd shoot the string!"[26]

Dave and Jo were Christian Scientists, which meant that unlike most of Hand's coworkers at Disney, he did not drink. But this did not impair their social calendar. "My parents used to do a lot of entertaining," recalled Judy.[27] Frequent guests were friends Phil and Betty Dike (head of the art department at Scripps College), artists Phil and Gail Paradise, Hardie Gramatke (author of *Little Toot*), director Ben and Bernice Sharpsteen, and animator Ward and Betty Kimball. Then, too, said Judy, "every Sunday after church we'd go to the Will Rogers Ranch, which is now a State Park, but wasn't then, and he would play [polo] with Walt Disney and Spencer Tracy, Gary Cooper, Will Rogers, and Wiley Post."[28]

But back at the studio, it was not all smooth sailing for Hand. While directing *Three Blind Mouseketeers* (1936), Dave "crossed Walt on something," recalled development head Joe Grant. "There was some arrogance on his part. . . . It could have been something very petty; I really don't know what it was. But everybody in the studio knew that he was letting him ride. That was [Walt's] technique: to let you go on your own, without any assistance. You'd flounder, because, after all, you were doing his bidding, you didn't own the studio." Disney left Hand alone, "to teach him a lesson."[29]

After six years of moving up, suddenly Hand's future was not looking good.

SNOW WHITE

Walt had pitched the idea for his first feature in 1934, at least a year before Dave fell out of favor. As the project gained momentum, Disney considered who would direct. Given where Hand now stood, it was no surprise he was not on Disney's list.

Walt had first considered directing *Snow White* himself, but perhaps because of troubles on *The Golden Touch*, thought better of this. According to story man Dick Huemer, animator Harry Bailey was next to be considered, which "was a dismal idea," said Huemer. Bailey "had been one of our old-time animators" from New York. Bailey was "just one of the boys, neither good nor bad, just a workman."[30] Walt soon reconsidered.

Animator Dick Lundy remembered the position was next offered to "a great big tall fellow, came from Alabama," whom historian Mike Barrier guessed to be story man George Stallings. "Walt wanted him to direct, and [Stallings] refused, and got in the doghouse because he did refuse," said Lundy. What had Walt seen in Stallings? "Don't ask me the workings of Walt's mind. I couldn't guess it."[31]

Top story man Bill Cottrell was next to be approached, a reasonable choice given Cottrell's skill and experience throughout the studio. "When *Snow White* was first started in production, Walt said to me, 'I want you to be the director of *Snow White*,' and I said, 'Fine, I'd like that.' But a few weeks later he came to me and he said, 'Dave Hand wants to direct *Snow White*. Do you mind?' Well, I didn't think that it was my position to object. I assumed that Walt wanted Dave to do it, so I said okay. So I was a sequence director instead of the overall director."[32]

Wherever the idea originated, Walt must have recognized he needed someone with strong organizational skills—one of Dave Hand's prime talents. "Dave at the time was considered Walt's best director and actually a logical choice for overall director of *Snow White*,"[33] remembered Dick Huemer. "And to give him credit, he really worked at it effectively."

Whatever offenses he'd committed in the past, Hand had abilities that outweighed the negatives. Dave was now officially the director of Disney's first feature.

THE ASSISTANT DIRECTOR

Assistant directors became a staple of all Disney filmmaking units. Jack Brunner described the duties of the job as basically being "everything that the director doesn't want to do. You pin up all the story sketches, and every dirty little job you can think of."[34]

Whereas directors seemed to come from the animation ranks, the eighteen or so assistants at the studio generally rose from the mail room, known at Disney's as "traffic." In terms of the job itself, recalled Brunner, "the first thing would be on the recording of the dialogue; you sit in on all the recordings and keep the punch numbers and keep track of all the takes." The assistant kept track of every bit of dialogue and sound effects that was recorded; music would be handled by the music cutter.

As the director determined roughly where the dialogue should be placed, "the assistant puts in all the dialogue readings—the modulations—on the exposure sheet."

They would also create a bar sheet, usually laid out in a tempo. "Scene one starts here, and it runs six feet and eight frames, and the dialogue starts four frames from the start, and you write what the dialogue is, and the punch number. That goes to the cutter so he can assemble a picture; he's got it right in front o him, on paper.

"That's another job the assistant director wil do; when he gets his bar sheets done, and th thing's all timed, he'll take the sketches of the storyboard and shoot those. He might say 'Shoot sketch number one for three feet, an the other one for 4:08,' and that's scene one. Then, as rough animation comes in, the assistant will "take out these sketches you've shot and you put in the pencil test; so eventuall you have a test reel," recalled Brunner.

Once the picture was nearing completion recalled assistant Don Duckwall, "it was the assistant director's job to find a theater—usually the Alex in Glendale or somewhere close like that—and you called the manage to get permission to sneak this thing between features at nine o'clock, say, and you would no tell anybody about that other than Walt, the director, the story man, and myself. You jus put the answer print under your arm and took it to the projectionist and you were there at nine o'clock, when it ran. At the end of the running, the group went straight outside the theater to the sidewalk, and that's where you heard from the boss, how he felt about it."[35]

SUPERVISING DIRECTOR

Though Hand was to direct, no one would dispute who was *Snow White*'s creative author. Disney built the plot, acted out characters, and guided design work. "Walt was in on every single move, every single thing that was done," said Dick Huemer. "You can't think of a thing Walt didn't okay in that picture." And "it was Dave's job," explained Huemer, "to see that Walt's directions were followed, to see that Walt got what he asked for."[36]

As the project came into focus, it was recognized that "one director could not have been expected to handle this entire picture as he would have of a short subject,"[37] remembered director Ben Sharpsteen. The picture was broken down into thirty-five sequences, with directors Wilfred Jackson, Bill Cottrell, Ben Sharpsteen, Larry Morey, and Perce Pearce overseeing each sequence according to their own strengths.[38] "Dave did not actually direct a sequence," recalled Sharpsteen, "but he was credited as the supervising director of the picture, and as such, he had supervision over all of the directors."[39]

It's easy to imagine the chaos in trying to relay changes and adjustments in characters and details from five separate units operating at once. Hand was passionate about this aspect: "I could go on for hours about organization. . . . It was a very strict organization; there was an organizational setup, and it took an awful lot of time and a lot of people to see that it worked . . . We couldn't have done it without organization; we just couldn't handle a thing like that without organization."[40]

But Walt didn't share Hand's passion for protocol. While he recognized the need for it, he was also comfortable ignoring it, leaving confusion in his wake. Hand explained that Walt might come in and see how a particular sequence was being laid out and not like it. Without checking with the director—whose instructions the artist was following and to whom the layout man reported to—Walt would order that the work be done differently. New instructions would then have to work back up the chain, and the pieces would have to be put back together. Hand remembered years later: "The kind of man Walt was, you couldn't expect him to care anything about organization, and he didn't."[41]

Fortunately, recalled Hand, "we had a vast Dictaphone system; we could call anyone with a button, never mind going through operators. This was before we went over to Burbank; this was on Hyperion. The director had about thirty keys he could push, to get anybody he wanted, and the animators had certain keys they could push—a not-as-big set of them. So it wasn't long before everybody in the studio who was concerned knew the signals had been changed. And that's how the studio was run."

Hand's involvement wasn't limited solely to organization. Animator Ollie Johnston said that Hand "was a big force on *Snow White*." He remembered: "Dave spoke up when he needed to. He knew he was not as creative as some of us, but he knew that he had good judgment, so he knew what to use of artists and our ideas. So as a director, he was great."[42]

Hand's supervision extended over the story department as well. Future Warner Bros. director Frank Tashlin remembered that Hand "would come over and look at our storyboards, and he would tear them to bits."[43]

Tashlin recalled Hand "would go in his expensive jackets with the padded shoulders—it looked like he wasn't walking; it was like the jacket was walking." Director Jack Kinney took to calling Dave "Shoulders."[44] Hand's assistant

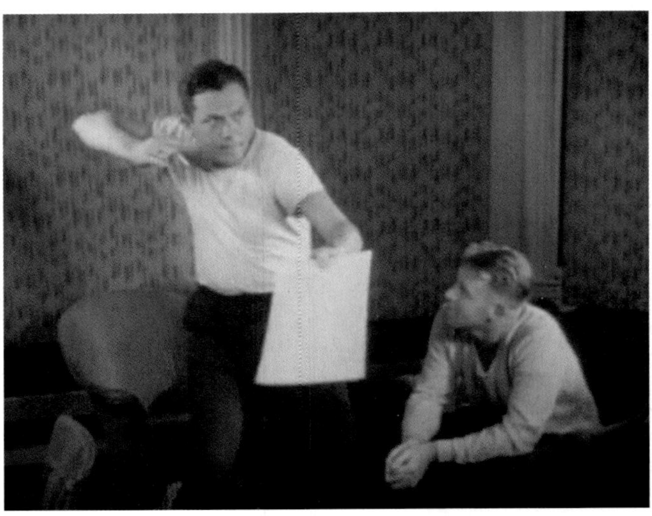

Hand acts out a scene for Ham Luske in a promotional film about the making of *Snow White*, shot on July 7, 1937.

Jack Cutting recalled that "there was a period there where he was riding high and getting important—we used to kid him and call him Lubitsch [after highly respected director Ernst Lubitsch]. And he would kind of squirm, but he kind of liked it."[45]

Hand was feeling his oats, enjoying the production and his involvement in it. He seemed to relish crossing swords with his boss, as he told the following anecdote several times:

> We had a meeting on *Snow White*, on one of the sequences, and the director is always in on a sequence when it's finally getting ready to be delivered . . . Walt was a marvelous pantomimist, a marvelous actor. If you said it to him, he would grump and walk away, but he was. . . . Anyway, I couldn't see the action getting completed in the time allotted. . . . I said, 'Walt, the animator can't do it in that time.' He said [Hand imitates Disney's grumpy voice], 'Hell, yes, Dave, you can do it in that time.' He got up and did it again—very good acting. I said, 'Well, it looked too long to me, Walt.' He didn't know it, but I had a stopwatch hidden in my pocket. A dirty trick. And I said to him, 'Walt, do it once more for me, will you, please?' Now, it was supposed to be done in thirty seconds—not thirty-two seconds—and he'd get up, and he'd go all through it . . . And he got all through and he said, 'There! You see, there it is—thirty seconds.' And I pulled this stopwatch out . . . I looked at my watch and I said, 'That was fifty-five seconds, Walt.' I learned a lesson. He didn't like that kind of thing; he didn't like that at all. He had an eyebrow that went up and helped to part his hair, and it went up and the other one went down. He had a very disturbing frown. He didn't say a word. He just turned and stomped out of the room.[46]

Hand had other eccentricities. He told animator Frank Thomas, "I can't be effective in an argument unless I'm mad." When hearing about a problem or situation, Hand would calmly ask for details. On hearing more, he would build into a state of fury until suddenly, remembered Thomas, "he would blow you out of the room!"[47] Even Walt worried when Dave was upset about something. As Thomas told it, "Walt said to me, 'Sometimes Dave would come to the office so mad he'd grab the corners of my desk and I'd look down and all the blood was out of his fingernails. If his fingers were white, I'd keep the desk between us!' He was half kidding about it, but Dave was bigger than Walt, physically. The kind Walt always said he liked: an aggressive guy who knew what he wanted and would fight for it. And Walt respected that. That's why he had Dave in his top position."[48]

On most occasions, however, Hand kept his anger in check, even when others caused trouble. Animator Art Babbitt, who was notorious for speaking his mind and going off his own direction when he thought it best, was called into Sweatbox No. 4 on March 3, 1937. It was the peak of production on *Snow White*, and Babbitt was still stubbornly presenting ideas for Dopey that were different from what was being asked. When Hand asked how he could help, Babbitt mockingly suggested that Hand "might animate it for me!" But a transcription of the meeting shows Hand calling Babbitt to task in a fair and straightforward way. "I think you are going off in your corner and taking it upon yourself to present something in the sweatbox which is entirely out of line or away from what we as directors have tried to follow through from the story conferences into the sweatbox. We try to give each animator the stuff the right way; work it all out with him so that he enters into it. When he leaves the room we like to feel that it is pretty much set as far as our mentality can go. Walt is above us in that, but we do the best we can." Hand continued: "You tell me you know I can direct and I say I know you can animate. Now that we agree that each knows his business, we must come to an agreement before we leave the Music Room. You must not go down to the drawing board and go against the direction without consulting with us. If you do, there is a loss because you have not talked it over the new way. If you have a new way, you should come back and talk it over and convince us that the new way is better. Then we are working in unison."[49]

Walt valued Hand professionally and must have enjoyed being around him outside the studio as well. Besides playing polo on Sundays, Dave and Walt were members of a club of business professionals who called themselves the Rancheros Visitadores. The group of businessmen would saddle up and ride off into the Santa Ynez Valley, camping and riding on the trail. Hand complained that they "might just as well have brought along tables and chairs," since "Walt would talk more and more about his new ideas, always ending with directions for me . . . upon our return to 'civilization.'" Whenever possible, Hand would hide out behind the oaks with his horse. "He was wearing me down," said Hand. "He didn't know anything else; he couldn't talk anything else but that studio."[50]

Throughout *Snow White*'s production, "no money was coming in," recalled story man Leo Salkin. With all the money tied up in *Snow White*, "the shorts were meant to sustain the studio while the feature was being done."[51] Since Disney needed to keep his full focus on the feature, he asked Hand to supervise shorts in addition to performing his role as supervising director. This meant Hand would approve story for the shorts, as well as production. Hand would direct eleven shorts while acting as *Snow White*'s supervising director.

Not everybody felt Hand's logical and reasoned approach was right for cartoons. "Dave Hand in my view had absolutely no sense of humor whatsoever," said Salkin. "You'd go through the whole storyboard in dead silence; and then Dave would say, 'Well, would you explain to me what causes that bump to come up in that rim?' And then one of us would say, 'Well, it's a cartoon gag, Dave, it just does it.' He'd say, 'That's not enough. There's got to be a logical motivation for that to happen.'" Salkin remembered that "those kinds of discussions would go on for thirty to sixty or eighty minutes, about the goddamned mechanical basis of the gag. Instead of saying, 'I can see that working, it's a funny gag, let's do it,' or 'It ain't funny, forget it, fellas.'"

It's unclear how long Hand was kept in the position of supervising shorts; Ben Sharpsteen took a turn at this as well. Likely Disney himself approved shorts whenever his schedule allowed.

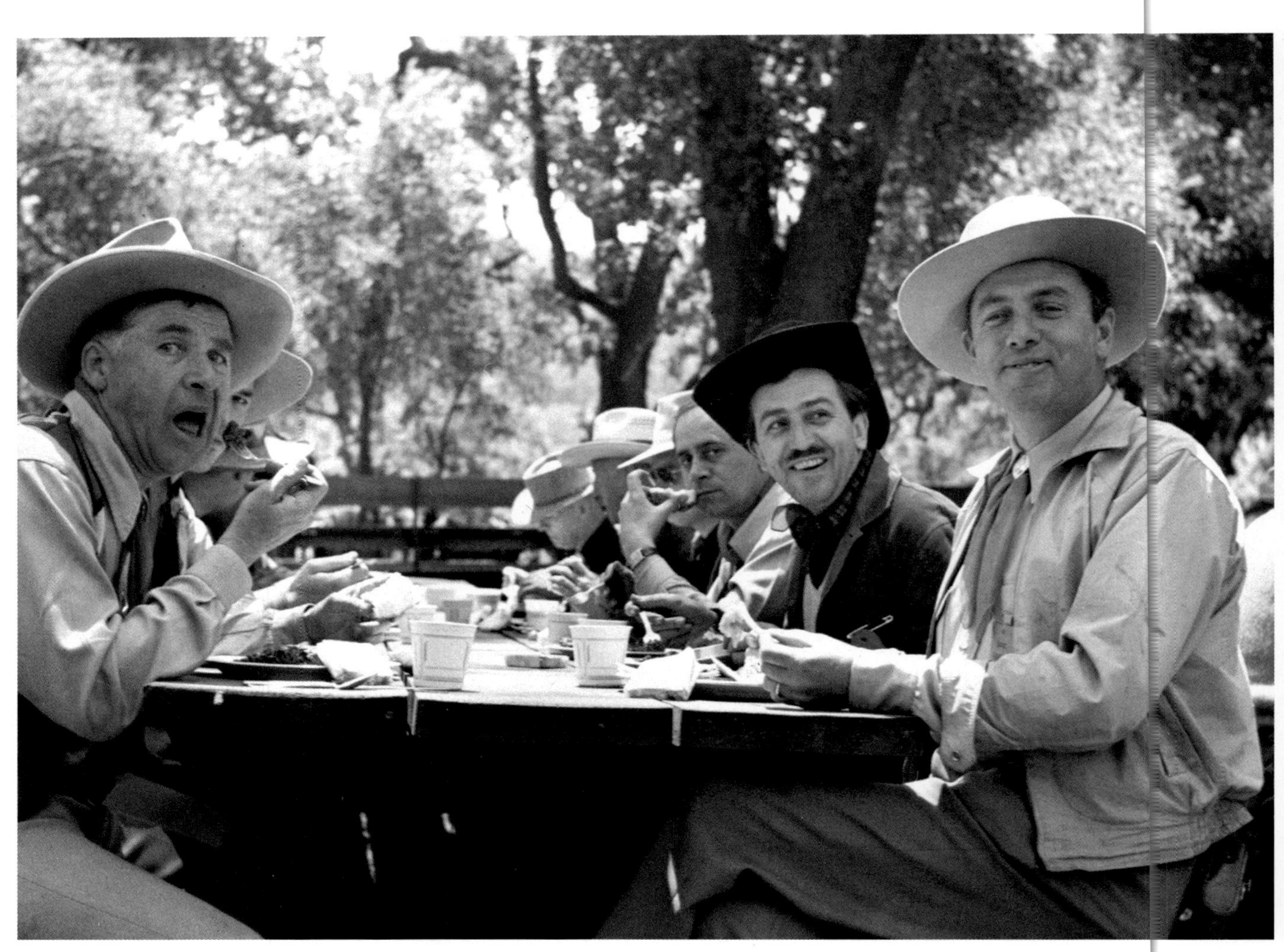

Hand (FRONT RIGHT) and Walt dine with the Rancheros Visitadores near Santa Barbara.

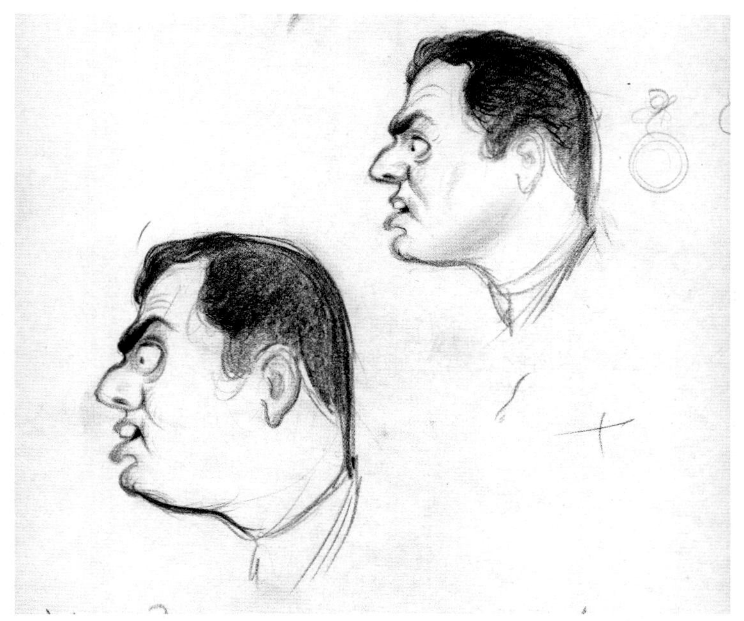

Hand's intensity is evident in these caricatures by Joe Grant, © Jennifer Grant Castrup. Hand and Grant admired each other and worked closely together.

Regardless, his lack of time led to a shift in the creative balance between Walt and his directors. Director Wilfred Jackson recalled:

> As Walt became interested in developing the feature, the first feature, he paid a little less attention to the shorts that were going through at that time. Suddenly, I found a lot more was up to me; I had a lot more latitude. There were more and more times when I would call Walt and say, "We need a meeting, we've got to make certain decisions." He'd say, "Well, what's on your mind?" I'd say, "Well, there's this and there's that," and he'd say, "Use your judgment." That didn't happen much before that time. So I'd go ahead, and if I was right, great, I wouldn't hear anything.[52]

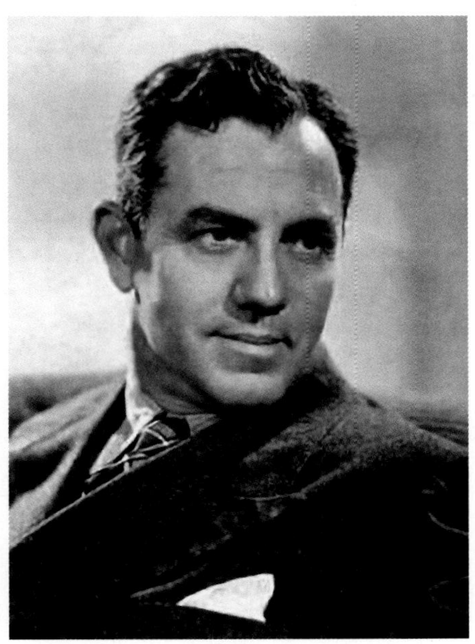

Hand, likely late 1930s.

The directors' creative responsibility would later continue to expand as Walt's interests grew. But for now, sequence directors completed their duties under Disney's leadership, timing out approved story sequences, working with the composers, and following through with animators.

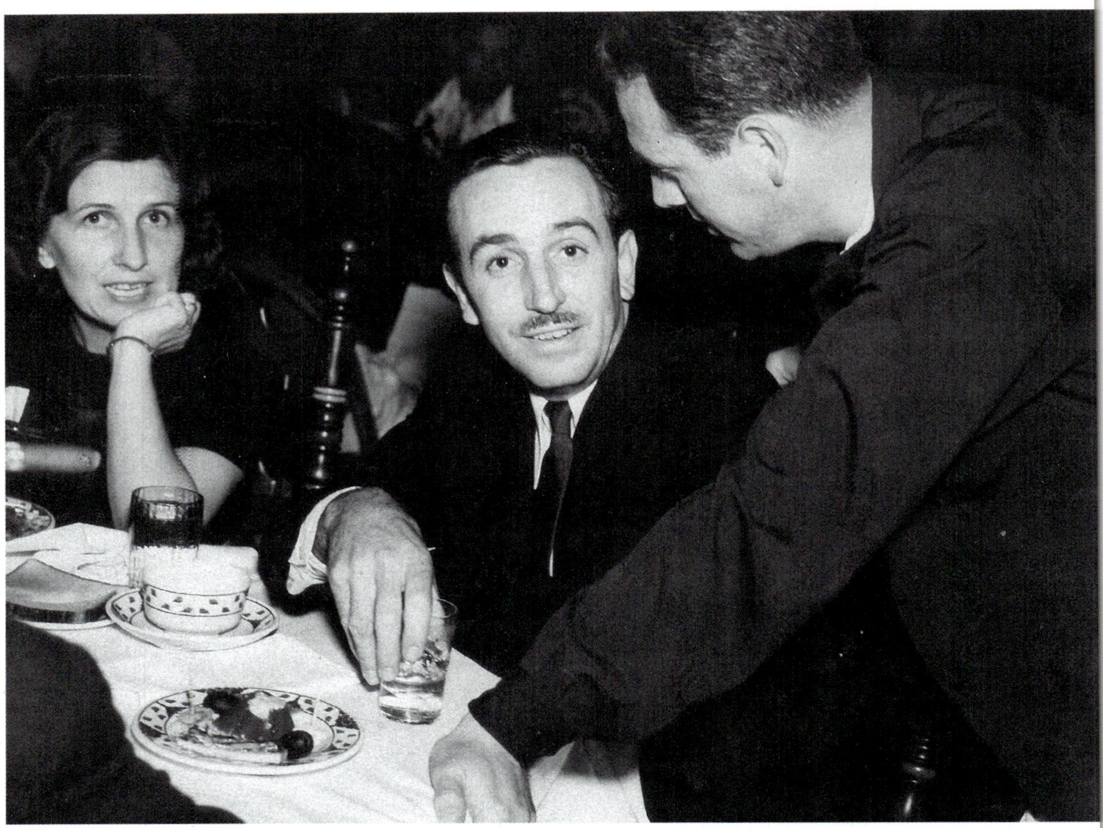

Lillian, Walt, and Hand share a celebratory moment at "Walt's Field Day" at the Lake Norconian Resort, June 4, 1938. Photo by Willis Pyle.

As production went into its last year, *Snow White* was still a long way from finished. With the studio in debt to Bank of America, Hand found his role becoming that of taskmaster: his missives to employees now were less about quality and more about faster, more efficient work. Long hours and unpaid overtime became the norm as everyone scrambled to finish.

When *Snow White* came out in December 1937[53], it marked just eight years since Hand had started at the studio as an animator. He was now supervising director of the year's most successful film. But some questioned his motivation. Animator Frank Thomas remembered Hand as "not searching for better ways nor driving himself relentlessly or trying to prove anything, as I saw him. He wanted to be on top of the heap! He wanted it to be a big efficient, envied heap."[54] Dick Huemer recalled that Hand "took it seriously: big man, second in command on *Snow White*, he was going to run the studio after a while."[55]

As Hand would soon discover, that position was already filled.

HAND THE PRODUCTION SUPERVISOR

"Walt always stressed organization at the studio," remembered director Ben Sharpsteen. "He persisted periodically in complaining that we had no plan for management and that we had to organize ourselves. But all the time he meant that he had to organize himself."[56] Animator Frank Thomas put his finger on the problem: "Walt was dead set against procedures. That was one of the troubles Dave Hand had with him. . . . The things Walt asked for you to do called for organization—you wouldn't get it done otherwise. And yet Walt hated organization. Just hated to be pinned down."[57]

With big plans for the future, Walt installed Hand as the studio's Production Supervisor, the "number two man" at the studio. (Interestingly, Hand was never credited on-screen as such, while Ben Sharpsteen, Joe Grant, and others received this credit on several films.) Dave's first job: organize the many projects already in the works, and bring some order to the growing enterprise. Dave had his work cut out for him.

Four months after *Snow White*'s release, Hand published a handbook titled *The Organization*, a fifty-eight-page manual—updated twice in the following months—with elaborate instructions as to the chain of command and process to be followed. The chart in it clearly shows Hand's passion for organization, though whether any of its dictums were followed is not clear.

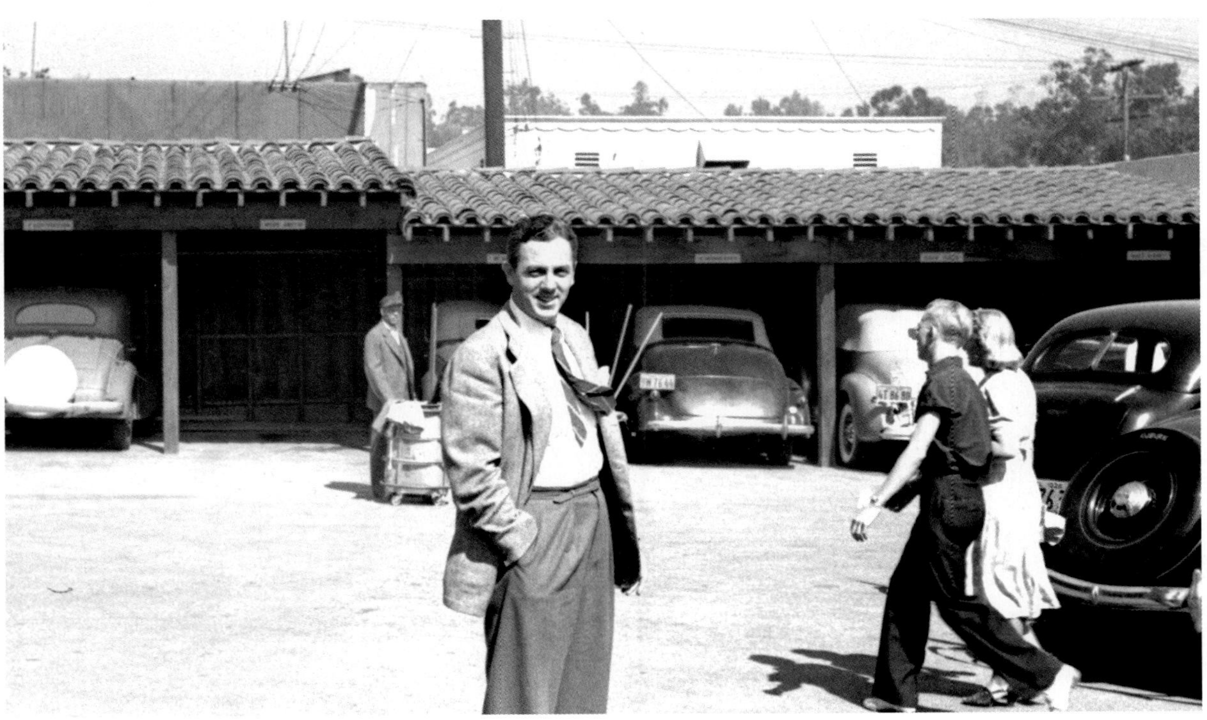

Hand in the Hyperion Avenue studio parking lot, circa 1939. In the back right is Hand's parking space, next to Disney's, with his Packard Super Eight Convertible Victoria. Hand bought one to match Walt's, which didn't go over well with the boss. Photo by Ward Kimball.

The stated goal of the manual was "to allow Walt to use his time exclusively in the creative end of production." Hand assigned himself both production supervisor and general production manager, attempting to establish a clear hierarchy: "Walt should not be contacted by his personnel on any item other than of a creative nature." The plan was set up so that "any or all of the above functions of Walt's can be taken over by the Production Supervisor [Hand] . . . upon Walt's designation or his protracted absence." Whether this was a power grab or simply an attempt to be helpful, Hand would find himself disappointed; Disney would seldom surrender this kind of authority for a decade or more.

Meeting notes from October 1938 show that Disney continued to engage in discussions over studio organization,[58] yet continued to make films the way he saw fit, leaving it to others to adjust. Walt's need for structure yet discomfort with it seemed in many ways to echo his relationship with Hand.

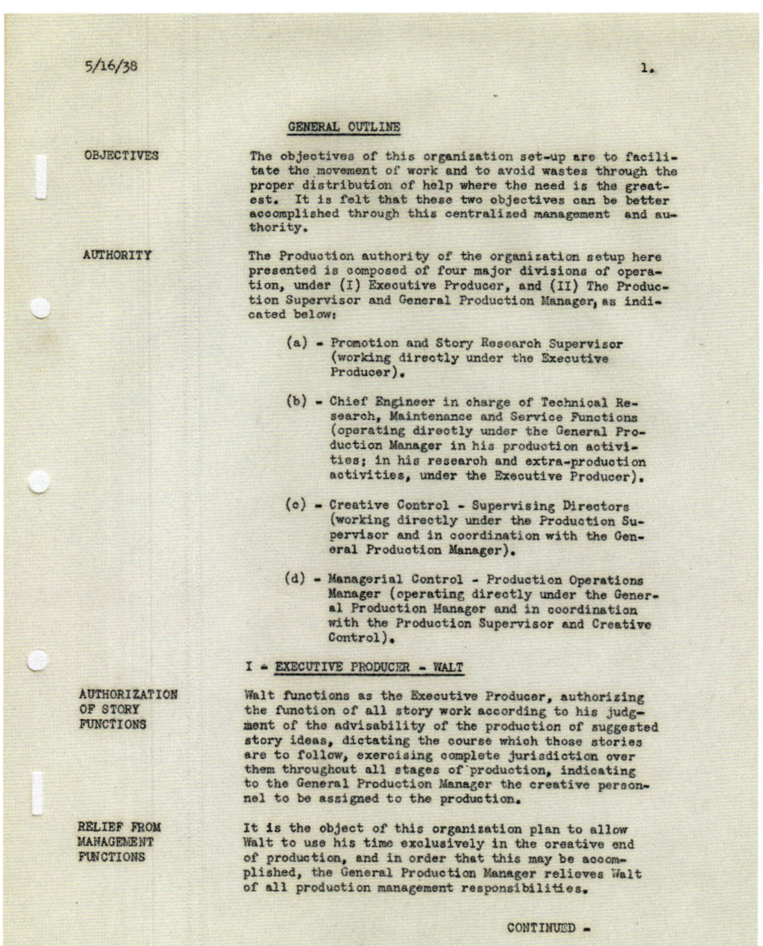

5/16/38 1.

GENERAL OUTLINE

OBJECTIVES — The objectives of this organization set-up are to facilitate the movement of work and to avoid wastes through the proper distribution of help where the need is the greatest. It is felt that these two objectives can be better accomplished through this centralized management and authority.

AUTHORITY — The Production authority of the organization setup here presented is composed of four major divisions of operation, under (I) Executive Producer, and (II) The Production Supervisor and General Production Manager, as indicated below:

(a) - Promotion and Story Research Supervisor (working directly under the Executive Producer).

(b) - Chief Engineer in charge of Technical Research, Maintenance and Service Functions (operating directly under the General Production Manager in his production activities; in his research and extra-production activities, under the Executive Producer).

(c) - Creative Control - Supervising Directors (working directly under the Production Supervisor and in coordination with the General Production Manager).

(d) - Managerial Control - Production Operations Manager (operating directly under the General Production Manager and in coordination with the Production Supervisor and Creative Control).

I - EXECUTIVE PRODUCER - WALT

AUTHORIZATION OF STORY FUNCTIONS — Walt functions as the Executive Producer, authorizing the function of all story work according to his judgment of the advisability of the production of suggested story ideas, dictating the course which those stories are to follow, exercising complete jurisdiction over them throughout all stages of production, indicating to the General Production Manager the creative personnel to be assigned to the production.

RELIEF FROM MANAGEMENT FUNCTIONS — It is the object of this organization plan to allow Walt to use his time exclusively in the creative end of production, and in order that this may be accomplished, the General Production Manager relieves Walt of all production management responsibilities.

CONTINUED -

Page one of Hand's organizational manual for the studio, May 16, 1938. Courtesy The Walt Disney Family Museum Library, Ward Kimball collection.

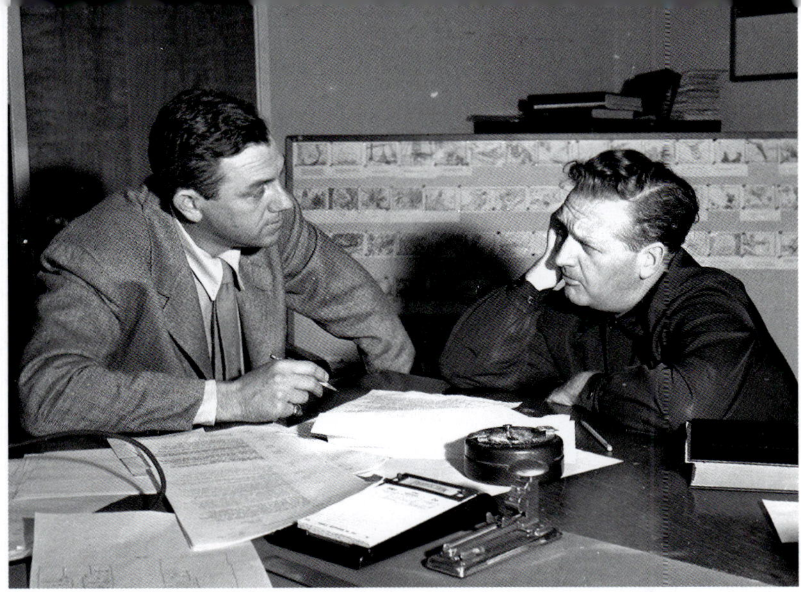

Hand (LEFT) and Perce Pearce discuss the progress on *Bambi*.

BAMBI

Bambi was originally planned as the second feature, but work progressed slowly, so *Pinocchio*—seemingly less of a challenge from an animation perspective—was moved in as the second feature.[59] *Fantasia* soon followed; two major undertakings were being produced at nearly the same time, followed by *Dumbo*, as well as the studio's continued diet of shorts.

Development of *Bambi* was under the supervision of Perce Pearce, a major story contributor to *Snow White*. He had been sent to develop the Felix Salten story and characters with a growing crew. In those early days of development, said story man Chuck Couch, "Walt stayed clear of that thing, completely. We were a separate unit, and he stayed completely away from it. It was strange. I think he may have looked at some of the running reels once or twice, but I doubt it."[60] Pearce developed quite a bit of charming material for *Bambi* but was slow in making decisions, laboring over details, seeming to prefer developing more material than crafting it into a single story. Pearce also liked to present ideas through beautifully rendered images shot on Leica reels, which took extra time and money. Chuck Couch recalled, "There were six crews on that thing, I think, and there were at least five men on each crew. We had made running reels, with the voices and all that. It was almost like a pose reel. The picture was way over length."[61] Disney soon realized that he needed to make a change. He brought in Dave Hand.

On August 17, 1939, Hand sent out a memo:

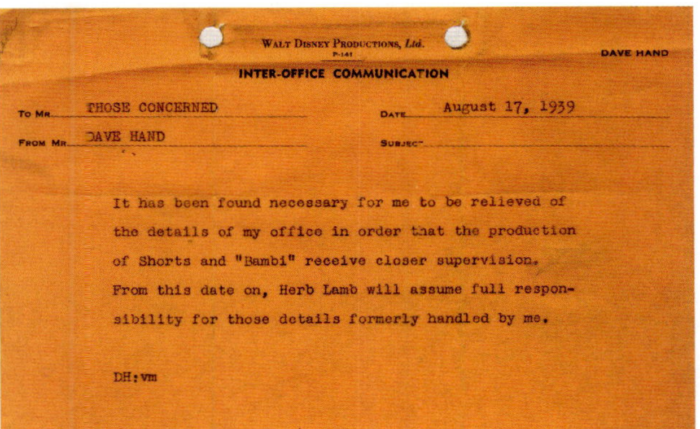

Walt Disney Productions, Ltd.
P-141
DAVE HAND
INTER-OFFICE COMMUNICATION

To Mr. THOSE CONCERNED — Date August 17, 1939
From Mr. DAVE HAND — Subject

It has been found necessary for me to be relieved of the details of my office in order that the production of Shorts and "Bambi" receive closer supervision. From this date on, Herb Lamb will assume full responsibility for those details formerly handled by me.

DH:vm

Couch agreed: "Perce Pearce had been heading *Bambi*, and my god, we wasted more time on that. Dave came over there and he took charge of things." Couch recalled that the work was "well done before Dave came on, but, well . . . there was so damned much material there that Dave came in and said, 'This will stay in, and this goes out,' and tied the whole picture together. I rather think that's what his job was." Hand shrunk the story crew to between seven and nine and made decisive cuts to the material.[62] "Dave just wound it up," said Couch.[63]

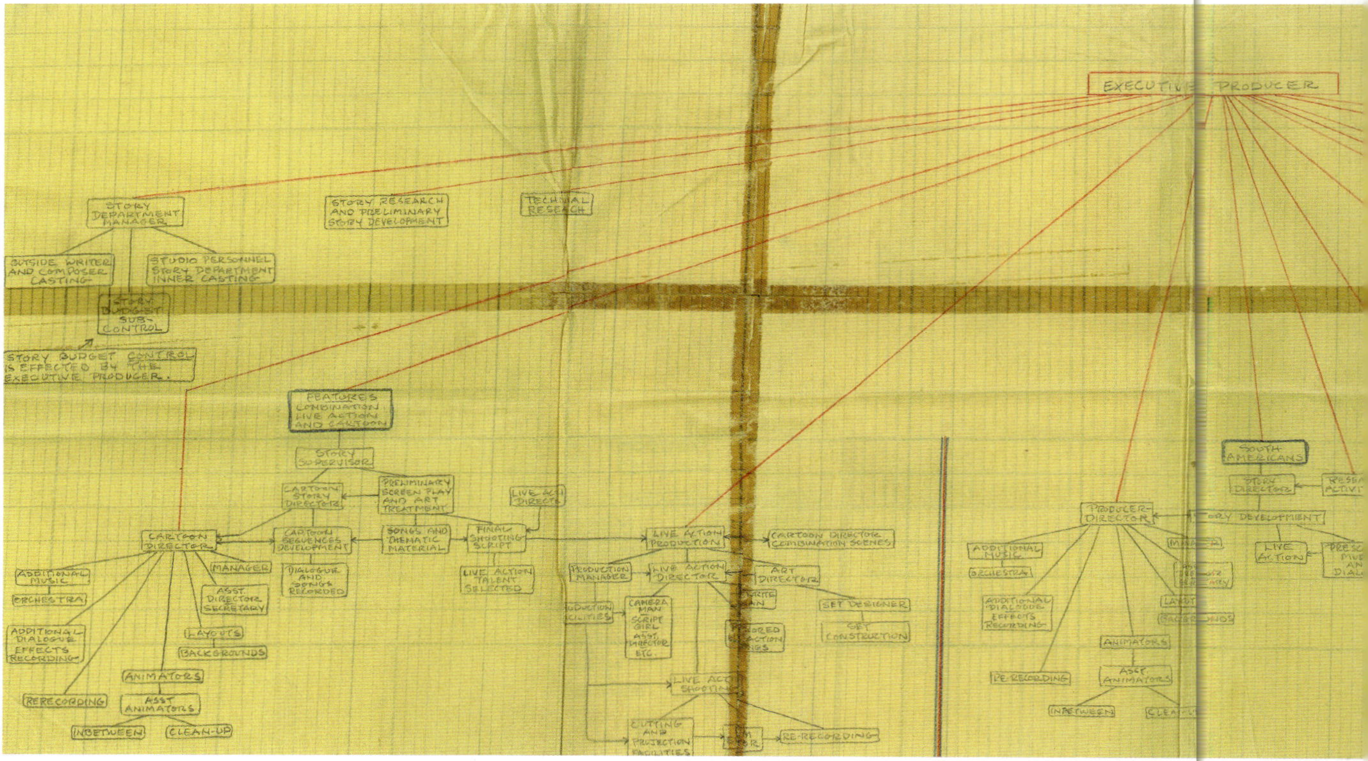

Additionally, Disney had outgrown its Hyperion Avenue headquarters, and a new studio was being planned in Burbank—an additional drain on Hand's organizational skills. But the new studio wouldn't be ready for some time, and as a result of tight space and an expanding workforce, work on *Bambi* was done at 861 Seward Street—the old Harman-Ising studio—4.6 miles from the main Disney studio at 2719 Hyperion Avenue.

One of Hand's jobs was to force decisions out of Walt, who would occasionally leave questions unresolved. Animator Frank Thomas mentioned Walt's dislike of closing doors; he preferred to keep things open-ended when he didn't feel he'd arrived at a strong solution. In a conversation with Hand, Thomas recalled:

> I always remember that showing of *Bambi* we had; we could run the whole picture in some form. And Walt had never made a clear decision on how to show the dead man in the charred forest. And you [Dave] said, "Goddammit, I'm going to force his hand. Make me a drawing of a guy burnt to a crisp." Because you'd said to Walt, "Do you want to

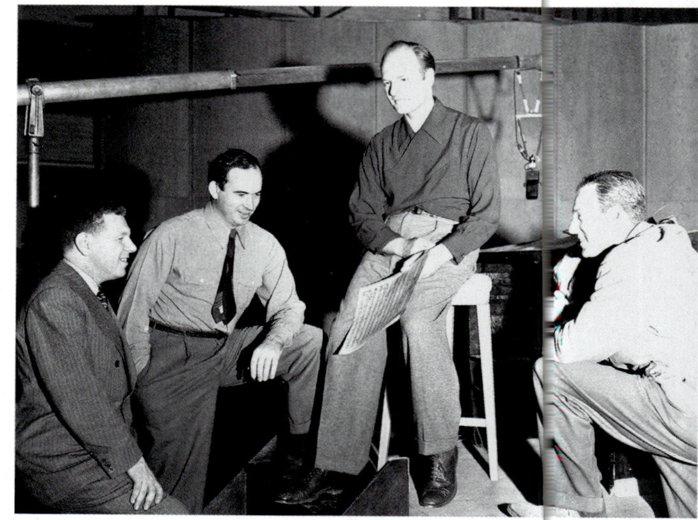

On *Bambi*, FROM LEFT: choral arranger Charles Henderson, composer and arranger Ed Plumb, conductor and arranger Alexi Steinert, supervising director Dave Hand.

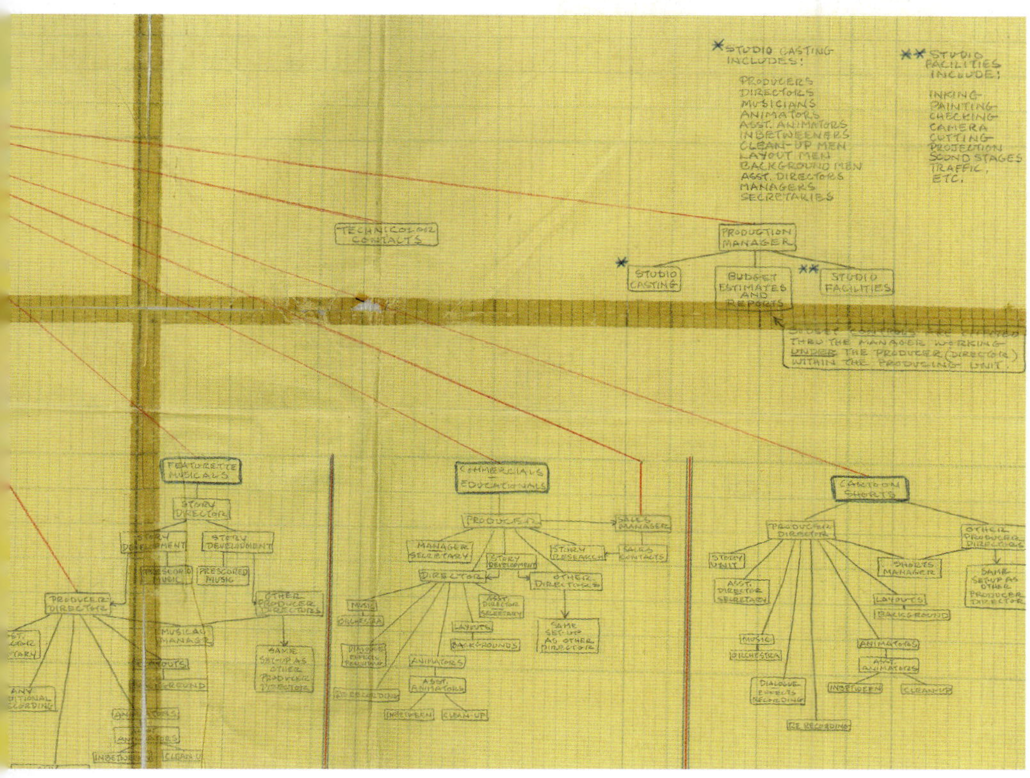

Hand's 1944 studio org chart provides a fascinating look into what was being planned at the studio: cartoon features, cartoon/live-action combo features, live-action features, South American films, featurette musicals, commercials, educational shorts, and cartoon shorts.

> just show a hand with a gun? Or do you want to show him charred? Or how do you want to do this?" And Walt said, "Well, uh . . . hell, you know . . ." and he kept putting off the decision. So you had someone do this drawing of this burnt corpse. You found out in a hurry what he wanted!

Hand supervised not just story and production, but the look and design as well. "*Bambi* was the first time I was aware of the director being interested in the style of the film, what style it was going to take," remembered layout artist Zach Schwartz.[64]

In fact, Hand claimed that "Walt Disney had practically nothing to do with the making of *Bambi*. At that very time he was enamored with the *Fantasia* Stokowski connection,"[65] and as a result, Disney "didn't look at it much; I don't know when he looked at it."[66] However, meeting notes both before and during production show Disney's heavy involvement in story as well as production. Disney had comments on pacing ("too slow"), color ("too much strong color, not enough depth"), and music ("too serious"; "needs more excitement and 'corn'") and had a lot to say about expense ("find ways to keep the cost down" by showing characters in silhouette).[67] What are we to make of both Hand's and story man Chuck Couch's memories of the lack of Disney's involvement with the film? Perhaps there was some truth to it, given the distance from Hyperion to the Seward studio. Likely also Disney's big-picture focus felt like such compared to his exacting oversight of *Snow White* and *Pinocchio*.

Bambi was released in the late summer of 1942 to mixed reviews, though today it is largely regarded as one of Disney's best animated features.

DIFFERENT PATHS

After *Bambi*, Hand worked on *Victory Through Air Power*, released in 1943, and was credited as animation supervisor. In 1944 he returned to his favorite activity—organization—and outlined a new set of ideas for studio structure on the back of animation exposure sheets.

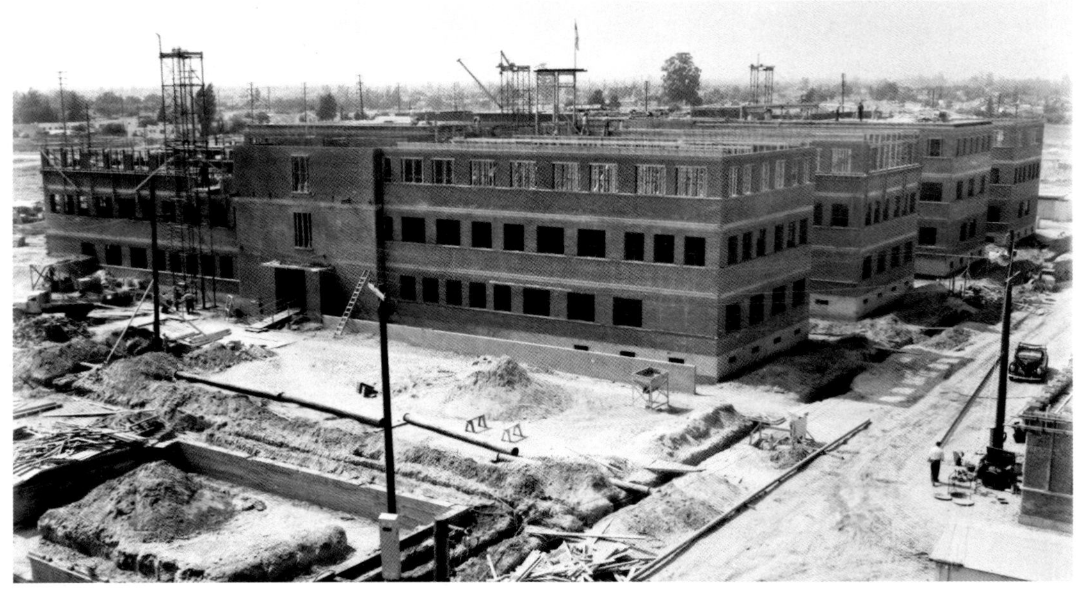

The Burbank studio under construction in early 1939.

Once again, as director/producer Ben Sharpsteen observed, Hand "entirely overlooked the simple thing I'm putting across to you, that that place was absolutely Walt's. Dave had the attitude that 'Walt gives me a job to do certain things, and outlines it that way, that's it—it's going to be that way.' But Dave would no sooner turn his back than he'd find out Walt had given part of his job to somebody else. Walt had no regard for protocol."[68]

But all this was a part of a larger problem. Walt had always sent conflicting signals in regards to Hand's organizational efforts; now he was sending conflicting signals about Hand himself.

"They fought a lot," said animator Frank Thomas of Walt and Dave's relationship.[69] This had always been true but had usually resulted in mutual admiration for their shared passion and abilities. But now Hand was feeling mistrust.

In his autobiography, Dave wrote:

> It is not my intention to dwell on the detail of the change that was taking place, but Walt's and my paths were beginning to go in different directions. The change was ever so subtle: anyone outside of our close working associates would have never noticed it, but it was definitely there.

"You have to remember that Walt's relationship with Dave more or less ended when he was the producer of *Snow White*," said story man Joe Grant. "Because Walt didn't know it was going to be the hit it was, and here's a man linked to it, with the credit that he had. Walt was pretty jealous in a sense of his position. Dave was ambitious, too."[70]

The delicate balance of ambition, tension, and pressure between Disney and Hand was beginning to crumble.

Not one to enjoy personal confrontation, Walt made a series of administrative decisions that would communicate his feelings. As the staff moved into the newly built Burbank studio, Walt decided to move Hand's office back by the story department, away from his own. And after the strike of 1941, when time clocks were installed, Hand was required to use them—even though he was part of the leadership team. "I think that that one decision ended my closeness to Walt," Hand wrote in his autobiography. "Not because of that decision, but because he insisted that I had also to be a part of the 'punchers.' That one move did more to my tiny ego than anything else I could possibly have thought up. That definitely became the beginning of the end of my connection with the Disney studio, and my loyalty to it."[71]

Story man Jim Algar later wrote, "I don't think I realized how mentally upset he might have been at the end."[72]

HAND LEAVES

On July 21, 1944, Hand went into Walt's office and announced he was leaving. Walt picked up the telephone and asked Roy to cut Dave's check. "Walt's ego would not allow him to ask me not to leave," remembered Hand.[73] "Fourteen years of building that studio with him, and that was the way it ended,"[74] said Hand's son, David Hale.

In the following days word came out that Hand had been hired by British industrialist J. Arthur Rank to create an animation studio in England. The news upset Walt, who assumed Hand had conspired to create a competing studio. Hand asserted he'd quit without knowing where he'd land. Though he did bring many lessons to Gaumont British Animation Studios, Hand left Disney's because he was unhappy.

"There was simply no direction for him to progress in the studio," reminisced Jim Algar to Frank Thomas. "I always felt that that was why Dave pulled out. He was like a man trapped under Walt, with the water rising."[75]

Looking back, Hand told animator Frank Thomas that he'd left because Walt was losing confidence in himself and his judgment. "Dave Hand had left right at the end of the war, because he said he saw that coming, that Walt had lost his confidence and he was a different man now with all these failures, and he just approached things differently."[76]

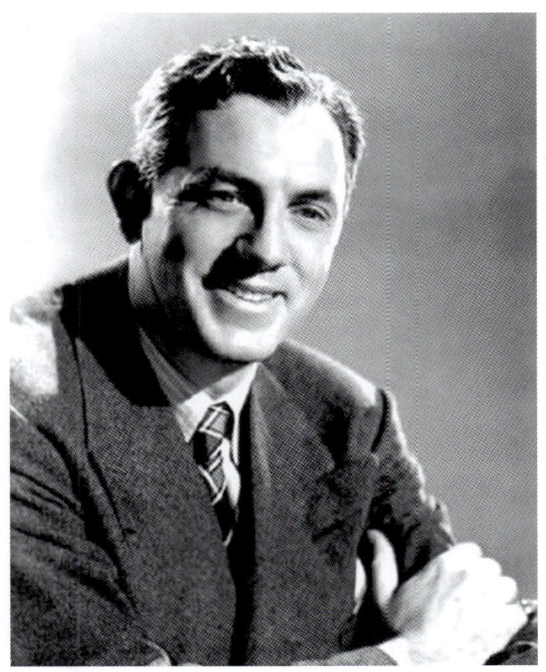

Dave Hand as managing director and production supervisor at Gaumont British Animation, Ltd., mid-1940s.

Then, too, as Hand said in an interview: "I was there, and I saw it, and I saw one man—who was a genius, no question about it—get the credit."[77] While Hand claimed that "it didn't bother me at the time," clearly it got under his skin.

Hand's ambition and desire for more responsibility were inseparable aspects of his personality that would not have a chance to flourish in his working with Disney. One can't blame Hand for wanting to continue to grow and challenge himself. At the same time, Disney knew what he wanted and did not see Hand as a partner. Walt was the boss, just as he was with others. As Hand realized, "the only interest Walt had in making pictures was to make them *his* way."[78]

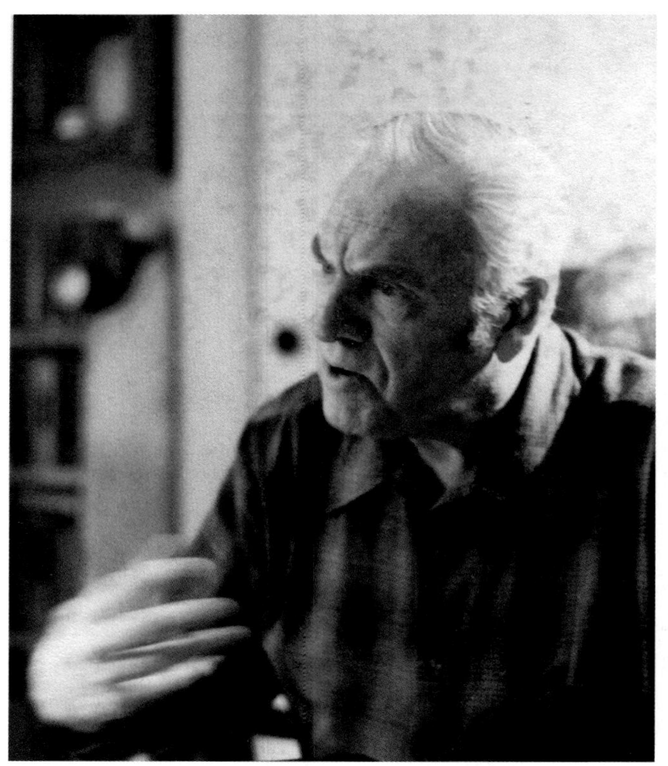

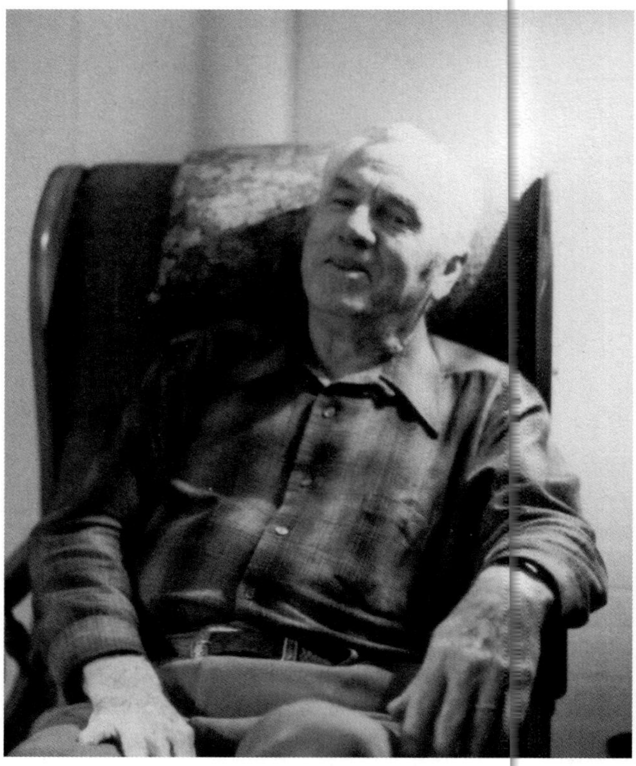

Hand's intensity and confidence are apparent even in his retirement, from these photos taken at his home in Cambria, California, in 1975 by Les Gibbard. Courtesy Ted Thomas.

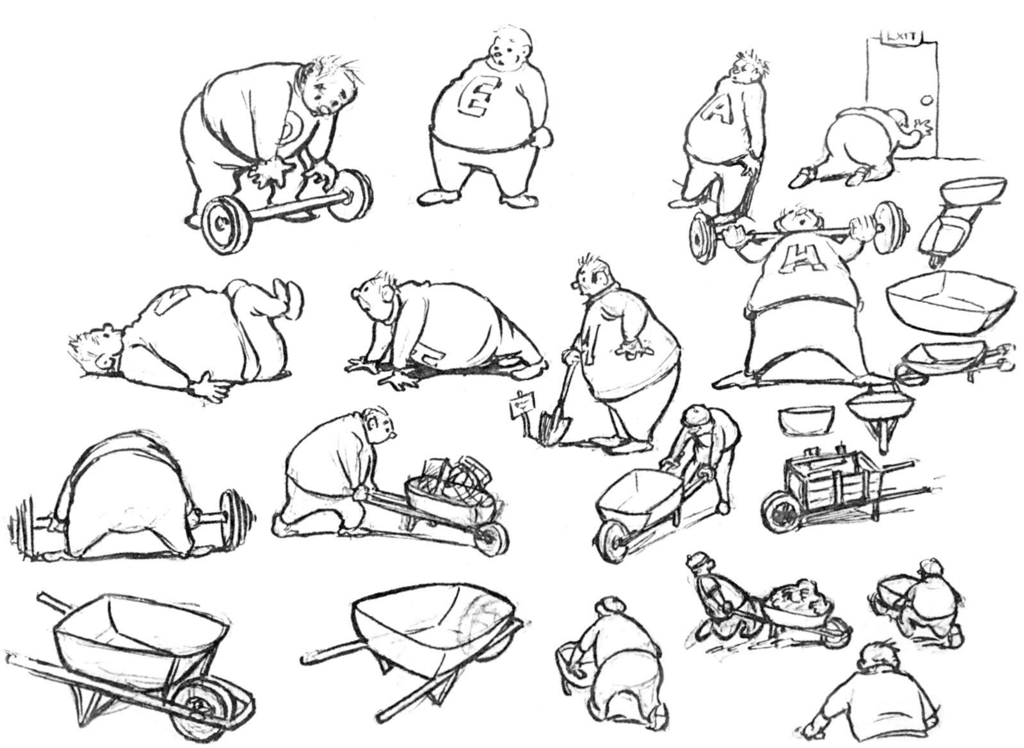

Drawing by Hand from later in his life. Courtesy Michael Barrier.

Hand built a studio in Britain nearly from scratch, producing several technically impressive but underwhelming shorts. "Hand's artists may draw like Disney but have not yet captured his sense of fun," opined one critic.[79] Hand's dream of making a feature fizzled when the studio went out of business in 1949.

Dave returned to the United States and made commercial and industrial films with the Alexander Film Company in Colorado and retired to Cambria, California, largely cutting himself off from his past. In his 125-page autobiography, *Memoirs*, Hand devotes a scant thirteen pages to his entire career at the Disney Studios, with only a handful of stories relating to Walt. He was honored with a Winsor McCay Award in 1984, and having died in October of 1986, posthumously made a Disney Legend in 1994. There is no record of any correspondence between Walt and Dave after his departure from the studio; sad, considering all they had accomplished together.

But perhaps this was the reason for Hand's barely concealed bitterness about his years with Disney: for him, it was a broken personal relationship. Yet for Walt, like his horseback rides into the country with the Rancheros Visitadores, it was always business.

Dave Hand—Disney Director Filmography

Disney Shorts:
- *Trader Mickey* (1932)[80]
- *Building a Building* (1933)
- *The Mad Doctor* (1933)
- *Birds in the Spring* (1933)
- *The Mail Pilot* (1933)
- *Old King Cole* (1933)
- *Camping Out* (1934)
- *Mickey's Steam Roller* (1934)
- *The Flying Mouse* (1934)
- *The Dognapper* (1934)
- *Mickey's Man Friday* (1935)
- *Mickey's Kangaroo* (1935)
- *The Robber Kitten* (1935)
- *Who Killed Cock Robin?* (1935)
- *Pluto's Judgement Day* (1935)
- *Three Orphan Kittens* (1935)
- *Mickey's Polo Team* (1936)
- *Three Little Wolves* (1936)
- *Thru the Mirror* (1936)
- *Alpine Climbers* (1936)
- *Three Blind Mouseketeers* (1936)
- *Mickey's Elephant* (1936)
- *More Kittens* (1936)
- *Magician Mickey* (1937)
- *Little Hiawatha* (1937)

Disney Features:
- *Show White and the Seven Dwarfs* (1937)—Supervising Director
- *Bambi* (1942)—Supervising Director
- *Victory Through Air Power* (1943)—Animation Supervisor

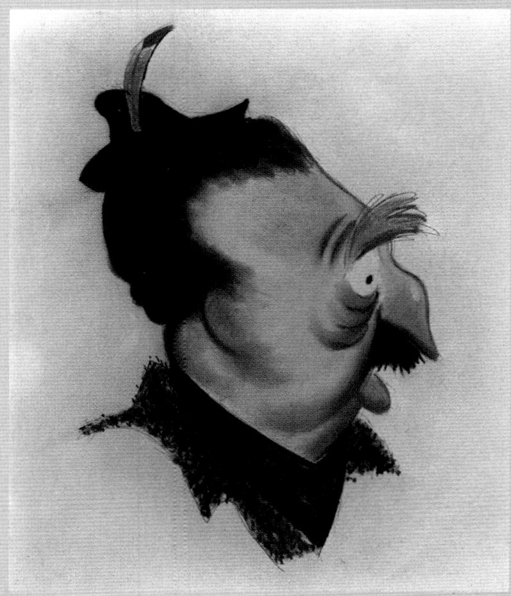

Caricature of Pearce by Bill Justice, 1952.

Percival C. "Perce" Pearce was one of those characters, like Roy Williams[81]: everyone who knew him or worked with him had a story to share. Animation director Jack Kinney, who worked for a time with Perce on *Bambi*, recalled others as saying that Perce was "the biggest flimflammer to rise from the ranks." Jack briefly summarized Perce's early career in a jaded manner: "Perce had started as a lowly in-betweener but by dint of research (stealing gags), a jolly ho-ho laugh, twinkling blue eyes, and unflappable ego, a manner of speaking up in story meetings, and other ploys, he had managed to get himself transferred to the Story Department."[82] There is no shortage of stories about the theatrics employed by Perce in deliberately and slowly lighting his ever-present pipe while pontificating in story meetings, but they proved effective with at least one member of the audience: Walt Disney. And more than just Walt, as noted by Frank Thomas and Ollie Johnston, in their book *Bambi: The Story and the Film*: "Next to Walt, Perce Pearce was the best storyteller and actor; he knew how to characterize the specific traits of an individual. He loved to get up and perform for us and even became identified with many of the cartoon cast on each picture."

Perce was born in 1899 in Waukegan, Illinois. He began cartooning at a young age and went on to study at the Academy of Fine Arts in Chicago. Ben Sharpsteen said, "The first that I knew of him was during the First World War. He was in the navy and he had a comic strip in the papers called *Seaman Si*. It soon went out, like many comic strips do, and I never heard any more about it."[83] Perce worked as a cartoonist at the *Denver Post* and news syndicates before he came to the Disney Studios in 1935. Ben recalled: "One day, Perce Pearce showed up at the studio and I interviewed him—he wanted a job. Because he had some experience in comic strip work, we decided to put him in on a trial basis. He developed quite rapidly and became a director."[84] Within a very short time span, he had moved into story on *Snow White* and then became one of its sequence directors, alongside veteran directors Wilfred Jackson and Ben Sharpsteen and fellow novices Larry Morey and Bill Cottrell. Perce ended up directing more footage than any of the other directors. Supervising director Dave Hand explained: "[H]e delegates to other people all work that is not essential for

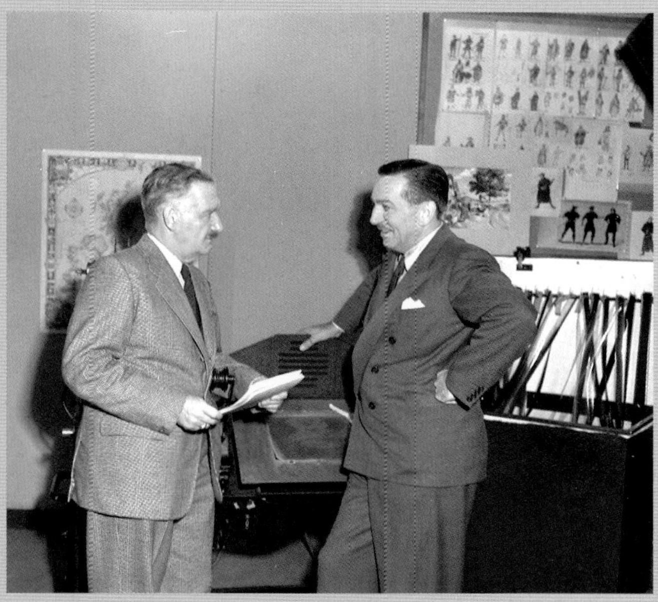

Walt and Perce in conference on *The Story of Robin Hood and His Merrie Men* (1952).

him to do. Offhand I don't know of any director who will do that . . . Perce has turned out more work in a short time than others because he is smart."[85] Perce acted out scenes involving many of the Dwarfs, and that also helped elevate him to a directing spot. "What won him that assignment was not an expertise as an animator, but rather his ability to bring out the personalities of the Dwarfs as he acted out a scene."[86]

On *Bambi*, Perce's acting found its way from behind the scenes and onto the soundtrack as the voice of the little mole who popped out of his burrow, squinted at the sky, and commented, "Nice sunny day!" before plunging back undergrond.[87]

Perce worked on story development on "The Sorcerer's Apprentice" segment of *Fantasia* and then was assigned to story on *Bambi.* He had a good deal of autonomy on the latter film, but the story development was

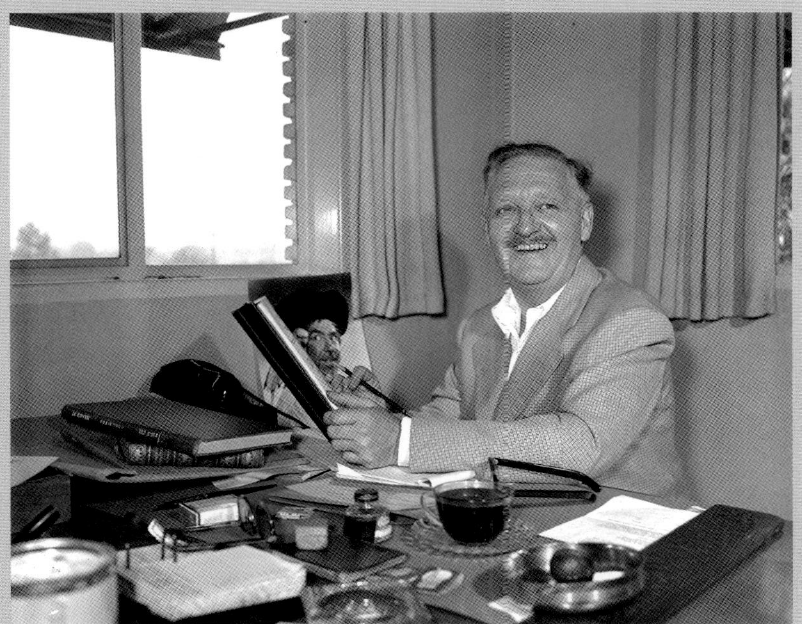

Perce at work on *Treasure Island* (1950).

progressing too slowly, and supervising director Dave Hand stepped in to move the production along. Perce continued to work on story with *Victory Through Air Power* and then transitioned into producing as an associate producer on *Song of the South* and *So Dear to My Heart*. As Walt diversified in the late 1940s into all-live-action films, Perce went with him as an assistant producer. Scouting locations for *Song of the South* and *So Dear to My Heart*, he did the same in postwar England for *Treasure Island*, becoming a producer on that film. He stayed in England through 1955, apparently driven by an issue involving taxes, producing *The Story of Robin Hood and His Merrie Men*, *The Sword and the Rose*, and *Rob Roy: The Highland Rogue*. At some point, he separated from the studio and developed some scripts for Twentieth Century Fox.

In January 1955, Perce asked to renew his connection with the Disney Studios, and Walt was receptive. In a February 9, 1955, letter, Walt said, "I am happy to know that you are interested in working with us again." Walt suggested that Perce could best fit in in the realm of television production, and Walt focused on a "kid show, aimed at the 5 to 12 age-level, five days a week, to be called the *Mickey Mouse Club Show*." He continued: "If this new show sounds at all interesting to you, perhaps we could work out something with you that would fit in with your own plans." Perce was interested and worked on a "London Correspondent" segment for the series and on eight-minute segments featuring Sooty, a popular puppet, created and operated by Harry Corbett, on British television.

Perce passed away suddenly on July 4, 1955. His unexpected death stunned his family and friends, most particularly Walt and his family. In a telegram to Perce's widow, June, Walt wrote that on hearing the news, he and Lilly and their family were shocked and grieved. Perhaps referring to a past conflict over the levels of success of some of the films Perce produced in England for the studio, Walt said, "While I had my little disagreements with Perce through [the] years I really loved and respected him." Walt made every effort to help June and her family through the loss. Perce had left his mark on the studio and an indelible impression on all who worked with him.[88]

Perce Pearce—Disney Filmography

Snow White and the Seven Dwarfs (1937) (Sequence Director)

Story development on *Fantasia* (1940), *Bambi* (1942), *Victory Through Air Power* (1943), and *Song of the South* (1946)

So Dear to My Heart (1949) (Associate Producer), *Treasure Island* (1950), *The Story of Robin Hood and His Merrie Men* (1952), *The Sword and the Rose* (1953), and *Rob Roy: The Highland Rogue* (1953) (Producer)

BILL ROBERTS

When we began researching directors for this book, the name Bill Roberts jumped out as someone we had not heard of. Ben Sharpsteen mentioned him in an interview, but didn't talk about him enough to leave a lasting impression. "He had had animation experience in Chicago and came to us as an experienced animator. From that, he moved into direction and was a very competent man."[89] Historian Mike Barrier said about Roberts, "Yeah, he's a mystery man. That's one that is frustrating to me because I don't know much about him at all."[90] The details of Bill's life are a bit sketchy at both ends, but we can fill in some of the middle, at least his years at the Disney Studios.

William Opal "Bill" Roberts was born in August 1899 in Jordan, Kentucky, the second son to barber William Alexander Roberts and Birdie May Watkins.[91] Roberts's 1918 draft card lists him as "Refrigerating Engineer," and later, he worked as a junior engineer in the maritime trade. He moved to California with his family in 1922 and married his wife, Lillian, in 1929. The couple are not known to have had any children. Census data shows Bill back in New York in 1931, working as an illustrator, and living in the Bronx through 1933.

Most of his colleagues at Disney referenced his "hillbilly" demeanor. Animator Shamus Culhane described Bill at the time they worked

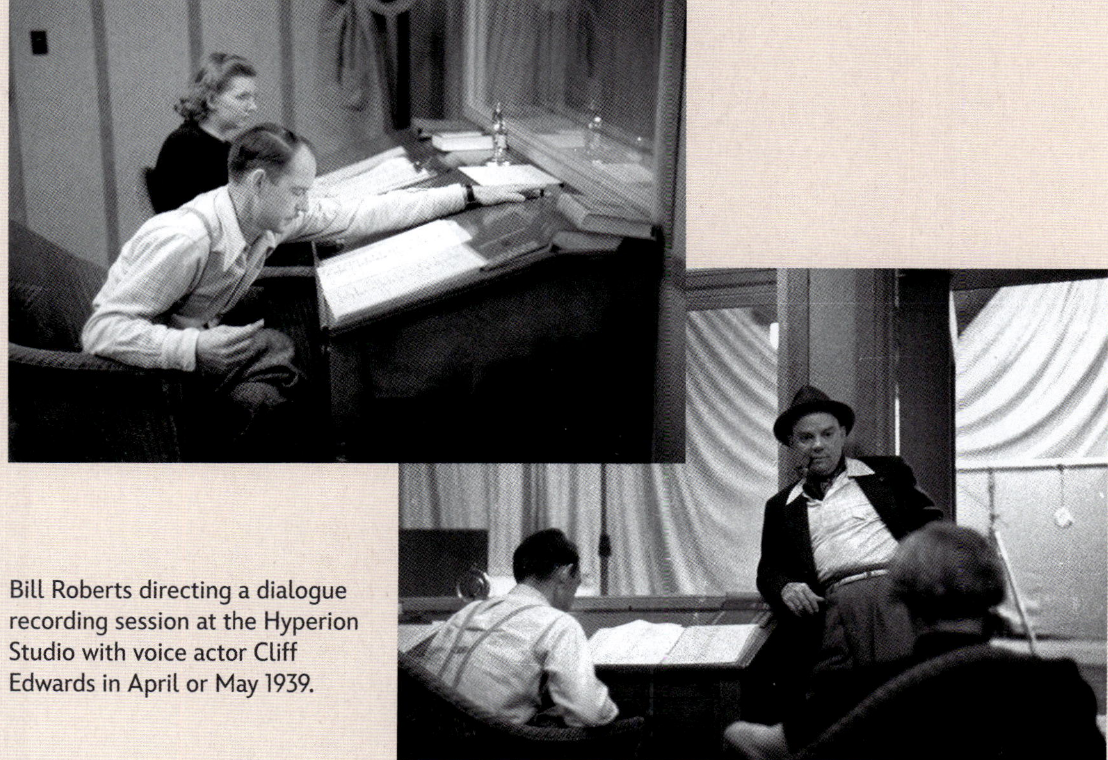

Bill Roberts directing a dialogue recording session at the Hyperion Studio with voice actor Cliff Edwards in April or May 1939.

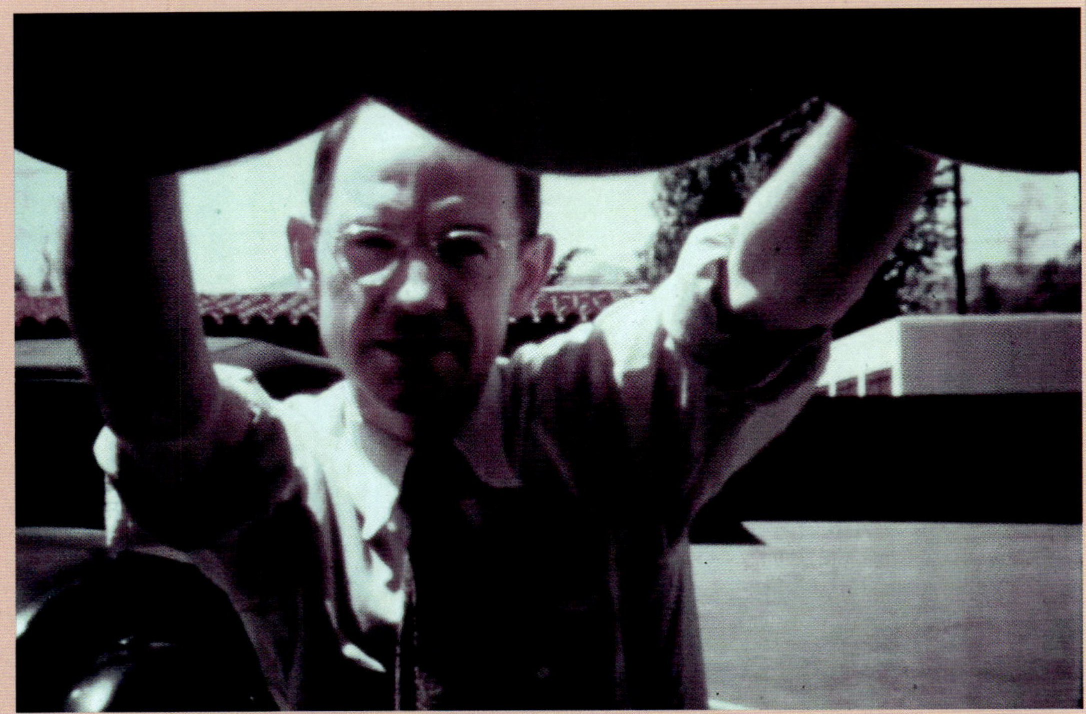

Roberts as seen in a frame from animator Gilles "Frenchy" de Trémaudan's home movie shot at Disney's Hyperion Avenue studio.

together in the *Snow White* era this way: "Bill was a craggy little man who peered at the world over a pair of wire-rimmed eyeglasses, and what he saw he didn't seem to approve of. He smoked a black stubby pipe that smelled as if it had been marinated in bilgewater. . . . I gathered from his picturesque vocabulary that Bill had been raised somewhere in the Appalachian Mountains. Bill sounded like comic strip character Snuffy Smith. He was the only person in the studio who called Mickey Mouse a varmint."[92]

Layout artist McLaren Stewart, a close friend and work colleague, added: "He had absolutely no formal education, to the best of my knowledge. I think he told me he had never worn a pair of shoes until he was like eighteen years old. A real hillbilly; and yet he was one of the keenest minds that I was ever in the presence of, and he was a very knowledgeable man when I knew him. He educated himself in art, music—he was an excellent musician, in the sense of knowing music, understanding it, working with it. He understood art; and everything he had learned completely by himself."[9]

Bill Roberts's pre-Disney years are vaguely documented, but he apparently worked at an animation studio and as a magazine illustrator prior to his employment at Disney in 1932. In his first five years at the studio, he animated on many shorts, including *Father Noah's Ark*, *Giantland*, *Gulliver Mickey*, *Who Killed Cock Robin?*, *Mickey's Polo Team*, and *Mother Pluto*. He was known as one of the best "Pluto men." Wilfred Jackson recalled a handout to Bill of animation on *Mother Pluto*. Everyone who had seen the storyboards laughed at a scene where baby chicks hatched from eggs hidden in Pluto's doghouse assume that Pluto is their mother. But Jaxon said, "The first time through it on the storyboards Bill didn't crack a smile. His strongest reaction was to nod his head approvingly at one point or another. I was a little disturbed. Didn't this new guy know a funny thing when he saw it? Would he be the right one to handle this kind of thing? I asked him what he thought of it, and after soberly considering it for a few minutes, he just said: 'I think I understand it all right. Let's look at the layouts and go over the way you've got it timed out.'"[94] Fortunately, Bill did understand the humor, and his animation proved that. Jaxon said in retrospect that he knew Bill's later approach to directing would be the exact opposite of Burt Gillett's, because "Bill would rather figure a thing out than feel it out the way Burt would."[95] Eric Larson thought Bill was fun to work with and did share some of Burt Gillett's qualities, although he was much less demonstrative. Along the way, future animator Milt Kahl became one of Bill's assistant animators. He and Milt had different animation styles; Milt described Bill as "one of the fast-action boys." But Milt said, "You learned something from everyone. Even if they didn't have something to teach you, it was stimulating."[96]

Bill seamlessly transitioned to feature animation on *Snow White*, also directing a few shorts, notably *Brave Little Tailor* and *Society Dog Show*.

On *Fantasia*, Bill was assigned to "Rite of Spring," working with Woolie Reitherman on the dinosaur scenes. He is said to have advised Woolie on animating a huge dinosaur: "just

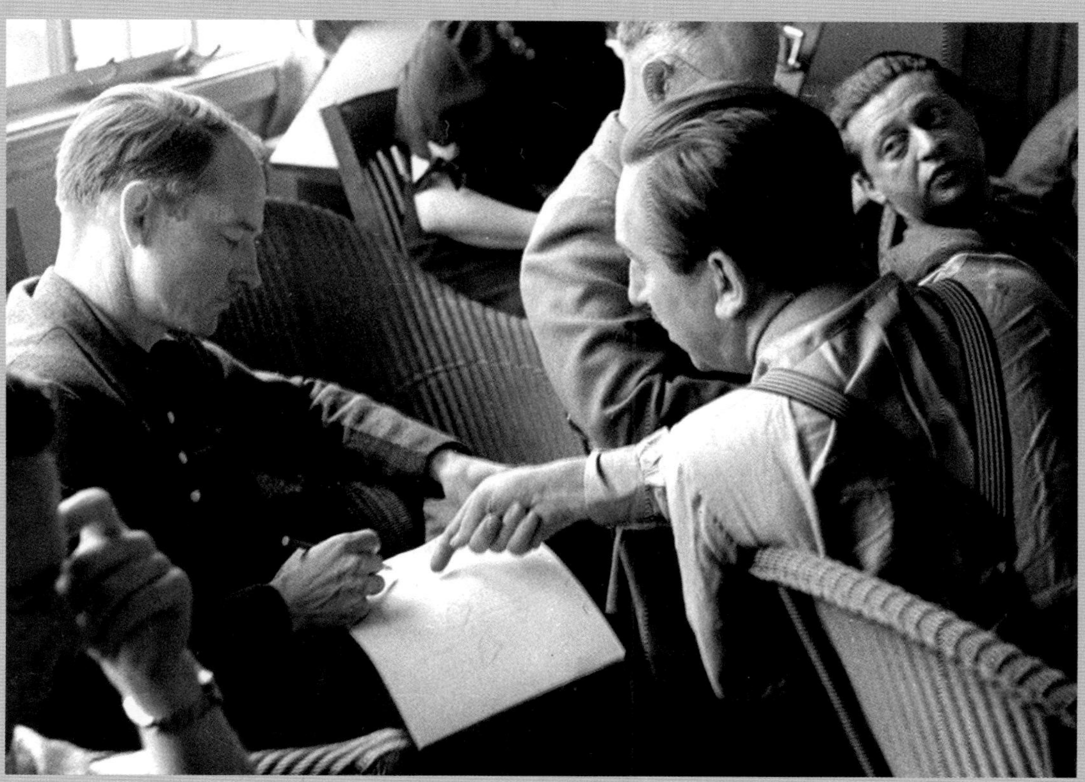

Roberts (LEFT), Walt, and Joe Grant in conference on *Pinocchio*, April/May 1939.

draw a twelve-story building in perspective, then convert it into a dinosaur and animate it."[97] McLaren said that production on this segment of *Fantasia* was exhausting even to him as a young man, and "it seems that Bill Roberts had a kind of a nervous breakdown; he had to stop and rest for a while."[98] Just when Roberts took time off is unknown, but he served as the union representative for one of the studio-supported unions in 1940, which undoubtedly added to his stress.[99]

Bill bounced back and was a sequence director on *Dumbo*, helming sequences with clowns as well as the "Baby Mine" section of the film. Story artist Bill Peet, who rarely had anything positive to say about his colleagues, told historian Michael Barrier that he thought Bill was a good director. "He kept that life in the thing, and he didn't try to really be creative. . . . He'd put a lot of guts into the thing. Like in *Dumbo*, that thing where Dumbo flies in the Big Top—the way he timed it, and the intercutting—it's a thing that gives you chills when you see it happen. The guy knew the business from way back. . . . Bill knew how to put it together. The difference between a scene that comes off strong [and one that doesn't] is sometimes a couple of feet here and there—really fine stuff."[100] Dick Huemer, also part of the interview, agreed.

Bill continued as a sequence director on *Bambi*, *Saludos Amigos* ("Donald Duck Visits Lake Titicaca"), and *The Three Caballeros* ("The Flying Gauchito" and "The Cold-Blooded Penguin"). On *Bambi*, Walt praised Bill, telling Frank Thomas, "You know, that guy is really good. He does great stuff—it's funny stuff, it's solid stuff."[101] During the war year Roberts directed some of the educational motivational shorts, including *The Grain Tha Built a Hemisphere* and *The Winged Scourge* but most notably *Reason and Emotion*, from a story by Dick Huemer and Joe Grant.

After the war, Bill directed "Mickey and the Beanstalk" for *Fun and Fancy Free* and he con tributed to a couple of shorts: *A Knight for a Day* (Hannah) and *Donald's Diary* (Kinney) Then he disappeared from Disney history. Bi moved into real estate and construction and according to Jack Kinney, was a very good businessman and reportedly became very wealthy.[102] He passed away at seventy-four in 1974 in Tulare County, California.

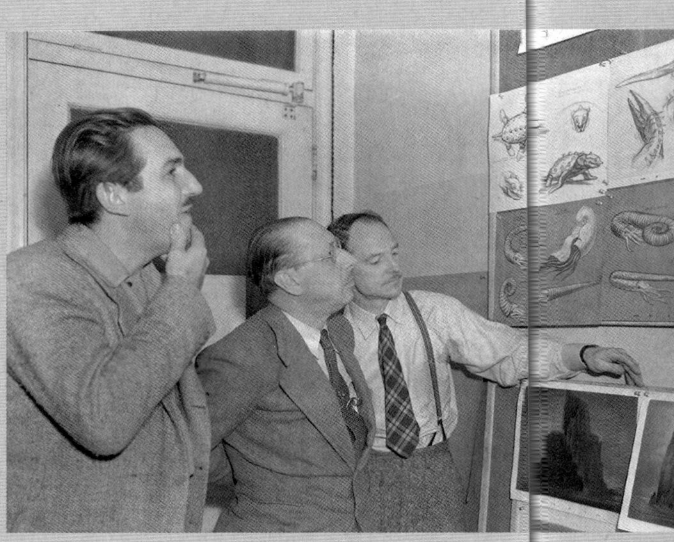

Walt, composer Igor Stravinsky, and director B l Roberts discuss the "Rite of Spring" segment of *Fa tasia*.

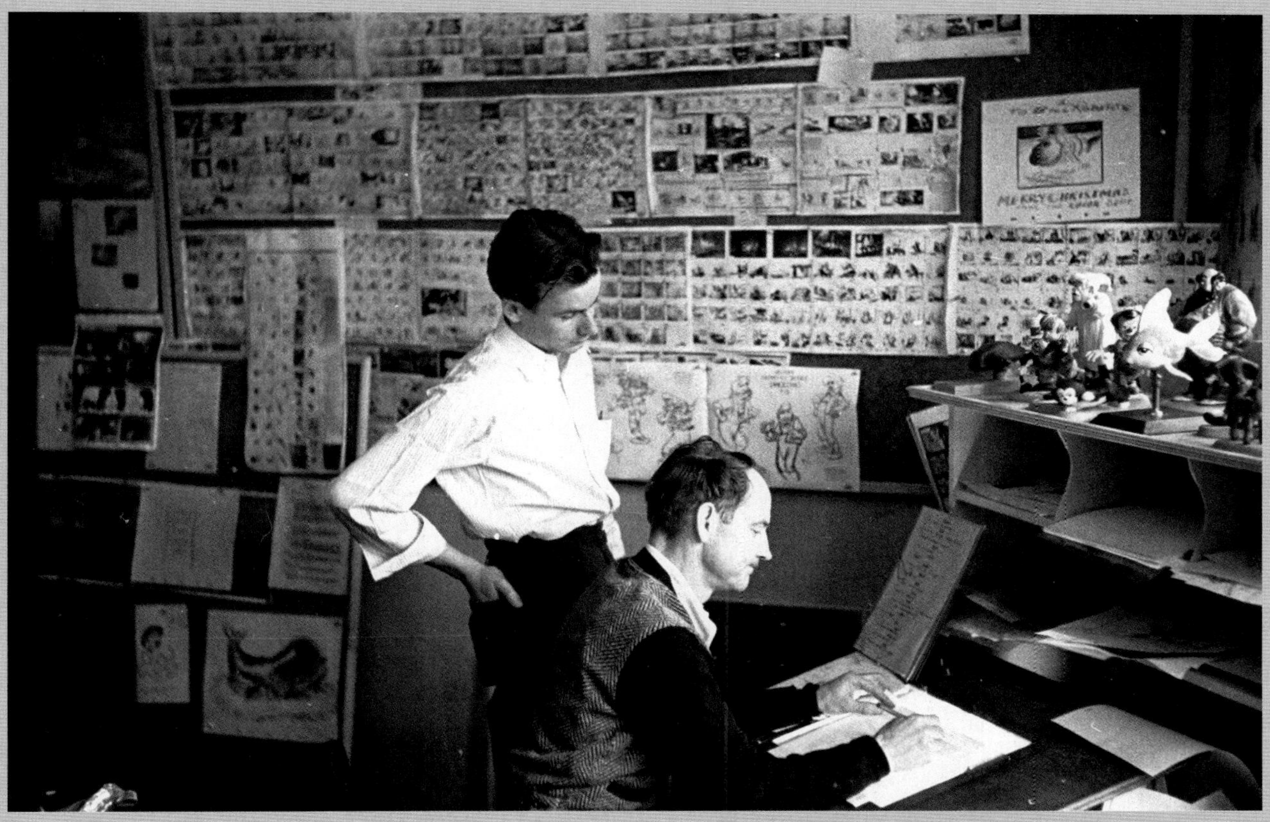

Roberts and a young Bill Peet (STANDING) at work on *Pinocchio*, April/May 1939.

Bill Roberts—Disney Director Filmography

Shorts and Training Films:

- *Mickey's Parrot* (1938)
- *Brave Little Tailor* (1938)
- *Society Dog Show* (1939)
- *Reason and Emotion* (1943)

Features:

- *Pinocchio* (1940) (Sequence Director)
- *Fantasia* (1940) (Sequence Director)
- *Dumbo* (1941) (Sequence Director)
- *Bambi* (1942) (Sequence Director)
- *Saludos Amigos* (1943) (Sequence Director)
- *The Three Caballeros* (1945) (Sequence Director)
- *Fun and Fancy Free* (1947) (Sequence Director)

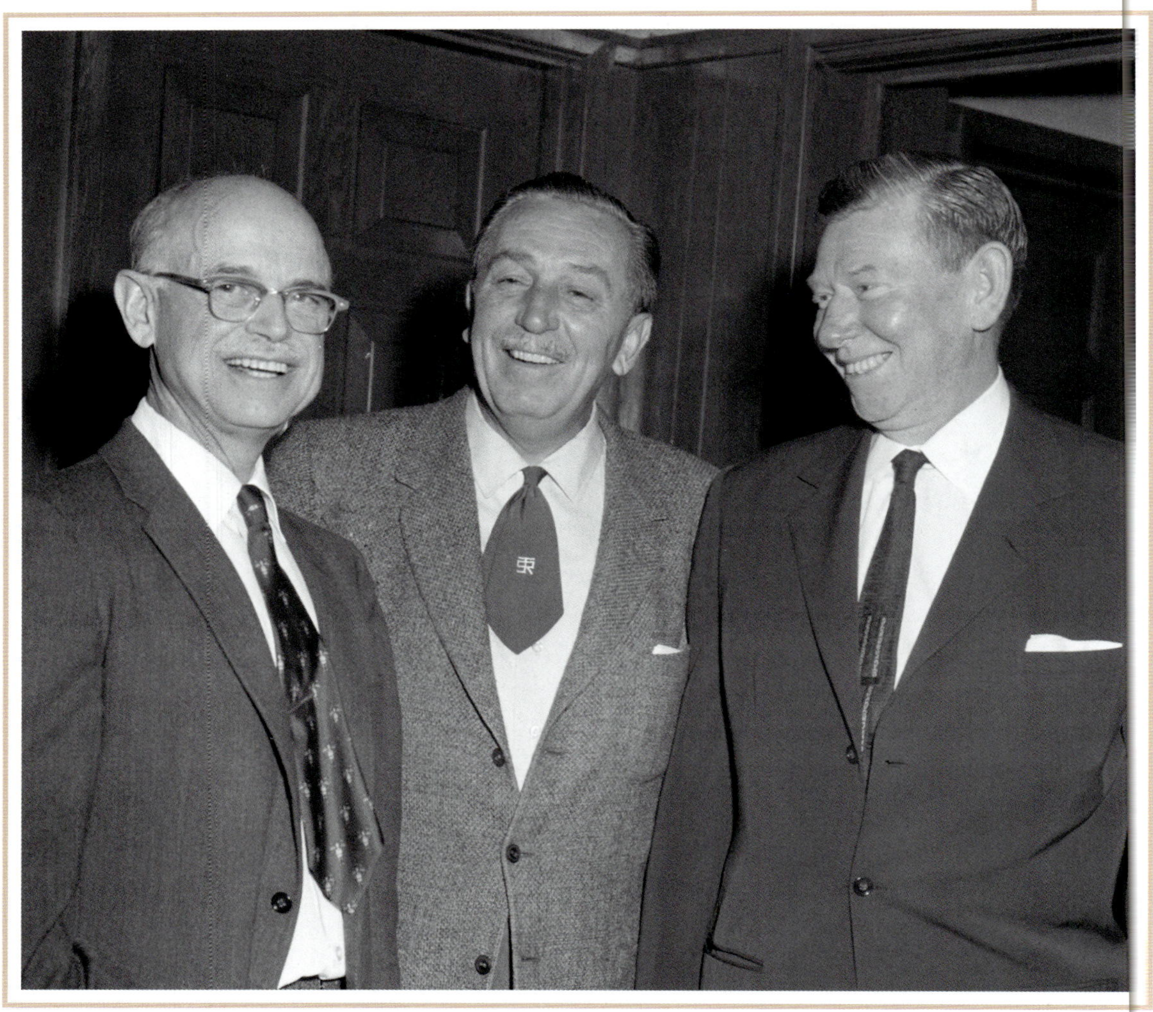

Ben Sharpsteen (LEFT), Walt, and Wilfred Jackson in the late fifties, toward the end of Ben's and Wilfred's careers at Disney.

CHAPTER 4

BEN SHARPSTEEN—THE ORGANIZATION MAN

"The big story of Walt and his success is that he was determined to make a superior product; he was determined to give the public more for their money than they thought they had paid for. He could not do that without demanding the utmost in effort from his people. To do that, he had to have a well-balanced organization."[1]

—Ben Sharpsteen

ATLANTIC
OCEAN
BRAZIL
ALGERIA
FRENCH WEST AFRICA
Motion Picture Hera
in Association with Fame
has the honour to present
This Award of Achievement
to
True Life Adventure
Selected by the Exhibitors
of the
United States and Canada
as
one of the top ten
Money Making Short Subject Series
of 1953
New York January 1, 1954

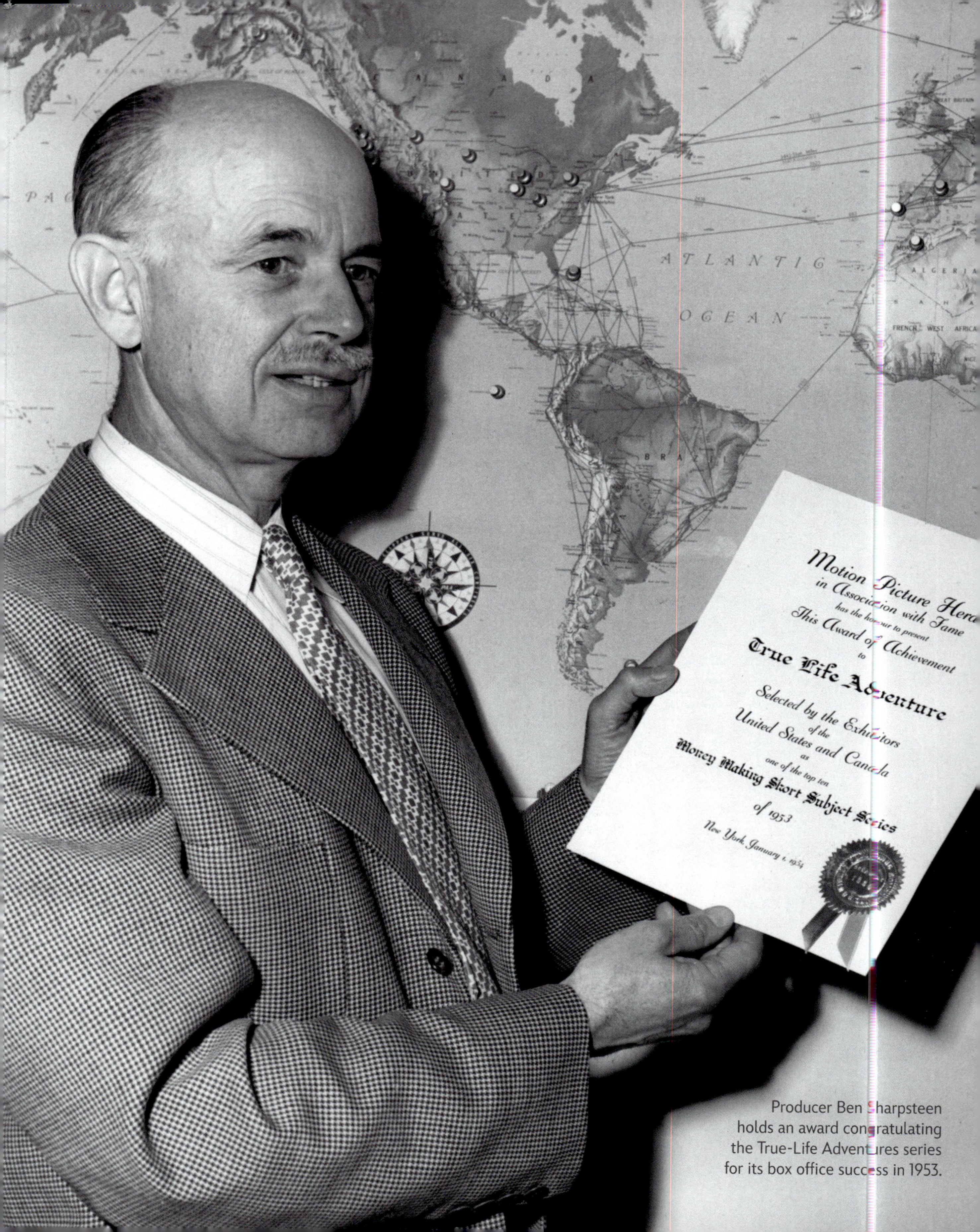

Producer Ben Sharpsteen holds an award congratulating the True-Life Adventures series for its box office success in 1953.

Looking back on his time as a middle school student, Ben, in a revealing comment, said, "I was always timid; I felt that I didn't have the talent required. I didn't realize that you could make up for talent by industriously applying yourself and learning from skilled teachers. . . . I didn't have confidence in myself."[2] This statement by Ben is a key to understanding his career. His lack of confidence in himself, and his overcompensating for it, at times colored his relationships, especially at the Disney Studios. Because Ben struggled through his early years in and out of the New York studios before landing what became a permanent job at Disney's, he believed that others needed to "pay their dues" and earn their way forward as he had done.

Maybe because of his Marine Corps experience in World War I, he put people through a sort of mental "boot camp," indoctrinating them in the ways of the Disney Studios and drilling into them how lucky they were to be at the studio and how imperative it was for them to be "eating, drinking, and sleeping animation." The most common term people used to describe Ben was "disciplinarian." He wanted people to take their job and their industry seriously, to be at their desk working during work hours, and to respect the hierarchy, however fluid it may have been, and especially to revere Walt Disney, as Ben did. Ben felt he was lucky to be working with Walt, and he wanted everyone else to feel the same way.

At the same time, Ben was concerned about what he termed the "fledgling animators": new staff members who might not be prudent in how they spent their money, in what kind of car they bought (Ben favored Fords), and in their dating choices. He was a father figure. Maybe a strict rather than a benevolent father, a father of the tough love variety, a surrogate father for these young men, often away from home for the first time. Ben's intentions were good, but his application was often heavy-handed. Ben's persona was that of a serious person, persistent and stern. Yet, ironically, in an interview late in life, he said, "Life is much too serious if you can't find something to laugh about. I always remember the funny things."[3]

EARLY LIFE

Benjamin Luther Sharpsteen was born the fourth of five children to William C. Sharpsteen[4] and Nellie Thompson in Tacoma, Washington, on November 4, 1895. The family moved to San Francisco in 1900, when Ben was five, and he was raised in nearby Alameda. Ben vividly recalled the exodus of survivors from San Francisco to Alameda after the earthquake and fires in April 1906. "From that moment, I developed a profound sympathy and understanding for those refugees, and as they made camp in a vacant lot, an empty barn or wherever they could, I listened in awe to their many and varied accounts of that terrible day."[5] A few years earlier, in 1903, Ben and his family started to spend each summer in rustic Calistoga at the northern end of the Napa Valley. Of those summers, which continued through Ben's twentieth year, he said, "I always remembered the succession of summers which became very dear to me, and as I have a great deal of loyalty and sentimental instinct within myself, I have cherished those things."[6]

Ben attended a football game between storied rivals Stanford University and the University of California at Berkeley ["the Big Game"] when he was fourteen or fifteen, and he said, "I was so inspired by that I came home and tried to draw some pictures of it from memory."[7] Despite his misgivings about his artistic ability, Ben said, "During my first year in high school, I became intrigued by the possibility of drawing something for reproduction. The obvious objective was the school newspaper, which was published semiannually. In my later years in high school, I contributed largely to the paper and I got a great deal of satisfaction from drawing. However, I did not feel that I had the talent to make a career in the art game, so when a representative of the Agricultural College at Davis spoke at a high school assembly, I was intrigued. A short time later, I applied for admission to this program."[8] Ben graduated from Alameda High School in 1914 and began attending classes at the University Farm [now the University of California at Davis] in September. While Ben was away from home for the first time during the holidays, his father sought to ease Ben's pangs of loneliness by presenting him with a copy of Charles Dickens's *A Christmas Carol*. Ben's father had been reading it to the family since 1897, and he hoped Ben would read it and so be with the family in spirit at the very least.

Ben spent two years in Davis and graduated in 1916. He said, "Although I was seriously pursuing a career in agriculture, I continued to draw pictures just the same. As editor of the college yearbook, *Agricola*, I contributed most of its illustrations and cartoons. Upon graduation, I pursued agriculture, but only as a laborer. While I was working on the grain-and-stock farm, I enlisted in the Marine Corps in 1917."[9]

JUST A FEW HOURS OF
LIGHT WORK IN THE MORNING
SHARP-1915-

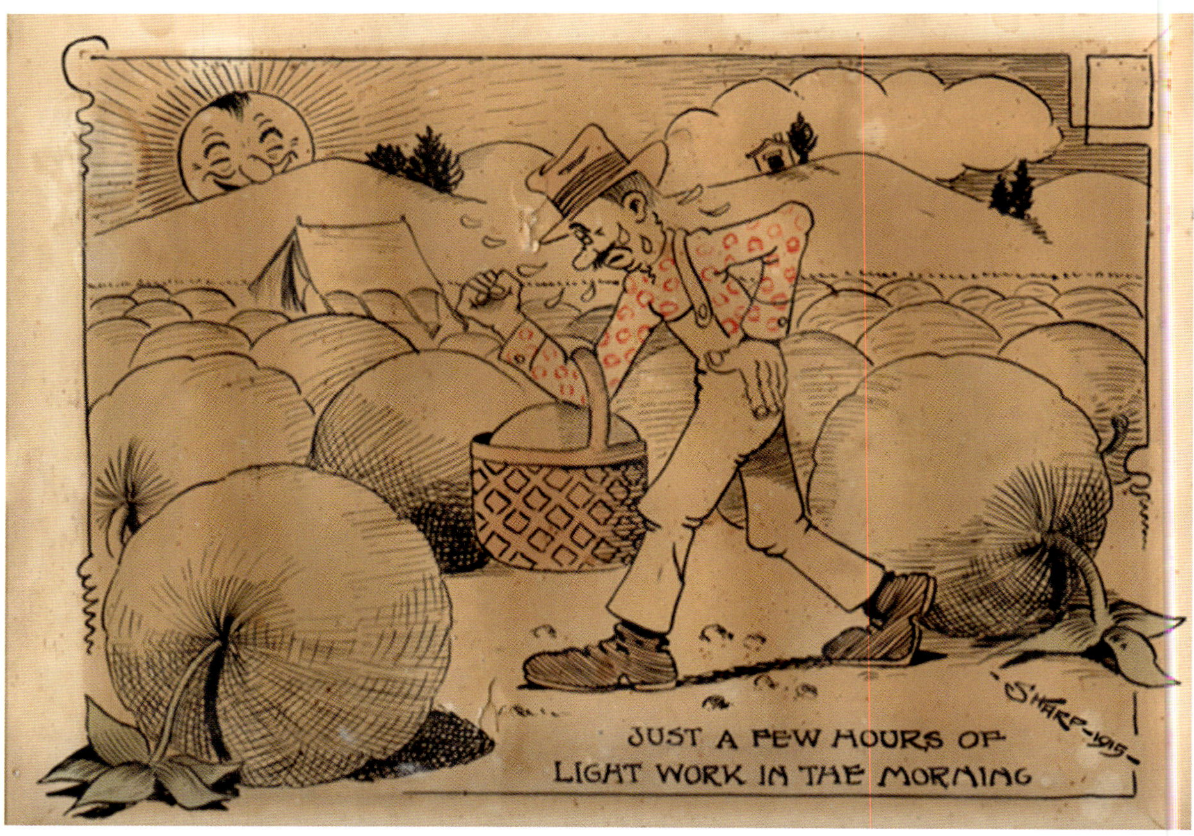

Early cartoon work by Ben Sharpsteen

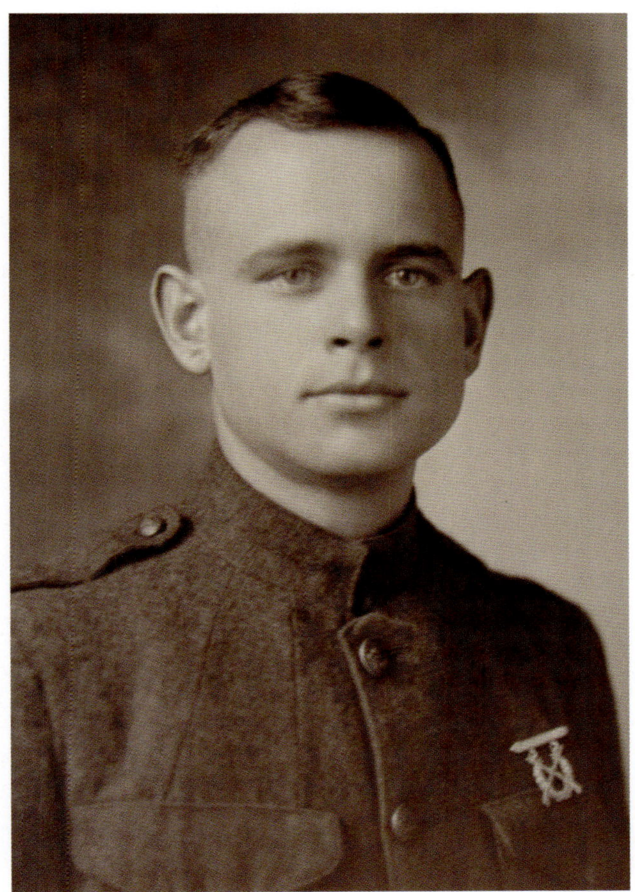

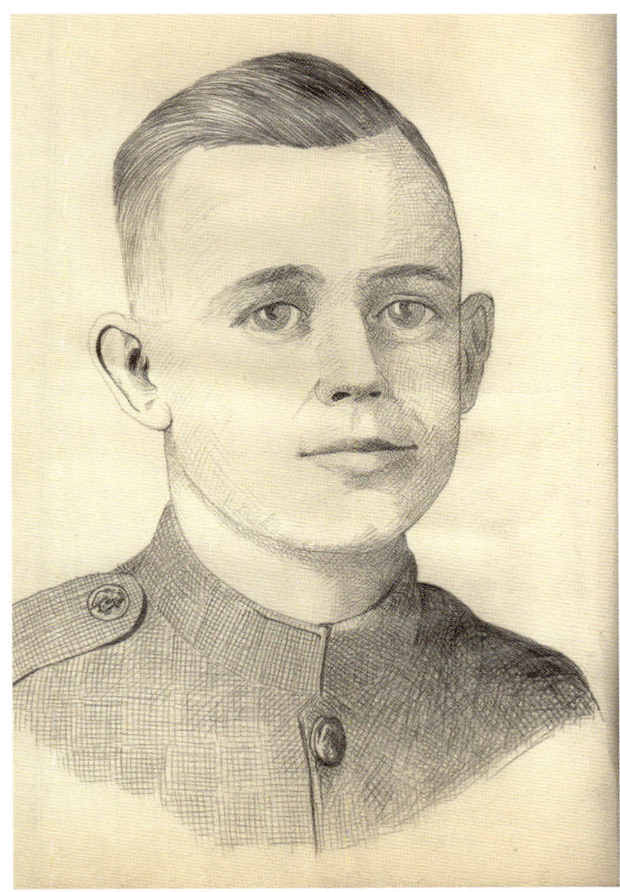

Ben in the Marine Corps in photo and self-portrait. Sharpsteen collection.

America had entered "the war to end all wars" on April 6, 1917. Ben's advance to the front took an unexpected turn. He contracted diphtheria, and while he was hospitalized, his unit was sent on. He and some other recruits were stranded and sent to different posts. Ben ran the post exchange in Guam, and in his free time, he drew. He said, "I wanted to apply myself to something, and naturally drawing was something I could do no matter where I was."[10] Ben captained a detachment of marines conducting bayonet assault training in December 1918 at Lake Merced in San Francisco. He was selected to go to the officers' training school on the East Coast, but before he could start classes, the armistice was signed and World War I ended. He was discharged from the Marine Corps in February 1919 in Virginia. Ben decided to take advantage of an opportunity to visit Washington, DC, and then to visit New York City and see what adventures might await him there.

Ben had met Bernice Thoburn in 1915 in Calistoga while she was on vacation with her family. They renewed their acquaintance in January 1920 in New York, where Bernice was enrolled at the Pratt Institute, and they married in December of that year. It was a union that would span sixty years.

PRE-DISNEY ANIMATION CAREER: HERE, THERE, AND EVERYWHERE

"I first entered the animation business in New York City [in 1919]. I started as an apprentice in an animation studio that was owned by Hearst Enterprises [Hearst International Film Service]. They had a license to handle all of the characters in the Hearst comic sections. When I first went there, I did menial things such as erasing pencil marks off of drawings after they had been inked, filling in places that should be black, and then doing the actual inking of the drawings after the animators had pencilled them. As the weeks went by, I was gradually given more important work and it was probably at the end of about six months that I gained the status of full animator, although I was by no means efficient."[11] Ben worked on the *Happy Hooligan*, *Silk Hat Harry*, and *Judge Rummy* series, among others. Ben fondly recalled those salad days in New York: "I lived in the YMCA and he [Walter Lantz] belonged to the YMCA—he lived at home, in the Bronx. We used to do calisthenics and jump in the swimming pool. The big thing was looking for places to eat where we could save a nickel or a dime at noontime. We'd walk long distances from the West Side to the East Side of town."[12]

Ben joined the Paramount studio early in 1921, working under animation legend Earl Hurd on the *Bobby Bumps* series. Even though his salary had jumped from ten dollars a week at Hearst to seventy-five dollars a week at Paramount, and he had "the very nicest of relations" with Hurd, he wasn't happy with the work he was doing there, so he left after five months.[13] (Ben and Earl will cross paths again later in our story.) His next stop on the New York animation circuit was at Jefferson Film Company and the *Mutt and Jeff* series, licensed to it by Bud Fisher. He stayed for over a year, until the studio closed up shop in June 1922. He worked under Burt Gillett at Jefferson.

California beckoned, and Ben said, "In the space of about three or four years, I came to the conclusion that perhaps I had better have some experience in the art game besides animation. So I came out and took a job with the *Oakland Tribune*, which I held for three or four years. I did a varied type of artwork there, anything the paper needed."[14] He was struggling to find artistic work that he could dedicate himself to and that had a future that would sustain him. He didn't find that at the newspaper. He said, "I left the newspaper because I had an offer from Max Fleischer, who had a cartoon studio in New York. He offered me considerably more than I was able to make at the newspaper, considerably more. So in 1926 we went back there. I worked for him for about two and a half years."[15] Ben animated on Koko the Clown in the *Out of the Inkwell* series. But the Fleischer Studio didn't hold the key to the future Ben sought—and maybe there was no future for him in this industry that seemed to produce mere fillers on a theater program, no more or no less than a serial or a newsreel, subservient to the main feature.

Back to California went Ben and his family—Bernice and sons, Jim and Tom—this time to San Francisco. "I came out to San Francisco to see if I couldn't develop a career in commercial artwork and illustration. I was a stranger and I had no contacts. I had to just tramp the sidewalks, looking wherever I could. I managed to get a little something to do to keep body and soul together."[16]

HOSANNAS FROM HOLLYWOOD

Walt Disney, flush with the success of his Mickey Mouse cartoons but anxious to rebuild his animation staff, was busy recruiting experienced animators from the New York studios. In a conversation with Burt Gillett, who wanted to come to Disney's, Walt asked if he had any recommendations to make. According to Ben, "Burt said, 'Well, there's Ben Sharpsteen out there on the West Coast. He's in San Francisco, I believe. I have his address, which I'll let you have, and you can write to him if you like.' That is how I happened to hear from Walt Disney."[17] Ben received a letter in March 1929 from Walt, pointing out that he was now making sound pictures, and he asked if Ben would be interested in working for him. Ben recalled, "Walt Disney was hardly more than a name to me; I had never really seen a Disney picture."[18] But because Ben was still struggling to find his niche in the art world and a secure future, "I decided to look into this prospect, so I took a train from San Francisco to Los Angeles."[19]

Ben's first meeting with Walt is memorable, because it was the beginning of a turnaround in Ben's career and the opportunity he had been dreaming of:

> I soon met Walt and we chatted informally. I soon found that we could have a conversation which was familiar to both of us. I recognized immediately that he knew the business. He informed me at that time of a succession of troubles that he had had [climaxing with his loss of the Oswald the Lucky Rabbit series]. Walt's conclusion from his experiences to date was that he would never be at the mercy of a distributor again. His whole salvation was in making a product that so excelled that the public would recognize it and enjoy it as the best of entertainment and that they would more or less demand to see Disney pictures. But Walt made a simple statement that "you can lick 'em with product," meaning that if you make your product good enough, they cannot deny it.[20]

Ben decided he would cast his fate with Walt. Ben was the first of the "New York" animators—animators with experience at the New York studios—to join the studio. He was followed in short order by Burt Gillett, Jack King, Tom Palmer, and Norm Ferguson. Other waves of animators with experience at the New York studios would join Walt's home-grown animators, and the synthesis of talent would help Walt raise animation from little more than a novelty to a twentieth-century art form.

As an experienced animator, Ben was paid $125 per week, more than Burt Gillett ($100); Ub Iwerks, the top animator at the studio ($90); Walt ($50); and Roy ($35).[21] Ben's lack of confidence in his own artistic abilities was evident from day one. "During the first day, I had occasion to see a few of the Disney pictures. My first reaction to them was that they were excellent, that is compared to animation as I knew it. There was something about those Disney pictures that were a cut above those of my experience, and I became concerned about

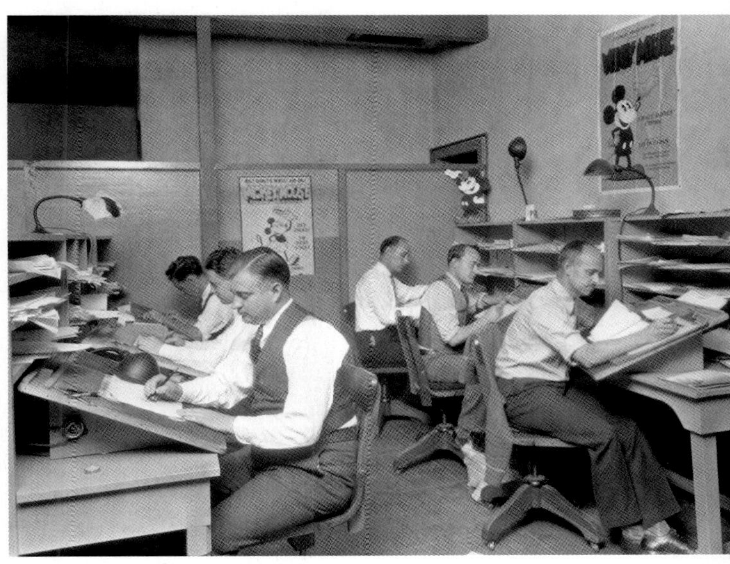

At Disney's: (LEFT FRONT TO BACK) Jack King, Norm Ferguson, Dick Lundy. (RIGHT FRONT TO BACK) Ben Sharpsteen, Merle Gilson, and Burt Gillett.

my ability to contribute to them."[22] Ben's first scene was on a picture called *When the Cat's Away* (1929). "It was a scene that I would have considered to be of a run-of-the-mill nature in importance, but I could see that he did not hold it that way. In Walt's estimation, everything that was done had to be executed with a great deal of thought toward finesse in order to make it better."[23] Despite his misgivings, Ben worked diligently as an animator. He was persistent and determined, and he animated on ninety-seven cartoons over the next five years.

THE ORGANIZATION MAN

As early as 1933, and for the next two years, Ben took it upon himself to be a recruiter of talent. This period coincided with his advancement to the role of subdirector and then director. Ben said, "I do not think Walt ever made a point of having me do it. I just went ahead and did it in an effort to get better people there than just the run-of-the-mill applicants who happened to pass by on the sidewalk. But like everything else, I made him aware of everything I was doing; if I did not make a point of it, I at least sent a copy of the letter to his office."[24] Roy Williams said in 1976 that in his view, Ben's screening of people is what made the studio what it is today.

By 1934, Ben was identifying himself in these letters as production manager. Michael Barrier explained Ben's adoption of the title: "Ben had so many different titles because Walt knew he could count on him to fill any hole that needed filling; and sometimes, I'm sure, Ben had to give himself a title (like the "studio manager" or something similar that you see in early correspondence) because a title was needed, and Walt had given him responsibilities but no title."[25]

PRE-DIRECTOR

Soon into Ben's animation career at Disney, he was assigned an assistant, Merle Gilson.

> With the misgivings that I held, I was surprised that before long, Walt pushed a new man on my hands as an assistant or an inbetweener. . . . It was only natural that to have an inexperienced assistant shoved on me who could not possibly improve the quality of my work was not easing my state of mind. Soon I found myself with not only one assistant, but with two assistants. I did not realize it at the time, but Walt had singled me out as one who would be willing to put in the time training a beginner. Walt was a keen judge of abilities and capacities.[26]

As the studio grew in both the quality and the quantity of its animation output, there was a constant need for more animators, and animators who could and would work in the Disney method. Ben describes a humbling indoctrination for both raw talent and veteran: "learning how to animate the way we did, learning how to pick your work apart, learning how to diagnose, learning to cooperate with others, learning to accept criticism without getting your feelings hurt, and all those things. We had a saying, 'Look, this is Disney Democracy: your business is everybody's business and everybody's business is your business.' If you did not have that attitude, you were not going to stay very long."[27]

The fast-paced schedule for the release of short subjects in the two series of cartoons (Mickey Mouse and Silly Symphonies) necessitated giving the directors all the help they could get. "So in the course of events, there were two of us picked out by Walt to supervise small numbers of beginners. The other man was Dave Hand. We each had small groups of green animators, maybe ten to twelve. By picking up the scenes ourselves from the director, we saved him a great deal of time, because we did all the coaching of these new men."[28]

By 1933, Dave Hand was added to the director ranks, and, Ben said, "The sole burden of handling these new men fell upon my shoulders. I would say I handled from ten to twelve but that is just a rough guess."[29] "Handling" these new men meant, he said, "I was to give them actual animation to draw and not to use them as merely assistants. We used this system for several months and got work out of people who otherwise would not have been too productive or valuable. And we were learning about the capabilities of these young men."[30]

In looking back, Ben believed that Walt had evaluated his strengths and weaknesses and, loath to let go of a loyal employee, found the first of many niches for Ben: "In diagnosing that I was particularly adept at handling green people, that sparked him into realizing that there was a place for me in his organization where he could profit from that."[31]

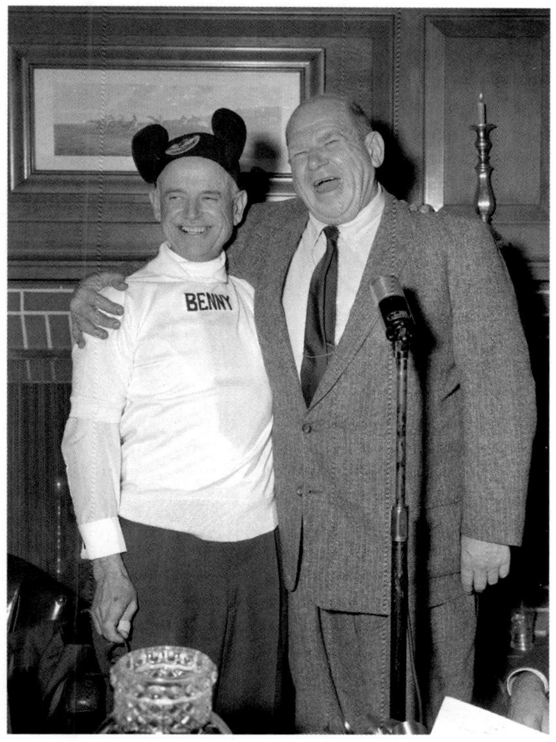

An alumnus of Ben's motley crew, Big Mooseketeer Roy Williams clowns with Ben at Ben's retirement party. Sharpsteen collection.

Frank Thomas and Ollie Johnston, in their celebrated book *Disney Animation: The Illusion of Life*, said:

> Ben Sharpsteen was chosen for this assignment because he was always worried and concerned and dedicated to the studio. He projected a father image and tried to raise his novices like his own children, counseling them on everything, from which car to buy [Ford] to which comedian to study. Ben was conservative and made us work on fundamentals until we were on firm ground before we could go ahead. He gave drawing problems to all the assistants and inbetweeners, not so much as a competition but so they could learn to talk over the difficulties and observe the variety of solutions."

Jack Kinney, an alumnus of Ben's training group, said, "Ben had quite a collection of characters working for him. Besides Roy Williams and me, there was Jack Cutting (who later supervised foreign dubbing when Disney went worldwide), Cy Young (who later became head of Special Effects), Ugo D'Orsi (special effects animator), and many others. We were housed in one large room. It was a motley crew, and Ben was a hard but fair taskmaster. He insisted on good draftsmanship, staging, and action analysis. You had to learn—no shortcuts, just do it right."[32] Ben noted that also among the artists he initially trained were Ham Luske, Fred Moore, Woolie Reitherman, Harry Reeves, Ken Anderson, Joe D'Igalo, and Hardie Gramatky.

Ben's self-appointed role as a father figure was part cheerleader, part disciplinarian, part caring parent. As a cheerleader: "I pushed the doctrine to these boys. 'You either learn how to draw or you got no place to go in here. If you want to make a career out of this, the sky's the limit. This man Disney is—no telling how far he's going to go.' And I preached the doctrine to them."[33] As a strict father figure: "Perhaps (to) one outstanding person I might say, 'Look, you'd better get hold of yourself. Are you in the business to get somewhere or not? Now, if you want to get wise to yourself and buckle down and take a little more interest . . .' Or I'd say to a fellow, 'Did you go to the preview?' 'Well, no.' 'Well, why not?' . . . I was guilty of paternalism, but it was done with the best of intent, and if you had to do it to jolt somebody, well, okay."[34]

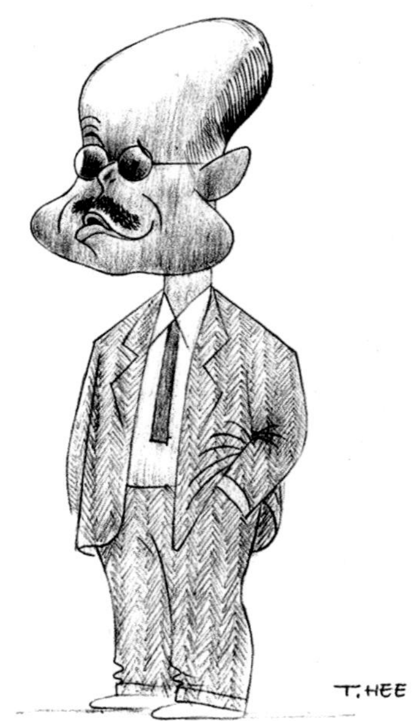

T. Hee caricature of Ben.

Milt Kahl experienced Ben's tough love approach: "They'd give you little bits of animation to try you out. The first really good chance I had was when Ben Sharpsteen gave me a sequence of two or three scenes in *Mickey's Circus*, which wasn't one of our better shorts. Talk about control: Ben asked me to pose the whole scene out to show him what I was going to do with it. I brought these drawings in to him, and he looked at them, and then he sat looking out the window for quite a while, and I thought, 'Oh, Jesus.' Then he finally said, 'All right, that looks pretty good.' I pretty near had a heart attack in the meantime."[35]

Positive, negative, or a combination of the two, no one seemed to be indifferent about working with Ben. Ken O'Connor, who trained under Ben and worked with him as a layout man said, "He was probably the most feared and hated man in the Studio. He was a very quiet man, never raised his voice, but jeez, if you did your hair the wrong way you suddenly found there was a knife in your back and you're out on the sidewalk. He wouldn't hesitate to fire anybody."[36] Bill Cottrell said Ben "was good for the organization, even if a lot of guys didn't like him."[37] Shamus Culhane also saw him as a tough but fair director. Chuck Couch said, "He was a well-intentioned man, but it was like you were a boot in a marine camp."[38]

But there was another side to him, too. Eric Larson said, "I always felt he had an appreciation of the problems of young people. He had a way of putting over points to you without making you feel uneasy. He had no ego at all, in my opinion. He was very honest and straightforward and fatherly, and very critical of things that you did, in a constructive way. He could get kind of nasty about it, but he tried not to discourage you in any way . . . Ben had a real warmth and understanding for people in difficulty."[39] Bill Tytla, recalled something Ben did that affected his long view: "In New York I first met Ben Sharpsteen. He tore out a page from a book on cartooning and gave it to me. I never forgot it—it was one of the most thoughtful things anybody ever did for me. Later on, I always remembered him from the old days. Some of the other men didn't like him—he was a hard taskmaster—but I always did. Because of what he did for me in New York."[40] Frank Thomas said, "Well, he was important. He wanted to help everybody, and he put up these signs all around the inbetween room where we all started: 'Does your drawing have weight, depth and balance?' He was behind all those things, I found out later, and I didn't even know what weight, depth, and balance was at the time. It wasn't until years later that I thought, 'Oh, that's what he was talking about!' "[41]

Aside from the immediate effect of completing more animation, the training of fledgling animators, as Ben liked to call them, helped inculcate what some would call the Disney touch. Ken O'Connor, hired by Ben, saw this phenomenon: "[Walt] got guys like Ben Sharpsteen in early to train animators. He trained Ben in what he wanted, and Ben was very receptive. And then he had Ben train animators and I think everybody trained everybody under them, assistants and the whole damn works, including layout, in the Disney way of thinking. I know Walt said one time that he didn't know what the Disney touch was. To him it was just a quality, just a touch of quality."[42]

TAKING DIRECTION

"While I was handing out work to beginning animators and Walt was probably giving me a couple of more men, he took the occasion to say, 'You know, I don't think that you need to feel you have to do any more animation.' Of course, I thought that if I was not going to animate, then was I worth keeping on the payroll? He could read my expression and he said, 'You can be just as valuable at that as at animation. I don't animate. I found out a long time ago that I could hire much better artists than myself.' This was an example of his clear thinking."[43] Ben began his career as a director helping Jaxon with *The Spider and the Fly* (1931). And then, when Burt Gillett left in 1934, Ben saw an opportunity. Ben suggested to Walt that he direct *Two-Gun Mickey*, and Walt agreed. For some, like Wilfred Jackson, the move from animator to director was not considered a promotion but maybe more of a consolation prize. Not for Ben: "Frankly, I was willing to step out of animation and leave it to the younger men, because I recognized the great challenge in the directing and producing of films. Many of the best animators were such specialists in their field that they were not necessarily qualified at direction."[44] But directing for Walt was no easy task. "We had a basic common problem, and that was Walt. Walt was the antagonist. He would take no excuses for a poor picture and he was prone to blame the director for a picture's weaknesses. He believed that a director should not only maximize all of a picture's possibilities, but he should also be alert to its weaknesses and then bolster them. That was difficult to do, because it implied that a director was aware of the weaknesses, and often he did not become aware of the weaknesses until after the animation had been completed. Walt would never tolerate redoing costly animation. Thus we had so many problems in common that we naturally confided in each other about them and we consoled one another."[45] Ben said that as a result, the directors developed much better analytical skills than they would have if Walt had analyzed their work in detail for them.

To compound their situation, the directors had to go ahead on their own and make decisions without always asking Walt beforehand. Ben said Walt didn't want directors bringing him problems without suggesting a solution or solutions. "As far as going ahead is concerned, that was part of Walt's policy: you went ahead on your own, you did not ask Walt's permission for every little thing you did. You learned to know the things that you should speak to him about and get his okay on. On the other things, you went ahead and you just had to wait until Walt discovered whether they were suitable and workable or whether they should be modified or thrown out completely. That was the lot you played."[46] Ben further explained, "I got accustomed to finding out the strategic time to advise Walt of something I was doing. Usually, if it was serious in nature, I'd tell him while I was doing it. He seemed to like it better that way, rather than saying, 'Is it all right with you if I do it?' He hated to be in that spot, of giving permission. So I thought it was better to start going ahead and doing it; then, if he saw some real objection to it, he could enter into it as much as he wished."[47]

Walt's vision for the cartoons dominated story development and production, and Walt focused a great deal of his attention on story development, deferring to the directors and animators some leeway in their work. Ben acknowledged this:

> I never felt hemmed in by Walt unless he expressed himself particularly on some facet of the production. I had such great faith in Walt's discrimination with ideas, and in his ability to think up ideas and to put them across, that I was constantly accepting his ideas. If Walt had been a director, however, he would have realized that some of his ideas were weak and he would have discarded them. As a director, I felt that it was my part to discard them. . . . Although I had as much freedom as I could hope for, I knew that it was a great responsibility as well. I could not just do anything that I felt like; I had to do something that would make the picture more acceptable. The payoff was in the audience reaction at the preview.[48]

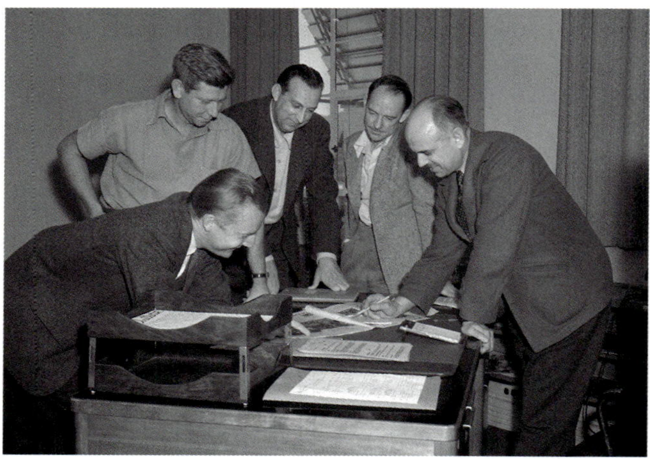

FROM RIGHT: Ben reviews work with Bill Roberts, assistant Paul Satterfield, Wilfred Jackson, and Jim Algar.

After *Two-Gun Mickey*, Ben directed *Mickey's Service Station*, the first cartoon to team up Mickey, Donald, and Goofy. A busy year for Ben—1935—also saw the release of *The Cookie Carnival*, *Mickey's Fire Brigade*, *On Ice*, *Cock o' the Walk*, and *Broken Toys*. *On Ice* provided for Ben a unique education on story structure when Walt visited him:

> *On Ice* was delivered to my room and I began planning its production. Naturally I assumed I would start at the beginning. Walt dropped in unannounced and he sat down and began looking at the pictures [storyboard]. He said, "This picture as it is is too long." Then he pointed to a section that was pretty far down in the picture. Donald Duck, being mischievous, strapped a pair of ice skates to a sleeping Pluto and then yowled liked a cat. Pluto woke up abruptly and in an agitated state, and as he took off in pursuit of the sound, he hit the ice and skidded around badly and so forth.

Walt said, "Here you've got a great situation. It isn't important how we lead up to the situation. This is the best part of the picture." Walt proceeded to describe the various ways that Pluto would try to get up on his feet again, only to flop down. He said, "Now after you get that done and you know how much footage it is, then you can go back and build your opening." It developed into the high spot of the picture. This experience was a revelation to me and a valuable lesson.[49]

Two hires Ben was particularly proud of and happy with were Earl Hurd and Ub Iwerks, who returned. Ben hired Earl when he was struggling with his career, and animation had, in effect, passed him by. He started in animation at the Disney Studios and soon moved into story. Ben said, "One of the most satisfying experiences I ever had in my life was to be able to return good to a man who had been so generous to me. It was the same feeling when I brought Iwerks back to the studio."[50]

BEN AND ME

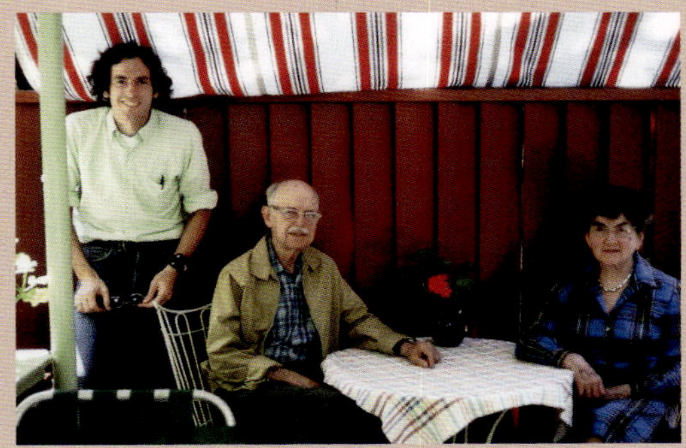

Author Don Peri with Ben and Bernice Sharpsteen at their home in Calistoga in the 1970s. Don Peri collection.

Ben Sharpsteen is the reason I am a coauthor of this book. My association with Ben enabled me to transition from being an ardent fan of Disney films and television and theme parks to becoming a Disney historian. My relationship with Ben is unique among the directors we are covering in this book, because even though I interviewed a few of them, I worked extensively with Ben from 1974 to 1977, recording twenty-one interviews, many of which he later deposited in the Walt Disney Archives, where they have provided history for many books about Walt and his studio. My connection with Ben and where it has led me was really a serendipitous outcome from what began as an autograph request. Unlike many historians, I didn't have a purpose in mind when I began this Disney odyssey, and I have been amazed and thrilled by all its twists and turns over the past fifty years.

The origins of my connection with Ben can be traced to the University of California at Davis. In 1972 for Picnic Day, an annual event at UC Davis, Ben Sharpsteen's painting of an old-fashioned picnic graced the cover of the Picnic Day program. I noted that the inside biographical blurb described him as a 1916 graduate of the University Farm—the research and science-based instruction extension of UC Berkeley located in Davis—and a former Disney animator, director, and producer, who was now retired and living in nearby Calistoga. I tucked away the program and thought nothing more about it. In 1973, I received a copy of Christopher Finch's celebrated *The Art of Walt Disney*. I had read a few Disney history books in the past, and I appreciated that this book included the names of many of the studio artists who had helped Walt attain his dreams. I retrieved the program to see if the artist, whose name I had forgotten, was mentioned in the book. He was, so in January 1974, I decided to contact him to ask if he would sign my copy of the book. I thought it would be exciting to meet someone who had actually *known* Walt Disney. I sent Ben a letter and he responded affirmatively. He suggested I call him for directions, because his place was out of Calistoga and easy to miss. In our phone conversation, he said, "You're not a writer, are you?" I thought that even then, former Disney artists, like Ben, were leery of writers who might be looking for something derogatory to publicize about Walt Disney. Even though at the time I was a graduate student in the English Department at UC Davis, I said that no, I was not a writer. My sister, Camille, and I visited Ben and his wife, Bernice, on February 1, 1974. What I thought would be a visit of an hour or two turned out to last for most of the day, with Ben telling us a great many stories and bringing out his Oscar for *Ama Girls* and a program from the premiere of *Snow White* signed by practically everyone in the studio. After lunch and our farewells, I said to my sister that I had misunderstood Ben; he was looking for a writer to help him capture his stories about his Disney career. On the following Monday—just three days later—I received a letter from Ben, in which he told me that he was delighted with our visit and had a proposition he wished to discuss. He hired me to help him write his memoirs, and over the next three years and twenty-one interviews, we explored his history and his analysis of Walt's success at creating an art form through his development and manipulation of his creative staff.

Over the years, I have come to appreciate more fully the golden opportunity Ben gave me to help him record his memoirs and to listen to firsthand accounts of life at the Disney Studios during its formative and golden years. And I think it was fortuitous for Ben that I came along when I did. Bernice told my mother that after my first visit, Ben told her, "That boy sparks me!" Fate drew us together and we both benefitted tremendously from our association. I will always be grateful to Ben for opening up the Disney world for me.

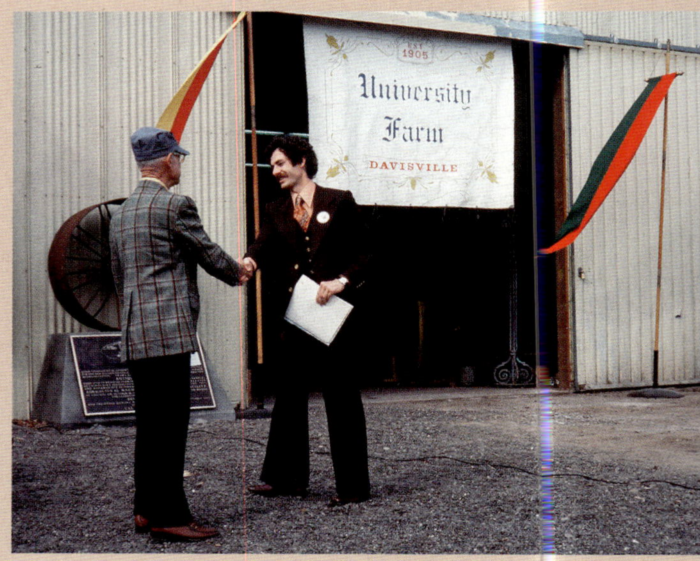

Ben and Don shake hands after Don introduced Ben at the dedication of the Antique Tractor Restoration Facility at the University of California at Davis campus. Ben donated half the funds for the facility. Don Peri collection.

THE CLASSICS

After Walt announced to his staff that they were about to embark on their first animated feature film, work on it started slowly but ramped up rapidly to a December 1937 deadline. "Perhaps I was the last director assigned to *Snow White* because I had been working with a preponderance of less experienced animators and naturally Walt did not want to open up the picture to inexperienced men until he felt that they could be properly controlled. That is how I happened to be involved in only the last stages of *Snow White*. I do not think that I worked on it for more than nine or ten months."[51] Ben's sequences included the Queen traveling to the Dwarfs' cottage, the Dwarfs chasing her, and her fall from the rocky cliff.

Snow White introduced the use of live-action reference footage to help the animators with depicting human figures. Ben said it also helped directors better convey to the animators what they were looking for in their scenes. "There always was a terrific chronic problem from the very early days of direction, from director to animator: how could the director explain the action he wanted to the animator. . . . With the live-action being employed for a specific purpose on a tough problem, like in *Snow White*, it spread very shortly, and it was decided that we would expand the use of live-action for handing work out to animators."[52]

Walt always liked the idea of having an organization to the studio, but he frequently overrode its dictates and did whatever seemed appropriate at the time. After *Snow White* another attempt was made to adhere to an organizational structure. Ben said, "Walt had decided that certain people would be in charge of this, and certain people would be in charge of that. I was in charge of the production of the short subjects."[53] Ben told historian Michael Barrier that he supervised shorts for about eight months after *Snow White* was completed, and then he moved on to the role

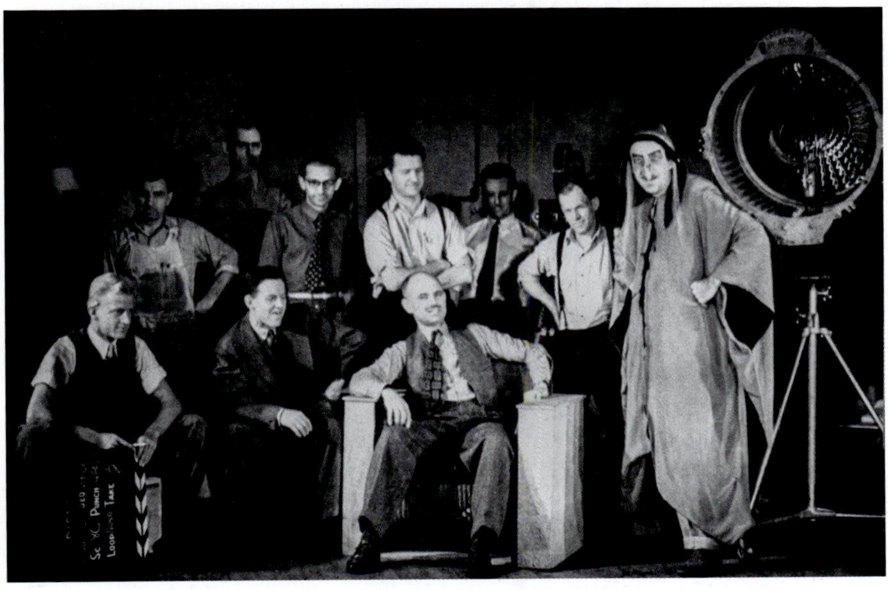

On the soundstage at Hyperion for *Snow White*. SEATED: Lou Debney (FAR LEFT), Norm Ferguson, and Ben Sharpsteen. AT FAR RIGHT, actor Don L. Brodie (also an occasional voice actor in Disney films) stands ready to perform for live-action reference as the wicked witch. Sharpsteen family collection.

of supervising director on *Pinocchio* and Dave Hand took charge of the shorts.[54]

Ben recalled, "He [Walt] told me he was going to put me in charge of the production of *Pinocchio*. In other words, I was to be the supervising director of it. Of course, I was very much flattered after the success of *Snow White*, but I realized that the story of *Pinocchio* was far afield from *Snow White* in universal interest. But that was just my nature to be skeptical."[55]

Ben had introduced Walt to the story of Pinocchio. "I personally recommended that he consider making a picture about Pinocchio, and I had a book that I let him have."[56] Walt also saw a local WPA production of *Pinocchio*, and Ben felt that inspired Walt.[57]

No feature runs a smooth path, and *Pinocchio* certainly had its challenges. "*Pinocchio* suffered from story changes. It was not an easy story to make. Walt kept making the story while it was being animated."[58] As the production neared completion, Ham Luske joined Ben as a supervising director to facilitate completion of the film. Even with this additional help, Ben said, "we came up to the point of previewing it and distributing it, and it was not long before we could see that it probably would not make its prospect on the first run."[59]

Walt's choice of *Pinocchio* did not have universal appeal within the studio, and Ben was criticized for suggesting it to Walt. Ben didn't believe that Walt actually disliked *Pinocchio*, because he always defended it.[60] But as *Pinocchio* earned less than a million dollars at the box office on its initial release, and the studio had to write off a million more of its cost, Walt's "misgivings had hardened into a feeling that *Pinocchio* should never have been made."[61] Ham Luske, in an interview a decade or so later, blamed Ben Sharpsteen for selling Walt on the idea of making *Pinocchio*, a film now considered one of the greatest of all time![62]

"THE SHAPING CREW"

A director's first job was to interpret and improve the layouts, cutting, and acting indicated in the story boards before handing out work to animators. With three features and multiple shorts in production, Walt evidently decided around 1940 his directors could use some help in this area—or at least a fresh eye.

In a conversation with production manager Ken Peterson, animators Ollie Johnston and Frank Thomas discussed a group "that Walt picked out to go around checking on things" which became known as "the Shaping Crew."[63] Art director and layout artist Ken Anderson mentioned the group "would go from music room to music room, shaping things,"[64] looking at the directors' work and offering alternate ideas and suggestions.

The group included:

- Walt
- Ted Sears—Head story artist
- Joe Grant—Head of Development (aka the Character Model Department)
- Bill Cottrell—Trusted story artist and writer
- Ben Sharpsteen—Supervising Director

It's unknown how often the group visited, or what scope of suggestions were given, but the organization doesn't seem to have lasted more than a few years. With work needing to be handed out and new ideas flying in the room, it's easy to imagine that more than one director may have agreed with story man Ted Sears's sardonic observation that "there is nothing worse than a fresh eye."

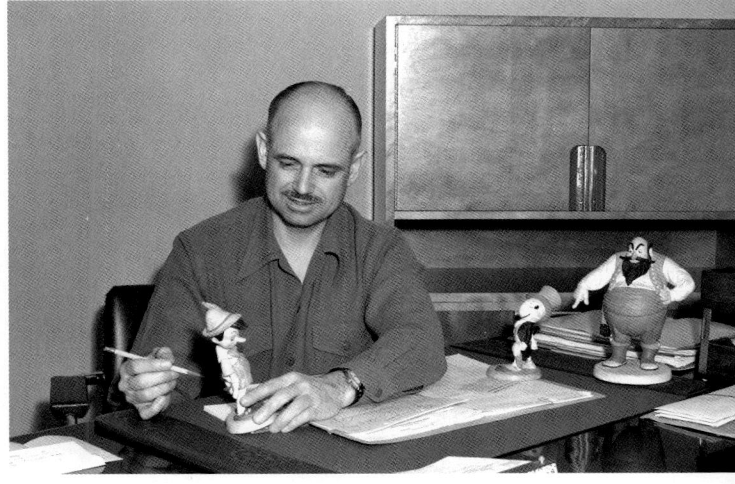

Ben during production of *Pinocchio*.

Despite the poor reception for *Pinocchio*, Ben was selected to be the production supervisor on *Fantasia*, so he was taking on more of the role of a producer, as he would for most of the rest of his career. *Fantasia* also turned out to be a disappointment in its initial release.

Dumbo began as not much more than a children's storybook galley Walt bought,[65] but through the talents of Dick Huemer and Joe Grant, it grew into a solid story that was perfect for an animated feature. Ben Sharpsteen was once again cast as the supervising director. After a string of disappointments at the box office, the production team on *Dumbo* was under a great deal of pressure. Ben said, "*Dumbo* was made at a very critical time. . . . Walt regarded *Dumbo* as a low-budget film that could be made with the available animators, and we had some very good animators available. He let me know very emphatically that this picture had to be made for $350,000. He subsequently raised that figure from time to time. When he first gave me that figure, I knew that he did not mean it, but I knew the spirit in which he said it. 'We've got a basic story here that we are going to put on the screen without any frills or gilding the lily.' Knowing Walt as I did, I knew this sentiment instinctively. But I also knew that he would not stand for any shoddy results. With all of this in mind, we organized our production."[66]

As story meeting notes attest, Walt was intimately involved with this picture, but he had many balls in the air. Ben said, "He was certainly active on it, but he had a great many things going on. . . . But never was there a time when Walt turned his back on that picture, such as he had on some other pictures."[67] Michael Barrier pointed out that Walt had help with the vision of this picture: "There are many hints in *Dumbo* itself, though, that other hands played a larger part in shaping it than was usually the case. Ben Sharpsteen supervised *Dumbo*, and in its economy and clarity, *Dumbo* recalls the best of the short cartoons (*Mickey's Circus*, *Moving Day*, *On Ice*) that Sharpsteen directed for Disney before he directed part of *Snow White* and supervised all of *Pinocchio*."[68]

As the next generation of animators thrived, Freddy Moore, once the top animator at the studio, was now sadly struggling artistically and with alcohol part of the mix. Moore was called upon to animate an inebriated Timothy Mouse. As Moore fought to produce work that would measure up to the escalating quality standards, Sharpsteen realized the effect could be achieved much more simply by implying the action off-screen, through sound effects. "As directors, we had to be discreet, since we worked day after day with the very men that we were correcting."[69] Ben and his story team altered the story so it would be easier for Freddy to animate. "It was a far better means of doing it than to have squeezed everything we could have out of the animator in some subtle manner."[70]

Dumbo had a running time of only about seventy minutes, but Ben felt compelled to edit it even further to tighten the story. "Then for me to cut another four and a half minutes out of the picture that was already too short, but it was something I did. . . . It was at a time when Walt Disney was out of the country, and he never saw the picture again until it was in release. As far as I'm concerned, he was never the least bit concerned of the four and a half

WALT AND *BAMBI* SEQUENCE DIRECTOR SAM ARMSTRONG

Ben Sharpsteen recalled an incident that happened during the production of *Bambi* that illustrated Walt's sometimes combative relationship with his directors. "One man [later identified by Ben as Sam Armstrong, primarily known as a background painter and layout artist prior to directing sequences in feature films] who was directing a sequence in *Bambi* had gone entirely too 'arty' on it. He did not particularly understand comedy situations or entertainment, but he was inclined to think mostly of the artistic impacts. As a result, his sequence had grown far too long. A great deal of expense had gone into such a sequence, and in desperation, Walt sat in the projection room with him and others in an effort to cut the sequence down, to cut loose from too much material that did not relate closely to the story line. In going through the sequence, Walt would say, 'Now you can cut here . . . now you ought to cut something out of this . . . now cut here.' After a little bit, the director complained, 'Well I think that I would be losing something if we cut that out.' Then he repeated again, 'Walt I think I would lose something if I cut this out.' Walt was exasperated. He said, 'You're telling me what you'd be losing. Here I am losing my shirt and you're telling me what you'd be losing!'"[71]

minutes that came out of it. But somebody had to do it and I'm convinced to this day that the picture is a far better picture for having those few little dull spots come out. It wasn't four and a half minutes in one spot. Nothing of the sort. It might be ten seconds now, three seconds there, and so forth. So naturally, a certain amount of stigma got associated with my employ there along those lines."[72]

When RKO salesmen complained that the film was too short for a feature, Walt defended Ben's editing choices: "No, that's as far as I can stretch it. You can stretch a thing so far and then it won't hold. This picture is right as it is. And another ten minutes is liable to cost five hundred thousand dollars. I can't afford it."[73] *Dumbo* was made for $812,000, considerably below the cost of the other feature films clustered around it, and it made a profit of $850,000. It helped the studio stay afloat at a critical time as World War II was about to descend on it and the nation. Founder of the Walt Disney Archives and Disney Legend Dave Smith said, "Ben showed his ability to not only stick to a budget but by proper casting of animators and a good story to come up with an excellent product."[74] In a 1974 interview with Dave Smith, Ben talked about how the features *Dumbo* and *Bambi* were very different from each other, yet both were Disney films. He said, "Walt could express himself through . . . well, almost anybody he picked up."

THE FORTIES

Dumbo opened shortly before the attack on Pearl Harbor and America's entry into World War II. With the military literally moving into the studio, Walt devoted most of his efforts to the production of military training films, and morale-building and health and sanitation films for civilian audiences at home and among the allies. These films helped the studio stay solvent as the European markets were closed for the duration.

The New Spirit was one of the key cartoon shorts that had an immeasurable impact on convincing the American taxpayers—many of whom were new to those ranks—to pay "taxes to bury the Axis." Wilfred Jackson and Ben Sharpsteen codirected that short, which was given an almost impossible deadline by Secretary Henry Morgenthau and the United States Treasury Department. Ben worked on a variety of films during the war, mostly educational films—sometimes with a propaganda twist—but also training films for the military. A June 26, 1942, memo from Ben to Walt is evidence of Ben's role as a producer on these wartime educational films:

WALT DISNEY PRODUCTIONS

INTER-OFFICE COMMUNICATION

P-156

TO MR. Walt DATE June 26, 1942

FROM MR. Ben SUBJECT

-2-

Walt, these are things I wish you would take care of in Washington:

1. Get an OK for us on the Corn picture.

2. Try to work out a solution for the Ever-Normal Granary. Get this in Bressman's hands as soon as possible upon your arrival there.

3. I think it advisable that you do not open for discussion the medical pictures, as I am convinced that we have exhausted, through conferences, the material on these pictures, and it is now up to us to make them.

4. Discuss the Amazon Basin with whoever is available, for general policies only. Let's see if we can't inject something in it like the Brazilian parrot as a master of ceremonies, to give the picture a thread of life. You will note that I have allowed $30,000 for this picture and I think we ought to make something out of the ordinary.

5. Check with Chester for bids on foreign versions for Food Will Win the War. He has all the dope. We expect to ship the print to them on July 17th.

6. The budgets for the six pictures are included herewith. The only change materially was with the Ever-Normal Granary which we have as much as decided should be an 800 foot picture instead of the 1200 feet we originally estimated.

There is no reason for coming down on any of the budgets as they are practically the same as were agreed upon when we were in Washington before.

I have included budgets on the other five pictures and arbitrarily figured them at about $50,000 apiece. That was because of the additional 20% in case you still make these pictures under a subsidy from the Coordinator's Office.

As the war ended, the studio tried to pick up the pieces financially and reset its course. Ben was the production supervisor on a number of films, including three "package" films, *Fun and Fancy Free*, *Melody Time*, and *The Adventures of Ichabod and Mister Toad*, and, in the fifties, two feature-length animated films, *Cinderella* and *Alice in Wonderland*. Winston Hibler worked with Ben in the early 1940s and continued on through *Melody Time* and the True-Life Adventure series of nature films. Winston recalled Ben in an interview with Richard Hubler: "When I first worked with him he headed up industrial-type films, then more cartoon features like *Johnny Appleseed* and *Pecos Bill*. He broke me in. . . . He was very tough, a strict disciplinarian, but I liked him very much. He taught me a great deal."[75]

TRUE-LIFE ADVENTURES

After World War II, Ben's next assignment came out of the blue. "In 1947, Walt spoke to me about doing something about Alaska. It was a new thought to me. I had not known that that was on his mind. 'What are we doing about it?' I said, 'Nothing that I know of.' 'Well,' he said, 'we should look into it.'"[76] The result was sending Alfred and Elma Milotte on an unspecified filming junket, selecting the footage of the seals on the Pribilof Islands, and turning that into a two-reel documentary, directed by Jim Algar, which won an Academy Award and ushered in the True-Life Adventures series and the spin-off People and Places series. Teamed up with Jim Algar and Winston Hibler, the True-Life Adventure series, in both short and long form, won eight Academy Awards. The People and Places series films won three Academy Awards. As a producer of both series, Ben also was in charge of research and the hiring of photographers.

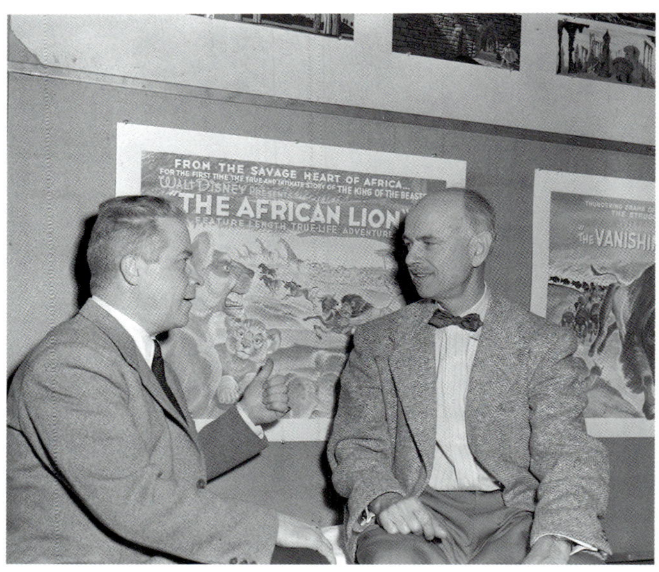

Publicity images for True-Life Adventures.

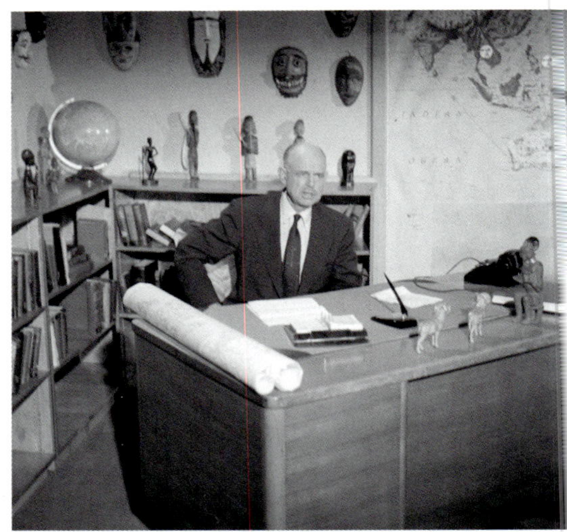

Ben on the first *Disneyland* television show, introducing "Adventureland."

A few years later, when the *Disneyland* television show premiered, Ben was on camera, introducing the Adventureland segment of the series.

WALT AND BEN

Working at the Disney Studios *was* working with Walt. He and the studio were one. Over a thirty-year career at the studio, Ben had many occasions to observe and interact with Walt on a personal level. Walt didn't want yes-men, but he didn't want people to throw cold water on his enthusiasm, either. It was a fine line to walk. Ben admired Walt for his accomplishments and allowed for the rough edge often used to achieve them. Ben summed up Walt and their working relationship:

> Walt was only one man. He was still the head of the business. He was still the prime mover of production. He was still *the* spark plug.

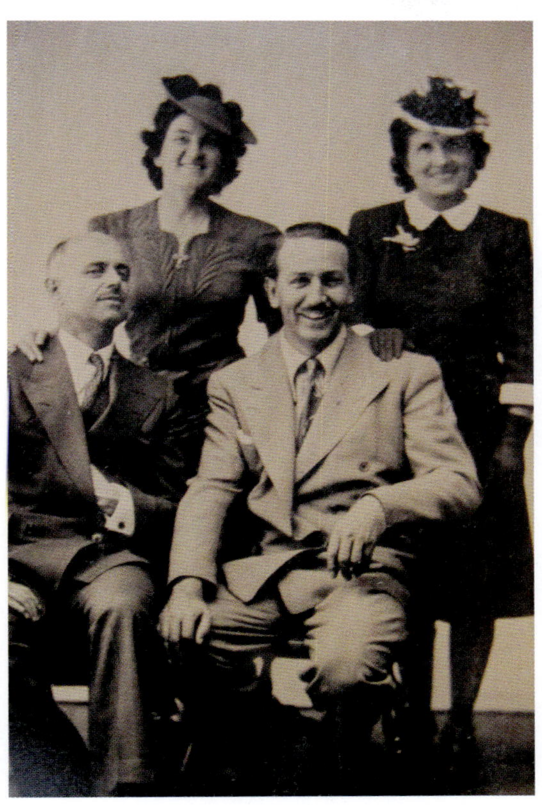

Ben and Bernice and Walt and Lilly pose for an antique photo at Henry Ford's Greenfield Village. Sharpsteen family collection.

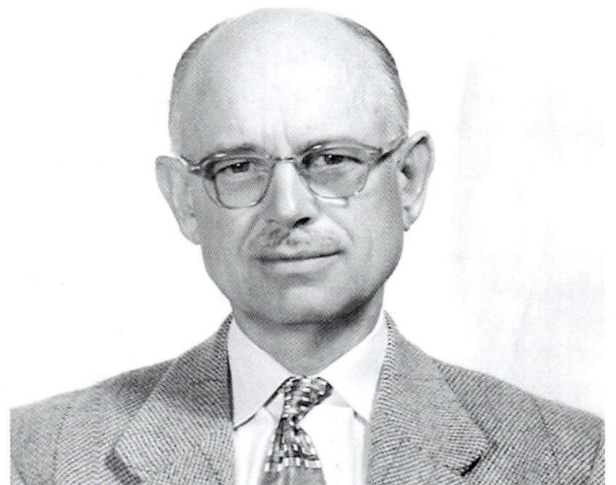

Sharpsteen in the late 1950s. Sharpsteen family collection.

> The whole movement of the organization was Walt Disney personally. He had to build an organization, but it was his judgment as to who was important in that organization. That exquisite organization of talent of which he could pull the strings and make this man do this and that man do that. . . . My personal reaction to Walt was that I never took him for granted. I never considered myself to be a sure thing at the studio. I always figured that what happened to others could happen to me. If I did not prove myself useful, I could be on the way out. And so in the process of terminating my long career of thirty years with him, I was rather amazed and pleased that his attitude toward me was as nice as it was.[77]

WHAT PRICE SUCCESS?

Health problems—most likely stress-induced health problems—seemed to have been a side effect of working as a director at the Disney Studios. Ben was not immune to them. In 1956, Ben sent Walt a memo in which he discussed his health issues: "I have developed a nervousness that somewhat alarms me. My cure has been to take frequent leaves from the Studio. These seem to be occurring oftener and for longer durations, and yet I hesitate to present a formal resignation. Perhaps an overlap is a better solution and Larry [Clemmons] might be a good prospect in whom I could impart my years of experience."[78] Ever the organization man, Ben continued, "With Larry handling the balance, I could gradually step out. Under this plan we can keep production up to a maximum

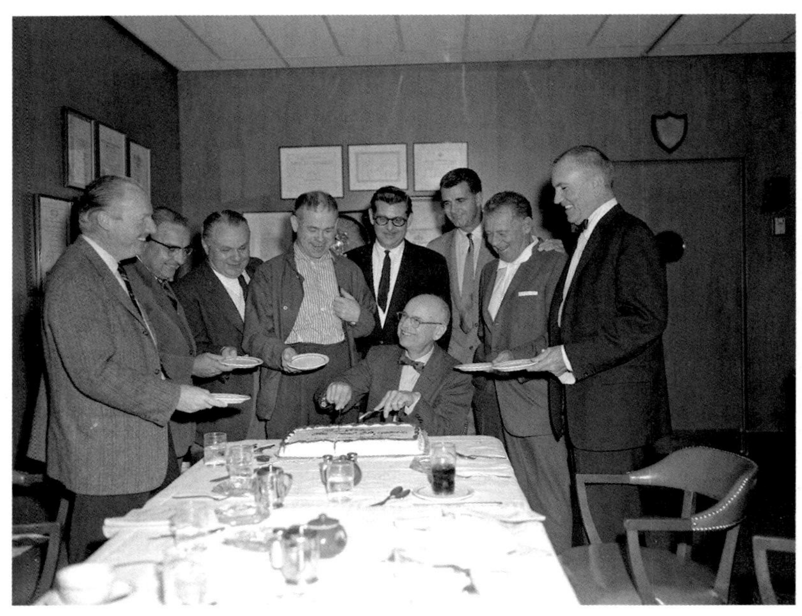

Celebrating Ben's thirtieth year with the studio: (FROM LEFT): Jim Algar, Erwin Verity, Gerry Geronimi, Ward Kimball, Winston Hibler, Card Walker, Ham Luske, and Bill Anderson. Sharpsteen family collection.

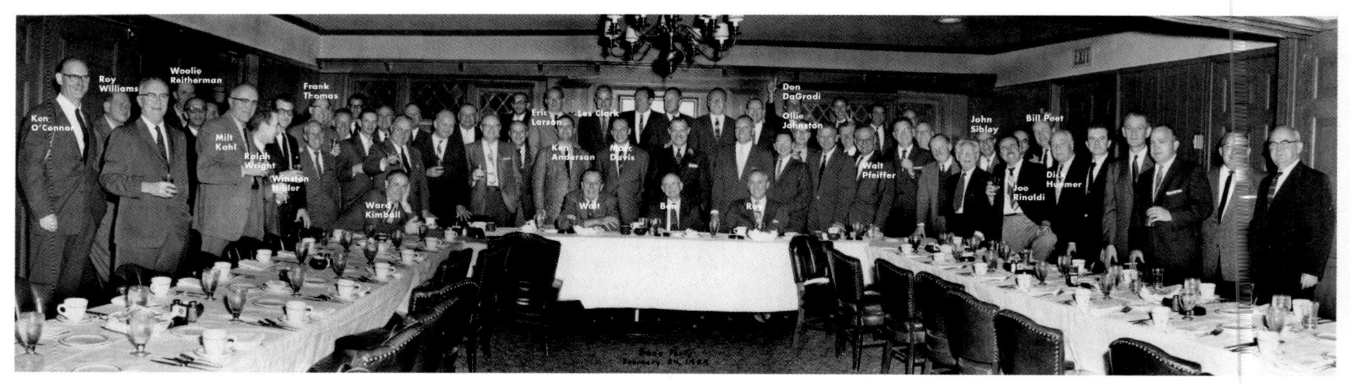

Ben's retirement party on February 24, 1959.

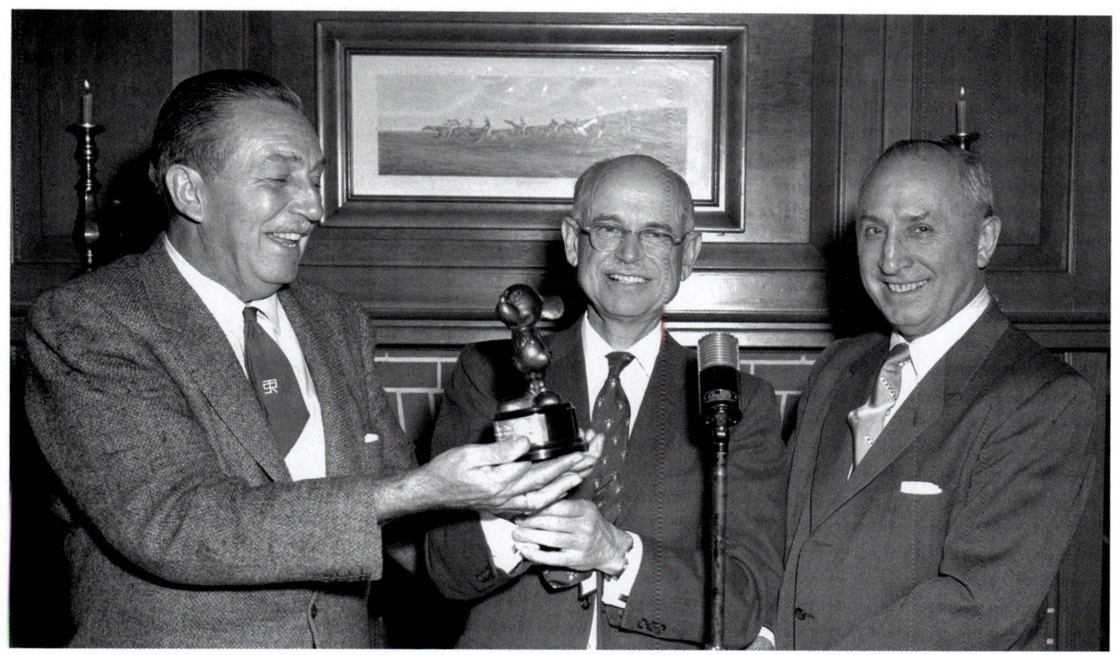

Walt, Ben, and Roy O. Disney with the Mousecar awarded to Ben at his retirement party. Sharpsteen family collection.

and my fading from the scene need occasion no upset whatsoever."[79] Earlier in the year, during one of Ben's absences, Walt had sent him a note saying, "Just wanted you to know we are all thinking of you and hoping that you will be feeling like a million in no time at all. Have a good rest . . . take it easy . . . the boys here are carrying through, so you have nothing to worry about. Everybody sends best wishes to you along with mine—"[80]

RETIREMENT

As Disney got into more projects and moved in varying directions, it seemed to hit long-time Disney employees the hardest. Ben found himself facing an uncertain future. Both Ben Sharpsteen and Wilfred Jackson, who left the studio in 1959, felt that they knew Walt less than they had earlier, when animation was the sole focus of the studio. Ben decided to retire. "On February 24, 1959, I was given a retirement party. Sixty-one people attended the very nice affair. Among the presents that I received was a watch inscribed 'To Ben from the Disney gang.' I felt quite honored by it all. It was a happy conclusion to a wonderful career for me," he said.[81] "The best present I had upon my thirty years' completion [was] when he [Walt] took the attitude that I could have stayed here as long as I wanted."[82]

In a rare gesture, Walt gave Ben the Oscar he received for *Ama Girls*. "I was called into his office by his secretary and I was very much surprised when she held it up to me and said, 'Walt said he thought you would like to have this.' I am very pleased to have it."[83]

AFTER DISNEY

Ben and Bernice decided to retire to their ancestral lands in Calistoga. After they established a home there, Ben suffered some serious health issues, which limited his physical activity.

"I had to plan my time in other ways. This led to my going back to perhaps my first love, which was drawing. I had always wanted to illustrate. In the days that I earned my living drawing, I was never fortunate enough to do anything of any consequence, that required a great deal of skill, and yet I wanted to try it."[84] Ben turned to his love of vintage cars, and his paintings graced the covers of the *Horseless Carriage Gazette*. Joe Grant said of Ben's paintings, "When he retired he did some of the most amazing drawings . . . I mean it was something that had been hidden in him all these years."[85] Ben said he was strongly influenced by Norman Rockwell, an artist he admired.

Twice a year, Ben and Bernice traveled to Southern California. They frequently visited old Disney Studios friends, like Wilfred and Jane Jackson, Dick and Polly Huemer, Jack and Camille Cutting, Ward and Betty Kimball, Ken and Mary Alice O'Connor, and Roy and Edna Disney. They also frequently visited Disneyland and the Disney Studios. One visit to the studio turned out to be their last visit with Walt Disney. Walt had just returned from St. Joseph's Hospital, where he'd had a lung removed and treatment for cancer. Ben was shocked at Walt's emaciated appearance and was going to cut short his visit with him, but Walt suggested they have lunch together. "It was perhaps the best conversation that I had ever had with him in all the years that I had known him. He brought many things to conclusion and into focus, many of his problems and how he had solved them. As the meal progressed, I felt that he was gaining strength and feeling like his old self again. Later that day, I was walking through

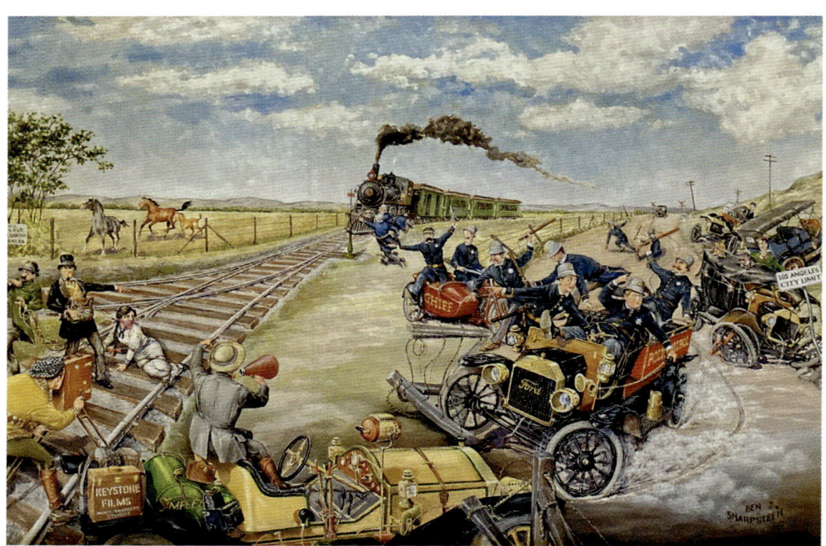

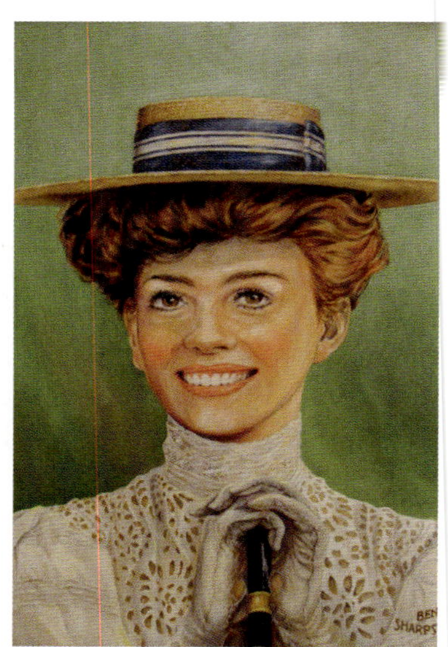

Ben's artwork after retirement. Sharpsteen family collection.

the main building and I saw Walt talking to another group of men about production problems. I was more convinced than ever that Walt was back in the groove. Naturally to hear only a couple of weeks later that he had died suddenly was a terrific shock to me."[86]

In June of 1967, at the commencement ceremonies at the University of California at Davis, Ben Sharpsteen received an honorary degree, Doctor of Humane Letters. This meant a great deal to Ben. What was equally moving for Ben was a letter from Walt Disney to then Davis chancellor Emil Mrak: "I want to say he was one of our valuable men. He played a very important part. . . . As time went on he became one of my good right hands in production. He directed a considerable number of cartoon subjects and was an important supervisor for us in feature films such as *Snow White*. In the forties we assigned Ben to the role of co-producer on the Nature Series we started at that time. From 1929 to 1962 when he retired[87], he was always a very active and integral part of the organization. . . . If anybody is worthy of an Honorary Degree certainly Ben Sharpsteen is."[88]

Ben Sharpsteen passed away in 1980 and was the recipient of a posthumous Disney Legends Award in 1998.

SHARPSTEEN
MUSEUM
DEDICATED TO
CALISTOGA'S
PIONEERS
AFFILIATED WITH
NAPA COUNTY
HISTORICAL SOCIETY

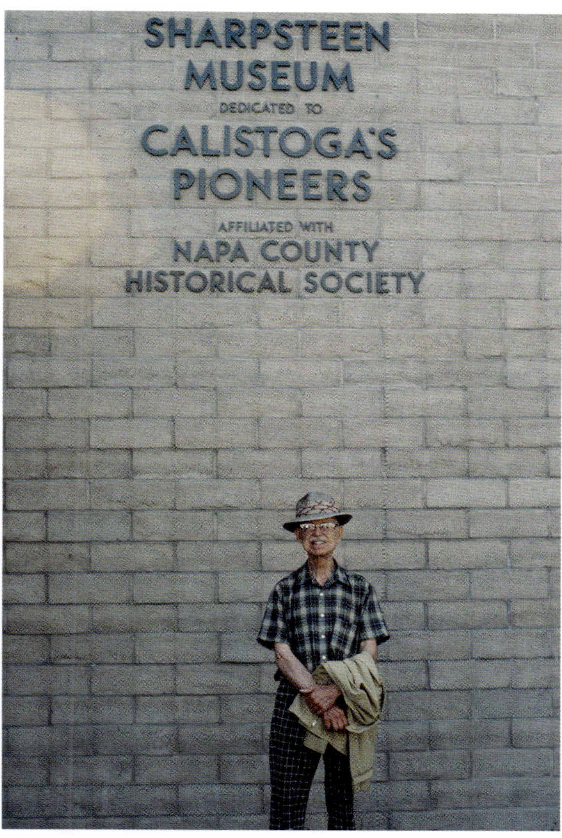

Ben loved Calistoga, and during his retirement years, he and Bernice donated the funds to help establish this museum and Ben recruited artists, including Disney's Ken O'Connor, to help give the museum the Disney touch. Don Peri collection.

A taskmaster, Ben was tough on others because he was tough on himself. His high standards and strong-willed opinions repelled many coworkers. Ben had a volatile relationship with Walt Disney. Although Ben was treated harshly by Walt at times, whether in a sweatbox session or before an audience of one kind or another, Walt relied on him. In their memos to each other, Ben's role as effectively a special assistant to Walt holds true. Walt knew Ben would be there for him, carry out any task, however challenging or unpleasant, and devote his energies to furthering the products of the studio. Ben's advancement and durability at the studio is testimony to his shrewdness, to his bending but never breaking as the winds of disharmony moved his way. His persistence and his unfailing loyalty were qualities Walt highly prized. Ben's huge retirement party was the only one like it during Walt's time, and he was treated with kindness and graciousness by Walt ever after. Ultimately, Ben found that his time at the studio defined his life and capped a successful and accomplished career for a timid artist who initially lacked confidence, but who industriously applied himself.

Ben Sharpsteen—Disney Director Filmography[89]

Shorts:

Two-Gun Mickey (1934)
Mickey's Service Station (1935)
The Cookie Carnival (1935)
Mickey's Fire Brigade (1935)
On Ice (1935)
Cock o' the Walk (1935)
Broken Toys (1935)
Orphans' Picnic (1936)
Moving Day (1936)
Mickey's Circus (1936)
Donald and Pluto (1936)
The Worm Turns (1937)
Don Donald (1937)
Moose Hunters (1937)
Hawaiian Holiday (1937)
Clock Cleaners (1937)
Pluto's Quin-puplets (1937)
Boat Builders (1938)
Mickey's Trailer (1938)
Polar Trappers (1938)
The Fox Hunt (1938)
The New Spirit (1942) (Codirected with Wilfred Jackson)

Features:

Snow White and the Seven Dwarfs (1937) (Sequence Director)
Pinocchio (1940) (Supervising Codirector)
Fantasia (1940) (Production Supervisor)
Dumbo (1941) (Supervising Director)
Fun and Fancy Free (1947) (Production Supervisor)
Melody Time (1948) (Production Supervisor)
The Adventures of Ichabod and Mister Toad (1949) (Production Supervisor)
Cinderella (1950) (Production Supervisor)
Alice in Wonderland (1951) (Production Supervisor)

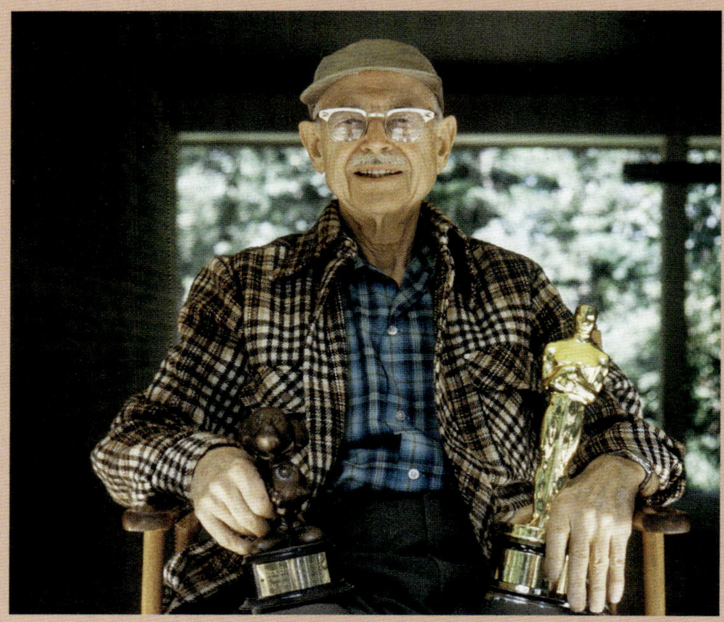

Ben at his Calistoga home with his Mousecar and his Oscar for *Ama Girls*. Don Peri collection.

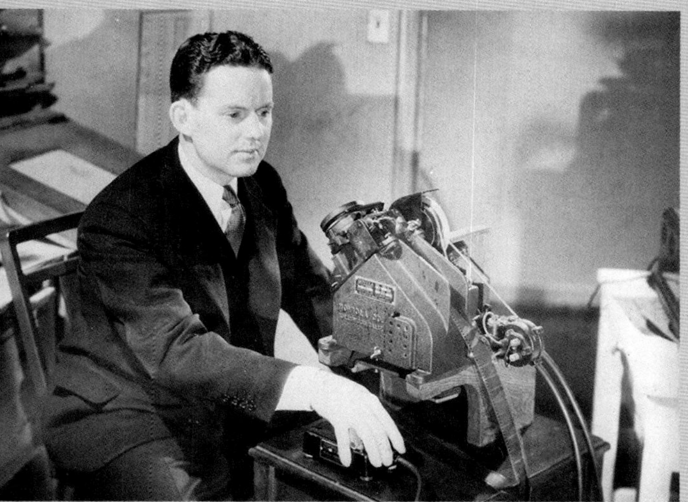

Fergy at the Moviola.

Almost all the directors covered in this book remained so once they left the realm of animation. Norman "Fergy" Ferguson was an exception. One of the most highly regarded animators at the studio, he moved into directing with the features, but after a falling-out with Walt, he returned to animation. By then, however, animation had progressed beyond his abilities. Ben Sharpsteen thought of Fergy as one of the tragic figures at the Disney Studios.

Norman Ferguson was born in 1902 in New York, and he always retained the fast-paced street vernacular of the New York of his era. He took business courses and studied commercial art at the Pratt Institute. While working as a camera operator at Paul Terry's Fables Pictures, Inc., Fergy discovered that a scene he was filming was missing some of its animation, so he completed the drawings. His work was successful, and he transitioned into animation. In 1929, he was part of the wave of New York animators that followed Ben Sharpsteen to the Disney Studios, joining Burt Gillett and Jack King, and soon followed by Dave Hand and Tom Palmer. Fergy loved watching vaudeville and theatrical performances, and he brought this broad type of humor to his animation. He quickly established himself as one of the top animators at the studio on the seventy-five shorts he helped create. His rough style of drawing helped advance the art of animation and the personality animation Disney became famous for. In *Frolicking Fish*, he animated a trio of fish singing and performing a vaudevillian soft-shoe routine. He introduced a fluidity that kept the animation alive: "moving holds." "In that scene there was a fluid type of action where they didn't hit a hold and move out of it. But when one part would hold something else would move," recalled Wilfred Jackson.[90] Walt was delighted with this innovation and insisted that it be adopted. In *The Chain Gang*, he created such a memorable character in one of the bloodhounds that it morphed into Pluto in later shorts, and Fergy was known as one of the top "Pluto men." Ben Sharpsteen said, "Fergy was successful in getting a looseness into the bloodhound that exaggerated its ability to sniff and to think."[91] Perhaps his most noteworthy achievement was in *Playful Pluto*, when Pluto engages in a mighty struggle with a piece of flypaper. Pluto's predicament and his thinking escalate with each movement to escape, and they are conveyed clearly to the audience. This was a milestone in the development of personality animation.

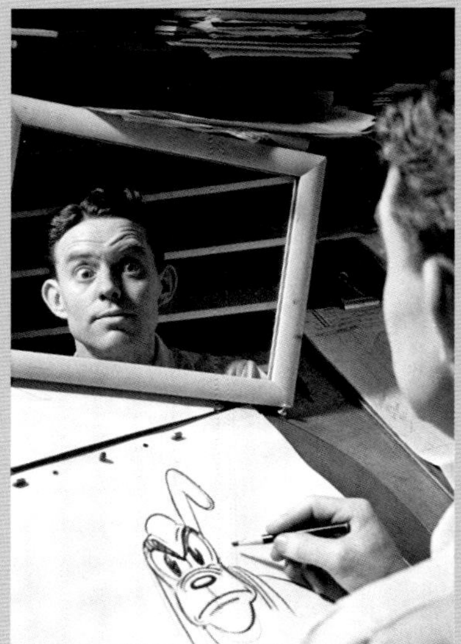

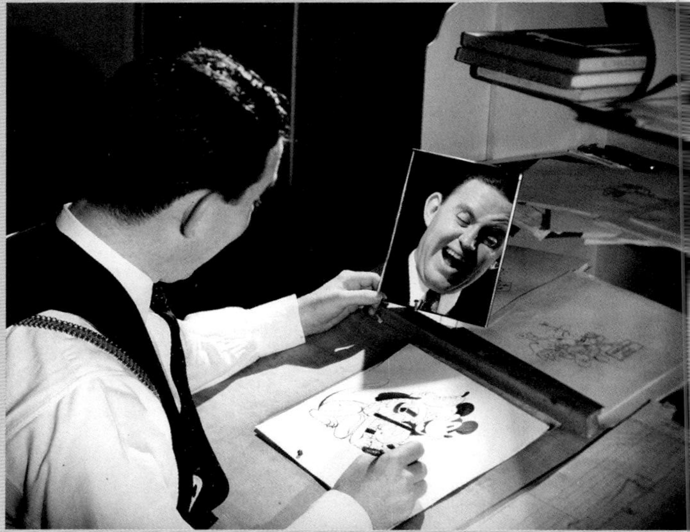

Fergy at his animation desk. His animation of Pluto stuck to flypaper was considered some of the first true personality animation by other Disney animators.

Fergy, Fred Moore, Ham Luske, and Bill Tytla were the titans of the studio and the mentors and inspiration for the next generation of animators, who would eventually become Walt Disney's Nine Old Men.

Fergy and Fred Moore were the lead animators on the highly successful *Three Little Pigs* but also served in this capacity in the disappointing short *The Golden Touch*. Ben felt that "it was apparent that Fergy had to have much more in his favor than just an ordinary story, that he needed the right sort of story preparation and the right kind of inventive gag work that was so necessary."[92]

Fergy was a supervising animator on *Snow White*, assigned to the Witch, and he and his animators created the first of the great Disney villains. He was an animation supervisor on *Pinocchio* (J. Worthington Foulfellow and Gideon) and on *Fantasia*—for which he codirected the delightful segment "The Dance of the Hours" with T. Hee—and a sequence director on *Dumbo*.

With the advent of World War II and the plan to create films under the Good Neighbor policy, Fergy's roles expanded. He oversaw a Latin American tour group from the Disney Studios—nicknamed El Grupo—a goodwill visit that doubled as a working trip, gathering story materials and visual images for the films to follow. Walt assigned Fergy as the supervising director of the most important films. As J. B. Kaufman said in his seminal book *South of the Border with Disney*, "He was an inspired choice; his intimate familiarity with the creative side of animation gave him a substantial background for supervision of the other artists." Fergy immersed himself in shepherding these films through their productions. On *Saludos Amigos*, Fergy oversaw sequence directors Wilfred Jackson, Jack

Kinney, Ham Luske, and Bill Roberts. On *The Three Caballeros*, for which he was both production supervisor *and* director, his sequence directors were Gerry Geronimi, Jack Kinney, and Bill Roberts. Fergy codirected with Eric Larson "The Flying Gauchito" segment for this film, and he even wrote the English lyrics to "Have You Ever Been to Bahia?"[93]

Something apparently soured between Walt and Fergy around this time. Ben said, "Whereas the pictures all turned out satisfactorily, there was evidently something occurred within Walt's relations with Fergy that were not to Walt's liking."[94] Dick Huemer contended that "Walt pinned some of the blame for the poor showing of *Saludos Amigos* on Fergy. I know they had several bitter arguments, which was very unusual."[95] But Ben said Walt was loyal to Fergy and wanted him to return to animation, where he had had such great success. Ben remembered Walt's admonition: "'Now we've got to get Fergy back to working the way he did in the old days.' Well that was the worst thing that Walt could ever say. I don't know how he could [not] realize that those days were past, gone, and could never come back again, and you could never use those days again. They weren't compatible with good animation. But Walt just was adamant, and he insisted, 'We've got to get Fergy working back in the ways he had before.' Of course, I was at my wits' ends, because I had no idea how that could be accomplished. All I knew was that Fergy was hopelessly behind and could never catch up with anything like some of our other animators could produce."[96] But Walt said, "Well he paved a great way for the studio and we've got to get him back to doing that."[97] So Fergy was assigned as a directing animator on *Cinderella* and the early features of the 1950s. Milt Kahl also witnessed Fergy's sad state of affairs: "'Fergy' had been directing for a long time and Walt got sour on him as a director and put him back into animation. And animation had passed him by. He was an awfully nice guy but he'd kinda of had it, I guess."[98]

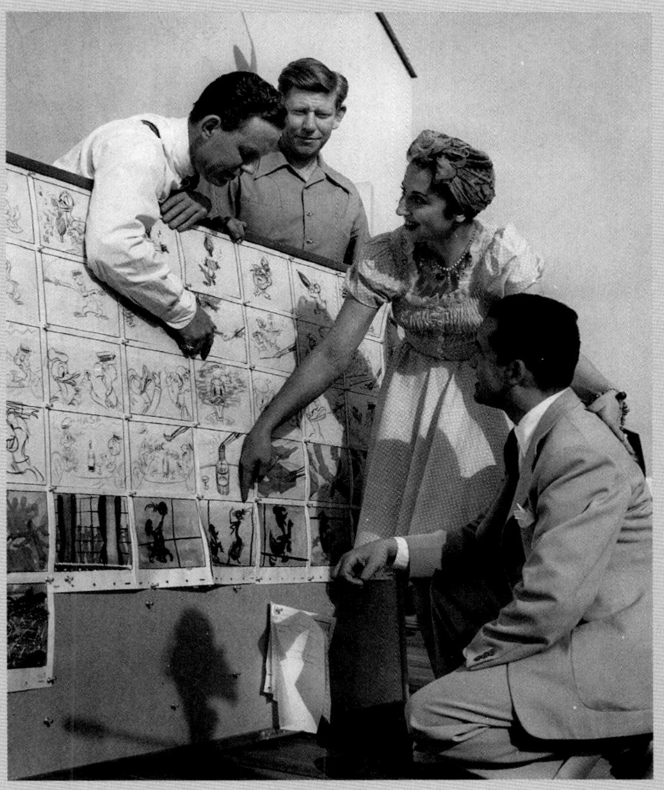

LEFT TO RIGHT: Fergy, Jaxon, live-action reference dancer Pilar Ferrer (seen dancing with Donald in the final scenes of *Saludos Amigos*), and Jorge Guinle, Nelson Rockefeller's point man for the Good Neighbor Latin American affairs unit during the 1940s. Dave Bossert collection.

Fergy was laid off from Disney in 1953 and went to work for Shamus Culhane Productions but was only there a short time before his long-standing diabetes led to other health issues. He died of a heart attack on November 2, 1957, in Los Angeles at fifty-five years of age. He was posthumously honored with the Winsor

McCay Award in 1987 and the Disney Legends Award in 1999. Jack Kinney, reflecting on the wave of New York animators that had arrived with Fergy, said: “They were all good, but Fergy was outstanding. He brought the characters to life. They breathed, they had weight, thoughts, real movement—and they were funny.”[99] Despite an unhappy ending, Norman Ferguson left an indelible mark on the Disney pictures that have enthralled audiences since their inception.

Norman Ferguson—Disney Director Filmography[100]

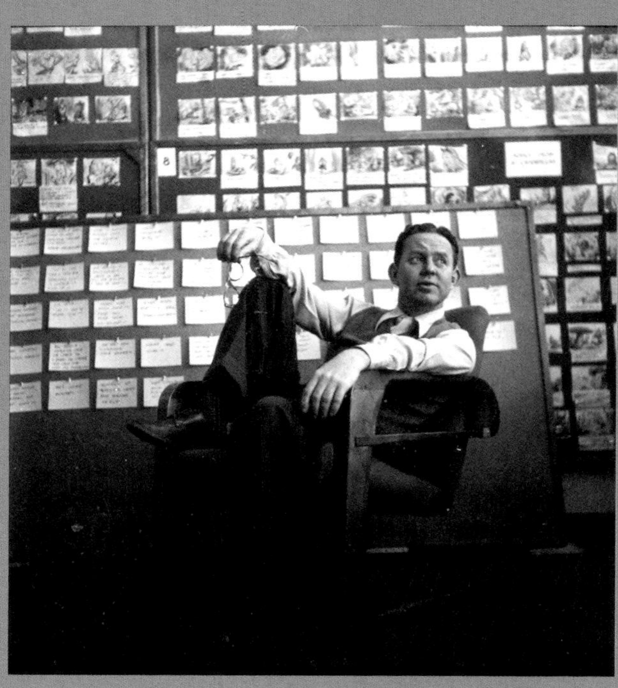

Pinocchio (1940) (Sequence Director)
Fantasia (1940) (Sequence Director)
Pluto’s Playmate (1941)
Dumbo (1941) (Sequence Director)
Saludos Amigos (1943) (Production Supervisor and Supervising Director)
The Three Caballeros (1945) (Production Supervisor and Director)
Cinderella (1950) (Directing Animator)
Alice in Wonderland (1951) (Directing Animator)
Peter Pan (1953) (Directing Animator)

A candid photo of Fergy at work, taken by Joe Grant. © Jennifer Grant Castrup.

THUMBNAIL SKETCHES
by
Larry Clemmons

BILL ROBERTS	Telegraph operator at a Kansas junction.
JAXON	The guy that won the spitting contests.
FRANK CHURCHILL	Fry cook in a lunch car.
BEN SHARPSTEEN	Leading dentist in a small town.
DAVE HAND	The fellow you never wanted your best girl to meet.
PAUL HOPKINS	Algebra instructor in a run-down military school.
PAUL ALLEN	Shoe clerk in a downtown department store.
HAZEL SEWELL	The teacher you took apples to.
JACK HANNAH	The fighter that never could get past the preliminaries.
JACK CAMPBELL	The slick "Black-Jack" dealer.
HARRY REEVES	Public enemy in any cheering section.
DON LUSK	A page in "Esquire" animates.
BOB WICKERSHAM	The kid your gang always tried to lose.
JOHN CANNON	The guy who throws the first pop bottle at the umpire.
ROY WILLIAMS	Bull in a china shop.
FRANK THOMAS	That nice boy you're allowed to play with.
"MAC" McGUGIN	The kid who racks up balls in a pool-room.
LES CLARK	House-party on Long Island.
HUGH HENNESY	A Franciscan monk.
HAM LUSKE	A Saint Bernard.
TED SEARS	Wilson Mizner reincarnated.
MILT SCHAFFER	The hands on a watch at six o'clock.
BILL SHULL	Floor-walker in a dry goods department.
ART BABBITT	"Red Flags in the Sunset."

-4-

One-sentence synopses of Disney coworkers by Larry Clemmons, published in *Mickey Mouse Deadline, the Disney Studio Monthly (We Hope) Magazine*, Vol 1, No. 1, January 1937. Price: five cents.

PART 4

“ALL OF A SUDDEN, WE HAD TO GROW UP”

1949–1961

1949–
1961

DIRECTING FEATURES

as Walt Diversifies

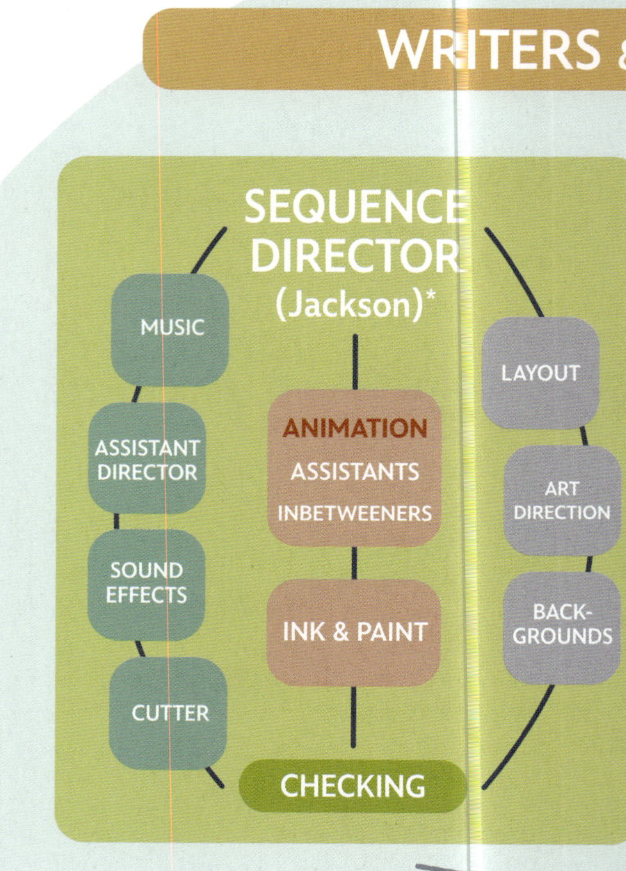

Each Sequence Director's job is still to previsualize and plan their sections of the film:

- Time out the action and cutting
- Collaborate with the composer
- Prepare work with the layout artist
- Hand out and supervise animation
- Review animation
- Supervise cutting

Directors now also guide the building of stories and characters, which Walt reviews and adjusts.

The Supervising Director position is eliminated; each feature is now directed by three Sequence Directors who report directly to Walt.

* Later replaced by Reitherm_n

Output: one feature approximately every two years

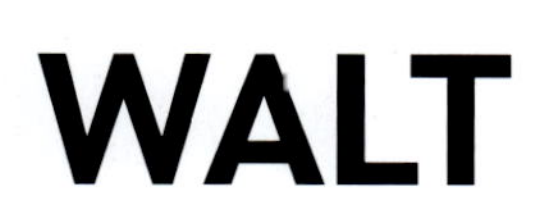

While Walt is still involved in guiding story and characters, his involvement in live-action, television, and theme parks leaves more and more responsibility to Directors to supervise story development.

TORY SKETCH

VOICE RECORDING

Story artists direct voice talent unless fixes or changes are required.

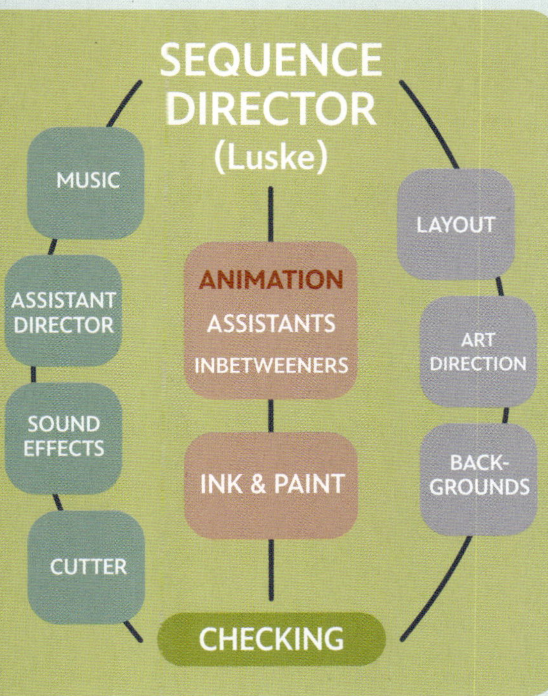

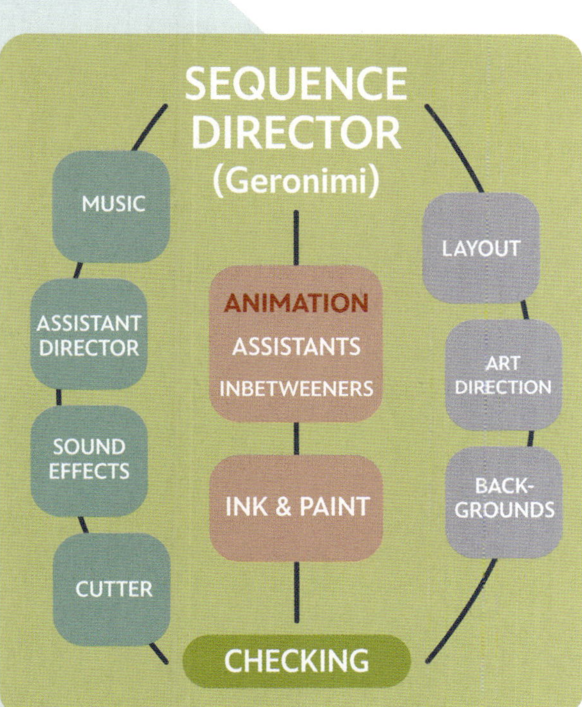

CAMERA

ANSWER PRINT

RE-RECORDING

FINAL FILM

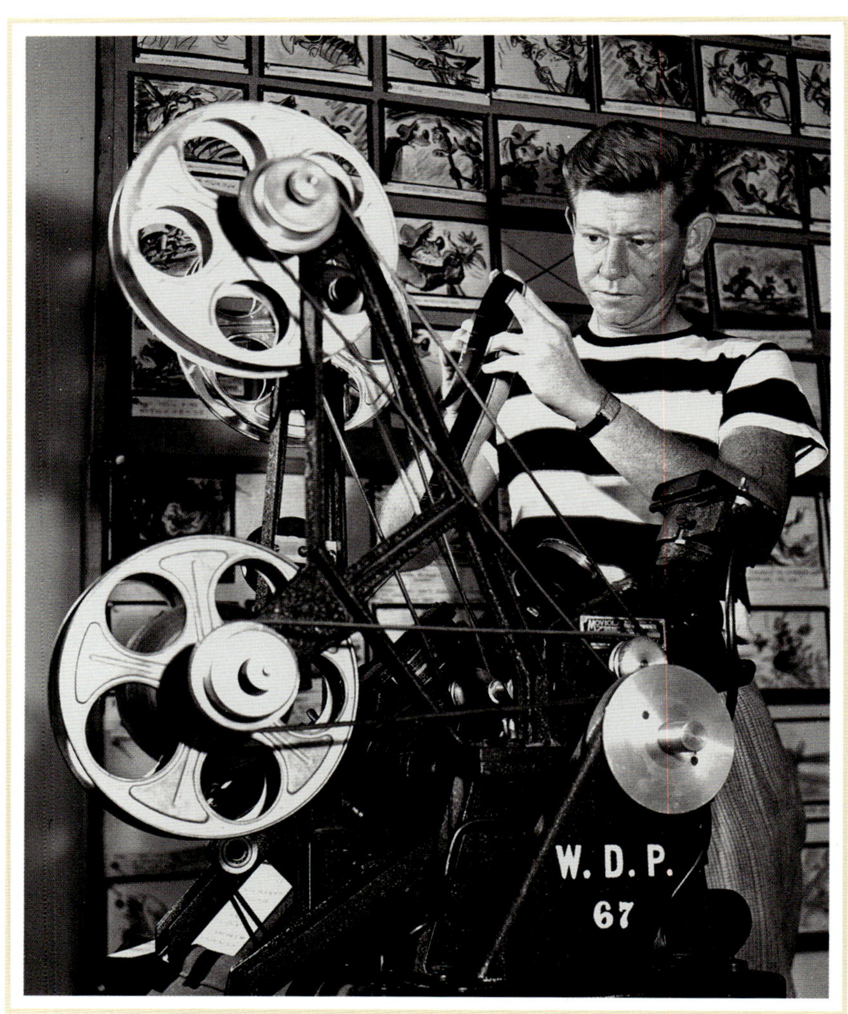

Jaxon reviews a section of *Song of the South*.

CHAPTER 5

WILFRED JACKSON—THE MUSICAL MAN

"I did animate for a few years, and when I simply couldn't keep up with the competition, Walt did the thing that was so characteristic of him: instead of kicking me out, he kicked me upstairs and made a director out of me. I had absolutely no qualifications to be a director, but Walt pointed his finger at me and said I was a director, so I had to try to be one. And I tried desperately to be one for years."[1]

—Wilfred Jackson

"Let me just settle this Jackson thing. He was the top director."[2]

—Animator Art Babbitt

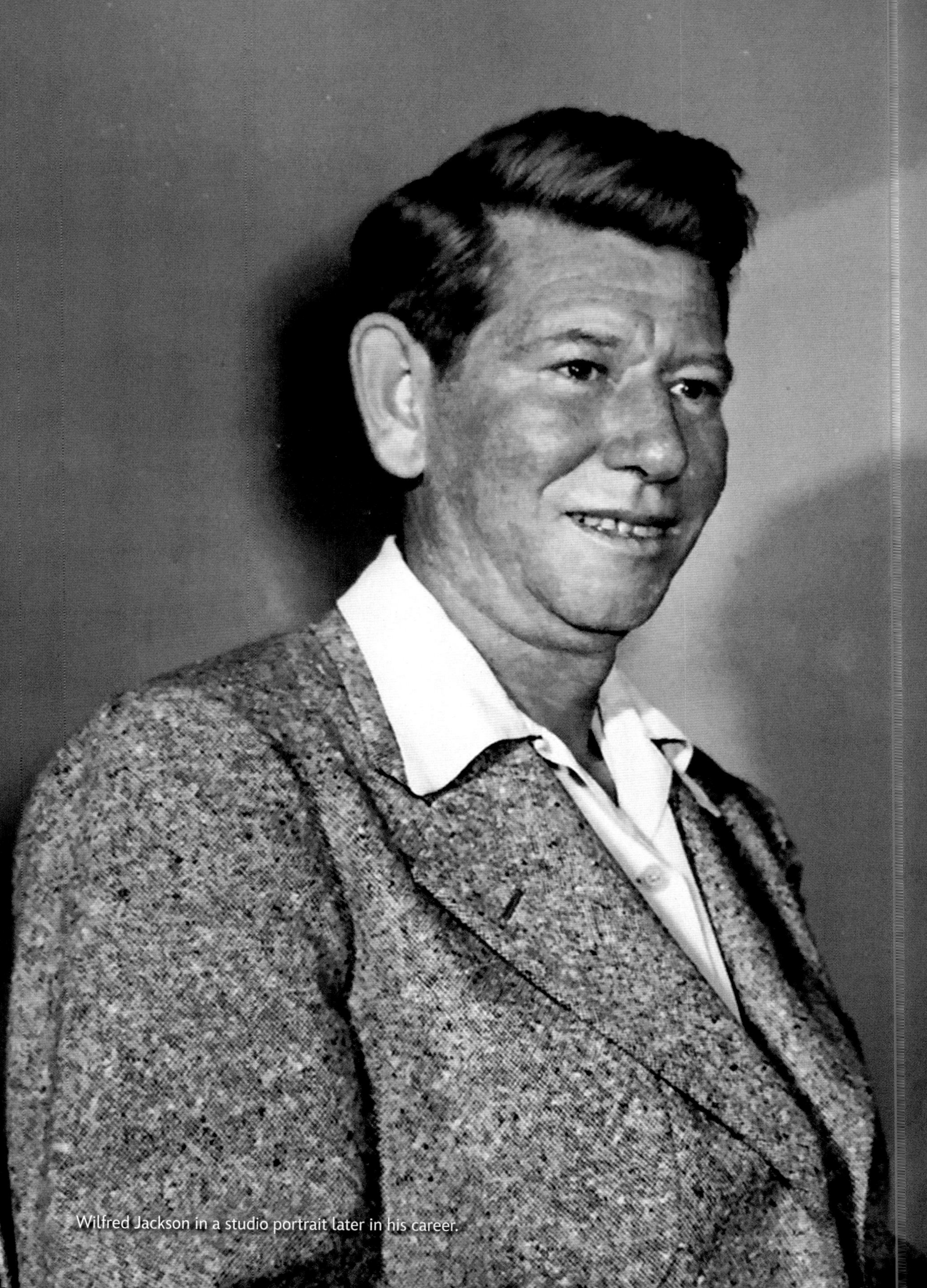

Wilfred Jackson in a studio portrait later in his career.

Wilfred Jackson loved animation ever since he first saw a silent cartoon as a child. After studying at the Otis Art Institute in Los Angeles, he wanted to become an animator, but he said he "didn't have the carfare" to get to New York, where the major animation studios were located. Wilfred discovered that Walt Disney was making cartoons in Hollywood, and his life changed forever the day he met Walt. After encountering the persistent but inexperienced Jackson, Walt decided to hire him on a temporary basis and try him out. So not only had Wilfred found a local studio where he could learn the animation business, but he had unwittingly hitched his wagon to the rising star of the one person, more than any other, who would transform the animated cartoon from a novelty, a filler on a theater program (a main feature sharing the program with a cartoon, a travelogue, a live-action short, a newsreel, etc.), into an art form. Wilfred was not just along for the ride, however; through *his* talent and *his* dedication, he helped Walt achieve his dream. Though keenly disappointed that he did not succeed as an animator and was "kicked upstairs" into the role of a director, he is nevertheless regarded by many of the animators who worked with and for him as the best director of Walt's Golden Age of animation. Didier Ghez stated in an introduction to an interview with Wilfred Jackson in Volume 7 of *Walt's People*: "Ask any of the Disney artists who worked with Walt who was the most respected of the animation directors and you will always hear the name 'Jaxon.'"

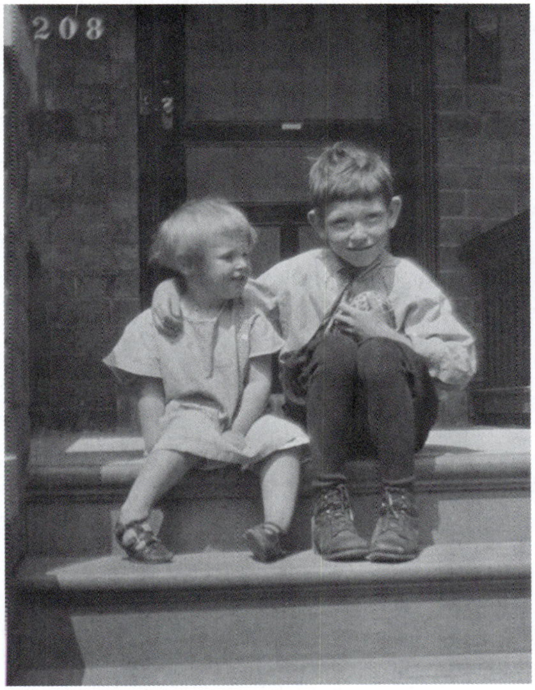

A young Wilfred with cousin Jeanne McLaughry Mahoney, likely taken in Chicago. Natha Horbach collection.

EARLY LIFE

Wilfred Emmons Jackson was born on January 24, 1906, in Chicago. Considering Wilfred's lifelong admiration for Walt, it is perhaps fitting that they were both born in the same city, less than five years apart. Wilfred and his parents moved to Glendale, California, when he was six or seven years old.

"Wilfred" was not an easy name for a young man in the early years of the twentieth century. Some schoolmates called him Winifred, and when his class read *Ivanhoe*, it became a tale of woe for him. So he chose to go by a variation he crafted from his last name—Jaxon—not only as a shield from teasing, but also as a name out of the ordinary. Years later at the Disney Studios, where everyone was on a first-name basis, most of the staff did not know that he had a name other than Jaxon, except for those few who called him Jack, Willy, Will, or Bill.

He grew up an only child in a family with a dad who stayed at home—due to ill health—and a mother who taught piano lessons. The family apparently did not have much money. But occasionally they went to the movies, and one time, Jaxon—let's call him by his preferred name—saw an Aesop's Fables cartoon. He said, "Boy, I went through the roof, that was the most wonderful thing I'd ever seen. That was what I had to do, there was no question about it."[3] He was bitten by the animation bug and made flip-books out of discarded stubs of Red Car transfer books and the corners of his textbooks (just like this book's coauthor!). He invented a comic strip called *The Adventures of Jim Coote*; it starred a stick figure character that was easy for Jaxon to animate.

Portrait of the artist as a young man: Wilfred Jaxon, with a career in animation just over the horizon. Natha Horbach collection.

During these formative years, he also developed a passion for music and film. These were the days of silent films with live music accompaniment. Displaying an intensity and thoroughness that was a prelude to his later directorial style, he sat through two or three showings of a film. He first sat in the middle of the theater for the best view of the film. At intermission, he moved to a seat directly behind the organist, "where I could look down at him in the orchestra pit to see everything he was doing or look up past him to see what he was watching on the screen. This man was one of my boyhood idols."[4] Later he had a chance to work with musicians like Frank Churchill and Leigh Harline, and Ollie Wallace, who had been a famed theater organist in the Seattle area before writing many Disney hit songs, and he said, "You can easily see it meant something very special to me to actually take part in putting together the action and the music for Walt's cartoons."[5]

Jaxon attended Otis Art Institute from September 1925 to January 1928. Through a contact at Otis, Jaxon learned that Walt Disney had an animation studio nearby in Hollywood. He called the studio, and Walt answered the phone! Jaxon brought his samples to show Walt. As he recalled, "Walt wasn't the least bit impressed with the samples that I brought and said very candidly that I needed to have a little bit more training before I would be able to go ahead. I was simply not a good enough draftsman."[6] After a lengthy discussion, during which Jaxon asked Walt to recommend art classes to learn animation (there were none), and offered to work for free or to pay Walt the

PALLETTE SCRAPINGS
OTIS ART INSTITUTE
MAY 20, 1927 LOS ANGELES CALIF.
OW! - GEE - GET OFF MY SUNBURN! WELL YOU MIGHT KNOW MY SHOULDER WOULD BE SORE! LOOK OUT NOW—!
AW- THAT AINT SUNBURN, THAT'S WHERE I BRUISED MY LEG ON A ROCK. HUH? WELL WATTA I CARE IF YOU BELEIVE ME!
WHAT WAS THE NAME OF THAT SUNBURN REMEDY AGAIN?
YEH, I GOT AWFUL RED, BUT I'M NOT REALLY SO SORE,- OW! - WELL, YOU DIDN'T HAVE TO TRY IT, GEE WHIZ!
I TOLD YOU NOT TO EAT SO MUCH! FOR LUNCH IF YOU WOULD ONLY LISTEN TO MY ADVICE—
SAY, QUIT KICK'N' THE BACK O' MY HEAD. HOW D'YA EXPECT ME TO DRIVE? DO YA WANNA ALL LAND IN THE DITCH?
AH SHUT UP!
SANTA MONICA
JAXON
BRINGING HOME THE BAKING, OR THE OTESIAN'S RETURN,
15

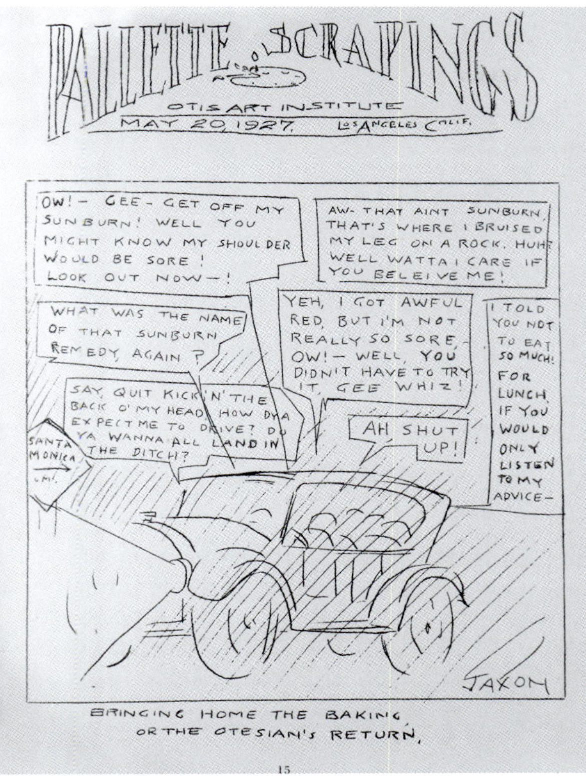

An example of Jaxon's work from Otis Art Institute. Natha Horbach collection.

cost of tuition to learn animation ("We couldn't do that"), Walt finally said, "Oh, hell! I'll hire you for a week to see if you can do anything worthwhile." Walt followed up with "After a week, I don't know if there's going to be a studio here."[7] It was a propitious beginning to a career of over thirty-three years, which started during the last week a group of animators worked at Disney before they left to work for rival Charles Mintz, who had exerted creative control over Oswald the Lucky Rabbit from Walt in a power play. Jaxon was employee number thirteen. The day he met Walt was Jaxon's lucky day.

While at Otis, Jaxon had met Jane Ames, also a student there, and she became the love of his life. In the spring of 1929, while he worked at the Disney Studios: "We just got married one evening and I went to work the next day as usual. You see, in the spring of '29 the little studio was awfully busy, and so I didn't feel secure enough to ask for time off."[8] The couple became a family with two daughters, Virginia and Barbara. They lived on three acres of land in Sunland and had a small beach house on Balboa Island, where they lived during their golden years.

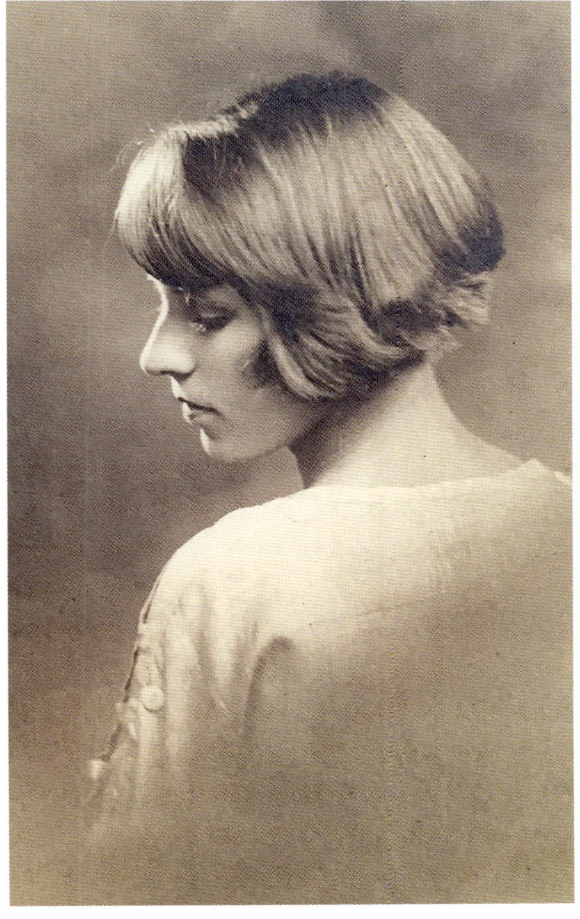

Jane Ames Jackson. Natha Horbach collection.

AS AN ANIMATOR

Jaxon began his career helping the janitor sort reusable cels (clear celluloid sheets). He graduated to painting cels and then began his climb up the rungs of the animation ladder. Jaxon felt in hindsight that with the studio's shortage of help after the Oswald defections, he moved from rung to rung too soon; he was always in the process of mastering one task when he was moved to the next, "like from painting to inking, from inking to inbetweening, from inbetweening to animation."[9] Jaxon recalled in a 1978 interview: "I didn't realize it, but I wasn't keeping up with the competition, with my animation. I really had a pretty good opinion of my animation and thought it was all right, and I wanted to animate a whole picture myself. I thought that would be a great thing, to sit there and see the whole picture go by, and every scene in it would be my animation."[10] But in a 1929 letter to Jane, he had doubts. "I am really worried about my animating—it is going so slowly. Walt is watching me closely, I know, for every morning and often, when I return from lunch, the drawings I have finished are not lying just as I left them. I am afraid that Walt will get the idea that my work is slowing down. . . . I saw that very thing happen to Johnny [Cannon, another young animator], and once Walt got the idea that Johnny wasn't learning as fast as he had started out to, everything was interpreted in its worst light, with the result that Johnny, although he was still working just as hard as he ever had—and was, I believe, advancing as fast as ever—was held back, and I was given a chance to go ahead. I have felt all along that I have been a special pet of Walt's, which is too important a thing to regard lightly, and what happened to Johnny must not be allowed to happen to me."[11]

INNOVENTIONS

At a gag meeting for an upcoming cartoon short, Walt told his staff of artists that he had just learned about sound-on-film. Walt said, "I wonder if there's a way that we could put sound with cartoons? I know how fast the film is going to go. The film is going to go ninety feet a minute. But how in hell do you tell how fast the music is going to go? How do you know how fast the sound is going to go?"[12] Jackson, still relatively new at the studio, spoke up. He knew from his mother's piano lessons how a metronome worked. "I can show you how fast music will go."[13] He brought in his mother's metronome and set it to tick once every eight frames or twelve frames. He played a tune on his harmonica, and Walt could see how fast the music went. It was on that basis that *Steamboat Willie* was planned.

It shouldn't be too much of a surprise that Jaxon succeeded as a director, because even from the very beginning of his career at Disney, he was innovative. In addition to his contribution to the synchronization of sounds, which, incidentally, became the industry standard and confounded rival studios for over a year, Jaxon invented what was first called a dope sheet and later a bar sheet. (SEE SIDEBAR ON PAGES 28–31.) The bar sheet also made its debut during the production of *Steamboat Willie*.

Filming pencil tests (animation was drawn on paper with a pencil before inked onto cels) had been one of the hallmarks of Disney animation techniques almost from the beginning. When Jaxon was directing, he came up with the idea to assemble multiple scenes together so that an entire sequence or even an entire film could be viewed for the flow of action and continuity. With the addition of sound effects

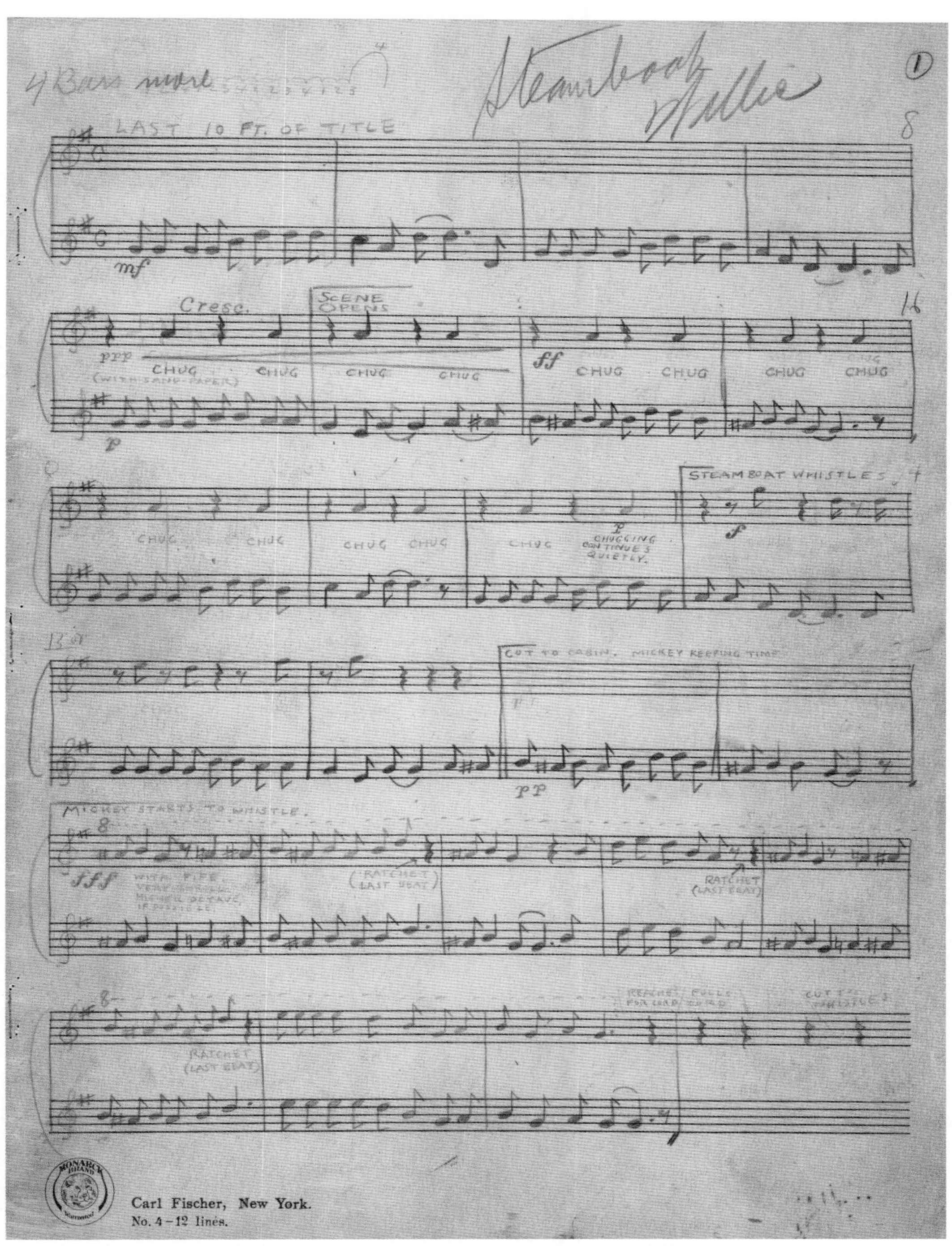

Jaxon prepared the music for *Steamboat Willie*, which became the de facto bar sheet, but with music staves. He marked the first 4 measures with an "8," which would make each measure 2 beats. A metronome setting of 180 would make this a 2-16 beat (though they hadn't formalized that signature yet).

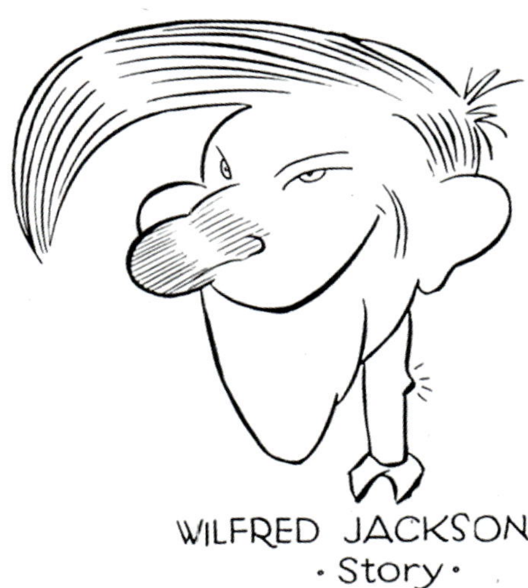

Jack King's 1931 caricature of Jaxon from *Motion Picture Daily* magazine.

and a dialogue track, synchronization could be checked as well. Jaxon called these "running reels" and put them together as soon as Walt had approved his timing of action, the musician's proposed scoring, and the layout man's staging of action. For a later, more refined version of the running reel, "we shot running test footage of the storyboard sketches, with each one timed so as to sync with the sound and indicate in a general way the action that was to be animated. This way, as the very first animation tests began to be cut into the reel, these test scenes could be viewed as part of the visual continuity of the entire cartoon picture."[14] The running reels helped both the director and Walt oversee the productions.

DISNEY DIRECTOR

Jaxon liked to say that he became a director through a misunderstanding: "I caught Walt in a real good mood one time and I said, 'Walt, if it should ever work out this way, I'd like it if you would let me handle a whole picture myself.' I didn't realize it at the time, but I had given him the wrong idea. When I said 'handle,' I meant 'animate.' But it meant 'direct' to Walt and we never did get this misunderstanding cleared up."[15]

The film turned out to be *The Castaway* (1931), a mishmash of discarded scenes from earlier shorts that Jaxon was tasked with weaving together into a coherent story. Walt was behind schedule, and this was an opportunity to test a new director and a new musician, Frank Churchill, on a less costly cartoon. (Frank Churchill went on to write the music for *Three Little Pigs*, *Snow White*, *Dumbo*, *Bambi*, and much more.)

Jaxon came up with a theme for his first short: "With the diversity that was there, the only idea I could come up with was if Mickey was on a boat like Robinson Crusoe that was shipwrecked on a desert island and a lot of stuff from the ship washed ashore. That might account for the fact that he had a grand piano, that he had some adventures with a lion and with a monkey, and I forget what else. It was a hodgepodge of stuff. That was the only way that I could see to tie it together. So Walt okayed that and we put it through."[16] Jaxon thought he was going to animate the whole cartoon all by himself, but Walt had other ideas. Every time Jaxon started to animate, Walt asked him to give the scene to an idle animator. Jaxon learned of his destiny when Walt said, "'Have you thought any more about your next story? You know, you're going to have a lot of men out of work. You're going to have to hand out some scenes to them.' That's how I discovered that I had become a director. So after that, I was so busy trying to keep scenes coming out to the animators that I didn't have much time for anything else."[17]

Jaxon said for a variety of reasons—his lack of experience, the quality and diversity of the available footage—"the result was not anything that overwhelmed the audience." His description of Walt and Roy in the theater lobby after the short previewed is cinematic.

> I went out in the lobby and there was Walt over in one corner. He had his overcoat all up around his ears and he had his hat clear down over his eyes and he had his hands in his pockets with his shoulders up around his ears. Roy was talking to him. There was a little crowd of animators around him and I walked unobtrusively past. I didn't stop, but on the way by, I could hear Roy saying, "But Walt, it doesn't look like a Disney picture. I don't know if we ought to release it." Walt said, "We've got to release it to meet our schedule, Roy." And Roy was saying, "But Walt—"[18]

Despite the preview reactions, Jaxon was now a full-fledged director. But he came into the role of a director without the training and expertise that others brought to that position. Burt Gillett, Dave Hand, Ben Sharpsteen, Gerry Geronimi, Jack King, Bill Roberts, Norm Ferguson—all had experience as animators at other studios

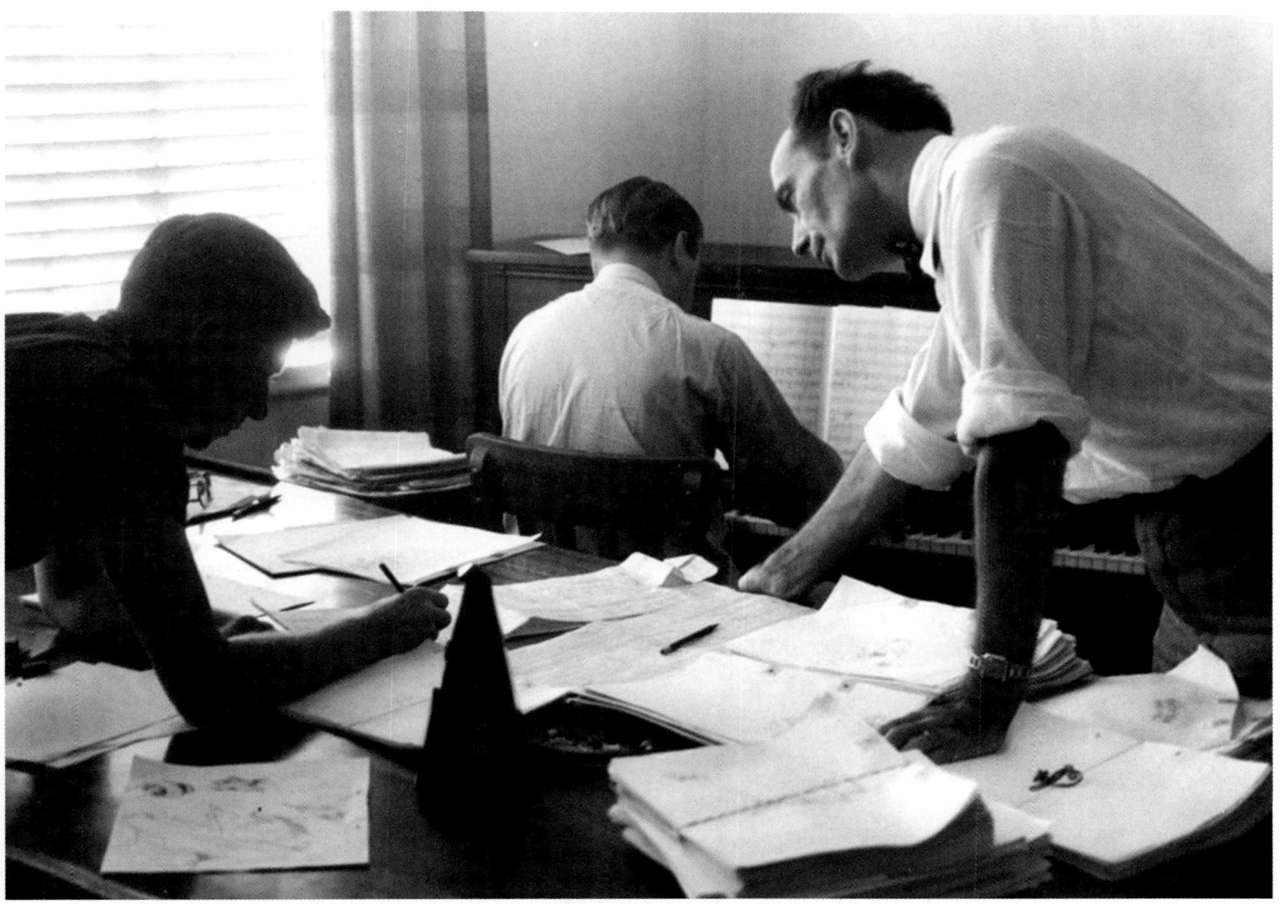

Jaxon (LEFT), Hugh Hennesy, and musician Leigh Harline. Note the metronome in the foreground.

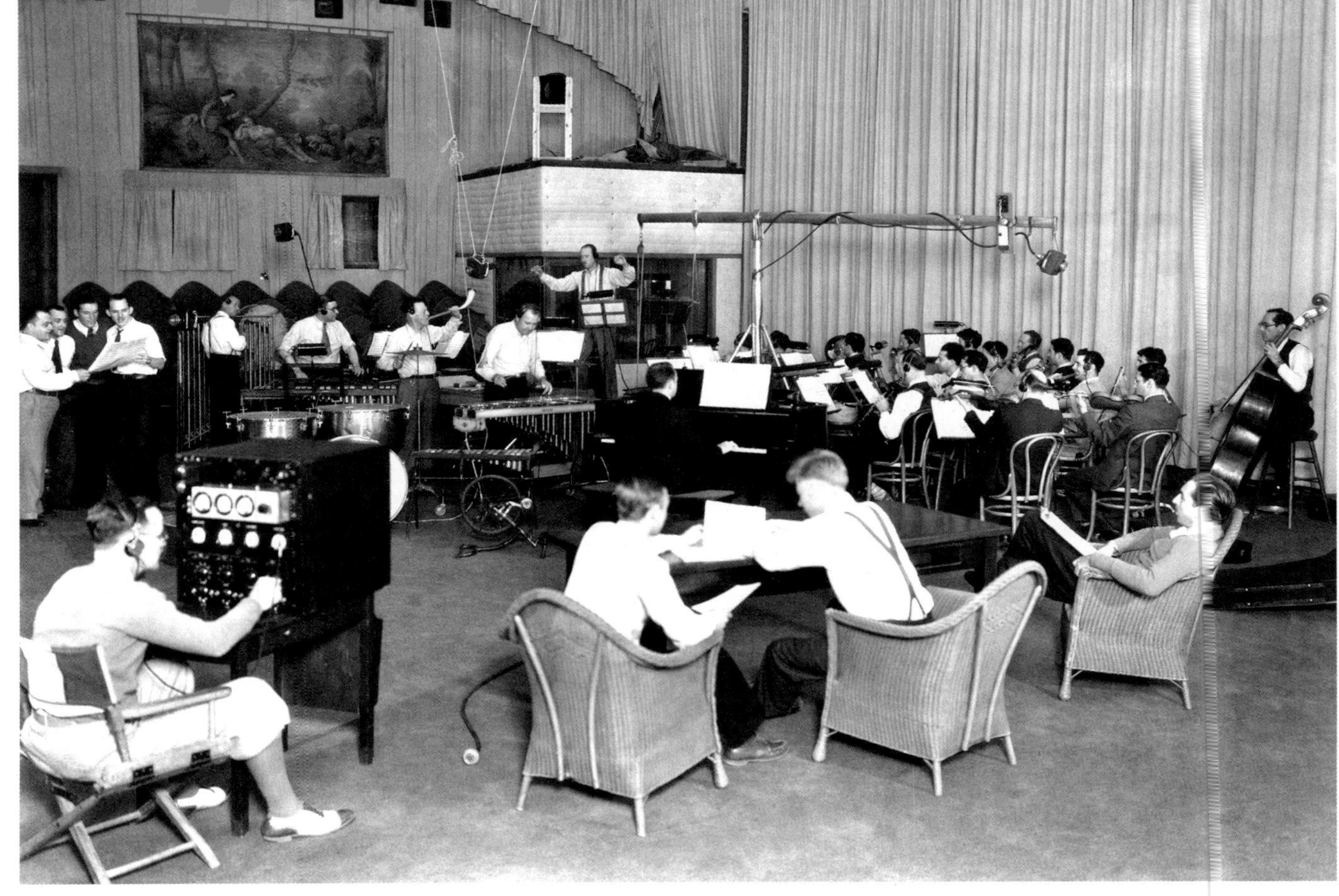

IN FOREGROUND: Audio engineer Bill Garity at mixing console, animator Earl Duval, Jaxon (with suspenders), Walt. Frank Churchill conducts.

before coming to Disney. Ub Iwerks, Ham Luske, and Woolie Reitherman had proven themselves as animators at Disney first, and Jack Kinney, Jack Hannah, and Nick Nichols had extensive experience both in animation and story work before becoming directors.

Jaxon said, "A director is supposed to have some ideas of his own about the picture he is directing, and we all did, too—that is, if we had enough time to think about it at our own speed."[19] He described himself as a "plough horse," in contrast to the other directors, who were "race horses." He said, "I could whip myself up and I could get to the finish line all right, if it didn't matter who got there first, but I did what I did by working harder and longer than the other fellows. . . ."[20] He could visualize his films on the screen and the central action as it related to the story, but he couldn't do it as fast as Walt could, and he often found himself thinking of how he should have responded only after Walt had made his suggestions and left the room. He sometimes reviewed footage before Walt saw it to try to level the playing field or, as he said, "it was more like giving a tortoise a short lead, or handicap, in a race with a hare."[21] (Jaxon, by the way, directed *The Tortoise and the Hare*.) His inability for quick analysis plagued him years later when he was assigned to television programming, with its high-speed demands.

A great deal of creative work was done before the animator began his work. Once the animator was ready to receive the assignment, collaboration between Jaxon and the animator became intense. "When the animator came in . . . I would go over with the animator, before I made the timing, . . . the layouts and get his ideas on it. If things in it didn't seem to suit him too well, we'd try to work his ideas and his feeling of presentation into it, to the extent that it seemed compatible with what I understood was wanted. So it was give and take, every step of the way."[22]

Coordinating the work of one animator with another or creating a smooth transition from one scene to another was a crucial task facing the director. Jaxon described this many-faceted challenge:

> From a director's point of view, it was not a simple thing to take a talented artist—who was good, and who knew it—and to somehow or other work with him and get a thing that would fit with what a musician could do, and would also be coordinated with what the other artists would do, so that there wouldn't be too much of a change of character, or timing, or feeling, from where one animator left off and another picked up on another scene, and at the same time, to try to get what Walt wanted on the screen, which wasn't always the easiest thing to understand, in the first place.[23]

He tried to reconcile excellent animation with the need for smooth transitions. This often led to clashes with the animators, and Jaxon recalled such a clash with the highly talented, but often contentious, Art Babbitt:

> I remember one time Art Babbitt got real exasperated, and we were in sweatbox,[24] and there were some things he just had to change, and he just didn't want to. Finally, I said, "Art, you've got to change them." He said, "I'm not going to." I said, "Well, then there's just one thing we can do. Why don't we get Walt in, and we'll let him decide this?" And Art said, "Oh, I'll do it, but you know, you just simply aren't qualified to be a director, Jackson." I said, "Well, Art, you're probably right, but since I am the director, what I say has to be done, whether it's right or not, so you've got to make the change." I worked with these people for whom I had so much respect for what they could do. They could do animation that I wouldn't be able to do, and yet I was in a position of having to tell them what changes to make. It was difficult.[25]

In deference to Art Babbitt, years later he told Disney historian Michael Barrier, "Let me just settle this Jackson thing. He was the top director."[26]

The relationship between director and animator was often contentious, despite the fact that the directors had all been animators once themselves. Wilfred Jackson told a story about Dick Huemer, who "used to come out of sweatbox mumbling, 'These doggone directors! You do a nice job of animation and they want the thing changed. You go into sweatbox and you can't win. You just can't win.' And I'd hear his voice going off down the hall. Then Dick got to direct two pictures [*The Whalers* and *Goofy and Wilbur*], and I heard Dick saying, as he came out of sweatbox: 'These lousy animators! You hand out a good scene to them and they turn in some

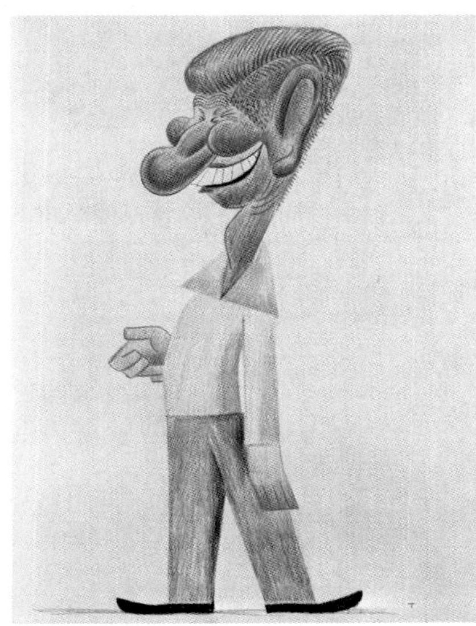

Jaxon by T. Hee.

other thing and then they don't want to fix it up. You can't win. You go into sweatbox with a bunch of animators and you can't win, you just can't win!' "[27]

THE DIRECTOR AS A CHOREOGRAPHER

Reflecting on the changing role of the Disney director over the decades, Jaxon theorized, "I wonder if it would not be fair to say that in the thirties a Disney cartoon director functioned more nearly as a choreographer than as a director since his attention was devoted so much to relating action to music, and then in the fifties, he was more fully functioning as a director, with a transition period somewhere in between."[28]

Jaxon loved to direct musical pictures. In a 1939 studio lecture, he distinguished between a musical score, which all cartoon shorts had, and a musical picture, as "one in which the action is planned to the music, as compared to a picture where the music is written after the action is completed."[29] In one kind of musical picture the characters play musical instruments; a classic example is Jackson's *The Band Concert*. Musicals in which the music was subservient to the action include *The Tortoise and The Hare*, *Water Babies*, and *Santa's Workshop*—all Jaxon films. He excelled at directing musical pictures. He explained why:

> I especially enjoyed working with the musicians in planning out and timing the pictures. Their music contributed so very much to the *feeling* of the picture. I wanted every part of my picture to be worked out in such a way that the music and action would enhance each other—not just the different elements running along parallel lines harmoniously, but a wedding of the two—a fusing of the two into a new thing that would become something more than just music plus action.[30]

CHANNELING WALT

All the directors were dedicated to bringing Walt's vision for a cartoon to the screen. Some were more than others, but this was inevitably their goal. Jaxon, as can be imagined, was particularly dedicated to fulfilling Walt's dream for his pictures:

> My own contribution to Walt, and to the studio, was not so much that I was a great idea man or had any particular talent or ability at direction. I think I was fairly successful in understanding what Walt wanted, and I worked awfully hard trying to get that on the screen. It did something to me as an individual: I had to suppress myself quite a bit. And I came out the other end of it a little bit lost when I dissociated myself from the studio, because I had tried so hard, for so long, to get what Walt wanted on the screen.[31]

He did go on to say that he put up the best argument he could when he disagreed with Walt, but would often give in. He said all the directors had their own creative ideas and wanted to include them, but in the last analysis, they knew they were making Walt Disney pictures. Walt was allowing him to be part of the creative world of the Disney Studios, and that was most important to him. "I thoroughly enjoyed the privilege of working closely with those wonderfully creative people as *they* would bring to life one part or another of a picture Walt had let *me* direct. For me, working at the Disney Studios in the thirties was like being a kid having Christmas every day of the year." He elaborated: "I think the outstanding thing about Walt was his ability to make people feel that what he wanted done was a terribly important thing to get done. We all wanted so much to please him with what we did, and to get what he wanted, in the pictures. It just seemed like the most important thing in the world. He was a very inspiring guy. I guess probably he was the best salesman in the world."[32]

A SHORT SELECTION

Wilfred Jackson directed thirty-five shorts. Most of the cartoon shorts were in the Silly Symphony series, and he directed three Academy Award winners: *The Tortoise and the Hare*, *The Country Cousin*, and *The Old Mill*. Jaxon stressed that the goal of fitting the music to the climax of *The Tortoise and the Hare* was a way of building excitement. Jaxon's short from the Mickey Mouse series, *The Band Concert*, has become a classic for its wonderful synchronization of action and music, and of characterization and music. In a lecture discussion about the scene in the short in which the music and action reverse in the middle of the cyclone, Jaxon pointed out the importance of building a gag to get maximum value:

> As I remember, the first time Walt talked about the story to me, that gag was in there, although I'm not sure about it. I think that the music suggested that gag. It winds up, stops, then unwinds. It is a natural if you listen to the music. I would like to point out something . . . I believe that if you came into the theater at the time the cyclone was first picking them up, you wouldn't get a laugh. It built up from the first of the picture. That mood—that the musicians in the band would play "William Tell" in spite of anything—carried through the picture had a lot to do with it being a funny spot towards the end.[33]

After the preview of *The Country Cousin*, Walt said to Jaxon, "That's a good picture, Jack." Jaxon said that a direct compliment from Walt was rare and "I don't think I came down out of the clouds for a couple of years."[34] The other Disney directors thought Jaxon was crazy to attempt to make *The Old Mill*, with no story and no characters to speak of. It was perceived as an experiment to explore something other than personality or character, and also a chance to test the multiplane camera (although because of scheduling conflicts, little of it was shot before the camera was used for *Snow White*).

ANIMATED FEATURES IN THE GOLDEN AGE

Jaxon said that the shorts directors took it for granted that they would be part of the directing pool on *Snow White*. He was one of the last directors assigned to it, because he was busy with *The Old Mill* and other shorts. Jaxon felt that this first feature was handled differently from any other feature at the studio. He explained why:

> The directors of *Snow White* didn't direct in the same way as they did on other pictures. In effect, Walt really directed that picture, he was so intensely involved in everything about it. And he was right in on everything that was done, right down to what color a character was painted. On *Snow White*, Walt was in on every last detail, it was Walt's picture, one hundred percent from beginning to end. That can't be said of any other picture that I've worked with him on after the very, very early Mickeys and Silly Symphonies.[35]

He said it was actually a step back in a sense, because Walt had been paying a little less attention to the shorts while the feature was in development, so consequently the directors had more latitude. But on this film, Walt was more intently involved. Jaxon said that various people made decisions on the film, but everything was reviewed by Walt before it got into the picture. *Snow White*, more than any, was a Walt Disney picture.

> If anybody wants to know what a Walt Disney picture is, I'll say, "Look at *Snow White and the Seven Dwarfs*," because that picture, while it lacks the superb technique of the later animation—it was the best we could do with the human characters, with what we had to work with, and the time we had to work on it—but in spite of that, the heart that's in the picture is the thing that Walt could put in a picture.[36]

Jaxon directed the entertainment sequence in which the Dwarfs and Snow White sing and dance at their cottage. He also had the last scenes of the feature, beginning with the "death" scene of Snow White and the Dwarfs reacting. That scene brought an unprecedented emotional response from many in the premiere audience, who had laughed and cheered earlier and now wept.

As the studio moved on to *Pinocchio* and the other films of the forties, Walt began to pull back. He said he never again wanted to work as hard as he had on *Snow White*, so he began gradually removing himself from day-to-day decisions and expecting his directors and staff of artists to take over more of the decision-making. As Jackson put it, "he was looking for a way of letting 'us mice' carry the ball ourselves, but with enough help and supervision from him to see to it that the pictures came out looking the way he wanted them to. He hadn't lost interest in the cartoons, but in time he began to become interested in doing some other things, too, and felt the organization could be set up in such a way as to eventually produce "Disney" cartoons almost on its own."[37] In place of Walt's intimate involvement, a team effort of story people, key animators, and other directors came into prominence. In the early forties, Dave Hand and Ben Sharpsteen, as supervising directors, played a strong role in these efforts, but as the decade progressed, Dave was gone, and Ben was busy with the True-Life Adventures. Jaxon felt that the substitution of a team's collective vision for Walt's vision became gradually apparent in the feature films:

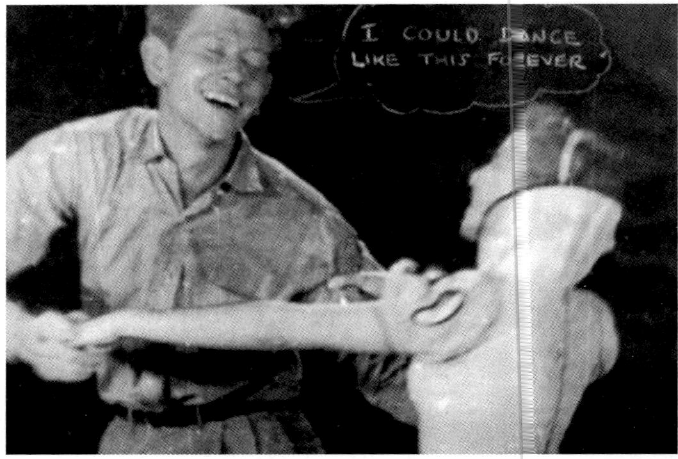

Reference footage of Jaxon and Marjorie Belcher (Champion) shot for *Snow White*. This showed up for years with gag captions provided by co-workers.

> And it's my personal opinion that this accounts a great deal for some of the difference in the spirit and the heart that you see in the pictures during the thirties—that gradually, it got a little less evident until it got to the point, in my estimation, where the Disney pictures became superb technically, but a little lacking in a joyous creative spirit you'll find in those early pictures. As time went on, it was more and more diluted by the influence of others.[38]

For *Pinocchio*, Jaxon directed the scenes of Geppetto carving the marionette, Pinocchio going to school, the marionette show, Geppetto awaiting Pinocchio's return, Stromboli imprisoning Pinocchio, and Geppetto searching for Pinocchio. He argued with Walt about the deletion of a scene where Pinocchio is teased at school because he is a wooden boy. Jaxon felt that Pinocchio being an outcast was "the guts

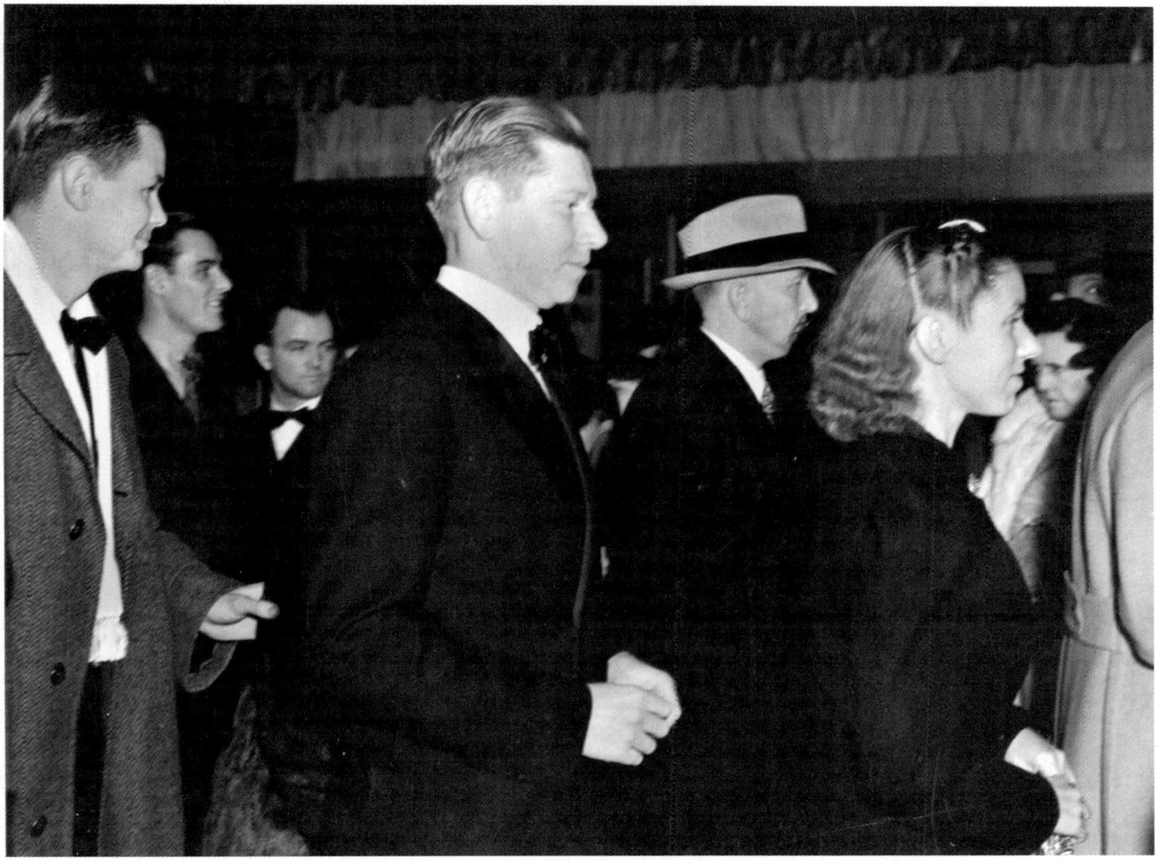

Jaxon and Jane in line for the premiere of *Snow White* (December 21, 1937). Natha Horbach collection.

of the whole story" and would have made his transition into a real boy at the end mean more. The scene was cut because the picture was too long, but Jaxon said, "I guess it was about the biggest argument I ever had with him, and about the best one I ever lost."[39]

Jaxon directed the powerful "Night on Bald Mountain" sequence in *Fantasia*, working with the legendary animator Vladimir "Bill" Tytla. Unhappy with live-action reference footage of *Dracula*'s aging Bela Lugosi (although Tytla may have captured Lugosi's expressions and fine gestures in his animation), Tytla convinced skinny Wilfred Jackson to take off his shirt and pose for him as the diabolical Chernabog.

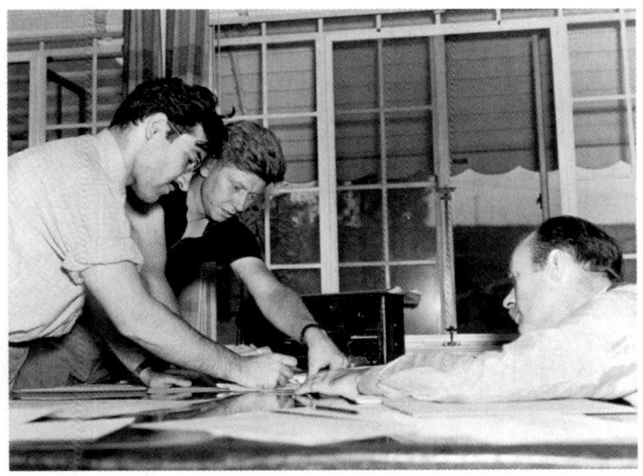

Animator Bill Tytla (FAR LEFT), Jaxon, and composer Frank Churchill on *Pinocchio*, circa 1938.

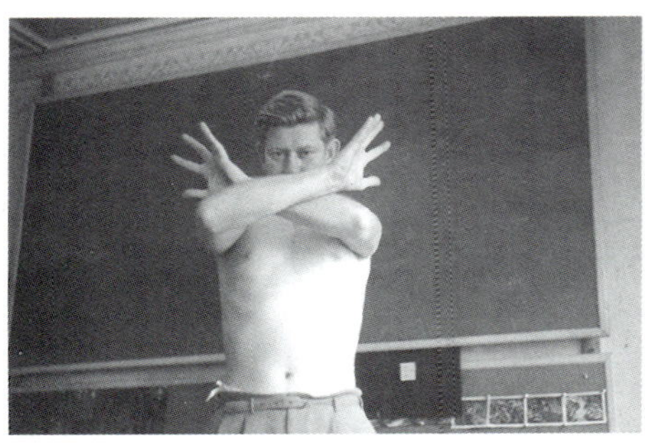

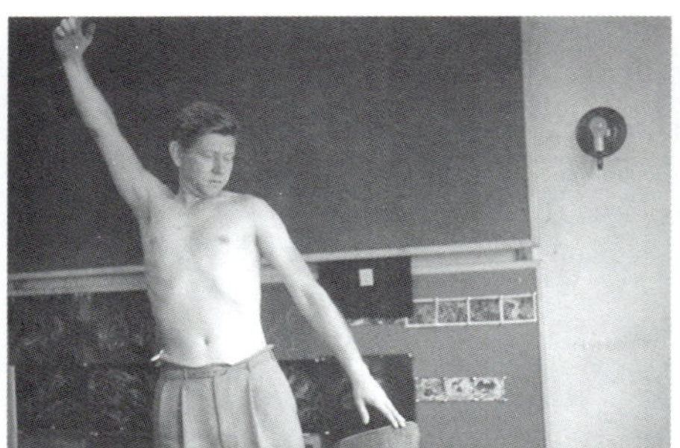

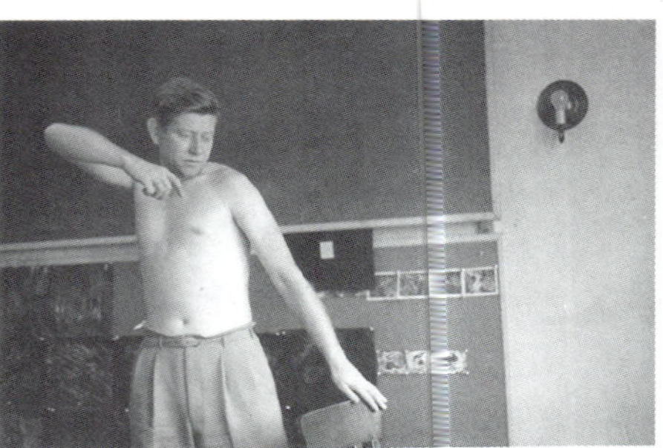

4-1-82

DEAR DON -

SEEMS KIND OF REDICULOUS TO THINK ANYTHING THIS SKINNY KID DID COULD SERVE AS AN INSPIRATION FOR WHAT BILL TYTLA DID WITH HIS ANIMATION IN NIGHT ON BALD MOUNTAIN DOESN'T IT?

PLEASE SEND THEM BACK WHEN YOU'RE THROUGH WITH THEM.

YOURS -

JAXON

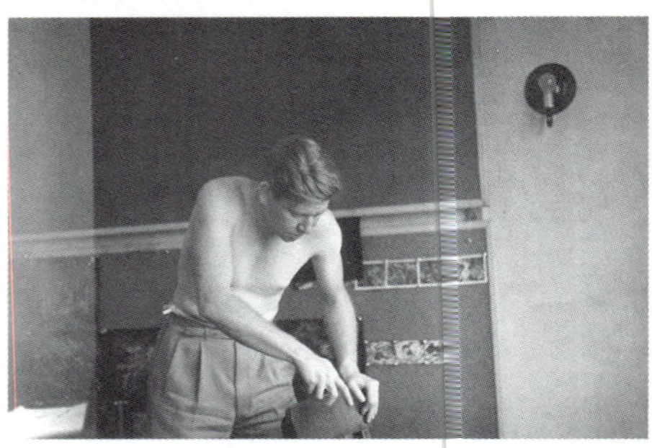

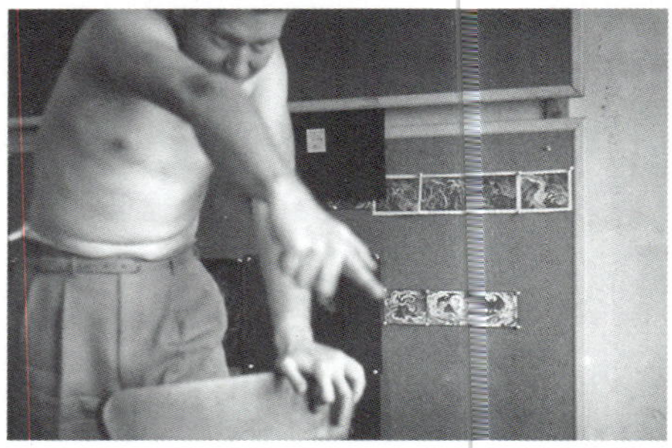

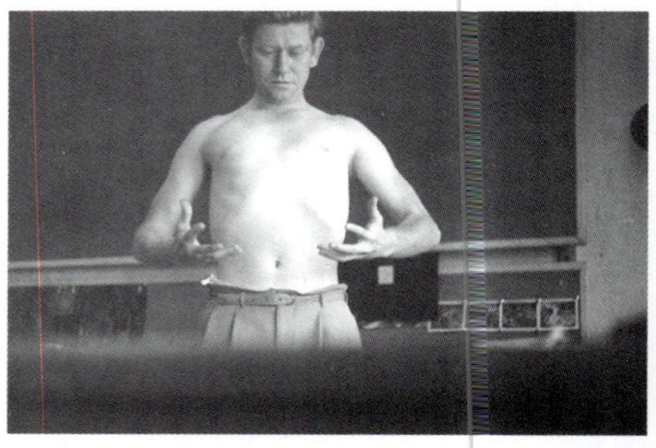

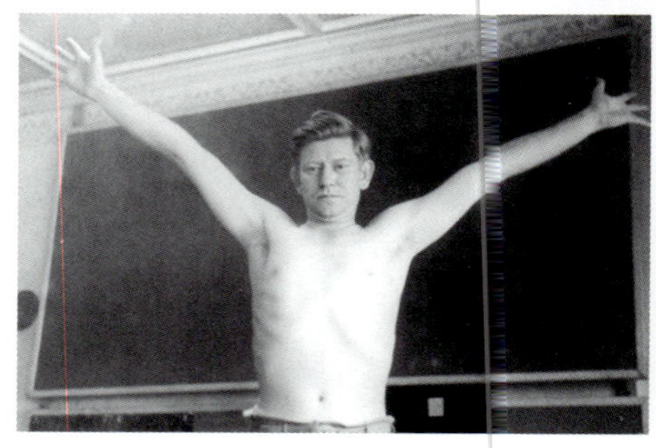

These photostats of a shirtless Jackson "went viral" at the studio and over the years took on a mythological stature, only recently brought to light in books and on websites, to the delight of all who have seen them.

Jaxon also directed the "Ave Maria" sequence, an unexpected additional assignment that came with orders to "get it out in a hell of a hurry and be sure not to disturb Stokowski's music because it was sacred."[40] Sacred or not, Jaxon was compelled to cut a repetitious musical segment that conflicted with the pacing of his story. He hit resistance at every turn (musician Ed Plumb "blanched") and resorted to devious measures to make the needed cut, physically removing the segment and asking the cutters to "repair" the film. When he showed the story reel with the revised music to Leopold Stokowski, the conductor accepted it, and a crisis was averted.

Jaxon next directed sequences on *Dumbo*. Bill Tytla served as an animation director, which took pressure off Jaxon. This new position enabled the studio to stretch the talents of the valuable top animators by having them animate crucial scenes and then oversee the work of other animators on the same character. The role was an important part of all future feature productions.

WORLD WAR II

As the studio plunged into training, health and sanitation, and educational films with the advent of World War II, Jaxon was equally swept up in the studio effort to do its part for the war effort. Impossible deadlines, highly sensitive subject matter, and limited animation techniques suspended the well-oiled Disney animation machine for the duration, and films were made with as much quality as time and circumstances would allow. On one film for the Royal Air Force, the subject involved the use of light patterns to aid bombers. It was a high-pressure assignment, and then, suddenly, it was canceled, and Jaxon had to burn everything related to the film in the presence of military personnel. Jaxon said, "I wept for a day and slept for a week. What I didn't know was that Ike [General Dwight Eisenhower] was planning to go into Normandy, and the pattern bombings weren't necessary anymore."[41]

The New Spirit was an important 1942 film for the U.S. Treasury to help motivate people—fifteen million new taxpayers, to boot—to pay their income taxes on time to support the war. Working under what in peacetime would have been considered an impossible deadline—four weeks for the entire production—directors Jaxon and Ben Sharpsteen and crew worked around the clock. Every corner was cut; sequencing of work was shortened or bypassed to reach the deadline.

Jaxon was concerned about how Walt would react. He felt that by their standards, the resulting film was very poor. Jaxon recalls the moment the lights came on in the screening room: "I didn't say anything. He didn't say anything. Finally, he turned around and said, 'Jack, ah. . . .' He rubbed his head. 'You know . . .

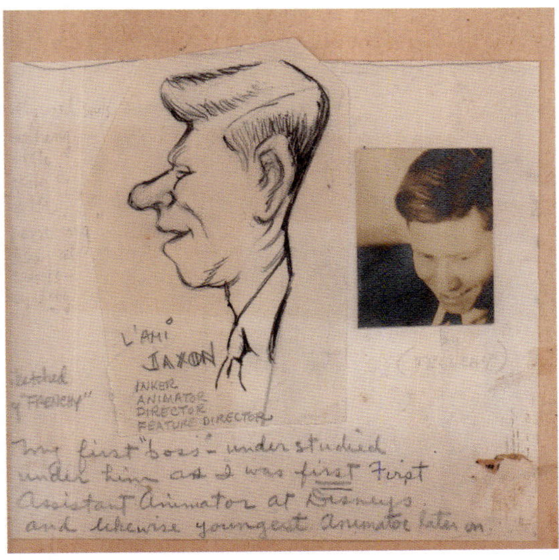

Caricature and photo by Jaxon animator Gilles "Frenchy" de Trémaudan from his sketchbook.

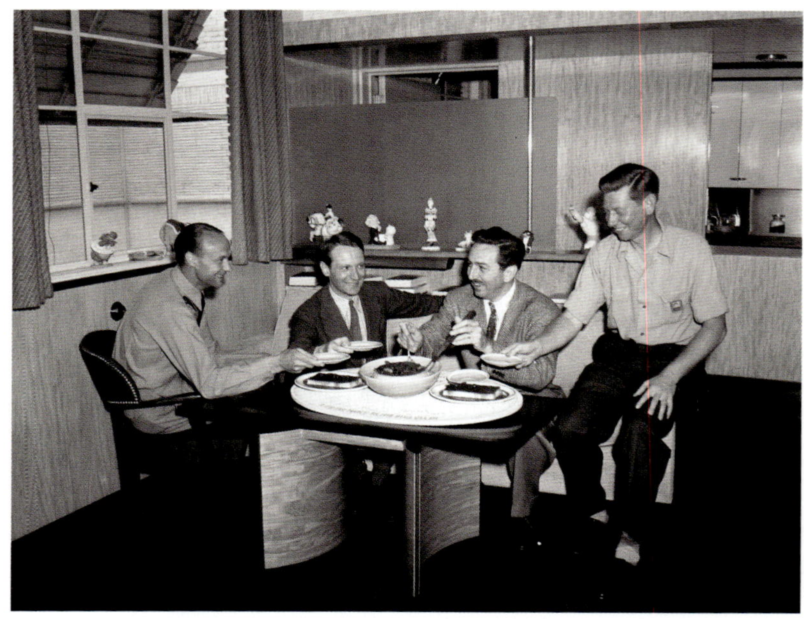

Walt and Jaxon (RIGHT OF WALT) and two unidentified people lunch in Walt's office.

Well, Jack . . .' He shifted in his seat. He got up and said with finality, 'Yeah.' And he walked out."[42]

During the war, Jaxon decided to start a work diary. He regretted not having started one years earlier. But for this decision, at this time, he wrote, "[I] began [this] diary because schedule and budget on US Navy Training films was getting all fouled up by circumstances over which I had no control—and I wanted some record of what was happening in case anybody started asking questions."[43] Jaxon kept this diary—not a daily record by any means—from 1943 until 1959, when he separated from the studio. Some of his entries are so typical of the emotional spectrum experienced by directors in a large studio that Pete Docter said, "If you changed the names and dates, they could have happened today." Emotional highs and lows are captured on paper, and Jaxon was frank about the disappointments and foreboding he was feeling as the studio moved on to television and what seemed like a myriad of other projects and he saw his opportunities and contributions waning. Jaxon's entry for March 15, 1944, is tantalizing and mysterious:

> [I] saw Walt [who told me] I am to pick up a short to get back into the swing (of directing) [and that the] organization must go ahead without depending on Walt. In five years he will pull free of it. Walt will be out of animation by '49.[44]

SONG OF THE SOUTH

Wilfred Jackson found his happy place when he was directing the animated sequences in the live-action/animated hybrid film based on Joel Chandler Harris's collection of folktales. He recalled, "I think that the happiest time I ever had working on any picture, after the first few early years, was on the *Song of the South*. That was a wonderful experience for me. I'll tell you why it was a wonderful experience: Walt was again very closely, personally involved with what we were doing. This was his first venture into live-action features and he was quite interested in the outcome. This meant that Walt was working very closely with us and this always made a thing really exciting."[45]

Jackson was especially impressed with the talents of actor James Baskett, who played Uncle Remus. His ability to synchronize his acting with animation to be added later was something Jaxon had never seen before. "I have never worked with any other actor, on combination scenes, who could do what old Jim Baskett did; and the man was dying."[46] Baskett received a special Oscar at the 1948 Academy Awards (the first Black male to receive an Academy Award) for "his able and heartwarming characterization of Uncle Remus, friend and storyteller to the children of the world." He passed away less than four months later at the age of forty-four.

Walt became aware of Mary Blair's style during the trip to South America to gather production material for *Saludos Amigos*, and he wanted her styling to be incorporated into these postwar films. Mary's style was wonderful for inspirational drawings for the films, but it was difficult to translate its flat two-dimensional style into fully rendered characters that populated Disney films at that time. Walt criticized Jaxon for not getting enough of her style into this film

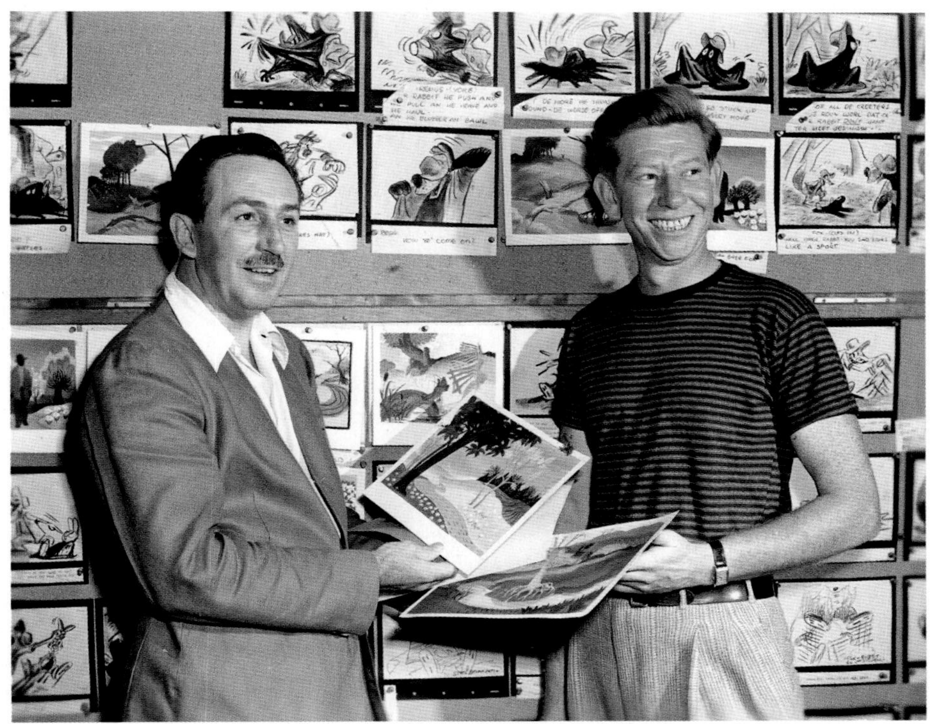

Walt and Jaxon on *Song of the South* in September 1946.

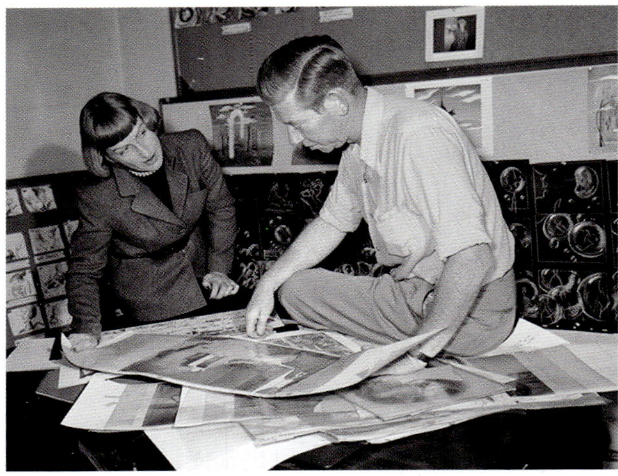

Mary Blair and Jaxon work together again on *Cinderella*.

but then getting too much of it into the "Johnny Appleseed" segment of *Melody Time*.

WORKING WITH WILFRED

By the late forties and early fifties, Walt's interests expanded outside of animation, and consequently more was asked of his directors as he was available less and less frequently. But Jaxon's strong work ethic enabled him to continue to work creatively within the confines of the studio system as Walt's presence was less intimate. Warner Bros. animator/director Bob Clampett likened the creative relationship between Walt and Jaxon to that of two storied figures from the live-action studios:

> [The relationship between Walt and Jaxon] sounds very similar to the way a director at Fox would work, like John Ford would work with [Darryl] Zanuck. Zanuck would set a story, develop the screenplay, assign it to John Ford, and then John Ford would make the film. Ford's work is considered very creative, even though he was handed a story, and Zanuck looked over his shoulder in certain respects. So, in some respects, I think you can consider a Jackson picture in the same context.[47]

Animator Milt Gray and Michael Barrier heard Jaxon's self-effacing opinion of his lack of qualifications when they interviewed him, and Gray observed, "It's amazing to me that the one guy in the studio who felt the least qualified is the one guy who ends up being remembered by everybody as the best, the most helpful, the most congenial—it's amazing." Jaxon responded, "It's odd to hear that, because there were complaints about me; there were animators who went to Walt and complained that I was too domineering, that I pushed them around too much, that I didn't give the animators a chance to do what they wanted to do." Gray continued: "What they [other animators] say to us is that sometimes you thought things out more thoroughly than they thought was necessary, but that you were also flexible, so they didn't mind. They felt that you were the best guy to work with." Jaxon replied, "Well, that's very flattering. I certainly had a respect for every one of them. Maybe that has something to do with it."[48]

Thoroughness is the most common term applied to Jaxon's approach to directing. Jaxon admits, "I think it is more likely to have been simply because I enjoyed doing it so much."[49] In interview after interview, whether it was Ken O'Connor, Lance Nolley, Marc Davis, or Eric Larson, they all used the word *thorough* in their descriptions of Jaxon. Frank Thomas and Ollie Johnston, in their book *Disney Animation: The Illusion of Life*, said, "Jaxon was easily the most creative of the directors, but he was also the most picky and took a lot of kidding about his thoroughness. Wilfred Jackson taught us thoroughness and the importance of detail."

Vitriolic story man Bill Peet said that Jaxon, with reference to their work on *Song of the*

South, was less respectful of the story man's work than other directors were—likely because Jaxon saw it as his responsibility to continue to improve the material as it went into production. While a few of his colleagues expressed a mix of both positive and negative opinions, the cumulative valuation of Wilfred Jackson is singularly high.

Walt Disney's Nine Old Men, among the kingpins of Disney animation, might be expected to harbor ill feelings about someone who directed their work and could be perceived as a barrier between Walt and them. But Jaxon won high praise from this group. Frank Thomas stated bluntly that "Jaxon was the better director by quite a bit but Dave [Hand] was the better organizer and driver."[50] Jaxon was particularly helpful for newly minted animators. Frank recalled, "When you were starting out to animate, he was also very helpful because of this thoroughness; he had thought it through, so you couldn't make a mistake. He was supporting you, and holding you in his hands, in effect, because everything had been thought out for you. You still had the problem of making the drawings, getting the appeal, getting the expression, getting the timing—all of these things you still had to do."[51] Ollie Johnston, another of the Nine Old Men, said, "We all wanted to work with him. I can remember I wanted to work with Jackson more than any other director when I started animating. I hoped for the day I'd get to work with him."[52] Milt Kahl, perhaps the most acerbic member of the Nine Old Men, said, "Jackson was one of the most highly creative directors we had. He really was kind of an old lady, but he had a better appreciation of entertainment and richness of character than any other director we had. . . . If you are working with somebody like Jackson, it makes it a hell of a lot easier, because there is a harmony there on what we can do. We'd talk things over and we'd find that we were in agreement; we'd agree on almost everything, we had very few disagreements. We had a few, but damned few."[53] Ward Kimball, known for his strong opinions, was effusive in his praise of Jaxon: "The only guys I really had any respect for were Willy Jackson, Ham Luske, and maybe Jack Kinney. . . . [Jaxon] thought everything out; he was intelligent. And he had a sixth sense of show biz. He had a good mechanical timing sense. You talk about meticulous sheets. That was all welcomed by me, when I was starting, until I got to the point that I felt my timing was better than anyone else's. And he was very nice and considerate and very patient with me. Jackson, in his meticulous way, was, for me and some of the other young animators coming up then, very good. We were fortunate. . . . He wasn't a great artist—and he would say that himself—but he was a great director. And I thought he was invaluable, [when] I, being a young know-nothing, he would almost tell

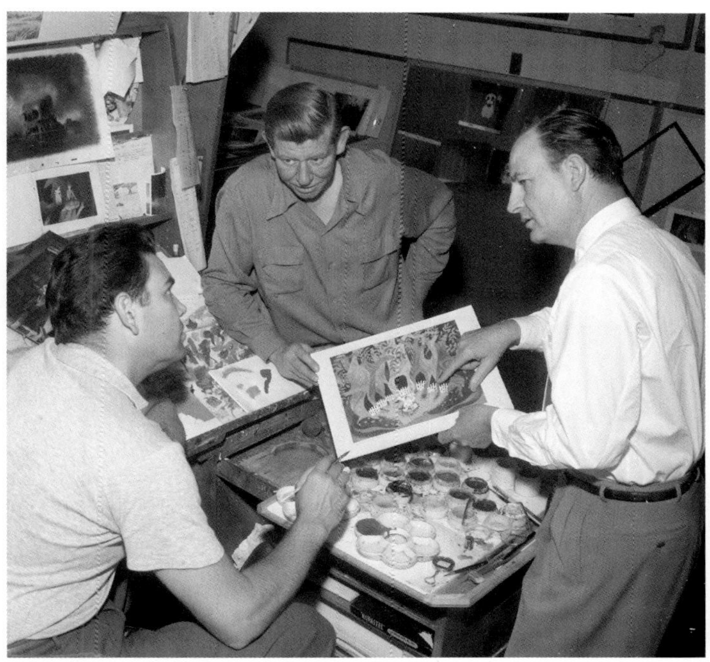

Jaxon in conference with Claude Coats (LEFT) and John Hench (RIGHT) for *Alice in Wonderland*.

me what he saw for every frame."[54] When Eric Larson began working with Jaxon, he said he was "like the soft breeze of summer."[55] He went on to say, "He was one of the best directors that ever crossed the path here, really, and very, very thorough."[56]

Ub Iwerks said simply that Jaxon was the most thorough director on the lot, and a real director; the others were coordinators.[57]

Fellow director Ben Sharpsteen appreciated the many facets of Jaxon's approach to directing: "He did a great job on almost all of the pictures we made there. I have many satisfying memories of working with Jackson; he was always an extremely willing and cooperative person. He certainly understood Walt, the way that Walt worked, and what he expected of people."[58]

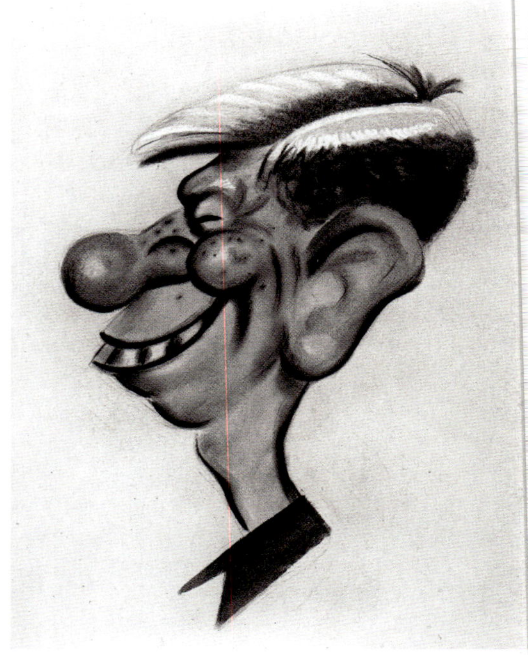

Jaxon, likely by Bill Justice, 1952.

FIFTIES FEATURES

With the exception of a short, *The Little House*, released in 1952, Wilfred Jackson was engaged in animated features throughout the late forties and early fifties, but now he was part of a trio of directors, teaming up with Gerry Geronimi and Hamilton Luske. This tripartite team would direct *Cinderella*, *Alice in Wonderland*, *Peter Pan*, and *Lady and the Tramp*. Interestingly, Jaxon (and presumedly Luske and Geronimi as well) were working on multiple films at once. Jaxon's diary entry in October of 1949 mentions that he is "still sweat boxing animation on Cindy, but mostly trying to get animation on *Alice* going." The fact Jaxon had brain space for two films at once is testament to his experience and professionalism. Jaxon would initially be the sole director on *Sleeping Beauty*, a troubled production with a less-attentive Walt, whose time and effort were pulled in many directions—live-action films, television, and a theme park in development—until Jaxon had a heart attack and was replaced first by Eric Larson and later by Geronimi.

The production of *Cinderella* introduced production changes that would continue on in feature animation. As noted earlier, dating back to *Pinocchio,* Walt withdrew more and more from day-to-day production decisions. Jaxon noted, "in the late Forties and in the Fifties, I went on ahead for a much longer time on my own, spending much more of Walt's money 'on spec,' before he decided whether or not to use anything at all of what I had done. This was a gradual change over the years. I think of *Cinderella* as the beginning of the time when I began to feel this change quite noticeably."[59] Increasingly the three directors had to communicate with Walt long-distance, as he was in England for two and a half months in the

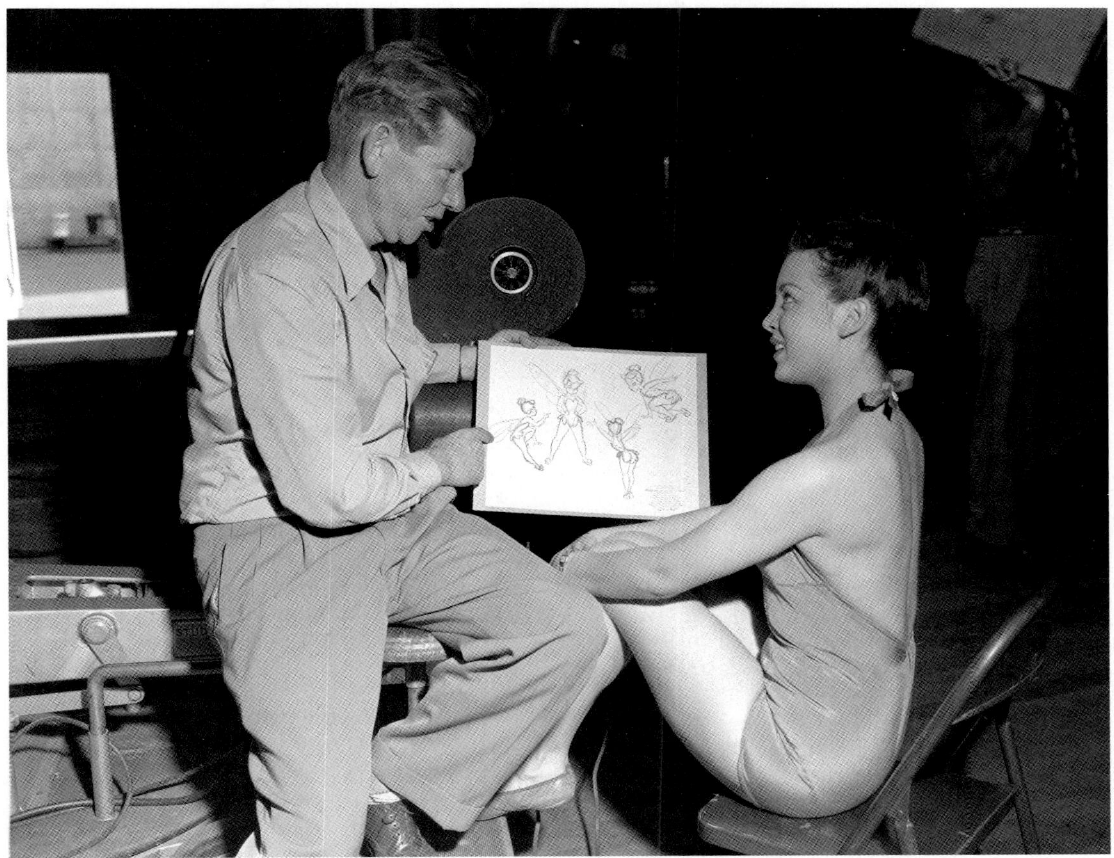

Jaxon and live-action reference actor Margaret Kerry on set for *Peter Pan*, February 1951.

summer of 1949 during the filming of *Treasure Island.* Walt was involved, though, with crucial stages of development.

Live-action reference footage was used extensively as a cost-saving device and to control animation. Songs were prerecorded as they had been before, but now the musician, in this case Ollie Wallace, composed his music, at least for Jaxon's sequences, after the animation was finished. For Jaxon, this was particularly a sad note (no pun intended); "It seemed to me that the time and effort I spent in pre-timing the action, working closely with the musician as he pre-composed the musical interpretation of it, was not only the very most delightful part of directing a cartoon, but also one of the most significant for [its] effectiveness."[60]

Jaxon wistfully recalled the pattern that became established with this first real animated feature after the war years:

> So when it came to *Cinderella* in a way, there was much more of a challenge for we directors who had come to Walt as raw kids who knew nothing and had kind of grown up in the business. Now we had to become better executives, we had to become better businessmen, we had to use much more of our own judgment on matters that would really pay off or not pay off in the pictures.[61]

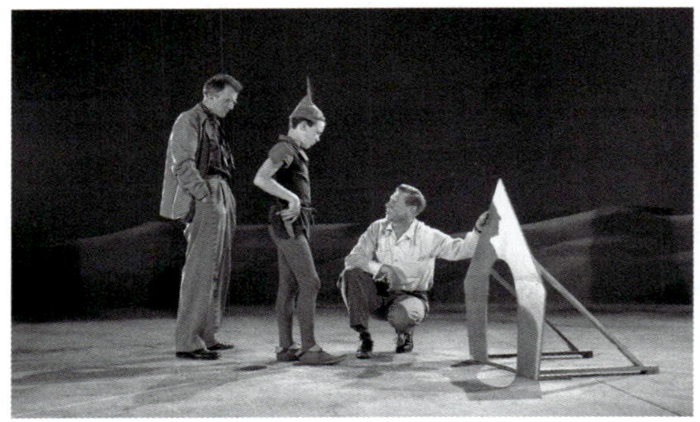

Milt Kahl (FAR LEFT), actor Bobby Driscoll, and Jaxon on live-action set for *Peter Pan* in March 1951.

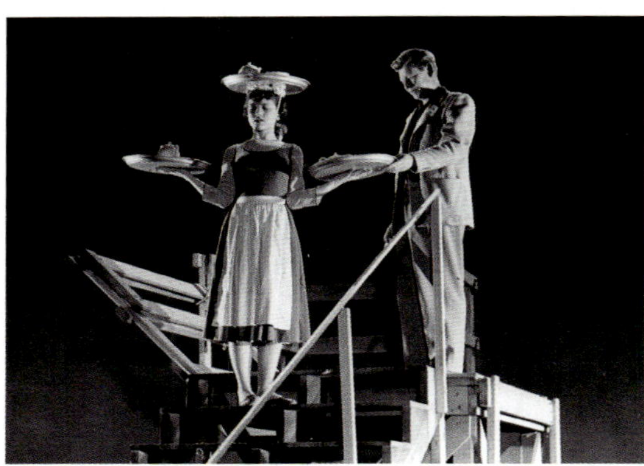

Actress Helene Stanley being directed by Jaxon on the *Cinderella* set, November 1948.

TELEVISION

In December 1953, Wilfred Jackson had a major heart attack. After his recovery and before he returned to work in 1954, Walt arranged for Jaxon and Jane to take an unprecedented three-month all-expenses-paid trip to Europe. Jaxon expressed his gratitude to Walt regarding the upcoming trip: "It's really quite overwhelming, Walt, to have all these people going to so much trouble to take care of me. I started out to express my appreciation for what you are doing for Janie and me, but it is becoming evident that I am not going to be able to find the words that would do it. I don't know how to thank you for all this, but I want you to know that I am deeply grateful."[62]

When he returned, he learned that he had been permanently replaced as the director on *Sleeping Beauty.* Walt had other plans for him. "When I returned, Walt said, 'I'm going into TV. I want you to help me on that.' What a nice way of saying, 'Look, old man, you're not up to this anymore. We'll have to put you out to pasture.'"[63] As Walt moved into television and other ventures and as he recruited his longtime directors to join him, he expected that they were capable of adapting and accepting new challenges. In his way, he was complimenting them because he believed that they could keep up with him and they were his loyal partners. Some could and did, but some could not and did not. The demands of television, with its voracious appetite for programming and tight deadlines, were at times overwhelming for Jaxon, but he did produce and direct thirteen television shows. He had spent a career trying to follow Walt's lead, but now their paths were beginning to diverge as Walt's interests expanded. "Everyone lives in his own world. Some worlds are bigger than others. Through the years his world got bigger and bigger. My world got just a little bigger. I couldn't see things he was looking at—they were always over my horizon."[64]

Jaxon was primarily assigned to television shows with themes and content that dealt with animation. The exception was the few occasions where he had to direct Walt's lead-ins for the television shows. Jaxon felt inept at this, but so did everyone else who directed Walt.

The Story of the Animated Drawing was one of the high points of Jaxon's television time. The program included clips from early animation. Many of the pioneer animators were still alive then and readily gave permission to use their cartoons. Most of the programming that Jaxon was involved with tied old cartoon footage together through new live-action or animation bridges.

Jaxon tried to be more flexible in this new medium, but old habits were hard to break. Animator Bob McCrea recalled, "I worked on the last TV show he did here. When we started the show, he said he was going to be very flexible. He was going to allow anything to get by that he thought . . . [the] public would accept. It never worked out that way. He had to hit every frame exactly on. I mean, he approached it just as if he was building a feature and of course it cost correspondingly."[65]

A PIECE OF MY HEART

Over the next five years, Jaxon made many diary entries describing the physical and emotional stress and the unhappiness he was experiencing. At the same time, and most likely not coincidentally, Jaxon was increasingly unhappy with working in television. On August 18, 1959, Jaxon sent what must have been a humbling and heartbreaking memo to Walt. Part two of the memo was titled "What to do with me." In this part of the memo, Jaxon stressed that he liked animation but not story work. In an understatement typical of Jaxon, he said, "I believe I have done reasonably well at directing animation in the past whenever I was backed up with good story work and had competent artists to help put it thru production."[66]

Jaxon was willing to take a leave of absence until there was an animation project available, and he said Walt favored his plan but wanted to limit the leave of absence initially to about four months. However, over the next two years nothing developed, and suggestions were gradually made that perhaps Jaxon could find work at another studio. In one entry, after it had been suggested to Jaxon that he consider freelance story work for television at home. He wrote, "I think I've just been fired, but the way they put it it's not easy to tell exactly when or why."[67] In a poignant note, he wrote: "For over two years I have been trying to find out if Walt would let me work on his feature cartoons. In Aug. 1959 he said he would—not later than Jan 1960—now I know he won't."[68] Jaxon retired from the studio in 1961.

In a 1976 interview with Michael Barrier, Jaxon reflected on what had transpired in the years leading up to his retirement:

> When I left the studio, Walt wanted me to do what I didn't want to do, and Walt didn't want me to do what I did want to do. . . . I had a feeling for quite a while that he just didn't know what to do with me. He didn't want me to . . . work with animation. He was trying to get people off of animation, and he already had me off of it, and he wasn't about to put me back on. It came to the point that I just had a feeling that Walt needed a little help

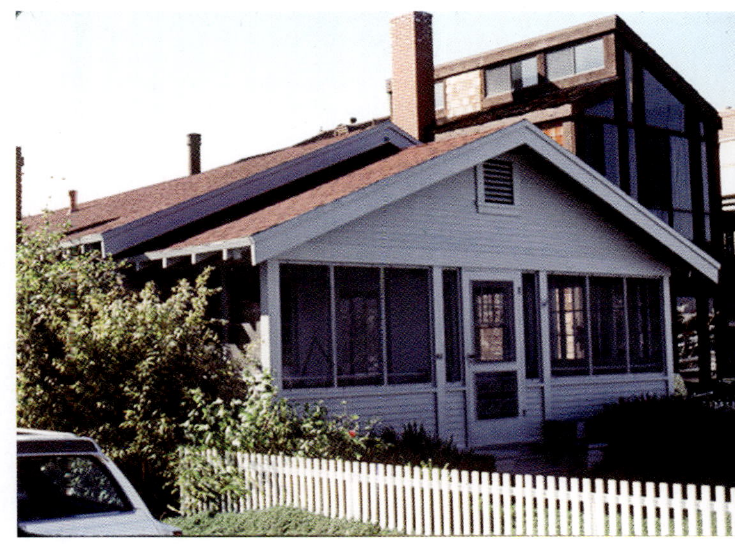

The Jacksons' beach house on Balboa Island in 1977. Don Peri collection.

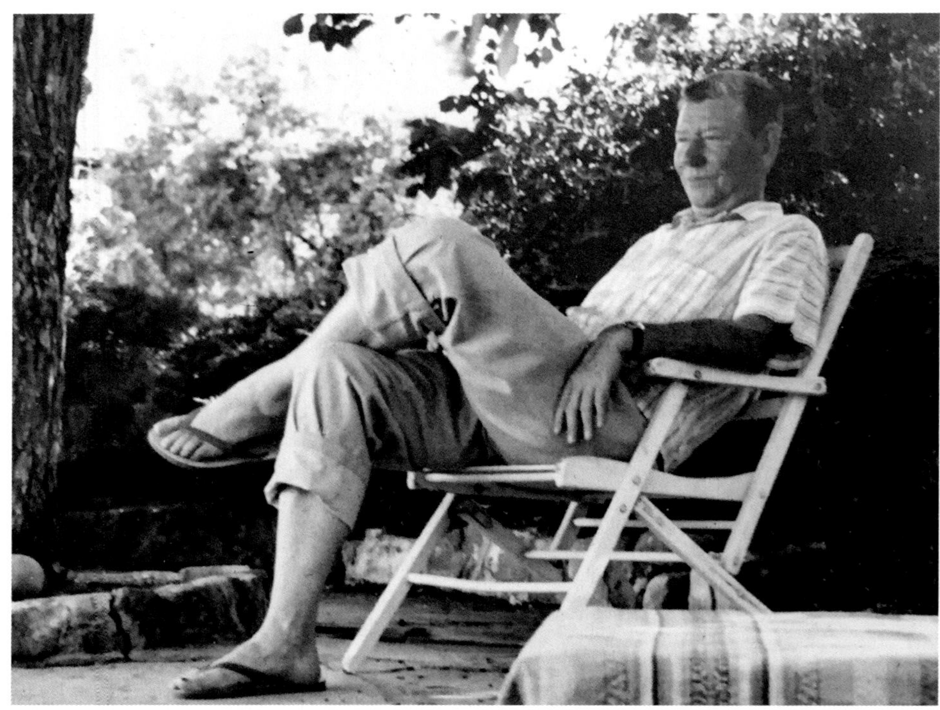

Jaxon in retirement. Natha Horbach collection.

> to let me go. . . . So the only thing to do was to get out, which broke my heart, really, but it was a matter of saving my skin. . . . The day I left, I left with no pension, no severance pay; I just cross-dissolved out. I have no feeling of anything but that I still owe Walt; he doesn't owe me.[69]

Wilfred and Jane moved permanently to their vacation home on Balboa Island and spent their remaining years quietly and happily together. Not forgotten by the industry he loved, he received a Winsor McCay Award in 1983. Jane preceded him in death by about six months. He seemed to live long enough to see her through a long illness, settle his affairs, and then join her. He passed away on August 7, 1988, and received a posthumous Disney Legends Award in 1998.

In his last years at the studio, in a way, Jaxon's heart had been broken twice: once literally and once figuratively, with his removal from animation. When he left the studio, he was only fifty-three years old. Late in life, he said he hoped someday he would be a real boy, echoing a theme from *Pinocchio*. He hoped to escape the insecurities that bedeviled him and to feel more secure and more at peace with himself, perhaps harkening back to a time when he was at the height of his creative powers doing the work he loved with Walt Disney right there beside him. He felt he had been very lucky in life. Having what turned out to be the premier animation studio practically in his backyard was fortuitous for him, but for Walt, too, because he hired a young man with little experience but big dreams and determination and a latent talent who practically willed his way into the animation field and, along the way, contributed enormously to the best of Walt Disney's animated films. If that isn't a Disney story, what is?

Wilfred Jackson—Disney Director Filmography

Shorts:

The Castaway (1931)[70]
The China Plate (1931)
The Cat's Out/The Cat's Nightmare (1931)
Egyptian Melodies (1931)
The Clock Store (1931)
The Spider and the Fly (1931)
The Fox Hunt (1931)
The Ugly Duckling (1931)
The Bird Store (1932)
The Grocery Boy (1932)
Barnyard Olympics (1932)
Mickey's Revue (1932)
Musical Farmer (1932)
The Bears and the Bees (1932)
Mickey in Arabia (1932)
The Whoopee Party (1932)
Touchdown Mickey (1932)
The Klondike Kid (1932)
Santa's Workshop (1932)
Mickey's Mellerdrammer (1933)
Father Noah's Ark (1933)
Mickey's Mechanical Man (1933)
Lullaby Land (1933)
Puppy Love (1933)
The Pied Piper (1933)
The Pet Store (1933)
The Night Before Christmas (1933)
The China Shop (1934)
The Grasshopper and the Ants (1934)
Funny Little Bunnies (1934)
The Wise Little Hen (1934)
Peculiar Penguins (1934)
The Goddess of Spring (1934)
The Tortoise and the Hare (1935) (Academy Award winner)
The Band Concert (1935)
Water Babies (1935)
Mickey's Garden (1935)
Music Land (1935)
Mickey's Grand Opera (1936)
Elmer Elephant (1936)
Mickey's Rival (1936)
Toby Tortoise Returns (1936)
The Country Cousin (1936) (Academy Award winner)
Mother Pluto (1936)
Woodland Café (1937)
The Old Mill (1937) (Codirector with Graham Heid, Academy Award winner)
Mother Goose Goes Hollywood (1938)
Golden Eggs (1941)
The New Spirit (1942) (Codirector with Ben Sharpsteen)
The Little House (1952)

Features:

Snow White and the Seven Dwarfs (1937) (Sequence Director)
Pinocchio (1940) (Sequence Director)
Fantasia (1940) (Sequence Director)
Dumbo (1941) (Sequence Director)
Saludos Amigos (1942) (Sequence Director)
Song of the South (1946) (Cartoon Director)
Melody Time (1948) (Cartoon Director)
Cinderella (1950) (Codirector with Ham Luske and Gerry Geronimi)
Alice in Wonderland (1951) (Codirector with Ham Luske and Gerry Geronimi)
Peter Pan (1953) (Codirector with Ham Luske and Gerry Geronimi)
Lady and the Tramp (1955) (Codirector with Ham Luske and Gerry Geronimi)

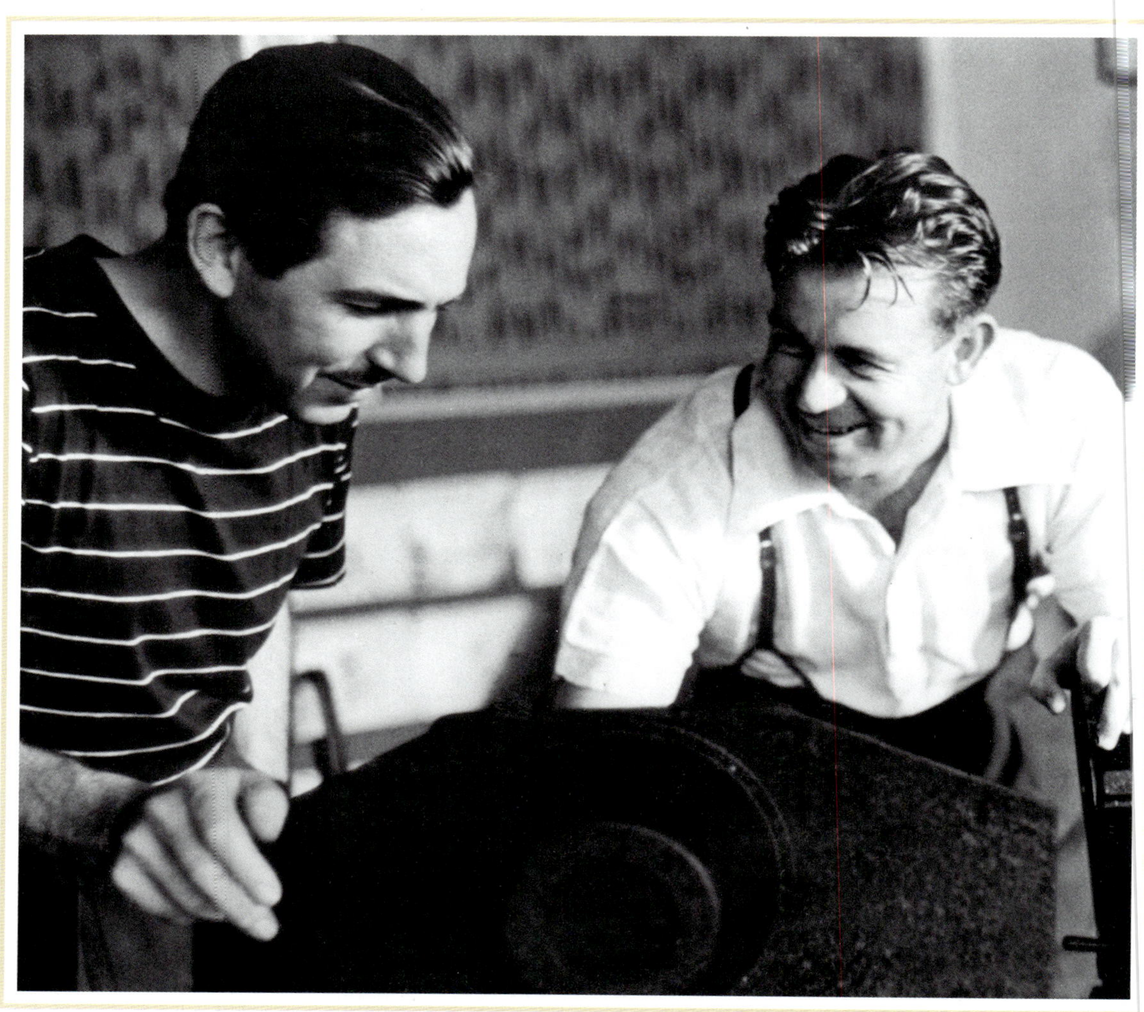

Walt and Ham review footage from *Pinocchio* on a Moviola in April or May of 1939.

CHAPTER 6

HAM LUSKE—A TEAM PLAYER

"Our actors are drawings. We cannot work on the inspiration of the moment, as an actor does, but must present our characterization through a combination of art, technique, and mechanics that takes months from the conception to the finished product. And we have to make the audience forget these are drawings."

—Ham Luske, studio lecture on character handling, Thursday, October 6, 1938

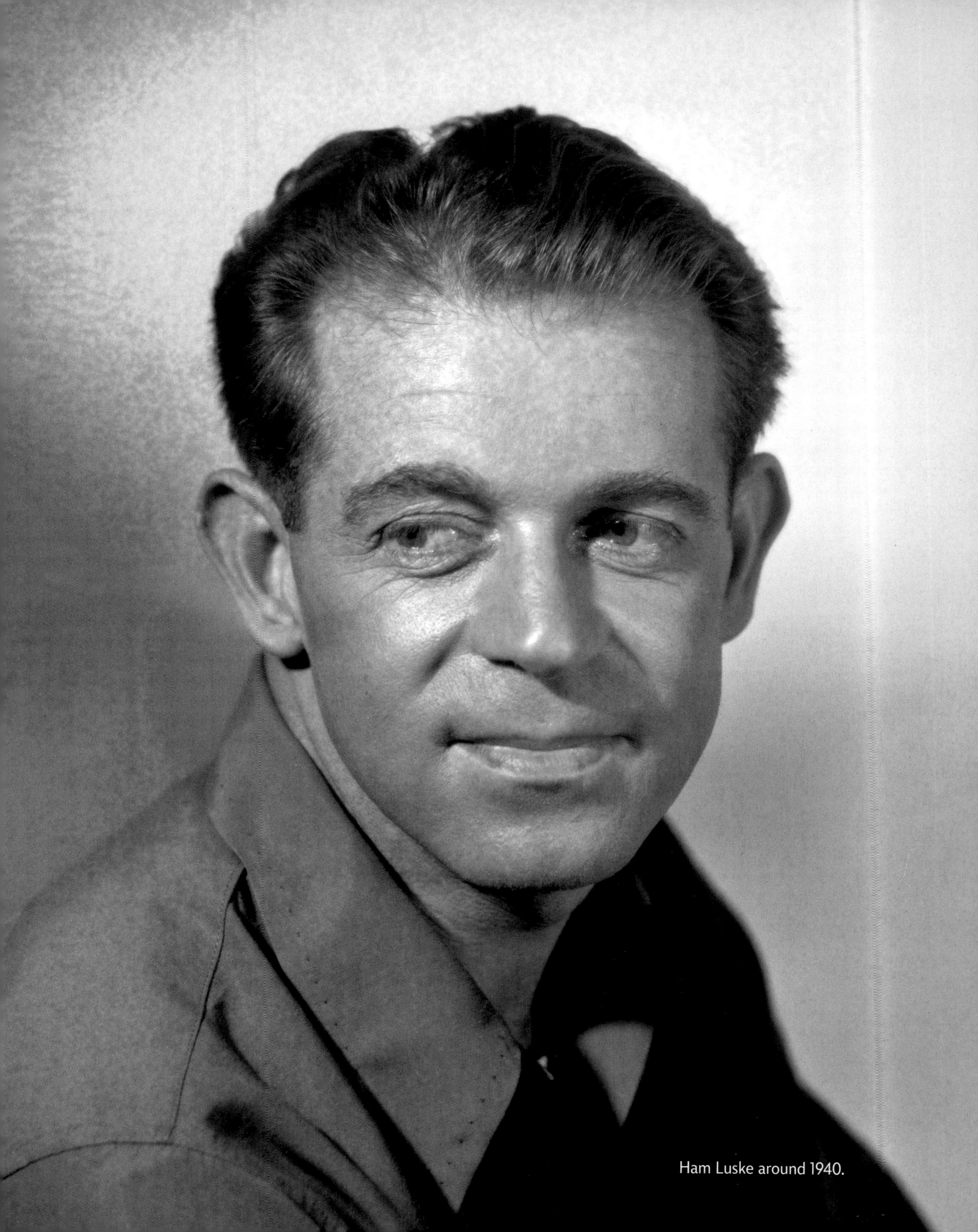

Ham Luske around 1940.

As the short films did before them, so too would features drop in Walt's priorities as he expanded his vision and interests. This in turn would mean big changes for the directors, who would increasingly need to anticipate for themselves what would likely please the absentee chief. Few did this better than longtime collaborator Ham Luske.

Eric Larson recalled that when he became an assistant to animator Ham Luske, Ham told him that they were now a duo and part of Walt's team. "No solos," said Ham. "You work for me, I work for you, and we both work for Walt."[1] Ham would spend his career at Disney rising to become one of the top four animators of the time (the others being Norman Ferguson, Bill Tytla, and Fred Moore), then as a director on features, special short subjects, and television programming. He was an invaluable member of Walt's organization, devoting himself to realizing Walt's ambitions for the films and programs that bore his name. Family members say that the studio was his life, and some colleagues felt that his early death, not long after Walt's passing, was the result of a broken heart. Ham's analytical abilities, his skill at working with and supervising young animators, and his intuitive understanding of what Walt wanted put him in an excellent position to help elevate animation to the unparalleled position it held during Walt's lifetime.

EARLY LIFE

Hamilton Somers Luske, described by one colleague as "a short, blondish, round-faced fellow with a slightly graveled voice which even in a whisper sounded like reveille,"[2] was born in Chicago (just like Walt Disney and Wilfred Jackson) on October 16, 1903. The family moved to the San Francisco Bay Area just before the devastating 1906 earthquake and fire, according to family members.[3] He was close to his mother—not so much to his father—who served in a variety of social services organizations and eventually was president of the Mother's Club for the Acacia Fraternity at the University of California at Berkeley, of which Ham was a member.[4] In the March 3, 1939, *Bulletin*, a Disney Studios house magazine, Ham said, "he doesn't remember when he wasn't drawing something or other." Although he never took any art classes, during his four years of high school in Sacramento he made "all the posters, signs, cartoons and miscellaneous drawings for the school paper."[5] He enrolled at UC Berkeley in 1922 and majored in "commerce" (business). There, in addition to

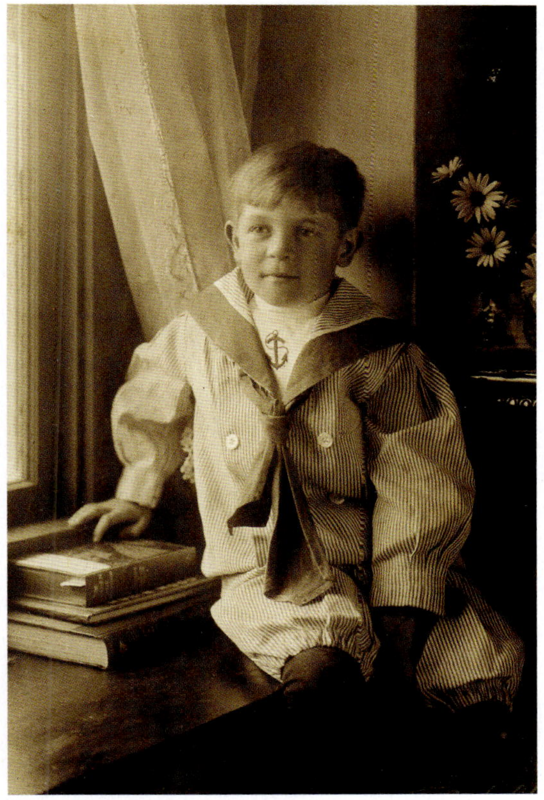

Ham Luske. Luske family collection.

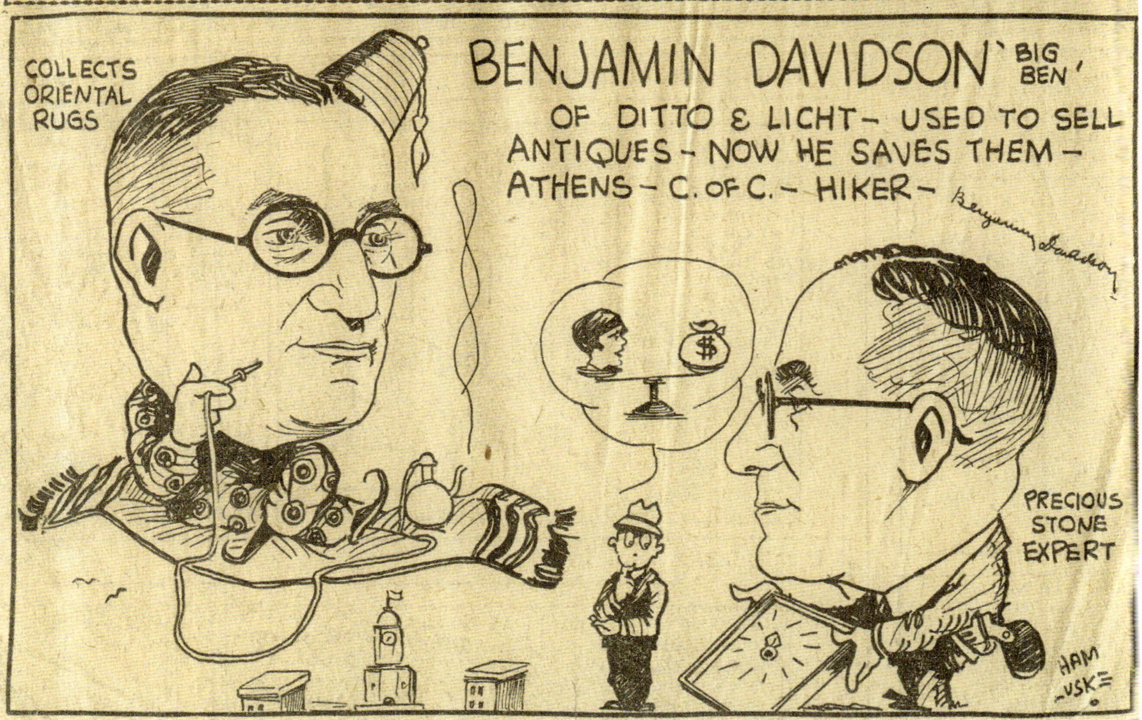

OAKLAND POST-ENQUIRER

Friday, Febru

mall Compared With

Men Who Are Building the East Bay—By Ham Luske

COLLECTS ORIENTAL RUGS
BENJAMIN DAVIDSON 'BIG BEN'
OF DITTO & LICHT- USED TO SELL ANTIQUES - NOW HE SAVES THEM - ATHENS - C. OF C. - HIKER -
PRECIOUS STONE EXPERT
HAM LUSKE

An example of Ham's early cartoon work for the *Oakland Post-Enquirer*. Luske Family Collection.

his fraternity, he was involved in a plethora of campus activities, including as president of the College of Commerce; secretary-treasurer of the sophomore class; art editor at the school newspaper, the *Daily Californian*; and contributor to the *California Pelican*, a college humor magazine.[6] Ham met his future wife, Frances (Frankie) Crabb, in 1924, and he graduated in 1926.

Ham spent the next two years at the *Oakland Post-Enquirer*, "doing illustrations for the sports section and the editorial page, and also contributing a daily sketch of prominent folk in Metropolitan Oakland."[7] One of his colleagues at the newspaper was a young man, six years Ham's junior, named Milt Kahl. In a few years, Ham would be instrumental in recruiting Kahl to the Disney Studios.

Ham said he left the paper to come to Los Angeles to get married. He spent a year working in the oil fields in Ventura. He couldn't stay away from drawing, and as a freelancer, he contributed to magazines, including the *Saturday Evening Post, Collier's*, and *College Humor.* He also worked part-time as an athletic instructor at public school playgrounds.[8]

Ham had a stint at a cartoon studio called Scoop Scandals, where he stayed until it closed.[9] According to Dick Huemer, Ham animated an amazing sample scene of somebody serving in tennis, but he was turned down by Charles Mintz.[10] Walt Disney hired him, and Ham joined the Disney Studios on April 6, 1931.

DISNEY ANIMATOR

Ben Sharpsteen, not known for lavishing praise, said, "Hamilton Luske is another person who did not receive the recognition that he deserved. He came to the studio during the early days of the Mickey Mouse series. He was not brilliant, but he was industrious and he accomplished a great deal of good animation."[11] Eric Larson agreed: "He was not the most accomplished artist in the studio but he was willing to work, to draw and re-draw the poses and attitudes he visualized and knew he needed to put the personality and action of his characters on the screen in a most appealing way. No one was a better analyst than he. He worked feverishly and with dedication to be a successful animator and later became an outstanding director."[12]

Ham brought something unique to the studio in 1931. "He was the first guy to come with a college education and the first guy to come with a feeling for movies and what should be in a movie—a front and a middle—and he knew all these things," Frank Thomas said.[13] In their book *Disney Animation: The Illusion of Life*, Frank and Ollie Johnston elaborated on this theme: "Ham had to struggle with his drawing, but he had a natural feeling for animation, story, and for what was entertaining. So, despite his lack of an artistic background, he had many things going for him. Perhaps it was his college training, or maybe it was just inherent in him to have a well-organized analytical mind."

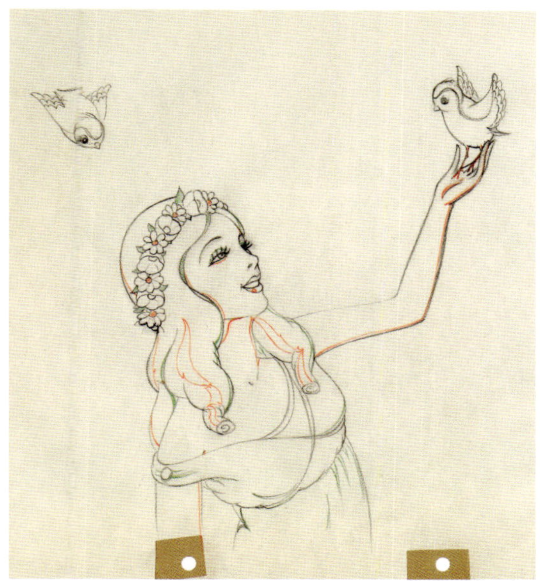

Ham modeled the movements of Persephone (from *The Goddess of Spring*, 1934) on his wife, Frankie.

Ham began his animation career at Disney animating animals on the short *The Barnyard Broadcast*. He worked on many shorts over the next few years. His breakout years began in 1934 when he was given the lead character Persephone in *The Goddess of Spring* (dir. Jackson). Even though he used both his wife and Eric Larson to model the character's movements (and Les Clark did the same with his sister, Marceil), the results were mostly dismal. Still, it was a learning experience for both the animators and for Walt, and they would redeem themselves a couple of years later with the character of Snow White.

Ham's first major success was animating Max Hare in *The Tortoise and the Hare* (dir. Jackson, 1934). Eric said, "Ham played a lot of tennis, so when he was given the chance to animate Max Hare in the tennis sequence of *The Tortoise and the Hare*, he knew precisely what he wanted to do."[14] The poses, held positions, timing, exaggeration of movement, all contributed to a

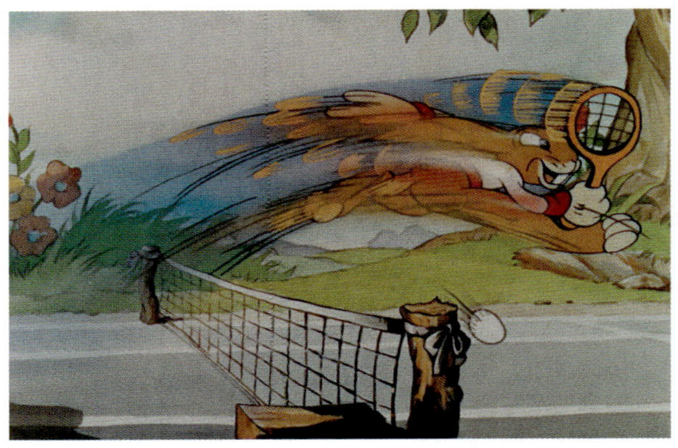

A frame from *The Tortoise and the Hare* (1934), showing Ham's groundbreaking use of speed in his animation.

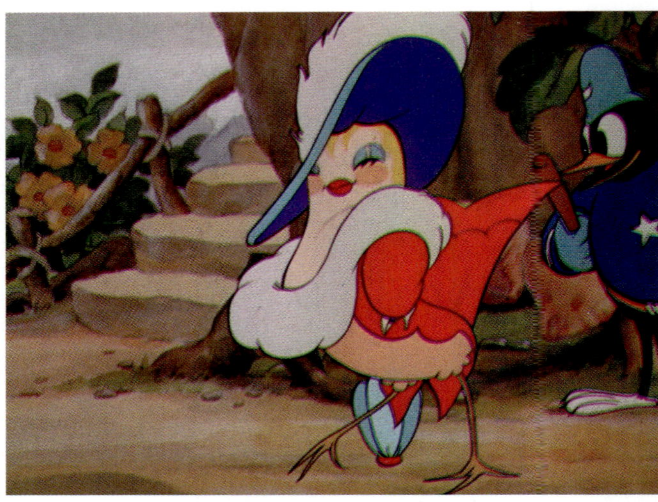

A pose from Ham's animation in *Who Killed Cock Robin?* (1935).

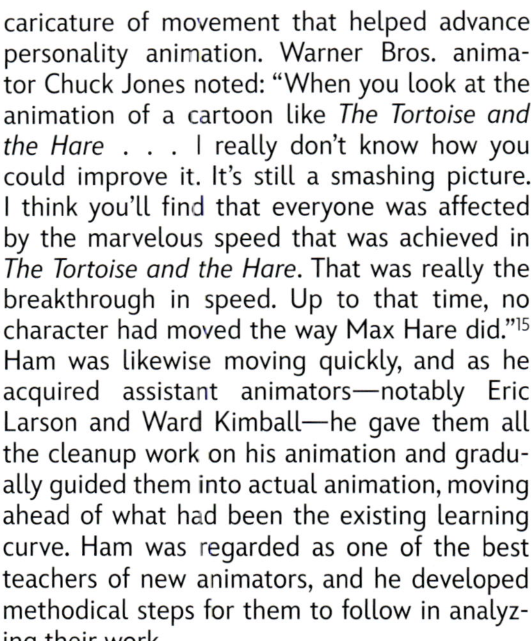

caricature of movement that helped advance personality animation. Warner Bros. animator Chuck Jones noted: "When you look at the animation of a cartoon like *The Tortoise and the Hare* . . . I really don't know how you could improve it. It's still a smashing picture. I think you'll find that everyone was affected by the marvelous speed that was achieved in *The Tortoise and the Hare*. That was really the breakthrough in speed. Up to that time, no character had moved the way Max Hare did."[15] Ham was likewise moving quickly, and as he acquired assistant animators—notably Eric Larson and Ward Kimball—he gave them all the cleanup work on his animation and gradually guided them into actual animation, moving ahead of what had been the existing learning curve. Ham was regarded as one of the best teachers of new animators, and he developed methodical steps for them to follow in analyzing their work.

On *Who Killed Cock Robin?* (dir. Hand), Dick Huemer praised Ham's analytical abilities: "He used to painfully analyze his action, like for instance when he did a scene in *Who Killed Cock Robin?*, that clever Mae West bit. The way he analyzed that problem—the dynamics of the action, the interplay of different parts of the body, the shifting of weight, the feeling of breathing and realism. These were things he put into it."[16] His caricature of Mae West was so good that Mae West herself wrote a complimentary letter to Walt.

With *Elmer Elephant* (dir. Jackson), Ham advanced the animation tool kit as he animated the lead characters, Elmer and Tillie. His scene of a tearful Elmer created a memorable and teaching moment for the animators. Woolie

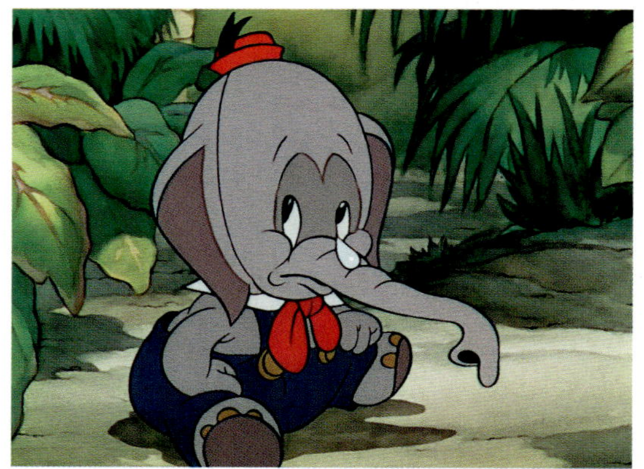

Elmer Elephant (1936), another noteworthy performance from Ham.

Reitherman recalled it: "When an elephant cried and he blinked his eyes, and the tear went down his trunk and into the water, that was a breakthrough for us. That here was a thing that was held without looking for a help drawing because there was movement in the eyes. These were the things that were the stepping-stones to a much subtler approach."[17]

SNOW WHITE—NEW DIRECTION

November 1935: Walt, in a memo to staff regarding assignments for the production of *Snow White*, stated: "From now on, Ham Luske is definitely assigned to *Snow White*."[18] His work would focus on the character of Snow White. Also in a memo that same month to animator Paul Hopkins, Walt elaborated on Ham's role: "It is possible that with the experience Ham will gain by the work he is now doing, plus his native ingenuity and ability, he will be enabled to handle all of the Snow White action, with the exception of the sequence when the dwarfs entertain her at night, which I intend Les Clark to handle."[19] Grim Natwick, of Betty Boop fame, had by this time joined the studio and was also assigned to the animation of Snow White. His depiction of her was of a more mature, sensuous figure in contrast to Ham's younger, more innocent girl. The two versions are evident in the final film, but Ham's dominates. Weathering this storm, he might have learned some valuable lessons about navigating conflicts that would serve him well later as a director.

That same month, Ham began filming and directing live-action reference footage of Marjorie Belcher, the teenage daughter of the owner of a local dance studio. As historian Michael Barrier said in *The Animated Man*, "Ham Luske, by directing the live action for Snow White, thus assumed control over the character greater than any he might have enjoyed if he had been only the lead animator. For scenes with dialogue, she acted in synchronization with the soundtrack, so that the timing of her action would match the timing of the dialogue." He went on to say: "In other words, Luske tried to make the staging and the timing of the live action as close as possible to the result desired on the screen. That way, the animators could concentrate on the details that live action might reveal, that is, how Snow White's dress moved and how the figure itself turned in three dimensions. The multiple filmings of each action became, in effect, pencil tests from which Luske and possibly Walt Disney himself could choose what they liked best."

Ham gave a talk on character handling on October 6, 1938, drawing from his experiences on both *Snow White* and *Pinocchio*. A substantial part of his talk was about the advantages of using live-action reference footage, which had begun earlier when background artist Mique Nelson had taken a series of still shots of Wilfred Jackson as the Sandman in *Lullaby Land*. Ham said that a top advantage to shooting live-action footage is that "it's making a character that is consistent throughout the picture," thus reducing the potential for variations in the look and movement of a character as it is animated by different artists. It also reduced miscommunication between the director and the animator. Ham said, "Heretofore our animators have been handed scenes without live action, and a lot depended on their getting the right interpretations from the director and carrying them out. The sweatbox was a pretty tough job in those days. Now the story has been discussed, any unnecessary business or any business not in character has been taken out. Then it's been acted and edited, and that is handed to the animator. He strengthens it and simplifies it—because an actor will put in faults like having two expressions where one will do—and that scene will serve its purpose in the picture, and the character will be what he is supposed to be and do what he is supposed to do." (Dave Hand, the supervising director of *Snow White*, following Ham's lead, began filming live action to assist the dwarfs animators, in late 1936 and early 1937.)[20]

Walt added animators Grim Natwick and Eddie Strickland to the Luske team animating *Snow White*, and over the years, there has been some controversy about who should get the most credit for the development and look of the title character. J. B. Kaufman, in *The Fairest One of All*, analyzed Ham's role: "During the two years following Walt's memo, Luske played a unique role in the making of *Snow White*: animating many key scenes himself, supervising a large unit of other animators, controlling virtually every appearance of Snow White as well as the animals and birds that surrounded her. Operating independently of the nominal sequence directors, Luske enjoyed an autonomy second only to that of Walt himself."

Ham's success with Snow White made him "too valuable," as Frank and Ollie saw it, for him to be confined to the animation board. "Even though he did some animation on the girl in *Snow White*, Ham was really a director on the picture. Walt felt that Ham's value lay in the influence he could have on the younger animators."[21] Ham's future as a director was set, but on *Snow White*, Ham was, as Ben Sharpsteen called him, "the man of the hour" on Walt's first animated feature.[22]

PINOCCHIO

Ham turned his attention to shorts after *Snow White* wrapped, with a codirector credit with Jack Cutting (who was later replaced by Geronimi) on *The Ugly Duckling*. *Bambi* was set to follow *Snow White*, but the story demanded a longer gestation, and *Pinocchio* moved ahead as the heir apparent. Ham was assigned several sequences, including those with the Blue Fairy. Ham's success filming live-action reference footage on *Snow White* led to a similar role on *Pinocchio*, where he directed the Blue Fairy sequences—again with Marjorie—and shot footage of other characters, including Jiminy Cricket. (Luske explained to the actor "that the Cricket was to be a combination of Mickey Rooney and W. C. Fields.")[23]

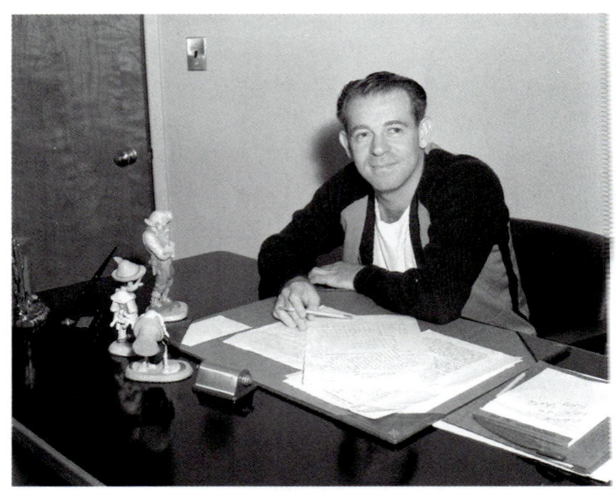

Ham as a supervising director on *Pinocchio*.

As the film moved through production, Ham joined supervising director Ben Sharpsteen as a co-supervising director. This new assignment only added to his workload; he still directed the sequences that had been originally assigned to him.

FANTASIA, THE WAR YEARS, AND THE FIFTIES FEATURES

His colleagues uniformly referred to Ham as a nice guy, understanding, and easy to work with. Story man Larry Clemmons said, "Ham Luske: Life is full of raised eyebrow surprises." But many also remembered him as a worrier. And one of his primary fears was that people working with him would be laid off and lose their

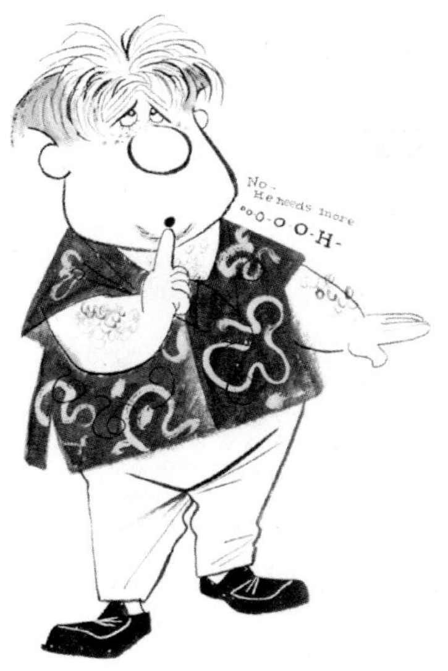

Ham as caricatured by Ward Kimball in the 1950s.

jobs. He remarked to biographer and journalist Bob Thomas in a 1956 interview that many artists had been brought in with the buildup in production on *Snow White*, and many had great expectations for their role at the studio. "When it ended, the Studio was loaded with talent and there was nothing to do. [Dave] Hand told me that we'd be making thirty pictures a year and that shorts would keep the artists busy meanwhile, paying no attention to the fact that a lot of features would compete with each other. . . . There was a period when people sat around doing nothing." Ham had become a director on the "Pastoral" in *Fantasia* and on *The Reluctant Dragon*. "Every week there would be a new batch of artists at liberty. Ben wouldn't have anything to do with them. I tried to take them on, but it was a horrible deal and I shudder when I remember it." Sagging box office receipts, the studio strike with accompanying layoffs, the advent of World War II, and the production of military training films and health and safety films were about to muddle the studio and its productions in unimaginable ways.

The Reluctant Dragon has a special place in the Luske family, because son James, at eight months old, appeared as the live-action model for the "Baby Weems" cartoon segment. But this was just the start. In the coming years, son Tom would be the voice and live-action model for Michael in *Peter Pan*. The family dog, Blondie, was the live-action model for Lady in *Lady and the Tramp*, and daughters Carol Jean and Peggy were voices of flowers in *Alice in Wonderland*.[24]

As the war years came on, Ham turned his talents south of the border as the sequence director on the Pedro cartoon in *Saludos Amigos* (1943). He directed a number of war-related shorts, including *Food Will Win the War* (1942), *Thunderstorms* (1943), *Air Masses and Fronts* (1943), *The Cold Front* (1943), *Flying the Weather Map* (1944), *The Howgozit Chart* (1944), and *Weather at War* (1944). He rounded out those years directing an entertainment short, *The Pelican and the Snipe* (1945), and an educational film, *Hold Your Horsepower* (1945). Postwar Disney saw the production of the "package" features as the studio tried to reestablish financial footing to make feature films again. Ham was a sequence or cartoon director on many of them, including *Make Mine Music* (1946), *Fun and Fancy Free* (1947), and *Melody*

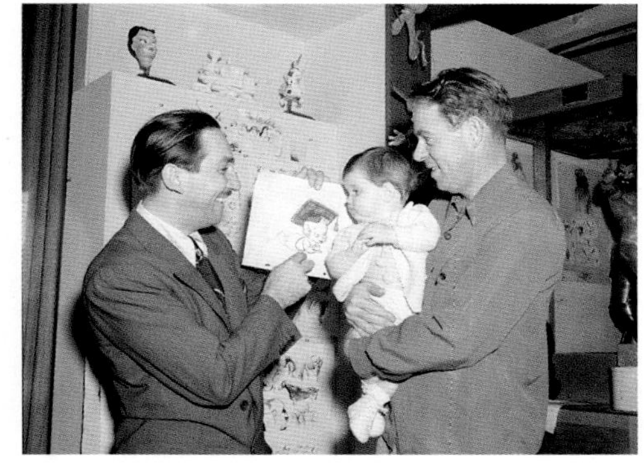

Walt, James "Jimmie" Luske, and proud papa Ham in January 1941 on the set of *The Reluctant Dragon*.

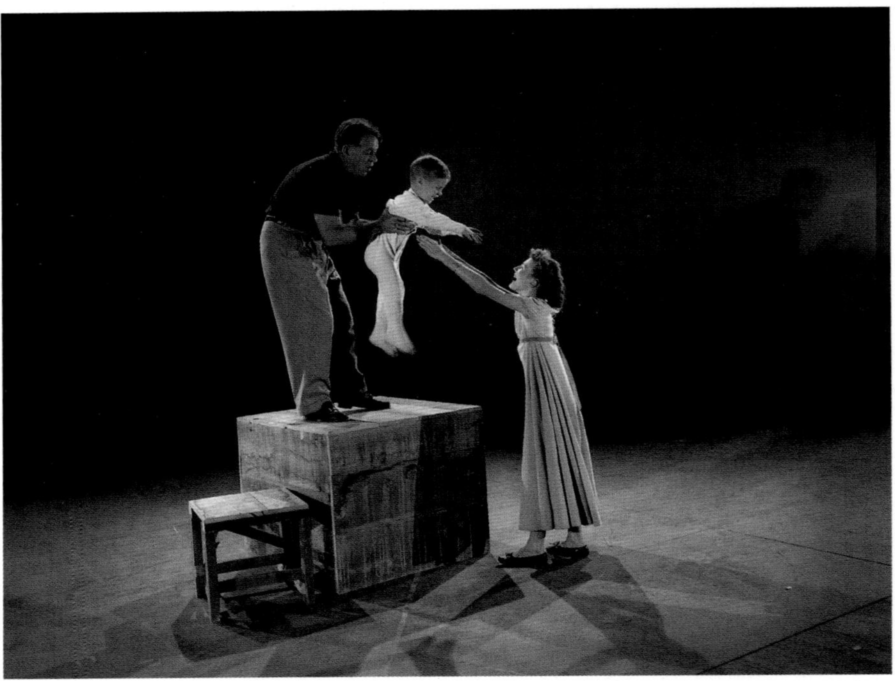

Ham, Tom Luske, and actress Kathryn Beaumont on the *Peter Pan* set in April 1951.

Time (1948). He then directed the cartoon segments on *So Dear to My Heart* (1949).

Once the studio restarted feature films, Ham joined Gerry Geronimi and Wilfred Jackson to direct the 1950s and early 1960s classic films *Cinderella*, *Peter Pan*, *Alice in Wonderland*, *Lady and the Tramp*, and *One Hundred and One Dalmatians* (with Woolie Reitherman replacing Wilfred Jackson). Increasingly, these three directors were on their own and making decisions without Walt's input as he diversified into live-action films, television, and a theme park. Walt had less time to be available for timely meetings, and the loss of his creative input was felt by all three. Live-action reference footage expanded greatly until virtually the entire feature story was filmed before it was animated. Ham defended this by saying: "Cartoonists, just like artists, must have living models to draw from. Otherwise, they'd be drawing what they think certain characters would do in a situation, not what they really would do."[25]

After the studio units making shorts were gradually disbanded as shorts were phased out in the 1950s, Ham, like the other directors, made a few special shorts, including the well-received *Ben and Me* (1953), the openings and closings for the *Mickey Mouse Club* (1955), *Donald in Mathmagic Land* (1959), *Donald at the Wheel* (1961), *The Litterbug* (1961), *Scrooge and Money* (1967), and ironically, *Understanding Stresses and Strains* (1968).

Ham's crowning achievement was directing the cartoon segments in Walt's megahit *Mary Poppins*. Ham, along with Peter Ellenshaw and Eustace Lycett, won an Academy Award in 1964 for Best Visual Effects. His family remembers his work on this film as an especially happy time for him.

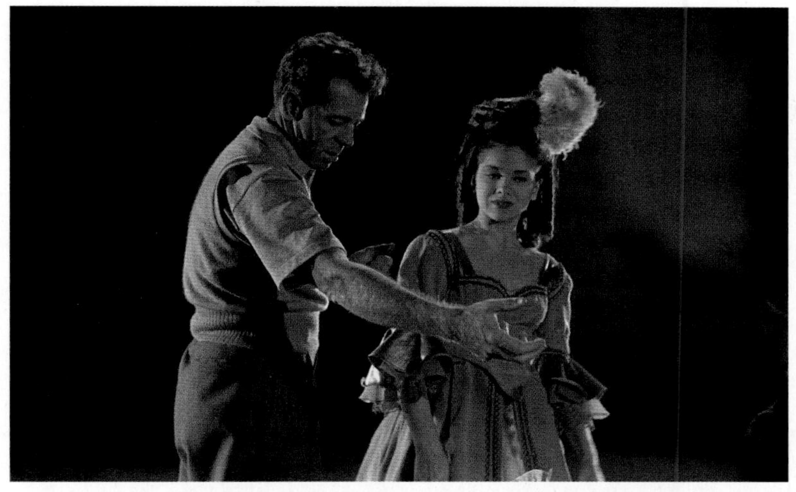

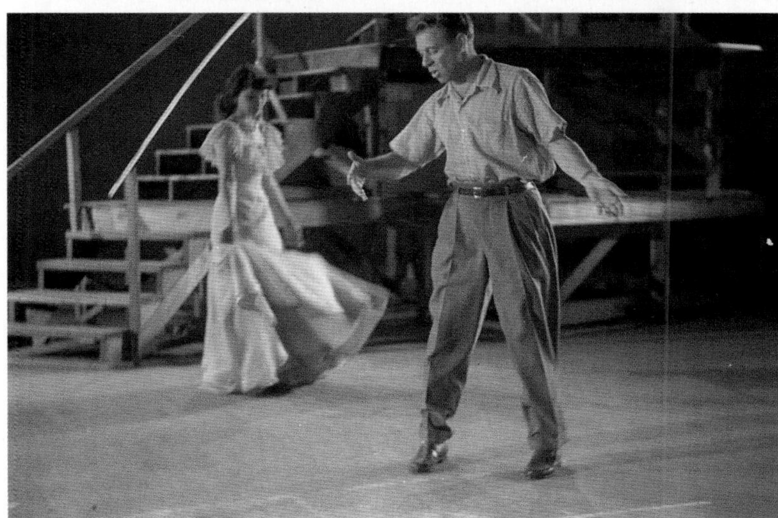

Ham directing Helene Stanley on the live-action reference set for *Cinderella*.

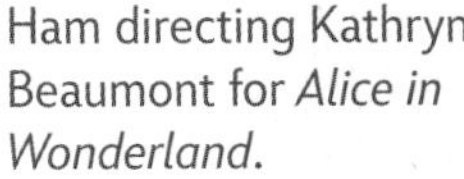

Ham directing Kathryn Beaumont for *Alice in Wonderland*.

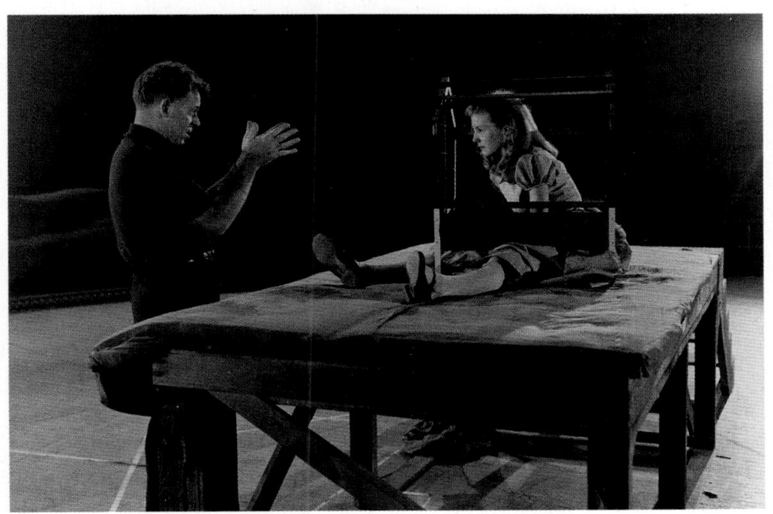

A SLICE OF HAM

Disney animators consistently credited Ham as a good director. One distinguishing characteristic was his ability to look at animation footage and very quickly analyze what was wrong. There was no hemming and hawing with Ham, as there was with some directors; once or twice through the Moviola and Ham knew what changes were needed. Wilfred Jackson thought that Ham's work as a supervising animator on *Snow White* led naturally to his role as a director: "Ham had the patience and perseverance it took to see this job through. I think, perhaps, those two qualities might well characterize Ham's approach to directing when he got into that. In order to get out all the footage on the Snow White character, Ham had a crew of other animators working under his supervision on the feature. So he was another one, like Ben, who seemed to sort of slip into directing later on by taking on the responsibility for what all the animators on a whole feature sequence were doing instead of only for what a group were doing on some one aspect of it."[26] Wilfred Jackson admired another ability that Ham possessed: "I had the impression that Ham, as a director, liked to work very closely with each thing each one of his crew was doing on his pictures. I noticed, for example, the way Ham would show with sketches of his own the suggestions he had for the animation character models, and for staging the cartoon business in the layout drawings when working with his layout men. And how he would go over one of his animator's pencil tests on the Moviola, sketching out animation drawings of his own to show the animator things he thought would improve the action. I envied Ham's ability to do this."[27]

Milt Kahl had an interesting take on Ham: "He was a good director. But Ham was a delegator. I always thought he retired the last fifteen years he was a director. Ham is sort of an enigma to me, still, when I think about him. He was awfully sweet; that was the word for him. An awfully nice person."[28] Others thought that as Ham settled into direction, he was not as intimately associated with the animators as he once had been. Frank Thomas and Ollie Johnston, in discussing who they would go to if they wanted to add a new facet to a character's personality, mentioned Ham, but with a caveat. They went to Ham in the early days, Frank said, but "as he directed more and more, he drew away from that aspect of things. Jackson was about the only guy, outside of other animators."[29] Frank reflected on the long-game evolution of Ham: "Well, he just sort of got pushed to the side, too. Walt gave him more and more of un-fun projects. Ham had sort of specialized in making things work. He liked to think that he could take a junky piece of film and make it usable. So Walt gave him all these junky things from Europe and things for TV and stuff like that and see what you can do with it, see what you can do with them. Ham found this much easier than the creative stuff he used to be so good at. One of the last lunches I had with him, we were kidding him about this and he kind of laughed and said, 'Yeah, I used to do that. I wonder what happened?' We said, 'We were wondering what happened. That was a lot more fun, what you used to do.' He just sort of laughed it off. He kind of realized he had grown out of that into something else, but he didn't have the stature or the contribution. In a different way, he was passed up the same as the others."[30] Michael Barrier, commenting on Ham in his later years, said, "I don't recall people talking about him as being a strong presence. He obviously had a presence because he was doing so much work. But were people feeling his presence as a director, with a certain point of view? Making himself felt? [He seemed like] somebody who was exceptionally strong at realizing Walt's ideas, that sort of thing."[31]

Perhaps this was partially due to a falling out between Walt and Ham, apparently over a personal issue, that set Ham back for a while. He eventually recovered, although evidently not to the same stature as before. Yet in later years someone once criticized Ham to Walt, who defended Ham by saying, "Don't belittle Ham. He helped build this studio out of nothing.[32]

Some of the assignments he received were not what they had once been, but this could also have been due to changing times and different priorities for Walt and the studio, especially with television programming.

"I sometimes wonder if Ham wouldn't really have been happier to have continued as an animator where he would have been in closer contact with the actual animation," theorized Wilfred Jackson. "Ham did not ever say so to me—but he probably wouldn't have mentioned it, anyway, one way or the other. He was not the sort of person to complain about doing whatever he was assigned to do."[33] Animator Burny Mattinson said that about a month before Ham died, the two of them and Eric Larson had lunch at the famed Alfonse's restaurant. At one point it was just Ham and Burny at the table. "I was amazed when he said, 'You know, every day I come to work and it's never really been satisfying, because all the time what I do is I give advice; I never draw anything or I never do anything.' But he said, 'I remember how nice it was when I was an animator. I left something every

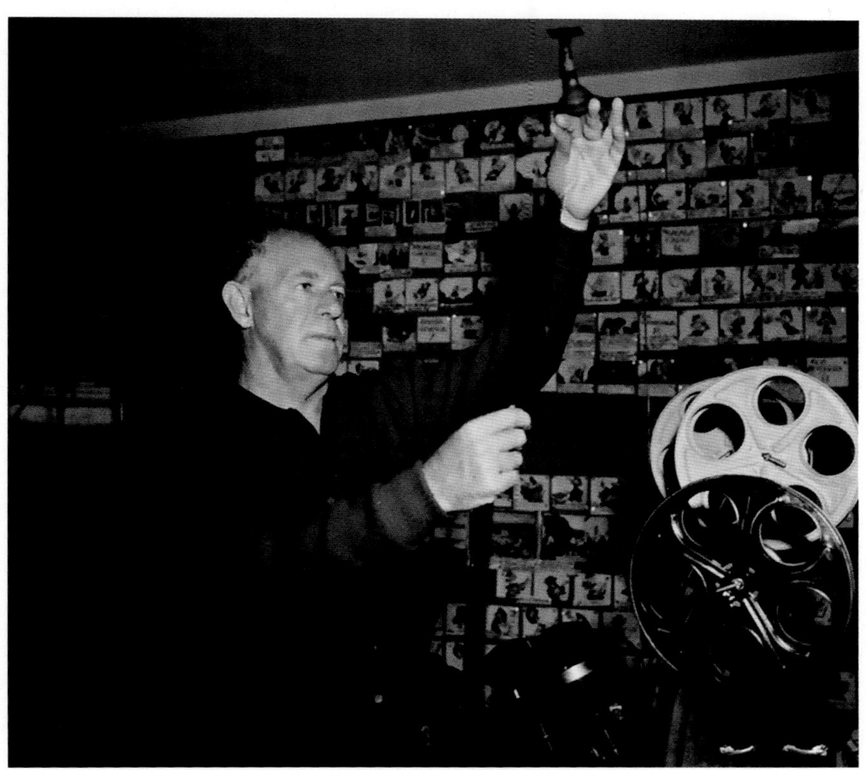

Ham reviews work for a *Disneyland* television program.

day that was part of me. But as soon as I became a director,' he said, 'I have nothing to show for it.' And I thought that was revealing. And I found it myself. I found when I directed a couple of things there, that I missed it: I missed drawing and putting down something every day."[34]

Even so, Walt could always count on Ham to give him his best work and to get the best out of those working with him. And Ham had that special talent that a few directors had, to be able to interpret Walt. Ken O'Connor recalled, "He taught me not to listen to what Walt said, but to read between the lines. He was an expert at it. I'd say, 'Well Walt said—' and he'd say, 'Oh, I know what he said, but what he means was this,' and he'd explain, because he was used to picking up the inferences between Walt's lines. I had the devil of a time because I'm sort of a literal, straight-forward person and I take what they say as being what they mean. You couldn't always do that with Walt. He sometimes was throwing out lines and sometimes just fishing. He couldn't express it perhaps or he expected you to do some detective work."[35]

Walt's passing saddened Ham, and he took it like the loss of a family member. Ham had had heart problems since he was thirty, and perhaps concerns about his role in the studio's future without Walt played a part in his early demise. Ham Luske passed away on February 18, 1968. He received a Winsor McCay Award in 1984 and a Disney Legends Award in 1999. Just a few years before his death, Otto Englander wrote in a letter to animator and *New Yorker* cartoonist Izzy Klein: "Ham is one of the few guys I know who have aged gracefully, without changing their basic attitude to life and people—especially people who work with him—he is always gracious, considerate and non-neurotic. Wish one could say that of some others. . . Most importantly, the title of producer-director didn't fill his noggin with helium."[36]

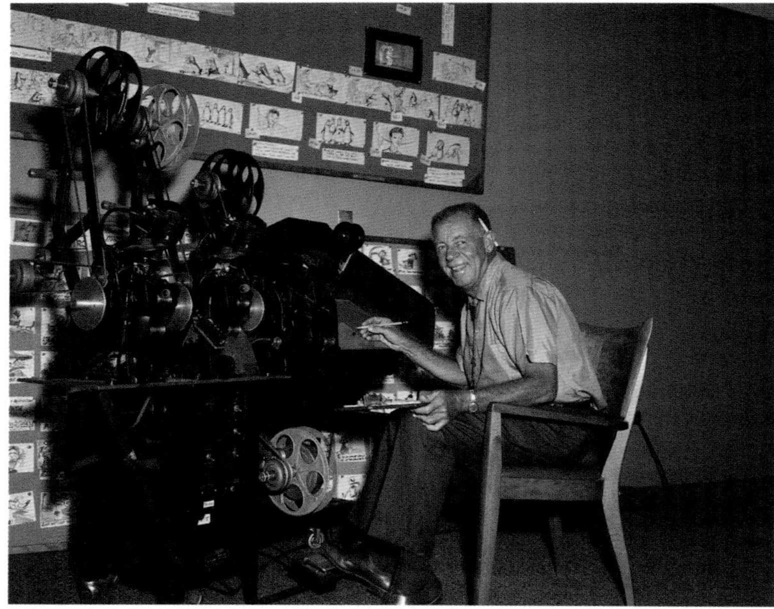

Ham at work on *Mary Poppins*.

Ham Luske—Disney Director Filmography[37]

Shorts and Training/Educational/ Specialty Films:

- *Thunderstorms* (1943)
- *Air Masses and Fronts* (1943)
- *The Cold Front* (1943)
- *Flying the Weather Map* (1944)
- *The Howgozit Chart* (1944)
- *Weather at War* (1944)
- *Weather for the Navigator* (1944)
- *The Pelican and the Snipe* (1945) (Animator and Director)
- *Hold Your Horsepower* (1945)
- *Ben and Me* (1953)
- *Mickey Mouse Club* openings and closings (1955)
- *Donald in Mathmagic Land* (1959) (Supervising Director)
- *Donald and the Wheel* (1961)
- *The Litterbug* (1961)
- *Scrooge McDuck and Money* (1967)
- *Understanding Stresses and Strains* (1968)

Features:

- *Pinocchio* (1940) (Co-supervising Director)
- *Fantasia* (1940) (Sequence Director)
- *The Reluctant Dragon* (1941) (Cartoon Director)
- *Saludos Amigos* (1943) (Sequence Director)
- *Make Mine Music* (1946) (Sequence Director)
- *Fun and Fancy Free* (1947) (Cartoon Director)
- *Melody Time* (1948) (Cartoon Director)
- *So Dear To My Heart* (1949) (Cartoon Director)
- *Cinderella* (1950) (Codirector with Wilfred Jackson and Gerry Geronimi)
- *Alice in Wonderland* (1951) (Codirector with Wilfred Jackson and Gerry Geronimi)
- *Peter Pan* (1953) (Codirector with Wilfred Jackson and Gerry Geronimi)
- *Lady and the Tramp* (1955) (Codirector with Wilfred Jackson and Gerry Geronimi)
- *One Hundred and One Dalmatians* (1961) (Codirector with Woolie Reitherman and Gerry Geronimi)
- *Mary Poppins* (1964) (Animation Director)

To give the reader a sense of where all this action took place, here is a map of the original Animation Building on Disney's Burbank campus, circa 1950. In general, the offices of the animators were on the first floor, with director units (director and layout) on the second floor, and Walt and many of the production, music, and—most notable—story people on the third floor.

These maps were created by and courtesy of Hans Perk, who did expert sleuthing to figure out who lived where—mainly via studio telephone directories.

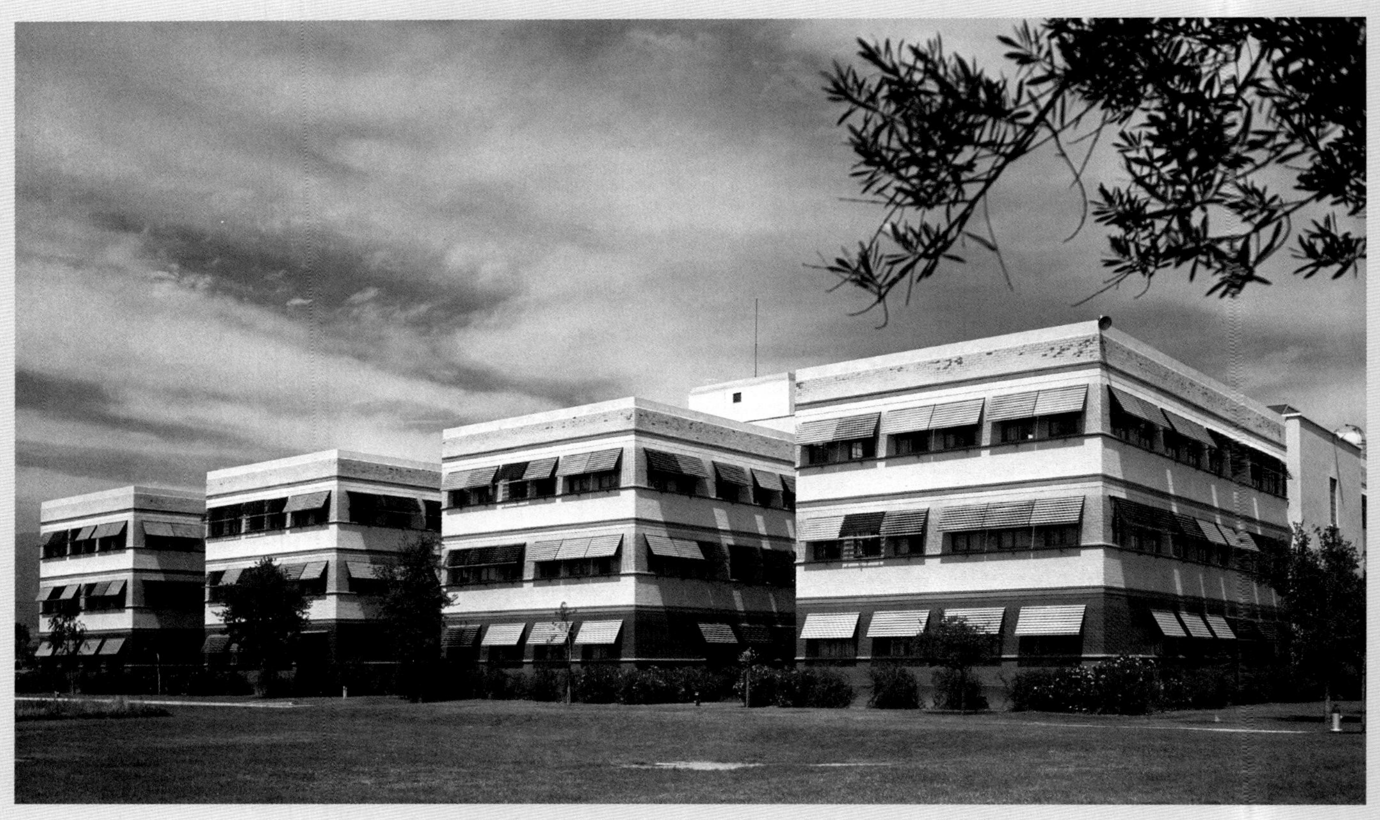

The Walt Disney Studios in Burbank, California.

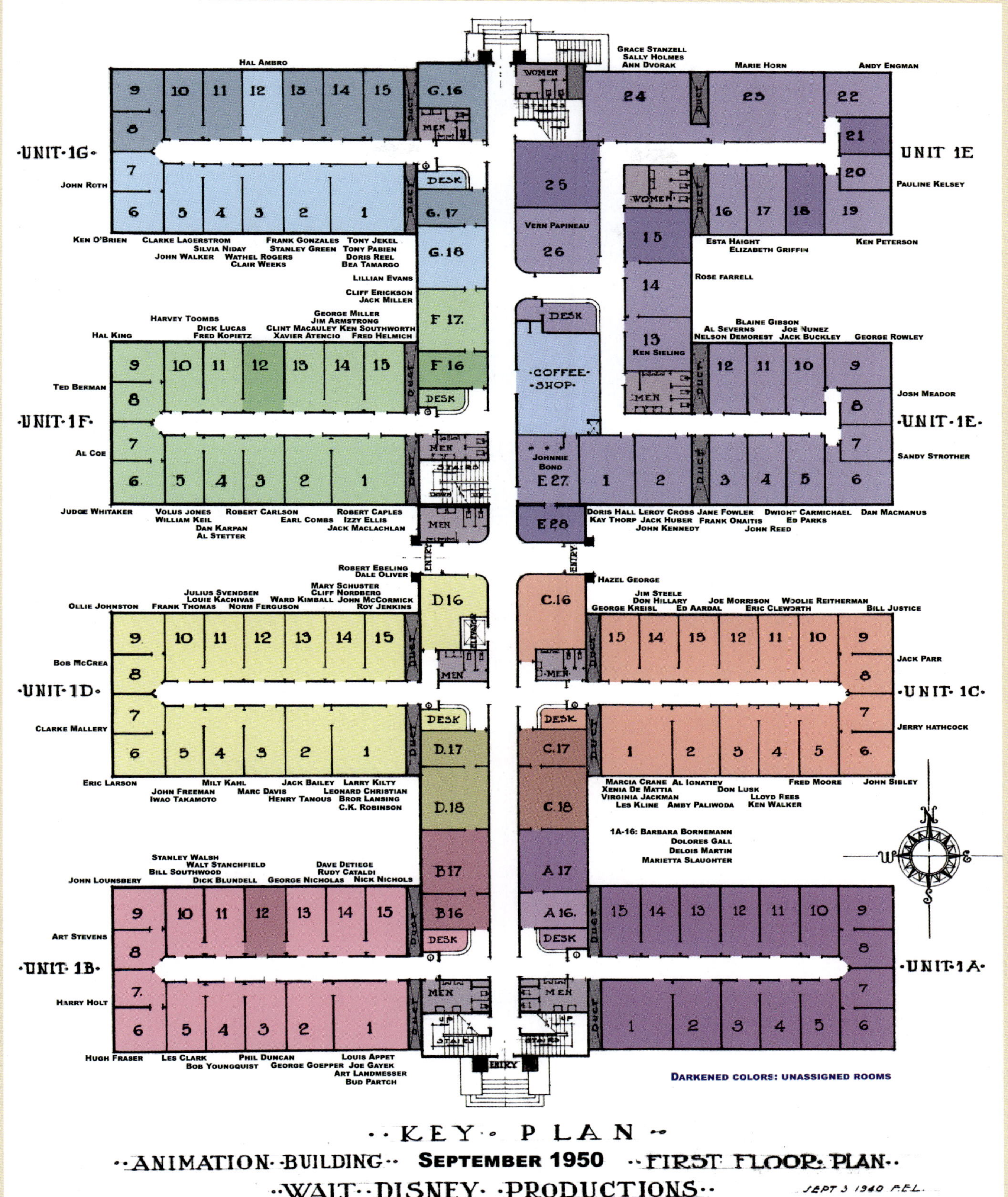

·UNIT·1G·
Hal Ambro
John Roth
Ken O'Brien
Clarke Lagerstrom
Silvia Niday
John Walker
Wathel Rogers
Clair Weeks
Frank Gonzales
Stanley Green
Tony Jekel
Tony Pabien
Doris Reel
Bea Tamargo
Lillian Evans
Cliff Erickson
Jack Miller
G.16
G.17
G.18
DESK
MEN
WOMEN
STAIRS
DUCT
Grace Stanzell
Sally Holmes
Ann Dvorak
Marie Horn
Andy Engman
UNIT 1E
Pauline Kelsey
Vern Papineau
Esta Haight
Elizabeth Griffin
Ken Peterson
Rose Farrell
Blaine Gibson
Al Severns
Joe Nunez
Nelson Demorest
Jack Buckley
George Rowley
Ken Sieling
Josh Meador
·UNIT·1E·
Sandy Strother
·COFFEE·
·SHOP·
Johnnie Bond
E 27
E 28
Doris Hall
Leroy Cross
Jane Fowler
Dwight Carmichael
Dan MacManus
Kay Thorp
Jack Huber
Frank Onaitis
Ed Parks
John Kennedy
John Reed
Harvey Toombs
Dick Lucas
Fred Kopietz
George Miller
Jim Armstrong
Clint Macauley
Ken Southworth
Xavier Atencio
Fred Helmich
Hal King
F 17
F 16
Ted Berman
·UNIT·1F·
Al Coe
Judge Whitaker
Volus Jones
William Keil
Dan Karpan
Al Stetter
Robert Carlson
Earl Combs
Robert Caples
Izzy Ellis
Jack MacLachlan
ENTRY
Robert Ebeling
Dale Oliver
Hazel George
Julius Svendsen
Louie Kachivas
Mary Schuster
Cliff Nordberg
Ward Kimball
John McCormick
Roy Jenkins
Ollie Johnston
Frank Thomas
Norm Ferguson
D16
ELEVATOR
C.16
Jim Steele
Don Hillary
Joe Morrison
Woolie Reitherman
George Kreisl
Ed Aardal
Eric Cleworth
Bill Justice
Bob McCrea
·UNIT·1D·
Clarke Mallery
Jack Parr
·UNIT·1C·
Jerry Hathcock
D.17
D.18
C.17
C.18
Eric Larson
Milt Kahl
Jack Bailey
Larry Kilty
John Freeman
Marc Davis
Leonard Christian
Iwao Takamoto
Henry Tanous
Bror Lansing
C.K. Robinson
Marcia Crane
Al Ignatiev
Fred Moore
John Sibley
Xenia De Mattia
Don Lusk
Virginia Jackman
Lloyd Rees
Les Kline
Amby Paliwoda
Ken Walker
1A-16: Barbara Bornemann
Dolores Gall
Delois Martin
Marietta Slaughter
N
W
E
S
Stanley Walsh
Walt Stanchfield
Bill Southwood
Dick Blundell
Dave Detiege
Rudy Cataldi
George Nicholas
Nick Nichols
John Lounsbery
B17
B16
A 17
A 16.
Art Stevens
·UNIT·1B·
Harry Holt
·UNIT·1A·
Hugh Fraser
Les Clark
Bob Youngquist
Phil Duncan
George Goepper
Louis Appet
Joe Gayek
Art Landmesser
Bud Partch
UP
ENTRY
Darkened colors: unassigned rooms
··KEY· PLAN·
··ANIMATION·BUILDING·· September 1950 ··FIRST FLOOR·PLAN··
··WALT··DISNEY··PRODUCTIONS··
··BURBANK · CALIFORNIA··
SEPT 3 1940 P.E.L.
Hans Perk 2021

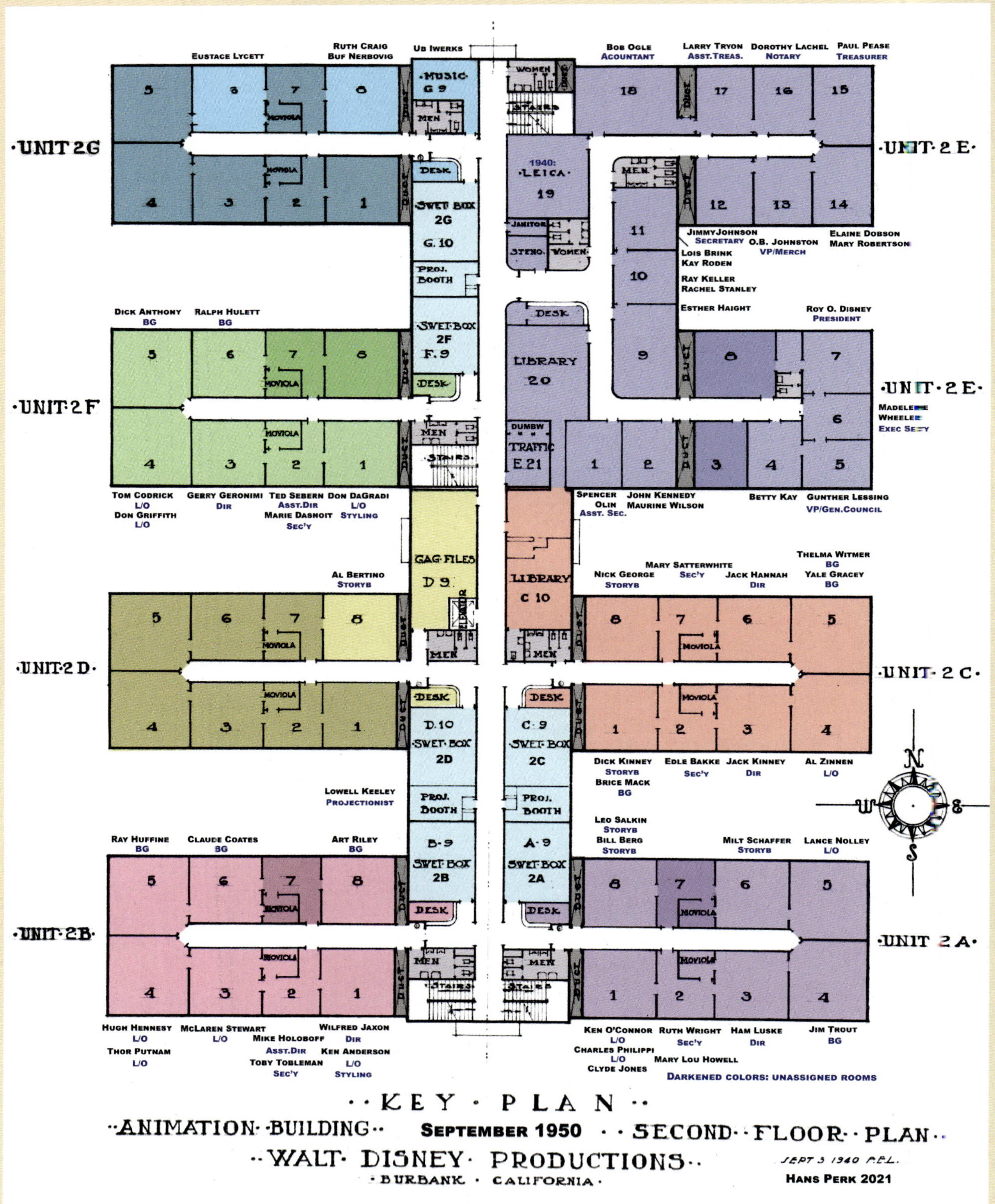

Eustace Lycett
Ruth Craig
Buf Nerbovig
Ub Iwerks
Bob Ogle
Acountant
Larry Tryon
Asst.Treas.
Dorothy Lachel
Notary
Paul Pease
Treasurer
·UNIT 2G
·UNIT·2 E·
Music
G 9
Women
Stairs
Men
Moviola
Duct
Desk
Swet Box
2G
G. 10
Proj.
Booth
1940:
·LEICA·
19
Janitor
Steno.
Women·
JimmyJohnson
Secretary
O.B. Johnston
VP/Merch
Elaine Dobson
Mary Robertson
Lois Brink
Kay Roden
Ray Keller
Rachel Stanley
Esther Haight
Roy O. Disney
President
Dick Anthony
BG
Ralph Hulett
BG
Swet·Box
2F
F. 9
Library
20
Dumbw
Traffic
E 21
·UNIT·2F
·UNIT·2 E·
Tom Codrick
L/O
Don Griffith
L/O
Gerry Geronimi
Dir
Ted Sebern
Asst.Dir
Marie Dasnoit
Sec'y
Don DaGradi
L/O
Styling
Spencer
Olin
Asst. Sec.
John Kennedy
Maurine Wilson
Betty Kay
Gunther Lessing
VP/Gen.Council
Gag Files
D 9
Elevator
Library
C 10
Al Bertino
Storyb
Mary Satterwhite
Sec'y
Nick George
Storyb
Jack Hannah
Dir
Thelma Witmer
BG
Yale Gracey
BG
·UNIT·2 D·
·UNIT· 2 C·
D.10
Swet·Box
2D
C·9
Swet·Box
2C
Proj.
Booth
Dick Kinney
Storyb
Brice Mack
BG
Edle Bakke
Sec'y
Jack Kinney
Dir
Al Zinnen
L/O
Lowell Keeley
Projectionist
Leo Salkin
Storyb
Bill Berg
Storyb
N
W
E
S
Ray Huffine
BG
Claude Coates
BG
Art Riley
BG
Milt Schaffer
Storyb
Lance Nolley
L/O
B·9
Swet·Box
2B
A·9
Swet·Box
2A
·UNIT·2B·
·UNIT 2 A·
Hugh Hennesy
L/O
Thor Putnam
L/O
McLaren Stewart
L/O
Mike Holoboff
Asst.Dir
Toby Tobleman
Sec'y
Wilfred Jaxon
Dir
Ken Anderson
L/O
Styling
Ken O'Connor
L/O
Charles Philippi
L/O
Clyde Jones
Ruth Wright
Sec'y
Mary Lou Howell
Ham Luske
Dir
Jim Trout
BG
Darkened colors: unassigned rooms
··KEY · PLAN··
··ANIMATION· BUILDING··
September 1950
· · SECOND· · FLOOR· · PLAN··
··WALT· DISNEY· PRODUCTIONS··
·BURBANK · CALIFORNIA·
SEPT 3 1940 R.E.L.
Hans Perk 2021

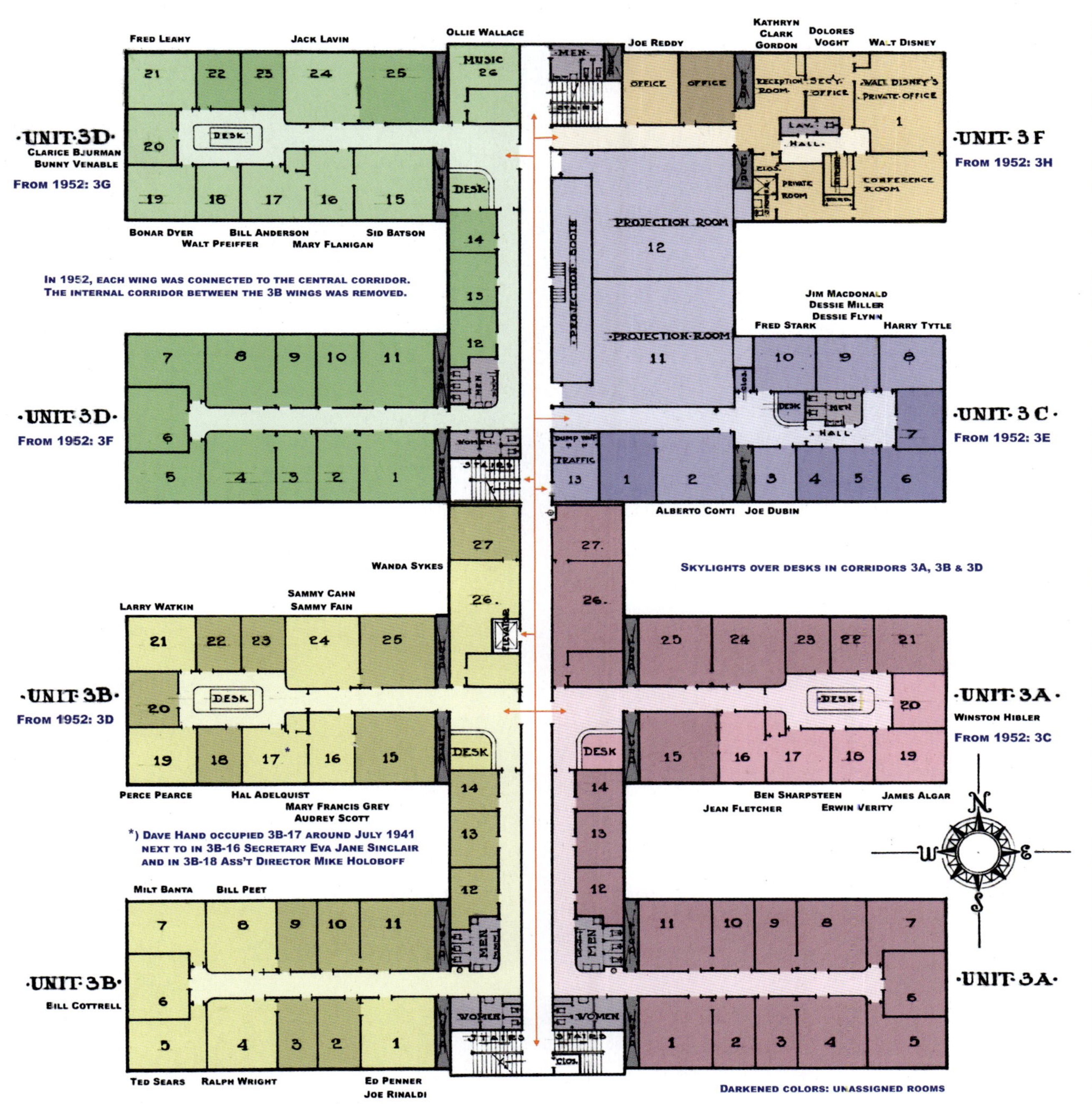
Fred Leahy
Jack Lavin
Ollie Wallace
Joe Reddy
Kathryn Clark Gordon
Dolores Voght
Walt Disney
Music 26
Men
Office
Office
Reception Room
Sec'y. Office
Walt Disney's Private Office
Lav.
Hall
Private Room
Conference Room
·UNIT·3D·
Clarice Bjurman
Bunny Venable
From 1952: 3G
Desk
·UNIT·3F
From 1952: 3H
Bonar Dyer
Walt Pfeiffer
Bill Anderson
Mary Flanigan
Sid Batson
Projection Room 12
Projection Booth
In 1952, each wing was connected to the central corridor.
The internal corridor between the 3B wings was removed.
Jim Macdonald
Dessie Miller
Dessie Flynn
Fred Stark
Harry Tytle
Projection Room 11
·UNIT·3D·
From 1952: 3F
·UNIT·3C·
From 1952: 3E
Women
Stairs
Dump Waiter
Traffic
Hall
Alberto Conti
Joe Dubin
Wanda Sykes
Skylights over desks in corridors 3A, 3B & 3D
Sammy Cahn
Sammy Fain
Larry Watkin
Elevator
·UNIT·3B·
From 1952: 3D
·UNIT·3A·
Winston Hibler
From 1952: 3C
Perce Pearce
Hal Adelquist
Mary Francis Grey
Audrey Scott
Ben Sharpsteen
Jean Fletcher
Erwin Verity
James Algar
*) Dave Hand occupied 3B-17 around July 1941
next to in 3B-16 Secretary Eva Jane Sinclair
and in 3B-18 Ass't Director Mike Holoboff
N
W
E
S
Milt Banta
Bill Peet
·UNIT·3B·
Bill Cottrell
·UNIT·3A·
Ted Sears
Ralph Wright
Ed Penner
Joe Rinaldi
Darkened colors: unassigned rooms
··KEY· PLAN··
··ANIMATION·BUILDING·· September 1950 ··THIRD··FLOOR··PLAN··
··WALT··DISNEY··PRODUCTIONS··
··BURBANK · CALIFORNIA··
SEPT 3 1940 P.E.L.
Hans Perk 2021

New employees coming to work in the mid-forties were handed a pamphlet written by Winston Hibler and Hal Adelquist (likely drawn by Tom Oreb) called *The Ropes at Disney*, which included these helpful maps, the first showing how to get around the lot and the second showing how to get around the organization.

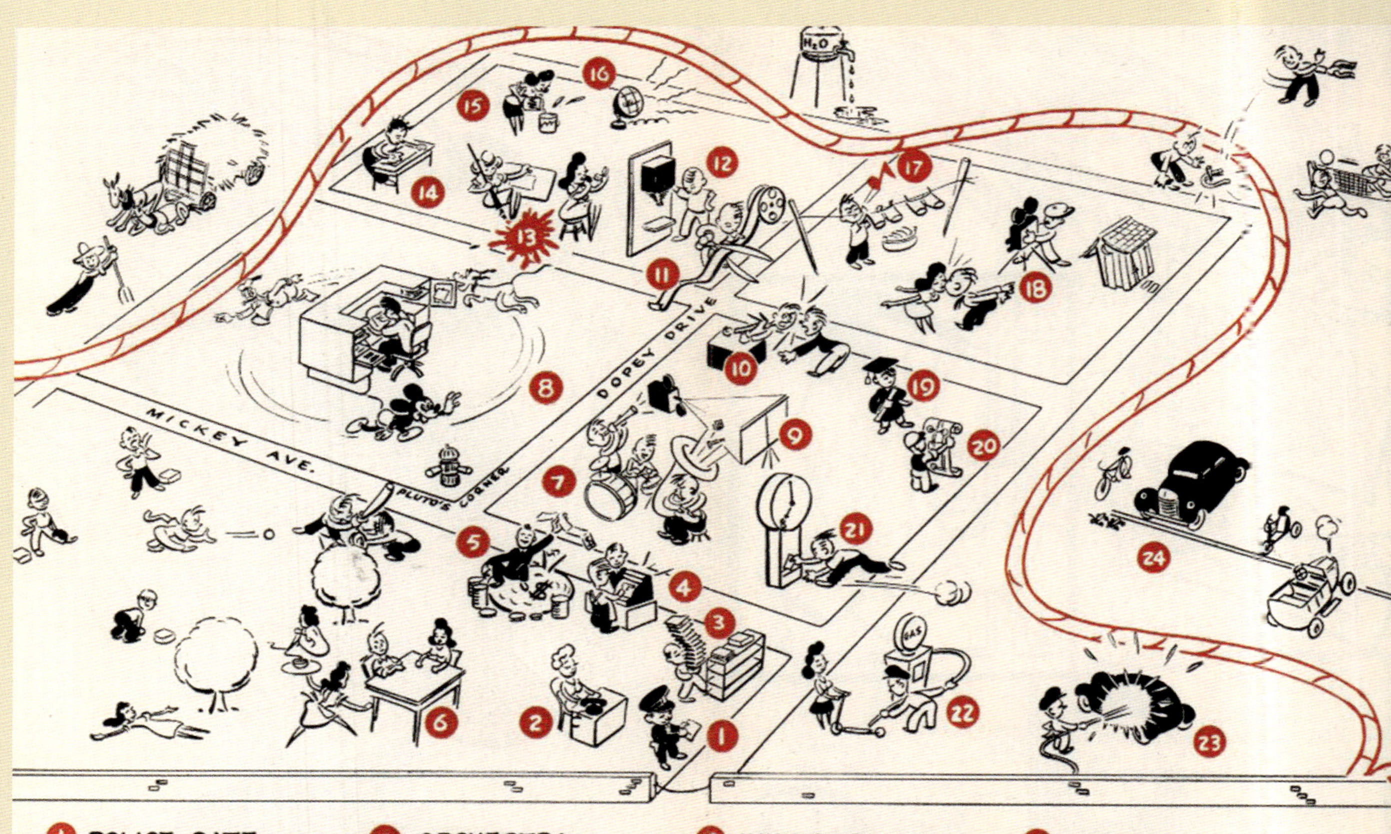

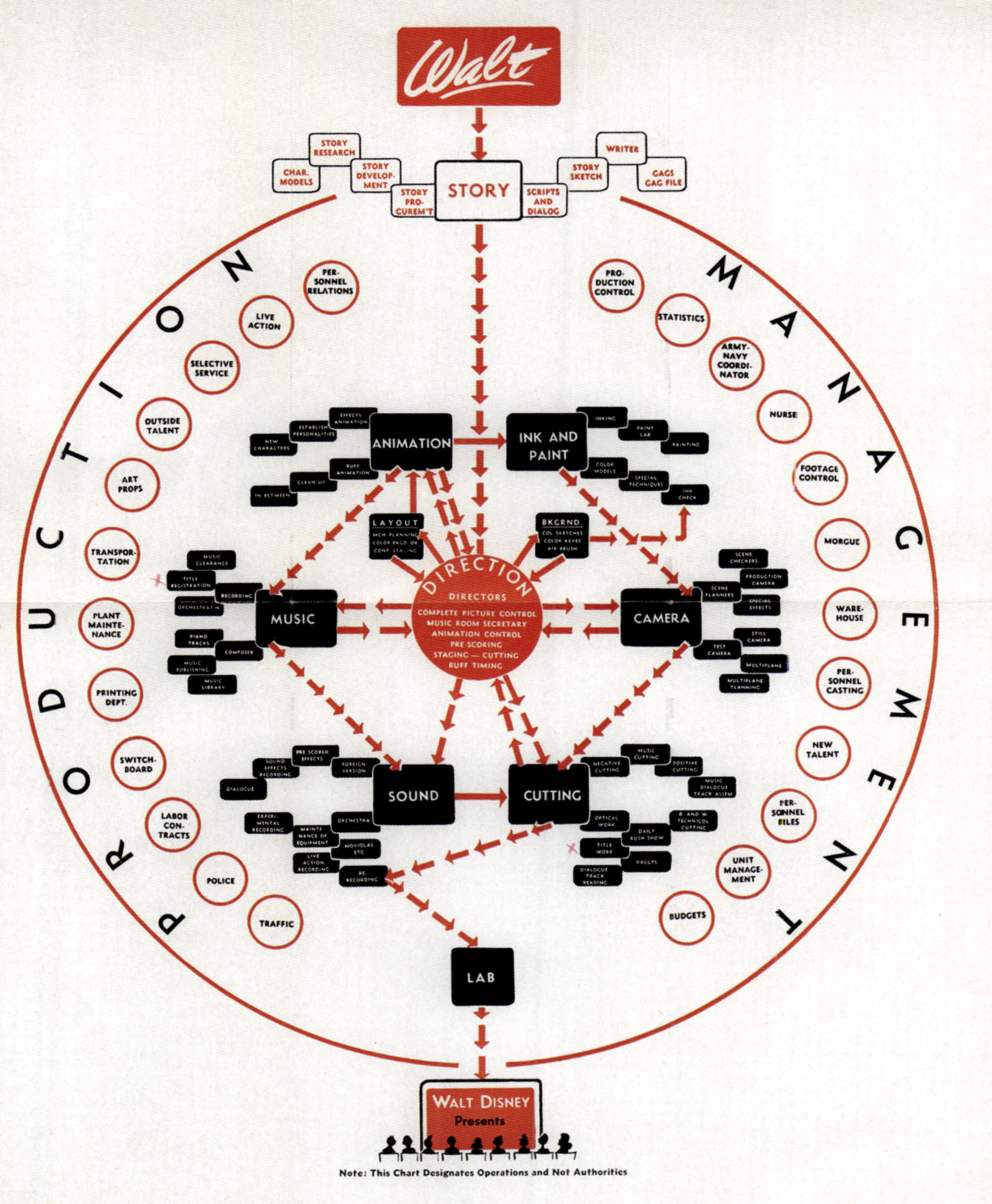

Walt
STORY
CHAR. MODELS
STORY RESEARCH
STORY DEVELOP-MENT
STORY PRO-CUREM'T
SCRIPTS AND DIALOG
STORY SKETCH
WRITER
GAGS GAG FILE
PRODUCTION
MANAGEMENT
PER-SONNEL RELATIONS
LIVE ACTION
SELECTIVE SERVICE
OUTSIDE TALENT
ART PROPS
TRANSPOR-TATION
PLANT MAINTE-NANCE
PRINTING DEPT.
SWITCH-BOARD
LABOR CON-TRACTS
POLICE
TRAFFIC
PRO-DUCTION CONTROL
STATISTICS
ARMY-NAVY COORDI-NATOR
NURSE
FOOTAGE CONTROL
MORGUE
WARE-HOUSE
PER-SONNEL CASTING
NEW TALENT
PER-SONNEL FILES
UNIT MANAGE-MENT
BUDGETS
ANIMATION
EFFECTS ANIMATION
ESTABLISH PERSONALITIES
NEW CHARACTERS
RUFF ANIMATION
CLEAN UP
IN BETWEEN
INK AND PAINT
INKING
PAINT LAB
PAINTING
COLOR MODELS
SPECIAL TECHNIQUES
INK CHECK
LAYOUT
MCH PLANNING
COLOR BACD OK
CONT STAGING
BKGRND.
COL SKETCHES
COLOR KEYES
AIR BRUSH
DIRECTION
DIRECTORS
COMPLETE PICTURE CONTROL
MUSIC ROOM SECRETARY
ANIMATION CONTROL
PRE-SCORING
STAGING — CUTTING
RUFF TIMING
MUSIC
MUSIC CLEARANCE
TITLE REGISTRATION
RECORDING
ORCHESTRATN
PIANO TRACKS
COMPOSER
MUSIC PUBLISHING
MUSIC LIBRARY
CAMERA
SCENE CHECKERS
PRODUCTION CAMERA
SCENE PLANNERS
SPECIAL EFFECTS
STILL CAMERA
TEST CAMERA
MULTIPLANE
MULTIPLANE PLANNING
SOUND
PRE-SCORED EFFECTS
SOUND EFFECTS RECORDING
FOREIGN VERSION
DIALOGUE
EXPERI-MENTAL RECORDING
ORCHESTRA
MAINTE-NANCE OF EQUIPMENT
MOVIOLAS ETC
LIVE ACTION RECORDING
RE-RECORDING
CUTTING
MUSIC CUTTING
NEGATIVE CUTTING
POSITIVE CUTTING
MUSIC DIALOGUE TRACK ASSEM
OPTICAL WORK
B AND W TECHNICOL CUTTING
DAILY RUSH SHOW
TITLE WORK
VAULTS
DIALOGUE TRACK READING
LAB
WALT DISNEY
Presents
Note: This Chart Designates Operations and Not Authorities

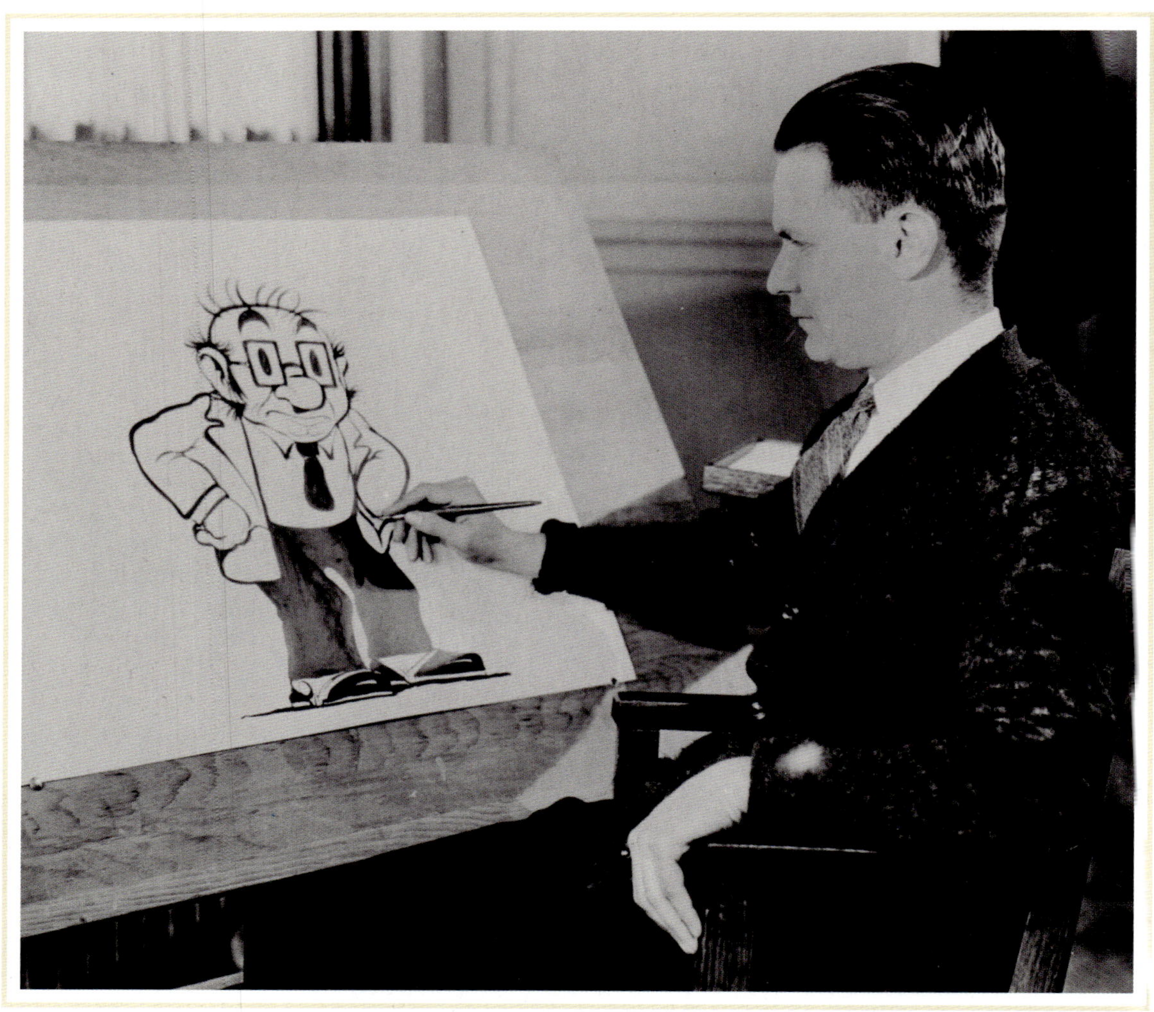

Geronimi at Bray Productions, inking Colonel Heeza Liar. Exact date unknown.

CHAPTER 7

GERRY GERONIMI—THE FIGHT FOR QUALITY

"What made it tough was this: Walt naturally praised those so-called Nine Old Men—and they knew it. They knew they were good, and they knew they had Walt's backing. That made it tough on directors."[1]

—Gerry Geronimi

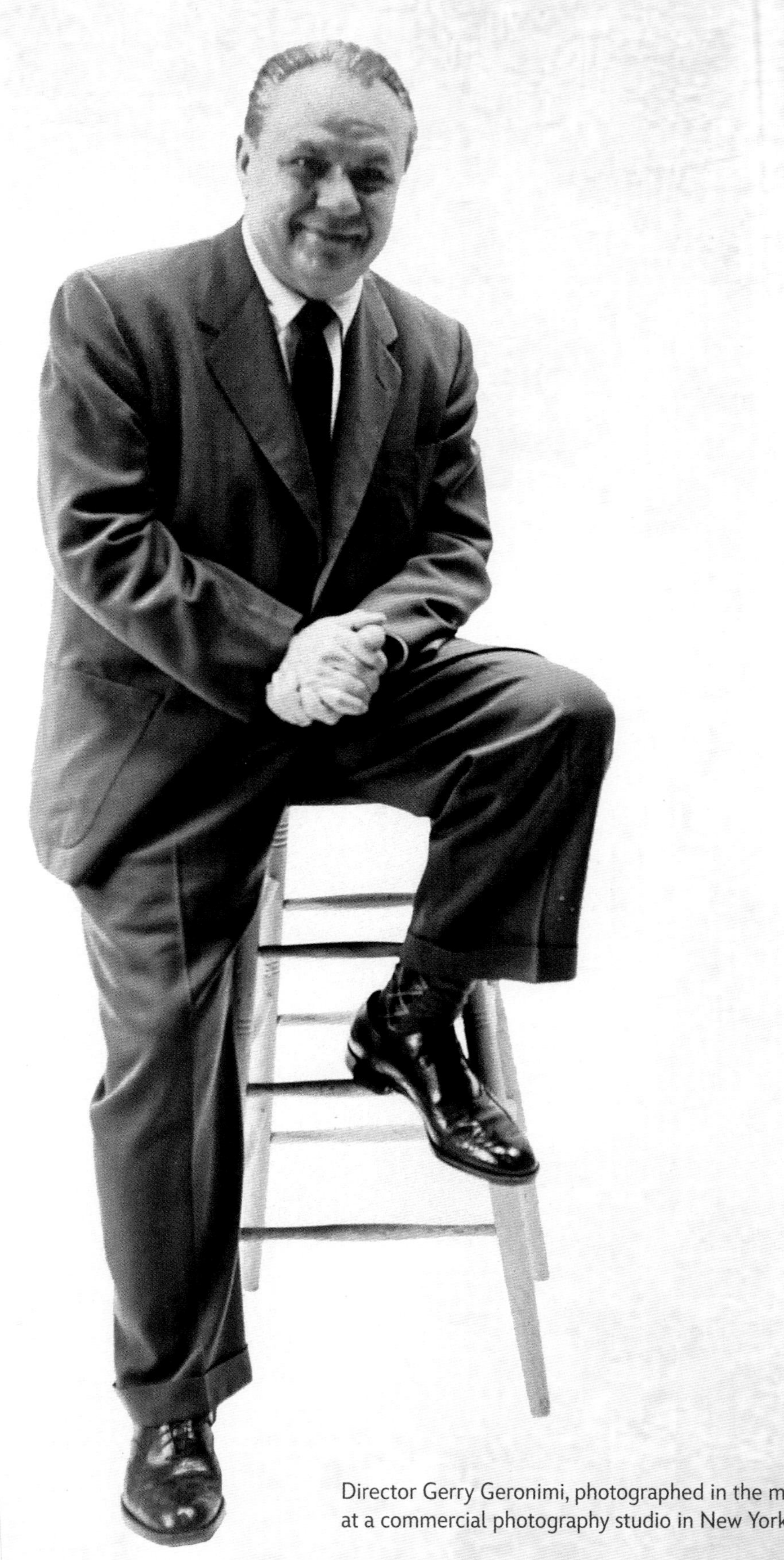

Director Gerry Geronimi, photographed in the mid-1950s at a commercial photography studio in New York.

Of all the director's responsibilities, one of the most important was the ability to work with animators. Walt saw animators as the stars of his studio. Top animators were treated well, were paid well (quite a few had higher salaries than directors), and were heavily involved creatively as to how characters would look and act. And like movie stars, they were also temperamental, with their own strong convictions and well-developed egos. It was the director's job to make sure their work improved on what Disney wanted—a subjective call to be sure, and an opinion not always shared by all.

No one seemed to ruffle more animators' feathers than director Clyde "Gerry" Geronimi. Coworkers called him "a tyrant," "impossible to get along with," and "one of the most hated guys around."[2] Yet he directed some of the very best sequences of the films he worked on, such as the storytelling and chase from "The Legend of Sleepy Hollow" segment of *The Adventures of Ichabod and Mr. Toad*, the spaghetti eating in *Lady and the Tramp*, and the slipper-fitting and rescue of *Cinderella*.

If Geronimi irritated his animators, that didn't seem to bother Walt. And as is often the case, there is more to all this than appears on the surface.

Clito Enrico Geronimi was born on June 12, 1901, in Chiavenna, Italy, a little village in the Italian Alps. The youngest of three, his father was a butcher, but hardships prompted a move to New Rochelle, New York, on December 27, 1908.[3] When the family arrived at Ellis Island, young Clito's name was Americanized to Clyde Henry. He would not run short on names: he would later go by "Jocko," "Butch," and his preferred moniker, "Gerry" (originally spelled "Jerry" but changed over time by friends and colleagues to match "Geronimi").

The Geronimi family arrived in an America not always friendly to Italian immigrants, who were seen by many as an impure race in service of a corrupt foreign power, and later associated with organized crime. Through the 1940s, Italian Americans were widely considered to be non-white. Between 1890 and 1920 in the South, an estimated fifty Italians were lynched.[4] Racist stereotypes were spread even through northern newspapers. "It is impossible to understand my grandfather without understanding the prejudice that existed towards Italian immigrants," wrote granddaughter Megan Hills. "He had to fight for everything. Nothing was handed to him."[5] Beyond how prejudice shaped Gerry, one wonders how much it drove how his coworkers saw and spoke about him, even years later.

Gerry's childhood was rough; he recalled street gang fights near his home in New Rochelle.[6] By the age of twelve it was necessary for Gerry to drop out of a New York public school to find a job.

Gerry was determined to get into cartooning and took night classes at Cooper Union and the Art Students League. After a brief stint retouching catalog photos for the Scientific Engraving Company, he did single panel sports comics for Hearst news, which got him started at William Randolph Hearst's new International Film Service. The work wasn't glamorous—Gerry started by erasing pencil lines from the inked drawings (characters were drawn on paper at this time, rather than the clear acetate sheets that would come later). But these were the formative days of the animation industry; it had been only three years earlier that Winsor McCay created *Gertie the Dinosaur*. Gerry was seventeen, and getting in on the ground floor.

At Hearst's, Gerry was assigned to a production unit under a fellow Italian named Walter

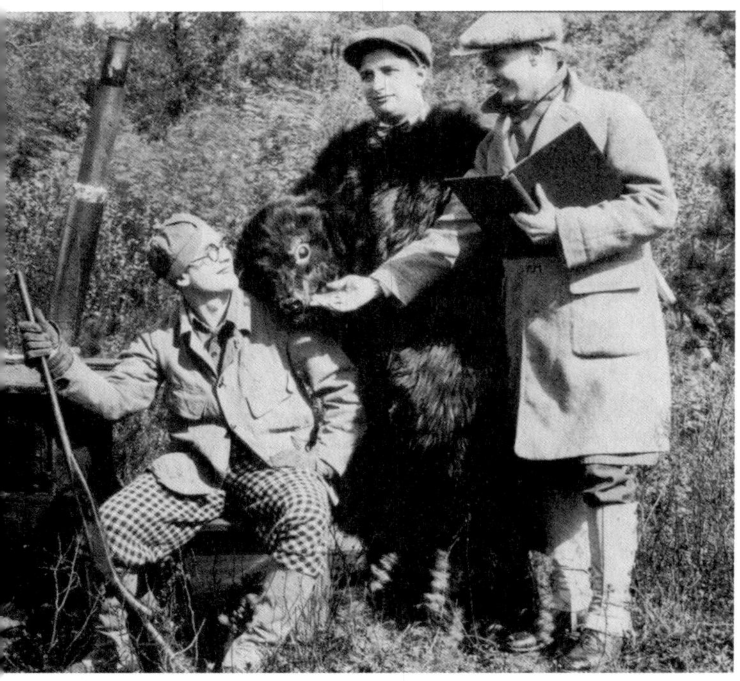

Geronimi (RIGHT) directs Walter Lantz (SEATED AT LEFT) for live-action segments at Bray Productions, where both animated on the Colonel Heeza Liar, Pete the Pup, Unnatural History, and Dinky Doodle films. The two arrived at Bray following Hearst's studio closure in July 1918, having first followed fellow animator George Stallings to his own short-lived studio. Geronimi delighted in telling the story of a short that involved Lantz's brother Al dressing up as a bear, only to be spooked by the sound of nearby hunters' gunshots.

Lantz (formerly Lanza, who likely changed his name to avoid being stigmatized as Italian), who would later create Woody Woodpecker. The two formed a friendship that would continue throughout Gerry's life. It was Lantz who gave Geronimi his first animation assignment—a train chugging into the station for a *Jerry on the Job* cartoon.

In these early days, animators were not only responsible for the movement of characters, but for the stories overall. "There were no storyboards," remembered Geronimi. "We had just a typewritten sheet, with an outline of what we were going to do."[7] As such, Gerry was the story man, layout artist, and animator all in one—experience that would come in handy later in his career.

By 1922 Gerry was seeing Elska "Alice" Jindrak, a New York fashion artist. The two had been dating for five years when Alice suffered a stroke, leaving her bedridden with her left side paralyzed for six months. After she traveled to Florida with her sister to convalesce, a flurry of cards from Gerry arrived to cheer her up. Alice taught herself to walk again, and would recover almost entirely.

In 1927 Geronimi's friend Lantz left for Los Angeles to set up his own studio and, after a few detours, invited Gerry to join him. Gerry was greeted in Los Angeles by a small earthquake, which "scared the hell out of me and I was ready to pack and head back to New York!"[8] But he soon found California life pleasant enough to send word back to Alice, and the two were married at City Hall in Los Angeles on September 15, 1929. Lantz was Gerry's best man.

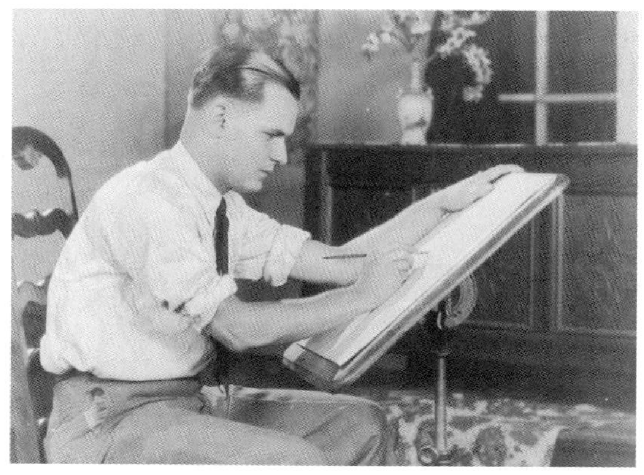

Geronimi in his late teens at his drawing board in New York.

No-46— FRI- JUNE-29-
I TRIED LETTING MY SMILE
BE MY UMBRELLA-DEAR
BUT I GOT ALL
WET!!
JERRY The PUP

NIGHT OF
JOON AN
LOVE
PLUNK
PLUNK
to my Valentine

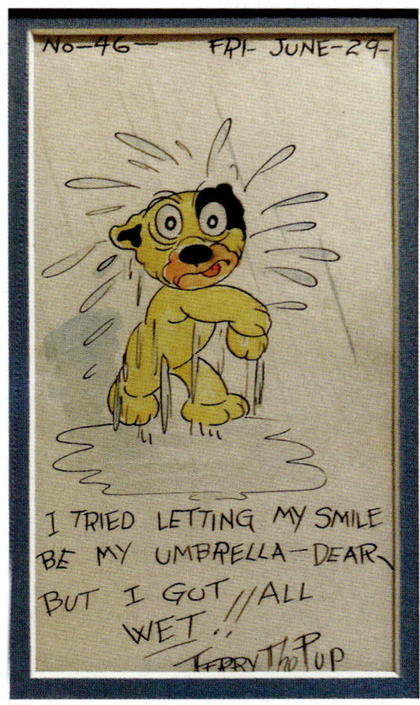

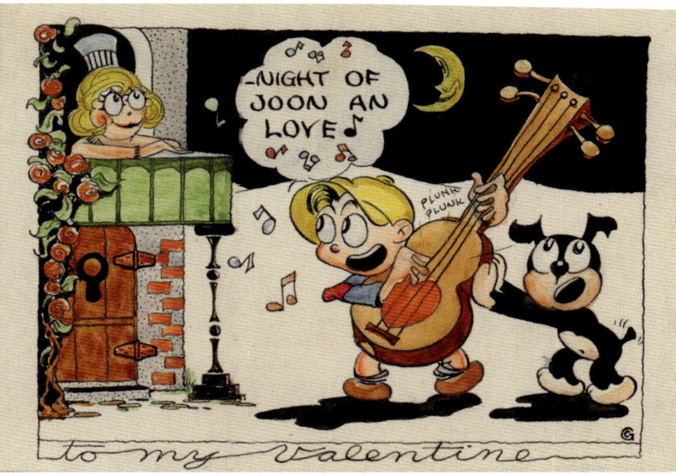

A few of the dozens of cards Geronimi drew for Alice.

Geronimi's first job in Hollywood was animating Oswald the Lucky Rabbit, the character Disney lost creative control over to producer Charles Mintz. An urban myth states that Lantz won the rights to take over the character in a poker game with Universal president Carl Laemmle. While the two did play cards together, it was Lantz who negotiated rights for the character in the wake of Laemmle's departure from the studio in 1936.[9]

Gerry had been with Lantz about a year when he was offered a job at Disney's, thanks to his friend Jack King. After a delicate discussion with Lantz, Gerry accepted Walt's offer. "It was probably the best move I ever made," reminisced Geronimi. "But you know, to this day, Walter says, 'Jocko, if you'd stayed with me you'd be my partner today.' I wonder. So I went over to Disney's as an animator."[10]

Working under directors Burt Gillett and Wilfred Jackson, Gerry remembered that he "didn't get big scenes to do at first," but was soon animating Donald getting twisted in the trees in *The Band Concert*, and Goofy's love affair with the boat's mermaid masthead in *The Boat Builders*. Geronimi animated on *Flowers and Trees*, *Lonesome Ghosts*, *Who Killed Cock Robin?*, and many others.

As *Snow White* moved into production, Geronimi found himself still cast on shorts, suggesting, as animation historian Hans Perk wrote, that perhaps Gerry was "not considered 'good enough' to animate on the feature."[11] Layout man Thor Putnam offered: "I remember Dave Hand going to four-letter words one time about Geronimi, when he was his animator, so I think that maybe he wasn't all that good."[12]

Perhaps Gerry felt himself falling behind. Or maybe after nearly twenty years working as an animator, Geronimi simply wanted a change.

"One night at a party at Jack King's, Walt was there," Geronimi recalled. "We had a few drinks, and I told Walt, 'You know, I'd like to direct.' He

HOLLYWOOD
SEASON'S GREETINGS FROM SUNKIST CALIFORNIA
NEWS
'ALLIE' AND 'JERRY' GERONIMI

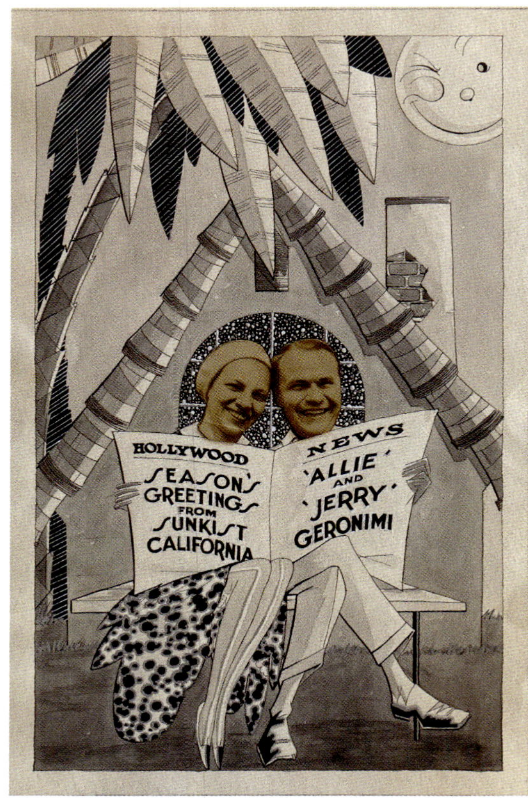

Geronomi's first Christmas card, 1929 or 1930.

said, 'I don't know, Butch, we'll see.'"[13] It wasn't long before Geronimi was assigned to direct *The Ugly Duckling*, after Jack Cutting stepped down in 1938.[14] The short won an Academy Award, and Gerry went on to direct *The Pointer*, *The Beach Picnic*, and some twenty other shorts.

In a later interview, Geronimi said he was originally set to direct on *Snow White*: "I was in a lot of story meetings, and I had a little sequence that I was going to direct. It was cut out; the picture was running too long. Then I went out to shorts."[15] Walt's near complete attention to the feature left Gerry with more autonomy than the directors of earlier shorts. It also meant he was held to task economically. Gerry developed a very successful way of working, making his the largest of the shorts units.

"We used to handle eight shorts at a time," recalled Don Duckwall, Gerry's assistant director. "We tried to kick one out every six weeks, and when one would go out, then we'd have a new story come in. We had a whole wing [of the Animation Building]—1B—and we were on Mickeys and Plutos."[16] Duckwall remembered: "Geronimi spent a good deal of time with the story people in developing these stories, which paid off in our bonus, because Geronimi was keeping them simple. Keeping simple backgrounds, simple layouts. He was really trying to get us into a formula where we could have some money left over even though [production manager] Herb Lamb was squeezing us down in the budget."[17]

Once storyboards were approved (either by Walt, Dave Hand, or Ben Sharpsteen, depending on Walt's workload) Geronimi took them to his music room. "I always worked closely with my head layout man," recalled Gerry. "We would sit down in front of the storyboard and work out scene for scene where to go into close-ups or long shots, where to pan, cuts, etc."[18]

But it was through supervising animator Charles "Nick" Nichols that Geronimi kept control over his shorts. Nichols would pose-test the picture, "doing the key drawings and the key poses," remembered Nichols.[19] Duckwall recalled that "Nick really controlled the action with his poses,"[20] and Geronimi would time out the action using a stopwatch, noting what should happen when on the exposure sheets. Layout artist Lance Nolley remembered that Geronimi was especially good at this. "He was a damn good director. He was a good timer: he knew how to time the stuff and he knew what he wanted."[21]

Armed with timing, recorded dialogue, and key drawings, Gerry would hand out the scenes to animators, going over each one in detail.

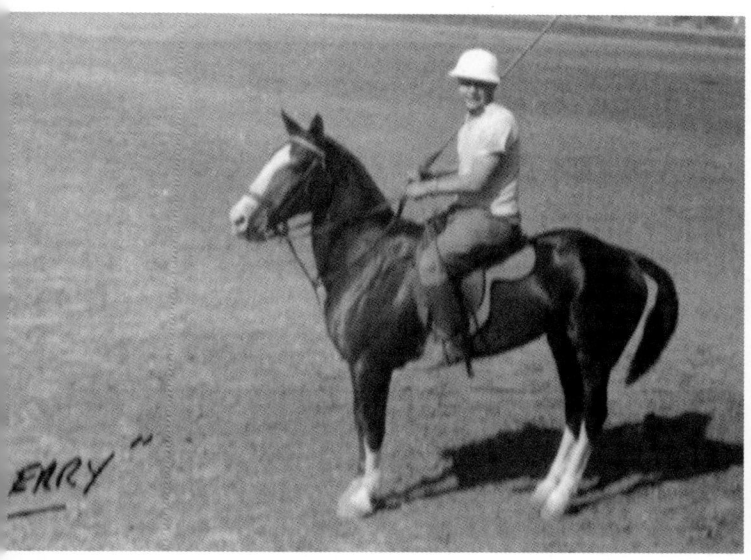

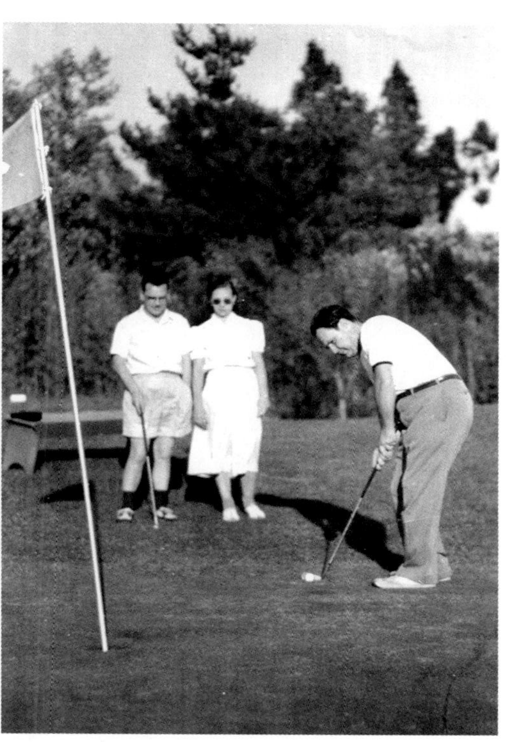

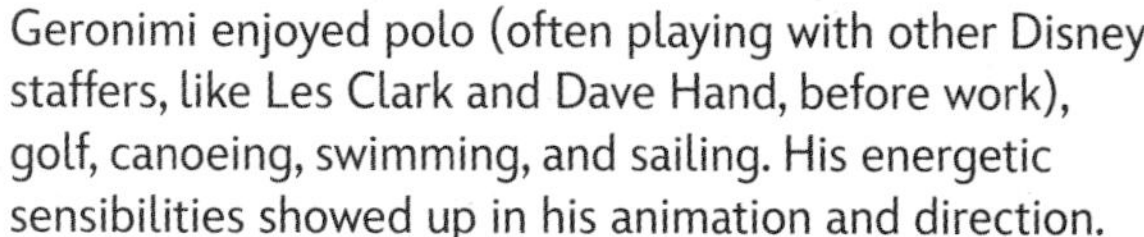

Geronimi enjoyed polo (often playing with other Disney staffers, like Les Clark and Dave Hand, before work), golf, canoeing, swimming, and sailing. His energetic sensibilities showed up in his animation and direction.

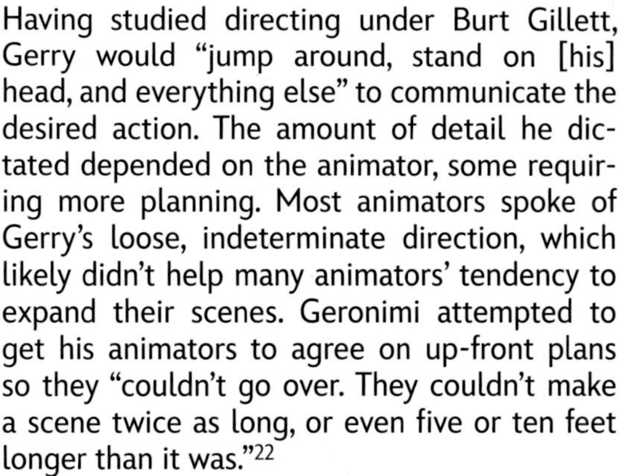

Having studied directing under Burt Gillett, Gerry would "jump around, stand on [his] head, and everything else" to communicate the desired action. The amount of detail he dictated depended on the animator, some requiring more planning. Most animators spoke of Gerry's loose, indeterminate direction, which likely didn't help many animators' tendency to expand their scenes. Geronimi attempted to get his animators to agree on up-front plans so they "couldn't go over. They couldn't make a scene twice as long, or even five or ten feet longer than it was."[22]

Though assistant director Don Duckwall was not an artist himself, he was encouraged to weigh in with suggestions because, "I might ask for something that he wouldn't" due to the fact that "I would not know how tough it was. But if I thought it would be better that way, I would ask for it and the animator might fool you and give it to you. That was typical of Gerry: he was like a football coach in some regards."[23]

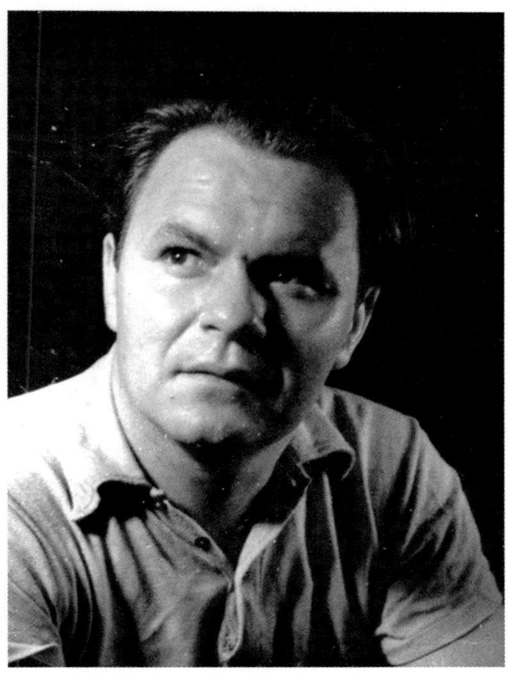

Geronimi in 1930.

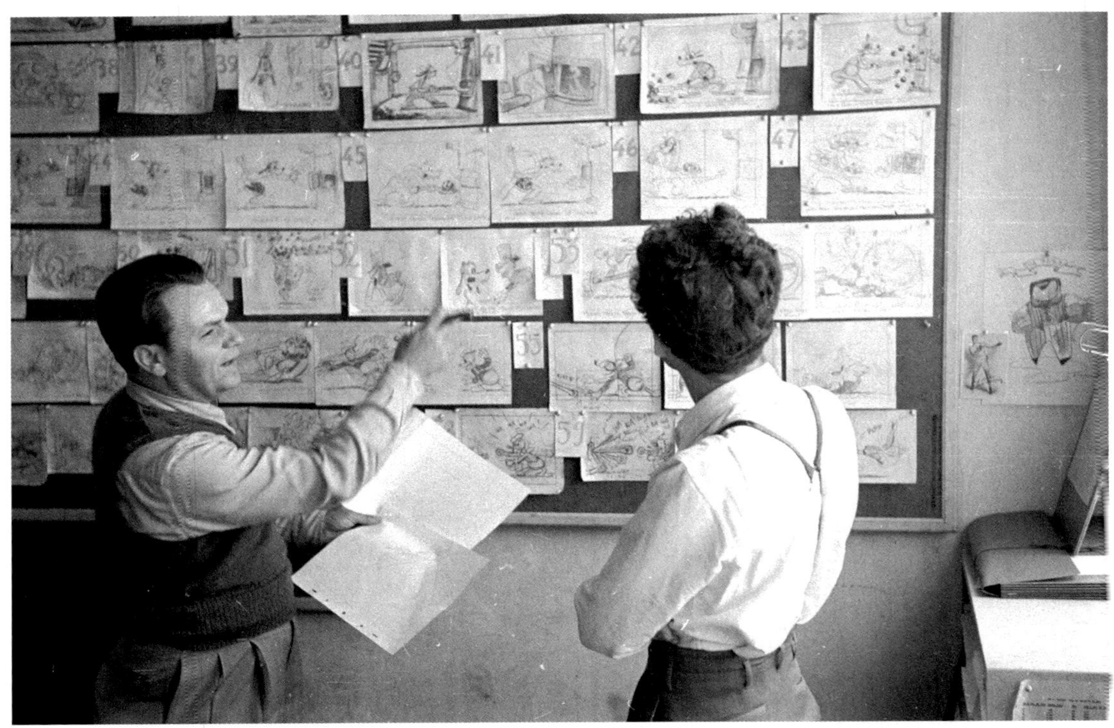

Geronimi at work on *Tugboat Mickey*, 1940.

As animators returned with rough animation, Geronimi would review each shot on the Moviola, a tabletop-sized film playback machine. Once a week all animation was cut together into a single "running reel," to be reviewed in context in a meeting called "sweatbox." The reviews took "from eight in the morning until five at night to get through all the shorts," remembered Duckwall. "What a headache!"[24] And as Geronimi recalled, "when the pencil test came into the sweatbox, that's when the hollering really started."[25]

Geronimi also worked closely with the composer, as well as "background artists, musicians, sound effects, in on all recordings, re-recording, dubbing, color models, etc. I was a stickler for accuracy."[26]

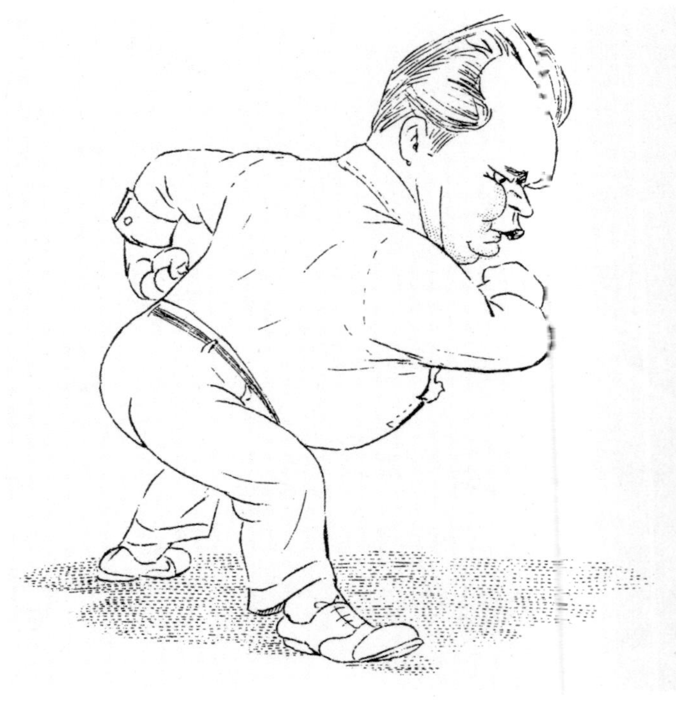

A caricature of Geronimi from a November 24, 1939, issue of *The Bulletin*, an in-house Disney employee magazine.

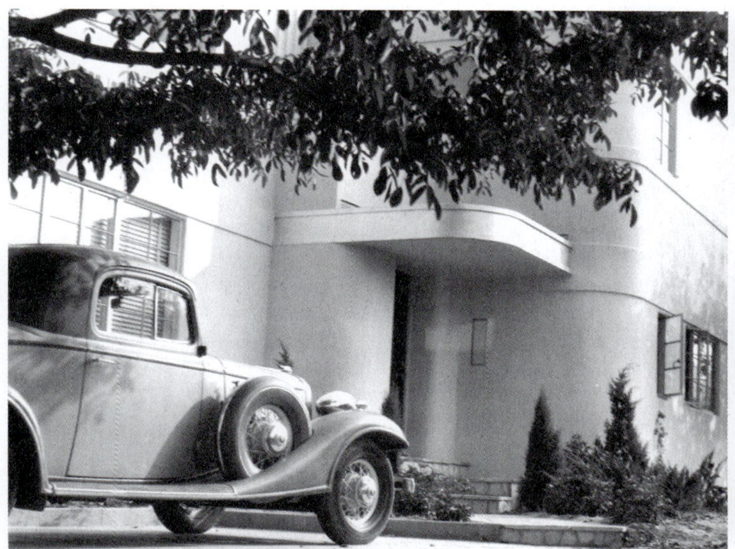

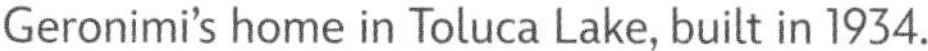

Geronimi's home in Toluca Lake, built in 1934.

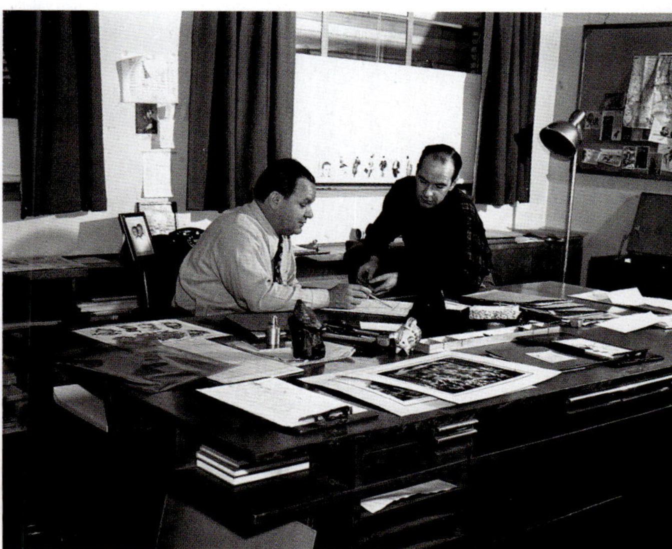

Geronimi in his music room with animator Ollie Johnston in 1946, working on "Casey at the Bat."

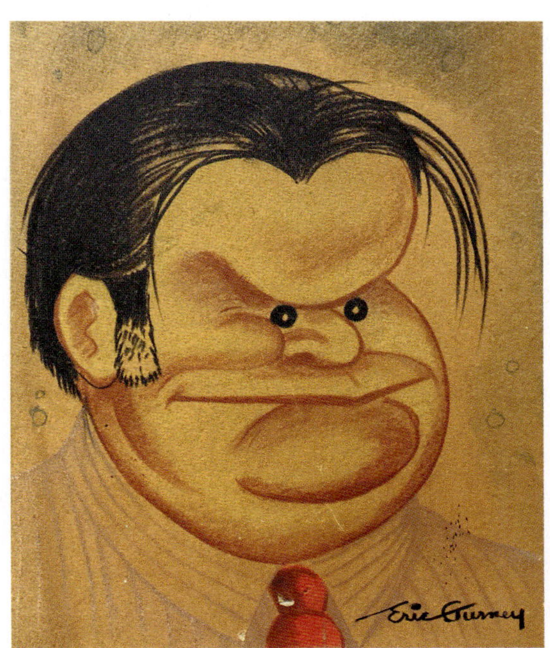

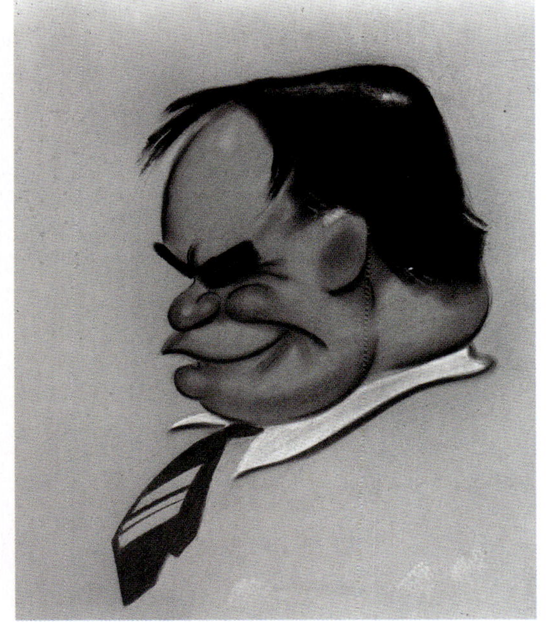

Consistent qualities emerge in these caricatures by story artist Eric Gurney (LEFT), around 1941, and Bill Justice, 1952.

For most people, working with actors epitomizes the job of a director. So it might come as a surprise that in most cases, Disney directors did not actually work with the voice talent. (It was certainly surprising to us!) Starting as far back as the shorts, directing voice talent most often fell to the story artist—which makes sense, given that the story artist was the person most familiar with the material and therefore most knowledgeable as to what specifically was needed from the actor. For her roles in *Alice in Wonderland* and *Peter Pan*, Kathryn Beaumont remembered working exclusively with story man Winston Hibler, whom she described as wonderful and patient. She also recalled being named "One Take Kathy"—though Hibler would often ask for "one more, for protection" (a trick modern animation directors use even today!). Actors were often recorded together, and scenes were recorded in a run, as opposed to one line at a time, so actors could get a flow going.

Once actors were recorded, the director then made a selection as to which "take" would be used in the film, and the assistant director would cut the dialogue into the film. If revisions or adjustments were later needed, it would be up to the director to record them. Again, this makes sense, because at this point in production, the director would be most knowledgeable as to what was needed.

After lines were recorded and edited, records would be pressed, and those would be played back as live-action reference was filmed. The same recording was used by animators as they crafted the animation.

This process changed under director Woolie Reitherman, who directed all actors from the start to the end of production. Then-assistant Don Hahn recalled that the usual session started with lunchtime, after which Woolie, story man Larry Clemmons, and the voice talent would head to Stage B on the Disney studio lot, where the sessions took place. Recording was done one actor at a time, though occasionally in pairs, one line at a time, if the actors had lots of scenes opposite each other. After ten or fifteen takes, all the dialogue was processed and reviewed by Woolie, along with a large crew of lead animators, in his office. Takes were selected, then edited together for review, like a radio drama, before being passed on to the animators.

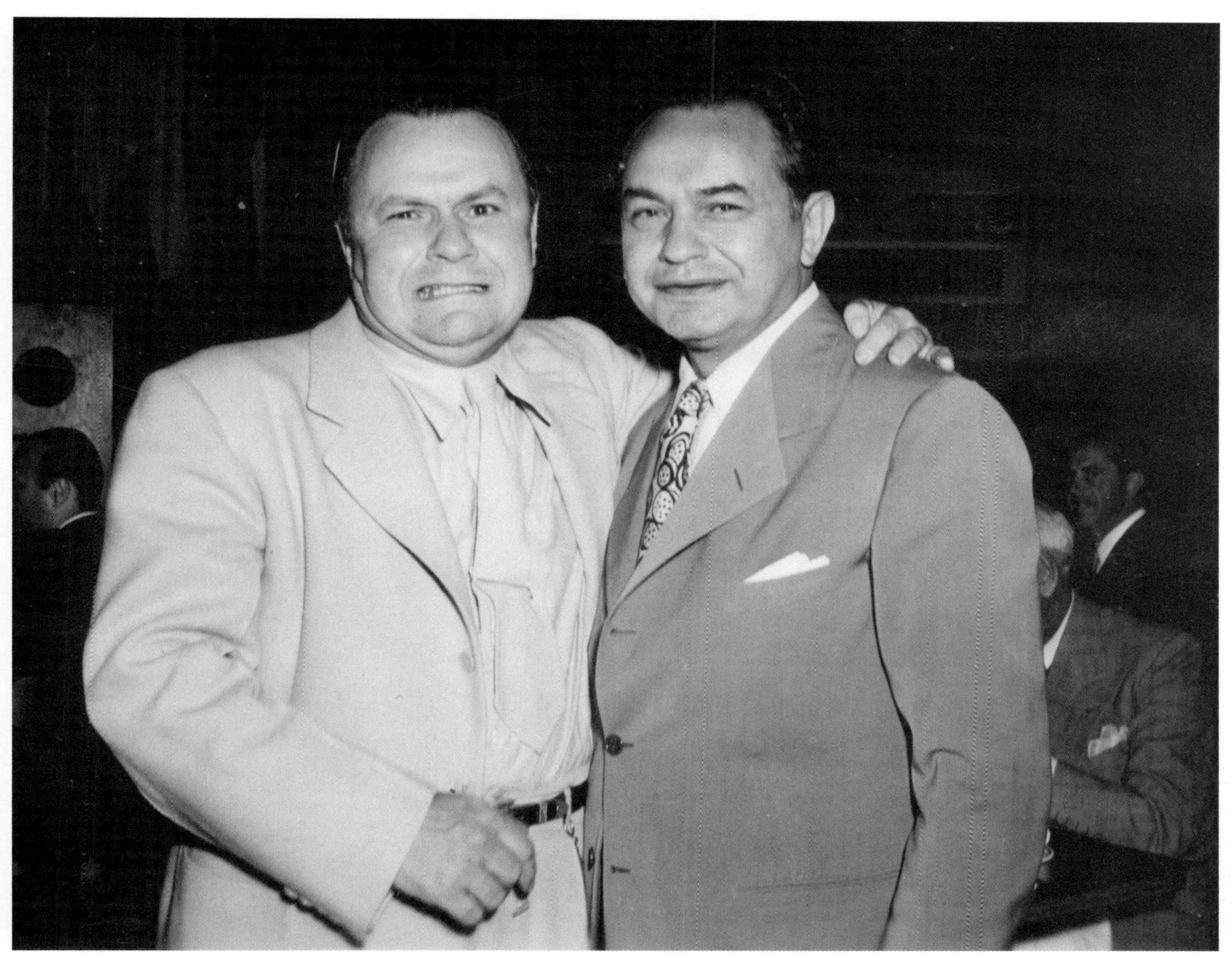

Geronimi was often teased that he looked like actor Edward G. Robinson. Unfortunately, where or when this photo was taken is lost to the ages.

PACKAGE FILMS

Geronimi transitioned from shorts to features with the 1943 *Victory Through Air Power.* Though he stayed a feature director, his work for a time would essentially be short subjects: "The Whale Who Wanted to Sing at the Met," "Casey at the Bat," and "Peter and the Wolf" within *Make Mine Music* (1946), and "Pecos Bill," "Little Toot," and "Blame It on the Samba" within *Melody Time* (1948). "Casey" and "Pecos" in particular show off Geronimi's snappy sense of timing, not just within scenes but the film overall.

Gerry's standout work from this time is *The Adventures of Ichabod and Mr. Toad*, for which he directed the dance, storytelling, and ride and chase. While some credit should go to the animators, this film is a masterful example of overall timing and pacing—both the purview of the director. "That was one we had to 'plus' a lot," he remembered. "We had to add a lot of business. Frank Thomas did the scenes of Ichabod entering the hollow—the scary stuff. Then, when the wild action started, it went to the wild man, Kimball."[27] Geronimi related to the work: "That's the type of animation I always liked to do when I was animating, with lots of guts in it.

"I worked very closely with Ollie Wallace, the music composer, on that. It wasn't pre-scored.[28] We'd have the pencil [reel] on Ollie's Moviola and we'd go over it, scene by scene. We got a wonderful score out of that, too—scary as hell." Singer and actor Bing Crosby provides narration for the film, as well as a singing voice for the title character, which provides a charm and counterpoint to the spooky tone. Funny enough, Geronimi wasn't fond of Bing: "I was sorry Crosby did the narration for it. Walt thought that maybe he would plus it, by having his name on it, but it was too much Crosby. I think it would have been better to have some-one who got more of that Halloween spirit

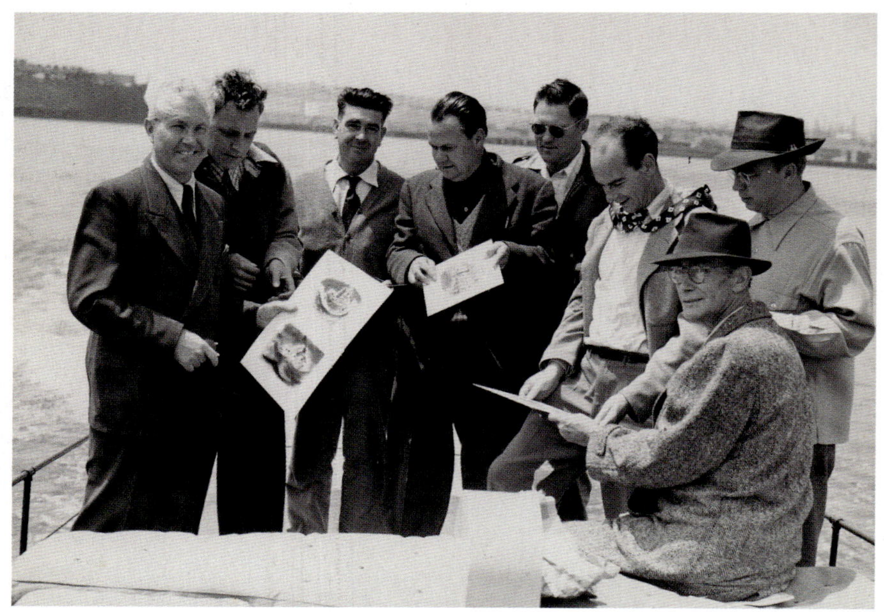

In the Los Angeles harbor to study boats and props for *Little Toot*. FROM LEFT: unknown, animator George Rowley, unknown, Geronimi, background painter Brice Mack, animators Ollie Johnston and Eric Larson. SEATED: layout man Hugh Hennesy.

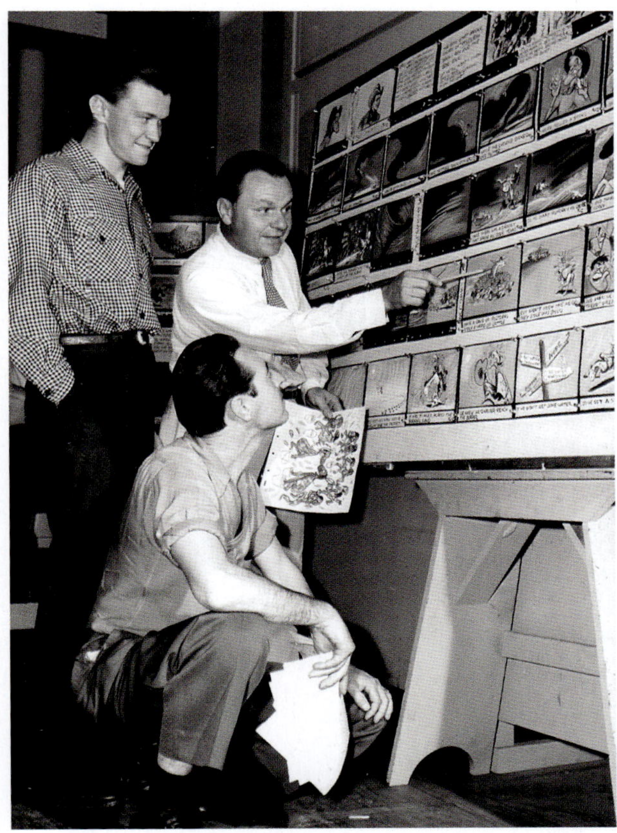

Geronimi (CENTER) at work on "Pecos Bill." KNEELING: Joe Rinaldi; STANDING: unknown.

into it." Geronimi also recalled that "recording Crosby was a little rough" because "he would say, 'Okay, the take is okay, print it.' He ran the show, and I didn't like it."[29]

There's no record of Walt's reaction to the short, but one can presume he liked the result: Geronimi would continue as a feature director for the next ten years.

THE RETURN TO FEATURES

"After the war, Walt was broke and heavily in debt," recalled animator Frank Thomas. "He had all these problems and could not get back on his feet. *Pinocchio* had not paid for itself, and *Fantasia* had not, and *Bambi* had not. Three big [expensive] blockbusters, and no money from them. So he was really in the hole and he was trying to make these package pictures [like *Melody Time*], which he didn't believe in as much as the experimental value. 'Maybe we can find a way here.' He was so disappointed that *Fantasia* had not gone over. So finally he realized, 'Well, the only thing the audience seems to like is a young girl in trouble, and people trying to help her out. So let's do *Cinderella* and try not to make it like *Snow White*.'"[30]

At the same time, Walt's interest in live-action films like *Treasure Island* meant that *Cinderella* would be made without the intense personal focus he'd given earlier features. Disney would rely on others to develop material, rather than working it up himself.[31] Wilfred Jackson, Ham Luske, and Gerry Geronimi would end up developing and directing the next four films: *Cinderella*, *Alice in Wonderland*, *Peter Pan*, and *Lady and the Tramp*, sometimes working on sequences from two different films concurrently. Disney knew he could count on these three to produce high quality while delivering on time and budget.

But Gerry's open-ended way of working grated on some. On shorts, Nick Nichols had drawn out key poses before handing out to animators; this was now left to each animator individually. Animator Ward Kimball was infuriated by Geronimi's inability to see the humor in his absurdly wonderful scene in *The Three Caballeros*, where Donald and José Carioca attempt to cut short an impossibly long note sung by Panchito. "A lot of times the animator would improve [the material he was handed] in spite of the director," asserted Kimball. "We always felt that's what we did for Gerry Geronimi, we saved him all the time. Whether we did or not, I don't know, but we'd like to believe it."

Assistant director Ed Brunner agreed, feeling that Geronimi's work "turned out good in spite of Gerry."[32]

The first problem, said layout artist Don Jurwich, was that Geronimi "didn't know what he wanted; he couldn't explain it."[33] Animator and assistant director Jack Cutting felt that Geronimi "was not very articulate," caricaturing Geronimi's speech as "dese" and "dose," concluding handouts with "You know what I mean, fellas."[34]

Without clarity up front, disagreements downstream were inevitable. Animator Ed Love remembered: "Gerry changed everything I did. I'd get a sequence, and I'd do it, and he'd throw it all out. I'd do it again, and he'd throw it all out. Then I'd shoot the first sequence, and he'd okay it. Honest to God, that's the way it would work." After this, Ed said, "I went and told Walt, 'I won't work with him.' I absolutely refused to work with him. I said, 'I don't have any trouble with anybody, but that man doesn't know what he's doing.' The funny part is, Gerry was a good personal friend of mine. That's the only time in my whole career that I had a problem with a director."[35]

Layout man Lance Nolley remembered: "Gerry was a little hot tempered. You know, he wasn't temperamental; he just had a temper. But he was a good director."[36] Animator Les Clark also defended Geronimi's approach. "Some directors were very loose in their directing, like Gerry Geronimi. The handout was really your first test. Where Wilfred Jackson would just patiently sit down and tell you everything he wanted, to every frame, or every foot or so. That was the difference between the two. Now, I don't mean any disparagement against Gerry Geronimi; he got some results. So did Jackson. I don't think that Gerry Geronimi actually had a visual idea himself of what he wanted as much as Jackson did. So, when he saw the first pencil test, then he got an idea what he wanted, and what he liked, and what he didn't like. Usually, working for Jackson, you came out pretty much right the first time. And yet Gerry turned out awfully good pictures; that was just his way of working. Jackson was slower, and took more time, so I guess economically, they were both about the same."[37]

Though his approach rubbed some the wrong way, Gerry's indefinite approach enabled animators to bring forward ideas of their own, which would not have been possible if everything were nailed down up front.

Still, some frustrated animators felt that Gerry wasn't able to diagnose when their work was improving on the material, and finagled ways to show work directly to Walt. Frank Thomas recalled that when he showed his scenes of Lady and Tramp eating spaghetti, "I did not cut my scenes of the last meatball into the reel until just before Walt was going to see it so Geronimi would not be upset by my changed continuity."[38]

Gerry knew what he was up against. "What made it tough was this: Walt naturally praised those he called the Nine Old Men—and they knew it. They knew they were good, and they knew they had Walt's backing. That made it tough on directors. Sometimes animators held the upper hand. But many a time, Walt would take your side, and say, 'No, Gerry's right,' or Jack's right, or Ham's right. After all, we were the ones who were close on the complete pix. Of course, the animators were in on the story meetings, too, and they had their own ideas, so you left it open, to give them a chance. You don't want to choke them and tie them up. But the sweatbox was always a hassle," he recalled.[39]

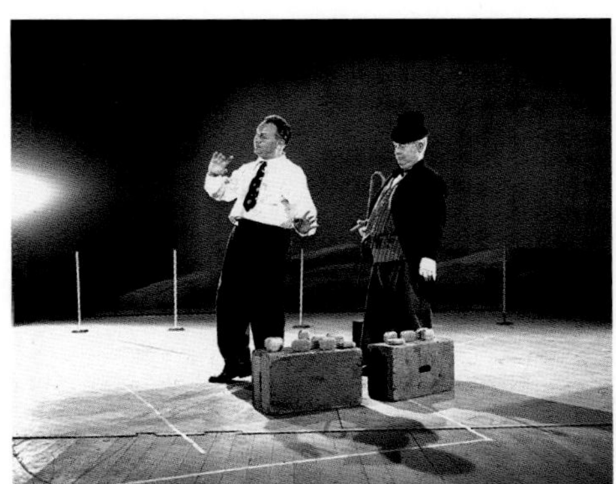

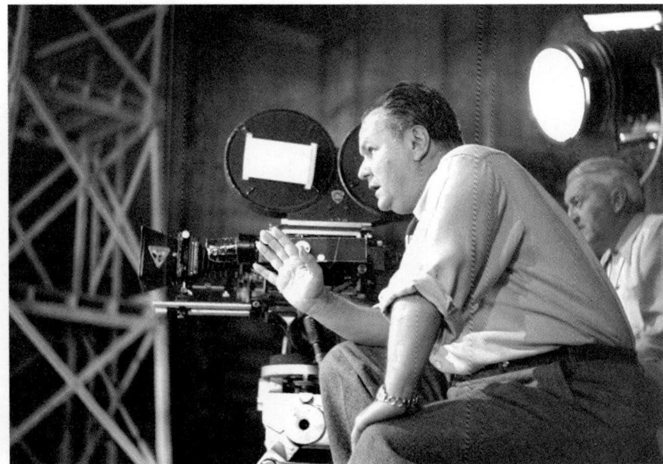

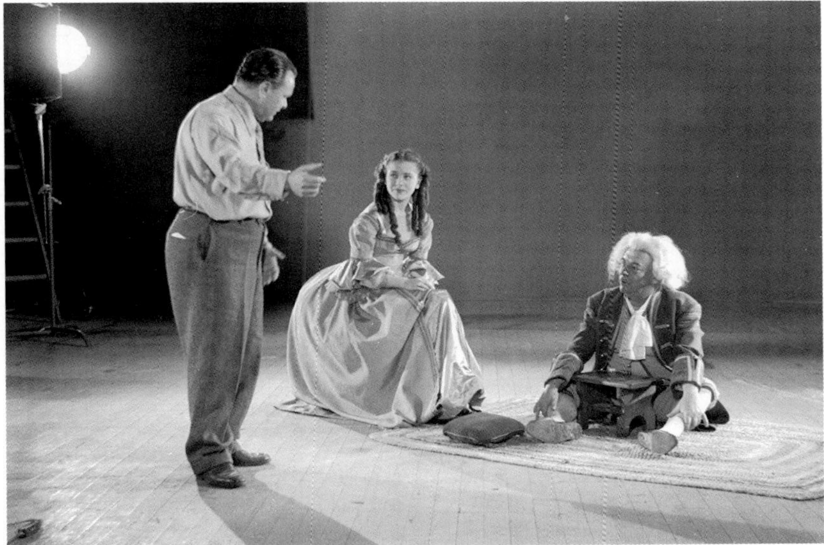

To save costs, live-action reference footage was shot for nearly all of *Cinderella*, *Alice in Wonderland*, and *Peter Pan*. The studio had followed this practice since the short films in the thirties, but not to this scale, and it occupied a large portion of the director's time during these films. Beyond being a valuable reference for the animator, it had the added benefit of forcing agreement between animator and director.

Animators weren't the only ones to complain about Geronimi's poor bedside manner. Eleanor Audley, who performed both the voice and live-action reference of Maleficent in *Sleeping Beauty*, remembered:

> When a take was over, he would say to everybody else on the set, "Well how was it with you?" And of course everybody would say it was fine, and he'd go, "Well, if you say so." Always made you feel as though you never did a good take in the whole picture. It was mostly he didn't want anything to come back to him. "Well, the boys said it was all right." I could have killed him![40]

So with all these complaints, why did Disney keep Geronimi on as director?

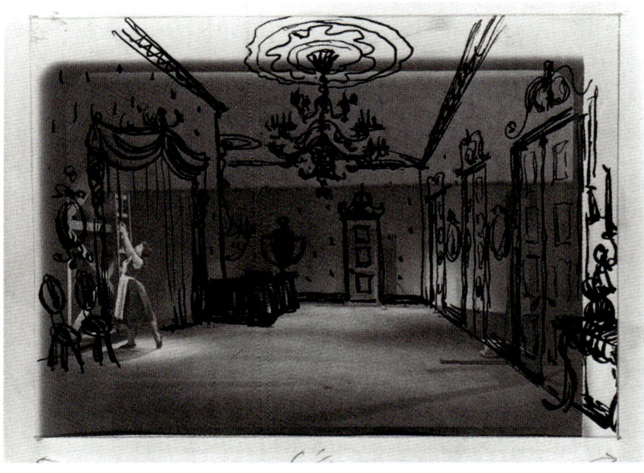

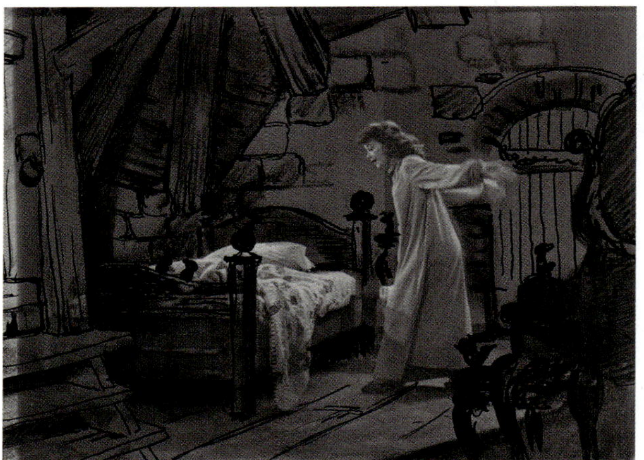

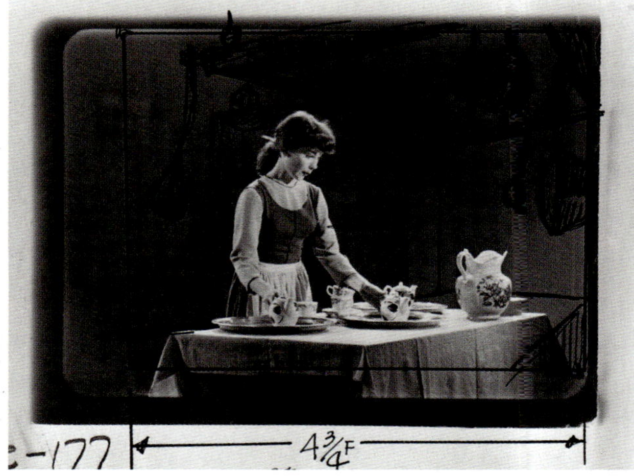

Camera setups were matched to layouts that had been drawn beforehand, and footage was printed out frame by frame and registered to animation paper to help guide animators. LEFT: Live-action actor Helene Stanley. BELOW: Actor Eleanor Audley.

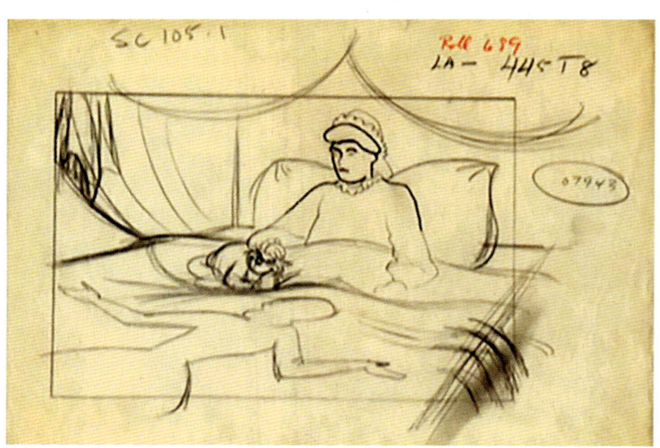

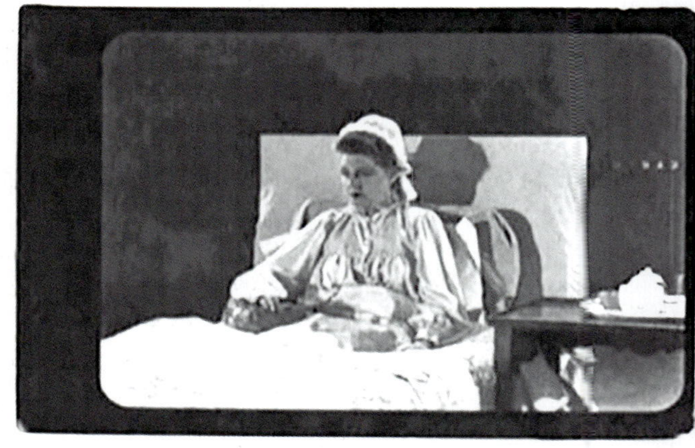

A direct tracing of each frame of the live action (called rotoscoping) results in a stiff and lifeless feel. Animators pushed form and movement to capture a stronger essence of the attitude and feeling, while following the acting suggestions from the actors.

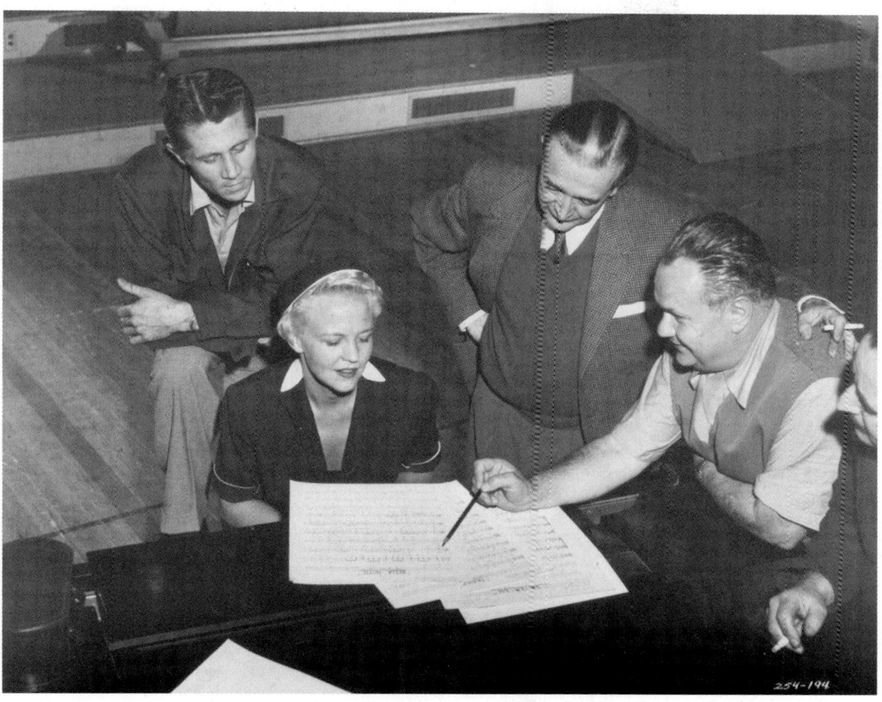

Joe Rinaldi (CROPPED AT RIGHT), Geronimi, story man Ed Penner, singer/songwriter Peggy Lee at the piano, and voice actor Lee Millar (Jim Dear and Dog Catcher).

For one, Walt felt that conflict in creative work was healthy. If a pairing of artists got along too well, one could almost predict Disney would split them up.

Then, too, Walt knew that many of his artists had big egos, and he could count on Geronimi to keep control. "Kimball was a tough nut to handle and Walt figured I could handle him," recalled Geronimi. "It's a funny thing about [Art] Babbitt, too, when he came back to the studio, to prove to Walt that he could not be fired, due to the strike. Walt asked me if I'd take him, and I said okay. Of course, Babbitt didn't stay long; he just wanted to prove a point. I always got along okay with Babbitt; he was a great animator."[41]

Most important, Geronimi's work was good. Animators, placing value on performance and draftsmanship, don't give credit to Geronimi's pacing, cutting, and camerawork. Watch the last twenty minutes of *Cinderella*, as the mice bring her the key so she can escape to try on the glass slipper. The animation is fine, but it's the camera choices and timing that make the film thrilling. Like notes within a song, each piece of animation can only mean so much; it is the relationship and placement of each against the other that gives it shape and meaning. Geronimi's work is strong, as difficult as some may have found him to work with. As assistant director Jack Brunner put it: "Gerry was a stinker, but he was a good director."[42]

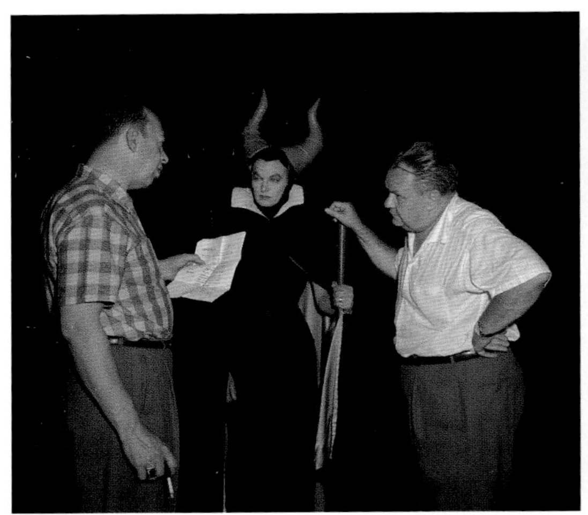

Animator Marc Davis (LEFT) and Geronimi work with Eleanor Audley to shoot live-action reference.

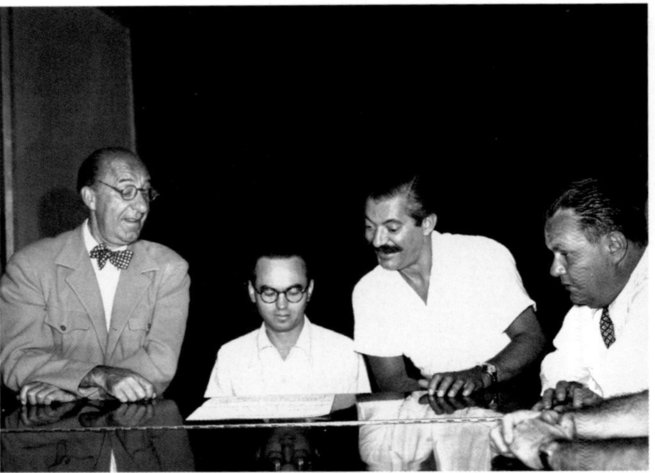

Ed Wynn (LEFT), composer Paul J. Smith, Gerry Colonna and Geronimi on right working out music for *Alice in Wonderland*.

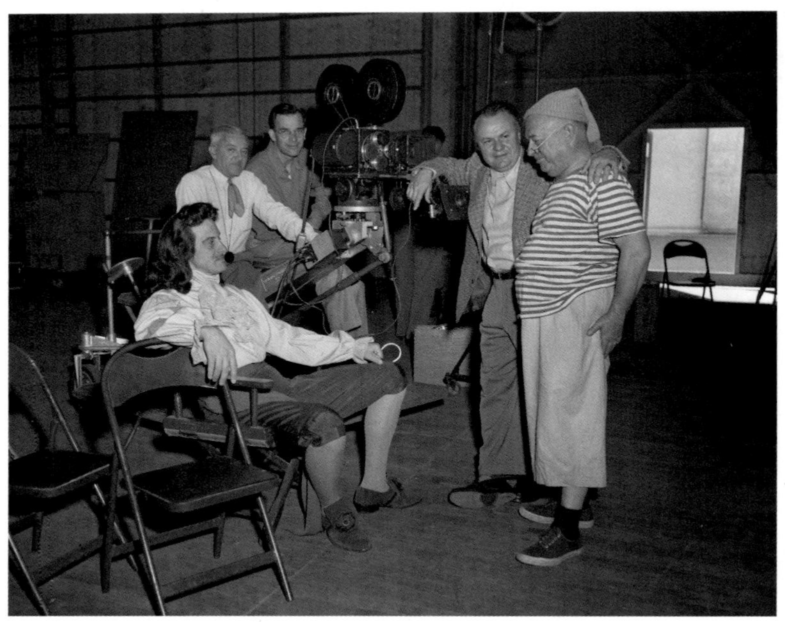

Sometimes voice actors did their own live-action reference, like Hans Conried (SEATED, LEFT) for Hook on *Peter Pan*. On the other hand, actor Don Barclay did physical movement for Smee, while the character was voiced by Bill Thompson.

THE LAST STRAW

Walt was determined to make *Sleeping Beauty* "a moving illustration." Wilfred Jackson began directing the pilot sequence in which the prince and the girl meet in the forest, but after health problems, Eric Larson was placed in the director's seat. An animator himself, Larson gave "prodigious notes," remembered then-assistant animator Floyd Norman,[43] which slowed progress. Animator Jerry Hathcock felt that the other directing animators, perhaps jealous of Larson's opportunity, didn't support him.[44] Disney himself was busier than ever with live-action films, television, and his newest mania, Disneyland—leaving *Sleeping Beauty* unattended for months. When he did show up, Larson seemed flustered, according to production manager Ken Peterson: "He was almost speechless when Walt was there." When Walt finally realized the pace and budget the film was racking up, he removed Larson and brought in Geronimi to corral the production as supervising director—which was similar to Dave Hand's role on *Bambi*. "I had to work with all the sequences," remembered Geronimi. In addition to supervising the picture as a whole, "I think Walt just wanted someone to oversee the whole picture, and tie it together."[45]

Gerry was sympathetic to the tough spot Larson had been in. "When you were assigned a sequence, at the beginning, on any of those features, you were bound to run into a lot of money, because [a lot of the work on pilot sequences] was always experimenting. The fellow who was on it always took the brunt of it, because he was trying to get the characters set—it was always expensive. His sequence always ran into money, and it was always a little tough on him."[46]

Geronimi's success finishing *Sleeping Beauty* led to another directing gig on *One Hundred and One Dalmatians*, this time with Ham Luske and Woolie Reitherman. But Gerry's reputation with the animators was not improving. Animator Fred Kopietz recalled: "We used to be close friends; we golfed together, back in the early Universal days, before he left Universal and went to Disney's. We got along great. . . . He was a nice guy and a lot of fun. Through the years at Disney's, with what success he had there, he got to be pretty obnoxious at times."

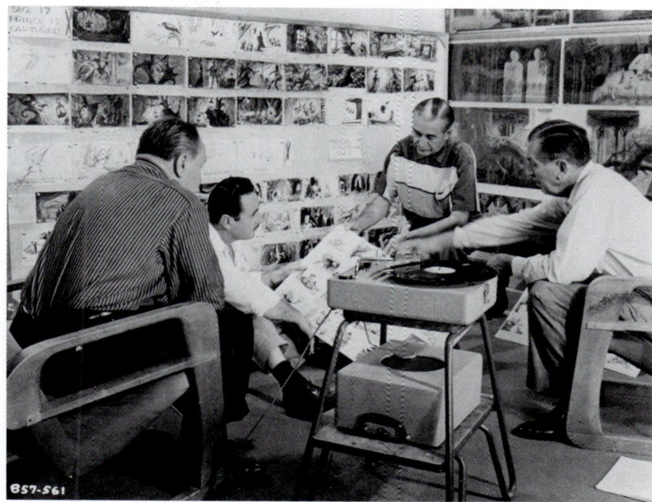

Walt Disney reviewing *Sleeping Beauty* boards with Geronimi (LEFT), story man Joe Rinaldi (MIDDLE, SEATED), and Ed Penner (RIGHT).

Several animators decided they'd had enough. "Finally we boycotted Geronimi, said we weren't going to work for him," remembered animator Ward Kimball. "The straw that helped break the back was John Lounsbery, the nicest guy you would ever want to meet, who was patient, and didn't want to hurt anybody's feelings, who finally went to Walt and said: 'I don't want to work with this man anymore.' And Walt thinks, if Lounsbery goes, there must be something wrong."[47]

Walt moved Gerry out of animation, and like other animation directors before him, into television. After some initial prep work, Geronimi was sent to Europe where he was to oversee production of *Almost Angels* and *Miracle of the White Stallions*, as well as *The Magnificent Rebel*, a biopic about Beethoven. It would be his last assignment for Disney.

While some took pleasure in rumors that Geronimi was fired, production coordinator Harry Tytle describes a dinner he attended in Europe where, after much work and travel, "Gerry started to appear strained."[48] As Walt described his vision for the opening of the Beethoven picture, "Gerry suddenly broke in with his New York accent and blurted, 'Dis is not for me, Walt!'" Walt initially assumed Geronimi disagreed with Walt's idea, but Gerry told Walt he wanted to return to animation and his unit. When Walt told him that wasn't possible, Geronimi resigned.

After nearly thirty years at the studio, Disney employment records indicate Geronimi resigned on October 24, 1959. But Gerry soon regretted his resignation, and on returning to California sent a note to Walt asking to come back as a director in the animation department. Walt sent a letter in response:

February 1, 1960

Dear Butch -

I have read your letter very carefully and noted what you say. I, too, am sorry that your many years here at the Studio had to end as they did, but it was your decision and I'm sure you will recall that when you made it I told you to think it over carefully. The choice was yours and I feel it is definitely a little late now for any reconsideration.

In addition to that, the way things are going here the cartoon end is being curtailed and so I don't see how you can hold any hope of coming back into the organization in that field.

With your many years of experience, I think you would be wise to try some of the other places where your experience would hold you in good stead and be of value to you.

I want to wish you luck in whatever undertaking you go into.

Sincerely,

Mr. Clyde H. Geronimi
10074 Valley Spring Lane,
N. Hollywood, California

WD:tb

Geronimi returned to his love of painting in retirement, 1971.

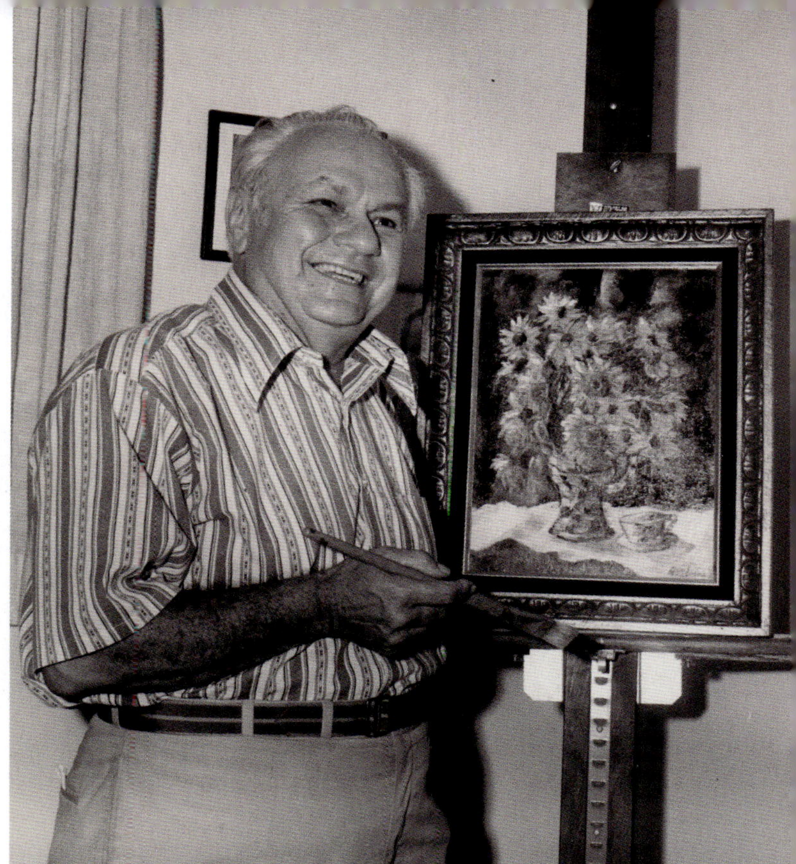

Upon leaving Disney, Gerry directed commercials and TV cartoons starring the Marvel Super Heroes for Steve Krantz, before retiring in the late 1960s. He died at his home in Newport Beach, California, on April 24, 1989.

In interviews conducted with many he'd worked with, Gerry Geronimi was often railed against throughout his retirement. But Gerry was consistently kind and gracious in return, even to his most vocal critics. Of Ward Kimball, who seldom missed an opportunity to criticize Geronimi personally or professionally, Gerry would only say that "Kimball was a damned good animator, but he had to be toned down." At the studio and elsewhere, Geronimi suffered much name-calling because of his heritage, but Geronimi didn't dwell on that, saying he'd had a good life and holding grudges didn't do any good. He retired just blocks away from lifetime friend Walter Lantz, and was honored with a Winsor McCay Award in 1978, and a posthumous Disney Legends Award in 2017. Gerry was kind and gracious years later as he recalled his work at Disney. Most important, Gerry's family members recall him as a sweet and loving family man who was fond of singing, sports, and his grandchildren, and who looked at his life with gratitude.[49]

THE END OF AN ERA

By the early 1960s almost all of Disney's reliable and proven directors had either quit, retired, or suffered health issues that would force their resignation. Even more troubling was the fact, even after a number of massive layoffs, that the animated films no longer seemed to pull in enough profits to make them worthwhile. Close advisers were calling for Disney to shut down animation entirely.

Walt would give it one last chance, once again redefining the role of the director in the process.

Clyde "Gerry" Geronimi Disney Director Filmography

Shorts:

- *Beach Picnic* (1939)
- *The Pointer* (1939)
- *Officer Duck* (1939)
- *Tugboat Mickey* (1940)
- *Billposters* (1940)
- *Pluto's Dream House* (1940)
- *Mr. Mouse Takes a Trip* (1940)
- *Pantry Pirate* (1940)
- *A Gentleman's Gentleman* (1941)
- *Canine Caddy* (1941)
- *Lend a Paw* (1941)
- *Pluto, Junior* (1942)
- *The Army Mascot* (1942)
- *The Sleepwalker* (1942)
- *T-Bone for Two* (1942)
- *Pluto at the Zoo* (1942)
- *Education for Death* (1943)
- *Pluto and the Armadillo* (1943)
- *Private Pluto* (1943)
- *Chicken Little* (1943)
- *The Big Wash* (1948)
- *Susie, the Little Blue Coupe* (1952)
- *The Story of Anyburg, U.S.A.* (1957)

Features:

- *Victory Through Air Power* (1943)—Sequence Director
- *The Three Caballeros* (1945)—Sequence Director
- *Make Mine Music* (1946)—Sequence Director
- *Melody Time* (1948)—Sequence Director
- *The Adventures of Ichabod and Mr. Toad* (1949)—Sequence Director
- *Cinderella* (1950)—Codirector with Ham Luske and Wilfred Jackson
- *Alice in Wonderland* (1951)—Sequence Director
- *Peter Pan* (1953)—Sequence Director
- *Lady and the Tramp* (1955)—Sequence Director
- *Sleeping Beauty* (1959)—Sequence Director
- *One Hundred and One Dalmatians* (1961)—Codirector with Ham Luske and Woolie Reitherman

"DIRECTING ANIMATORS"—ARE THEY DIRECTORS?

By now hopefully it's clear what a director does. But if you've watched the credits of any Disney film, you've probably noticed the credit Directing Animator. What's up with that?

Directing animators were lead animators. Though they themselves still animated key scenes, they also supervised a small group of animators working under them—usually younger artists or those deemed to need extra supervision. The roots of this practice stretch back to the early thirties, when Walt saw Hand's and Sharpsteen's ability to get more and better work from junior animators. Uncredited at that time, lead animators would soon be given prominent credit on the features. But confusingly, the actual title would change from film to film:

Snow White—Supervising Animators

Pinocchio—Animation Direction

Fantasia—Animation Supervision

Dumbo—Animation Directors

Bambi—Supervising Animators

Fun and Fancy Free—Directing Animators

Was there a difference between these roles? Not that we've been able to determine. After ten years of adjustments, the title Directing Animator would remain, from *Song of the South* (1946) through *The Rescuers* (1977).

But, that's not the end of the story. Stay with us! As with most everything at Disney, the actual job changed through time.

On *Snow White* and early features, lead animators would pick up scenes from the sequence directors and hand out work to the animators working under them. While these leads worked with their team members to improve quality, scenes would be approved by the sequence director, giving them the final word.

Later, after Walt's death and Woolie's deputization as the solo director, directing animators grew to become almost like the sequence directors of old. Each was trusted with the development and supervision of large swaths of the film, giving them sizable (though not final) authority over their sections of the film.

STORYTELLING TOOLS—A TIME LINE

It would be nearly impossible to set up and pass along plans for an animated film without previsualization tools. These developed along with technology and the ingenuity of the filmmakers.

1910 | 1920 | 1930 | 1940

1910s–1920s

Early cartoons are only loosely planned; most is left to the animator(s). In some cases, outlines are typed up to describe shots and action of the cartoon, occasionally accompanied by thumbnail drawings.[50,51,52] (Also see Chapter 1, pages 8 and 10.)

1920s

Ub creates proto-story/scripts for Oswald and the first two Mickey films which contain sketches accompanied by a typewritten outline, giving everyone a vision of the staging, style, and action of the film to come.[53] (Also see Chapter 1.)

Late 1920s

The storyboard is invented by Ted Sears, enabling multiple artists to previsualize and easily change the story as it was being created.[54] (Also see Chapter 1, page 14.)

1930s

Boards are routinely "told" to Walt in a story pitch. Story artists point to drawings while acting out the characters' movement and dialogue.

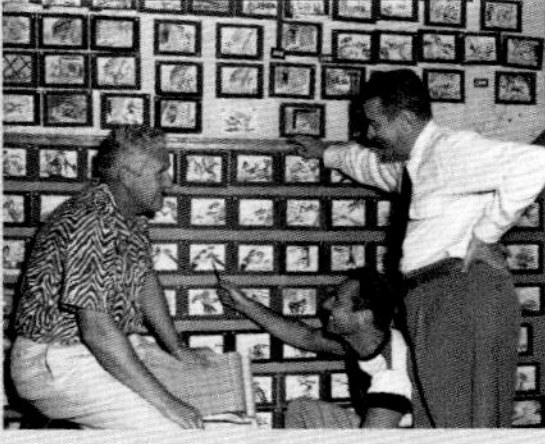

About 1936

Wilfred Jackson first edits together rough and cleaned-up pencil tests, layouts, and storyboards for missing scenes in order to check continuity and timing of the overall short. He calls these "running reels."[55]

1937

Jack Kinney invents the concept of the Leica reel for *Brave Little Tailor* (directed by Burt Gillett but credited to Bill Roberts, as Gillett resigned during its production) in order to get a feel for the staging, action, and timing of the as yet unmade film. Bill Garity likely did the actual technical work of creating the strip. And while originally just a film strip advanced by hand, accompanying sound was soon added, along with the ability to advance the images automatically. Leica reels are used extensively on *Snow White*, *Fantasia*, and *Pinocchio*.[56]

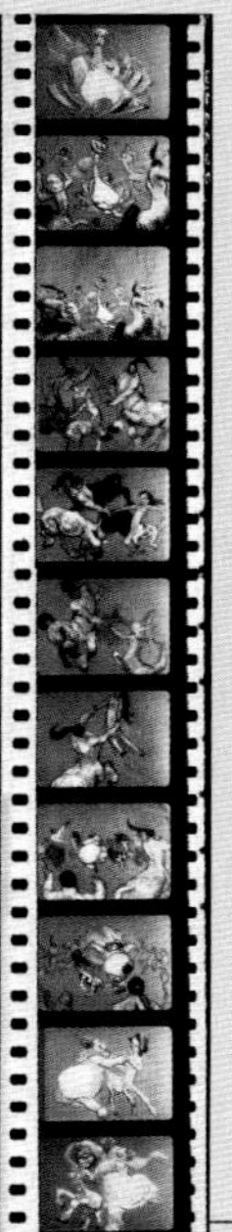

A Leica reel for *Fantasia*.

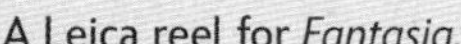

About 1940

Jack Kinney claims Perce Pearce produced a very expensive and creatively disastrous Leica reel for *Bambi*, causing Walt to demand a halt to their use. But in his 1944 diary entry, Jaxon notes he's building Leica reels for shorts indicating they were still used at that time.[57]

Mid-1940s

Sequences are approved by Walt by listening to a live story pitch. Boards are then timed out by a director who cuts them together with dialogue and music, building story reels one sequence at a time. (Note: "running reels" are distinct from "story reels" in that the former is a snapshot of the final film as it's being made, whereas story reels initially contain no animation and are a planning tool.) When possible, Walt would see these and approve overall timing, though in the late forties and fifties directors often soldiered on in Walt's absence.[58]

1950 | 1960 | 1970 | 1980 | 1990

About 1957
Bill Peet writes script for *One Hundred and One Dalmatians*. Though synopses and outlines had been written since the silent days and partial scripts had been written for *Cinderella* and *Peter Pan* in the late 1940s, this was the first one to have been written in the traditional live-action script format *and* supported by Disney as an approval gate before boarding. Likely inspired by efficiencies Walt witnessed in live-action production, it was a short-lived experiment; no other Disney film would have a similarly approved script until *The Great Mouse Detective*.

1966
Walt Disney dies.

About 1975
By the time of *The Rescuers*, Woolie cuts together running reels consisting of ruff animation, blank picture with radio play dialogue, and some storyboards. Some sequences are boarded, while others are just started by directing animators (for example, Frank Thomas started animating the organ scene inspired only by development sketches).[59]

Early 1980
The Great Mouse Detective is written, then built as story reels (first pitched, then cut in edit) one sequence at a time. The whole film was built and screened before animation started—a first at Disney, so far as has been determined. All initial dialogue was production dialogue: no scratch until changes were instituted. (Mike Gabriel recalls John Musker doing great Basil scratch.)[60]

About 1988
The Little Mermaid has an approved script and was cast with final actors, recorded, then boarded. Again, all production dialogue for first pass: no scratch.

Late 1980s
The Rescuers Down Under built in similar way: written, cast, recorded, boarded, etc.

1993
Toy Story is the first film with its reels built entirely using scratch actors. It is the first animated film to be edited nonlinearly, meaning for the first time it is possible to watch or edit any portion of the film by skipping to that section immediately rather than scanning through the entire reel of film.

PART 5

“YOU PRETTY MUCH HAD FULL AUTONOMY”

THE SHORTS GROUP

1936–1957

1936–
1957

SHORT FILM DIRECTORS

The Short Director's job is still to previsualize and plan the film, essentially editing it before it is made:

- Time out the action and cutting
- Collaborate with the composer
- Prepare work with the layout artist
- Hand out and supervise animation
- Review animation
- Supervise cutting

The Director (with the Story Man) also develops stories, which are pitched to Walt for approval.

The Short Director occasionally (though not always) works with the key animator to come up with poses and timing to guide other animators.

As in the early days, the Director has two key collaborators: a musician and a layout artist.

Output: twenty shorts every year, from three units

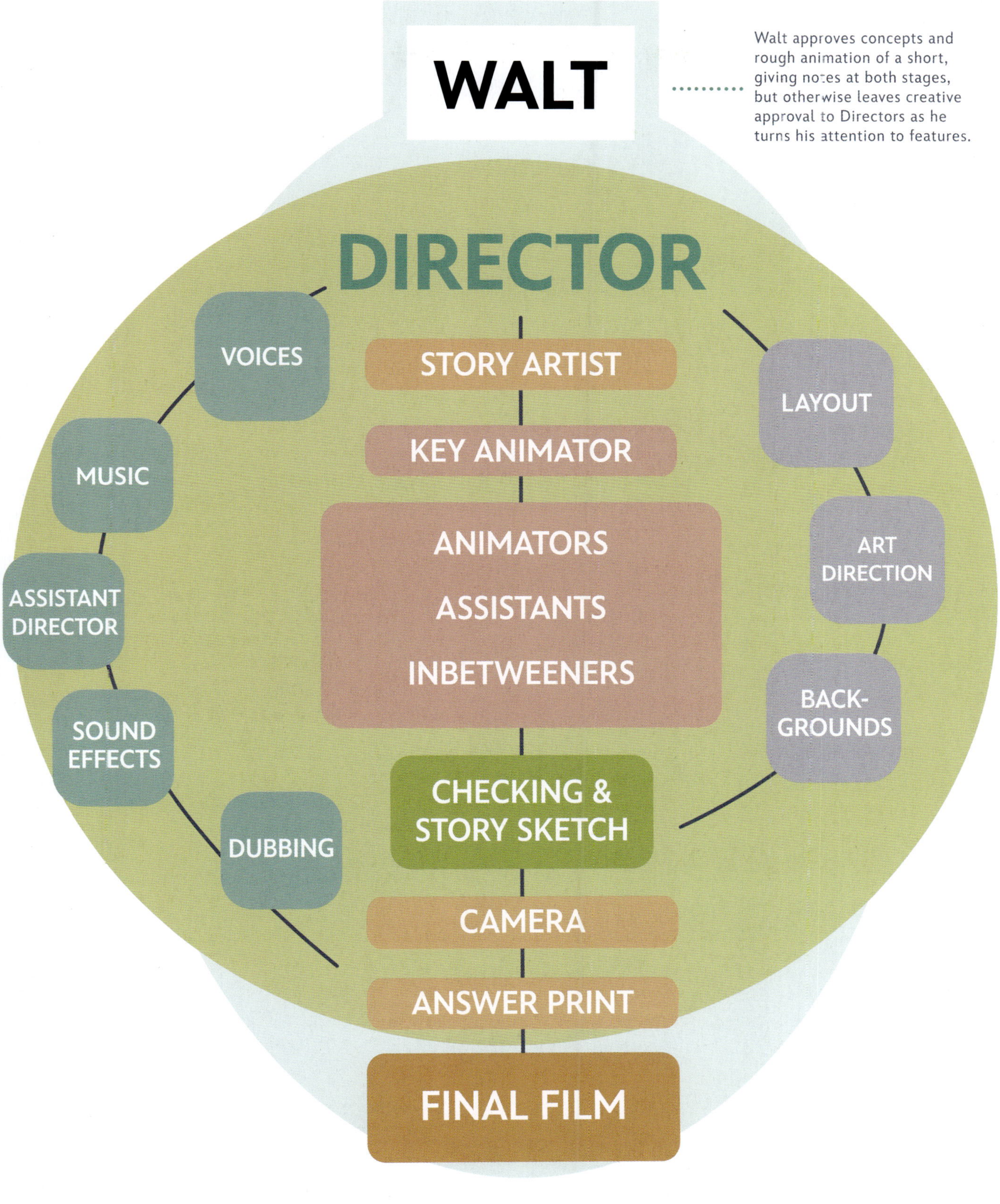

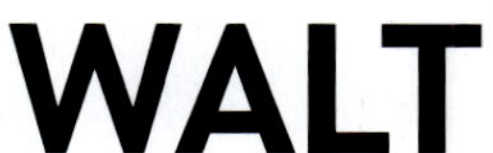

Walt approves concepts and rough animation of a short, giving notes at both stages, but otherwise leaves creative approval to Directors as he turns his attention to features.

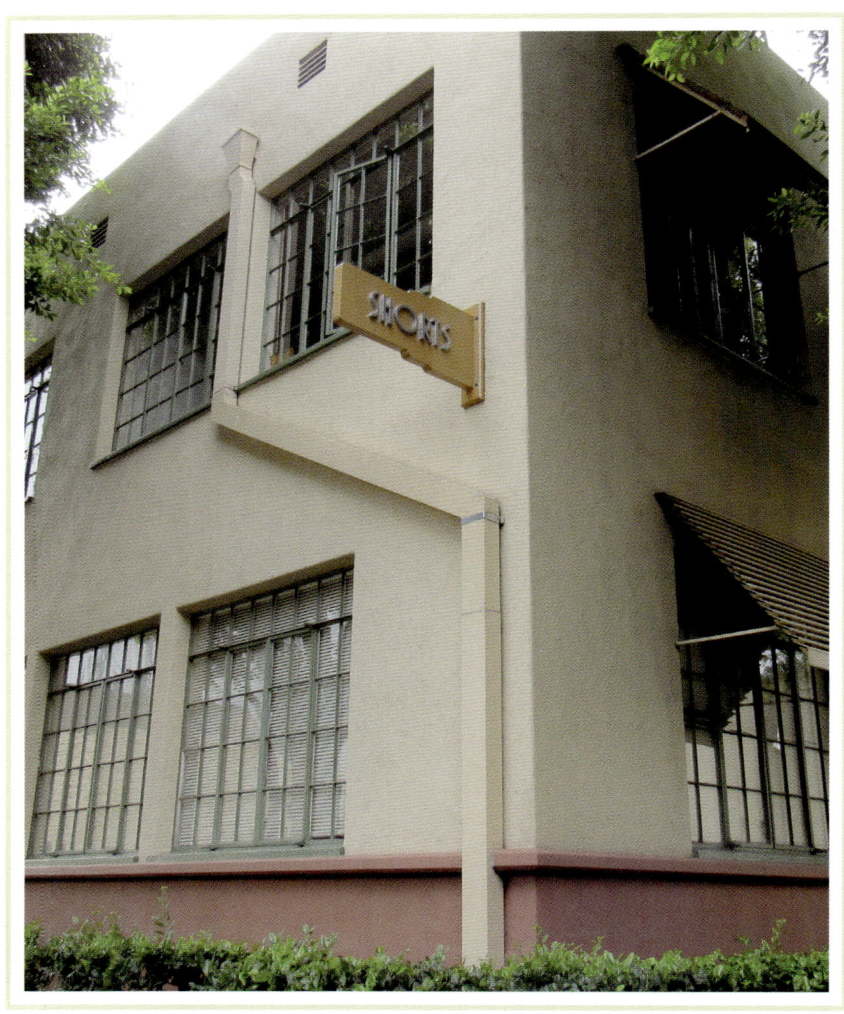

The Shorts Building at The Walt Disney Studios in Burbank. Ironically, once the shorts were moved to Burbank in 1938, none were produced in the building. Don Peri collection, 2017.

CHAPTER 8

THE SHORTS DEPARTMENT—KING, HANNAH, NICHOLS, AND KINNEY

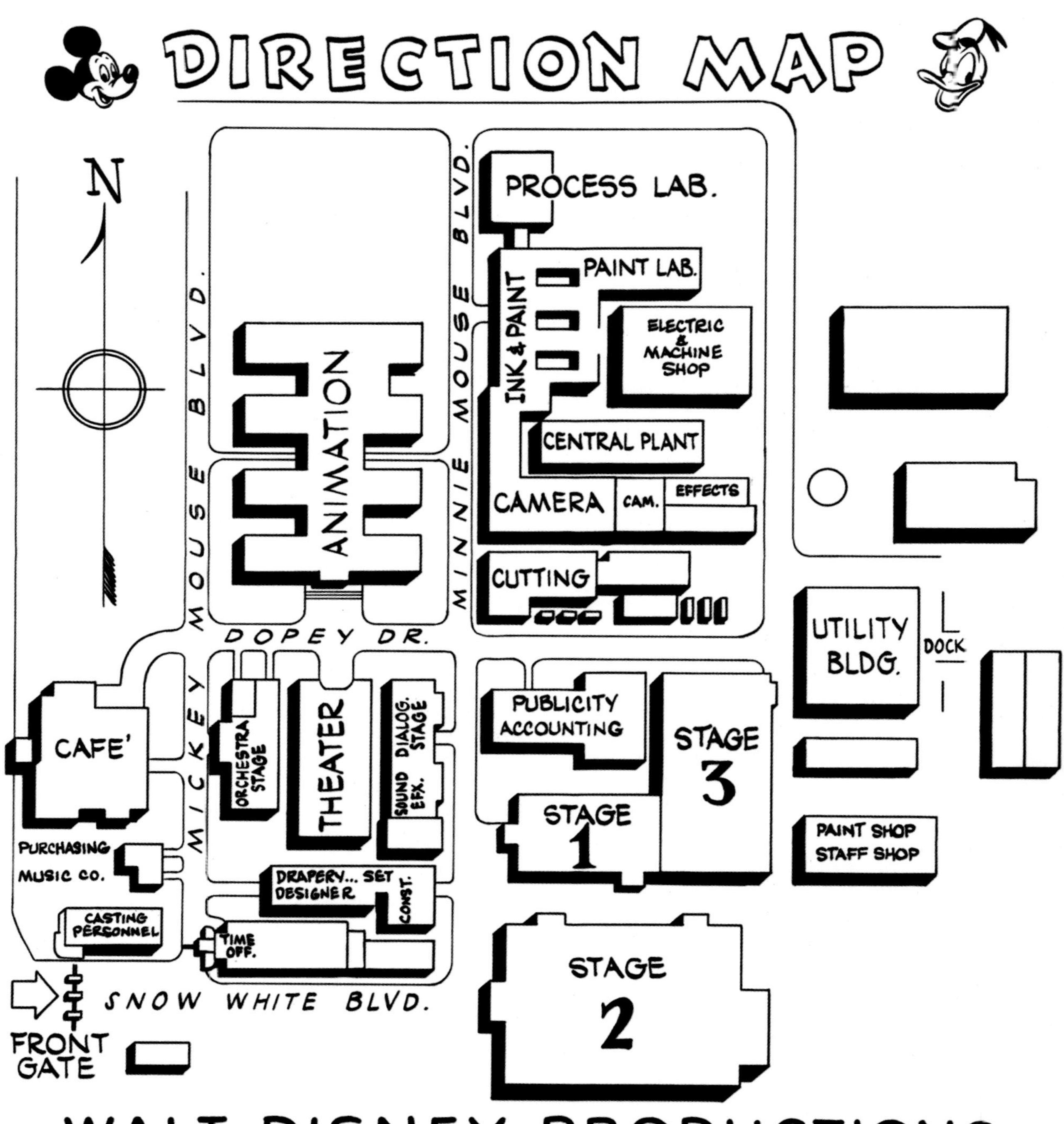

Map of the expanding Disney Studios in June of 1955.

Since the founding of the studio, Walt had made his name on shorts. The incredible artistic and technical innovations of both the Mickey and the Silly Symphony series had pushed the art form, each film looking to top the last. In less than a decade, Walt had grown his short films from run-of-the-mill to the gold standard in animation. But as shorts failed to return profits at the box office, Roy suggested the studio instead make a feature. He'd calculated that a single live-action feature fetched higher rental fees than the equivalent length of several shorts. And once Walt became engaged with the many possibilities of *Snow White*, shorts were doomed.

It was a slow decline—nearly two decades, thanks to their ability to turn a profit for a time. But creatively, shorts would never again be the juggernaut they once were.

Disney's employees knew this. Walt's infrequent appearance in the shorts department signaled their lowered status. Just as telling, a reward system was instated giving bonuses for shorts that, yes, were of good quality, but also came in below budget. When working on shorts, "you were doing your double darndest," recalled assistant Don Duckwall, "not just for bonuses; you were working to get yourself on a feature."[1]

True, compared with other studios, the Disney shorts were still top notch. Disney continued to set the bar for polish and technique. But with rare exceptions, their shorts just weren't as funny as those made at Warner Bros., nor as creatively innovative as those at UPA. Compared with Disney's own growth of the previous decade, most of their shorts of the forties felt tepid and rote.

It's easy to imagine why: Walt had strong creative opinions, yet no longer spent enough time in the shorts division to be a part of their creation. Risks taken that didn't pay off with approvals would result in lost time and revenue, and ultimately a loss of faith in leadership. Largely, the directors of Disney shorts were confined to repeat what had already worked.

There were exceptions; with the right combination of luck, timing, and hutzpah, a few directors would take advantage of the circumstances to make a few funny, ingenious shorts that reflected their own sensibilities and taste.

THE OLD GUARD

Snow White unlocked a passion for feature-length storytelling in Walt, and he couldn't go back. But neither could he abandon the shorts: during the feature's production, they were the studio's only source of income. They would need to be made—but on budget, and with limited oversight from Disney.

Walt at first leaned on Jackson, Sharpsteen, and Hand, his trusted collaborators who knew how to deliver the quality shorts Disney became known for. But Disney also wanted their help on his feature. Rather than choose, he split their time. In the two-year lead-up to *Snow White*'s December 1937 premiere, Jackson directed six sequences for the feature while also directing six shorts, including *The Old Mill* and *The Country Cousin*, both of which won Academy Awards. Sharpsteen directed ten shorts and eight sequences, and Hand directed eleven shorts while acting as *Snow White*'s supervising director.

But following *Snow White*'s release, Hand and Sharpsteen moved up to supervise other features, and Jackson would become Disney's top feature sequence director.[2] For shorts, Walt would need to find others.

So followed a period of experimentation between 1939 and 1943, ramping up to as many as six units,[3] trying directors from various backgrounds.

- Wilfred Jackson's assistant **Graham Heid** directed *Wynken, Blynken and Nod* (1938) and, along with Sam Armstrong, the "Raindrop" sequence of *Bambi*. That he did not continue is little surprise, due to, in his own words, "I am neither an artist nor a cartoonist, so animation was really not very interesting to me."[4]

- Ham Luske's assistant **Ford Beebe** directed two propaganda shorts using existing characters to encourage Canadians to buy war bonds: *The Thrifty Pig* and *Seven Wise Dwarfs* (both 1941), as well as codirecting "The Pastoral Symphony" section of *Fantasia*—all of which, according to Ollie Johnston, Frank Thomas, and Ward Kimball, didn't work out well.

- Dave Hand's assistant **Jack Cutting** directed *Farmyard Symphony* (1938) and *The Ugly Duckling* (1939) along with Gerry Geronimi and Ham Luske, but it must not have been wholly satisfying, as he went on to supervise the foreign dubbing for the majority of his career.

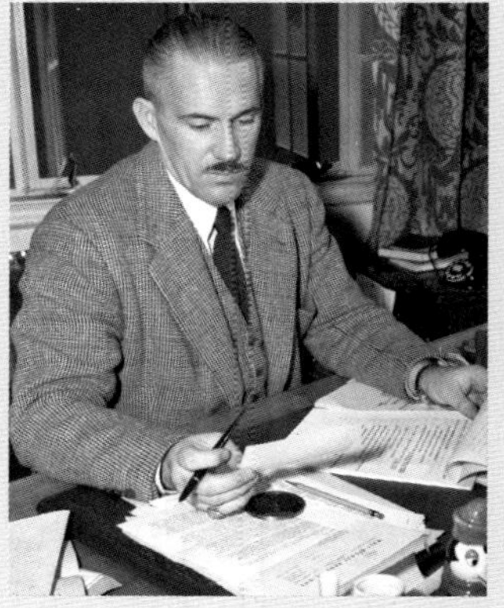

Photo of Jack Cutting in January 1947, taken for a publicity trip to Rio.

- Story man **Dick Huemer** directed *The Whalers* (1938) and *Goofy and Wilbur* (1939). It's uncertain how Disney felt about his abilities as a director, but likely his strength as a story brain was missed; he and Joe Grant became a powerhouse team, developing new story material for *Fantasia*, *Dumbo*, "Baby Weems," and much more.

- Animator **Riley Thomson** directed six shorts between 1940 and 1942. Production manager Don Duckwall described Riley as "a rough, tough, hard-to-bluff type of blustery Irishman" and mentioned that his father was a guard at the studio. Why Riley didn't continue directing is mysterious, as his work included the charming and stylish *The Little Whirlwind* (1941) and *The Nifty Nineties* (1941), though perhaps his skills as a draftsman and animator outweighed his contributions as a director.[5]

- **Dick Rickard** was one of a half dozen "idea men who had radio writing experience" but no experience with animation. Under Ben Sharpsteen's guidance, Rickard directed *Ferdinand the Bull* (1938) (though Sharpsteen credits Ham Luske for its success)[6] and *The Practical Pig* (1939) before Rickard "fell upon the skids" and "evaporated out of the business."[7]

- Ever the experimenter, Walt even attempted a short with no director at all, *Mickey's*

Amateurs, helmed by a small army of story artists and animators. "The picture," recalled Sharpsteen, "turned out to be an extremely weak one." (See Gillett chapter, page 38, for more information.)

There were several directorial experiments that did produce longer-term successes:

- Story man and animator **Dick Lundy** directed nine Donald shorts from 1939 to 1943.
- Animator **Bill Roberts** helmed three shorts (*Mickey's Parrot* [1938], *Brave Little Tailor* [1938], and *Society Dog Show* [1939]) before becoming a sequence director on *Pinocchio*, *Fantasia*, and *Dumbo*. (See sidebar on Roberts, page 79.)
- Animator **Ham Luske** directed *Mickey's Surprise Party* (1939) before being moved on to *Fantasia* and *Pinocchio*. With the exception of *The Pelican and the Snipe* (1944), Luske stayed in feature direction until Walt moved him to television. (See Chapter 6.)
- **Gerry Geronimi** began as a shorts director in 1939 with *Beach Picnic* and went on to direct twenty-seven shorts, dozens of feature sequences, and television. (See Chapter 7.) "I think you would find that the Geronimi unit was probably the most successful of any," remembered assistant Don Duckwall, due to Geronimi's ability to prep several shorts while others were in production. "We kept the most number of shorts going [at one time], and we spread our costs."[8]

THE CULTURE OF SHORTS

For some, Walt's seemingly irrational selection of directors was "very aggravating," said Ben Sharpsteen. "Walt would force these people in." But what did he see in them? "I don't say that Walt had pets; he didn't have yes-men. But he did have people that he, from time to time, thought quite highly of." Also, said Sharpsteen, "I think that Walt felt there was entirely too much emphasis placed on the word 'director.'"[9]

Despite Walt's own feelings, some worked out while others didn't—which seems to indicate that there was a unique value to the director, and a specific skill set required. Four men would prove they had these skills, and would remain the core of the shorts group for the rest of its existence.

Following the completion of *Bambi*, another feature that was not a box office success, and with profits shriveling during wartime, changes would take place throughout the studio. For shorts, as Jack Kinney recalled, "They thought, the shorts are costing too much, let's cut them down in footage, and instead of having Mickey and Pluto and Goofy and the Duck in one picture, let's break them up." (Fewer characters on-screen meant less drawing, and faster production.) Separate units would focus on each character: Jack King handled the Ducks—with Jack Hannah picking up his own Donald series in 1944—Nick Nichols got the Plutos, and Jack Kinney got Goofy. Mickey cartoons, increasingly difficult because of the restriction that the character be well-behaved ("He was a Boy Scout; you couldn't do anything with him!" complained Kinney), were made more sporadically.

King, Nichols, Hannah, and Kinney would become the spine of the shorts department, with only occasional exceptions, from 1942 until the shorts unit was disbanded in 1956. While Kinney would hop between features and shorts through much of his career, the others would stay exclusively in shorts.

Nichols remembered: "The whole idea behind a lot of the stuff was, they used the shorts to keep the doors open while they were doing the features, number one. Number two, the shorts were a training ground for animators that would eventually end up on the features. Number three was that there was a lot of competition between the short units . . . You all tried to make a funnier cartoon than the last guy and sometimes it was hard to do."[10]

"There was a certain amount of jealousy between units," agreed Kinney. "There had to be, that's the way Walt set it up, you're in the bowling alley."[11]

Each of the shorts directors spoke proudly of their tricks and systems to save time and produce under budget, subjects seldom discussed by feature directors. This was because "if you did a picture under $35,000, you got a piece of change back," said Kinney. Budget was not just an abstract thing, but dictated how much money you took home. "Everybody on the thing, not just the director, but the story guys, and the animators, and everybody else." No such reward system was ever set up on the features.

Another common theme was how seldom they saw Walt. "He would leave us pretty much alone," recalled Nichols. "If he didn't figure that it was going to work with the public as a good cartoon, why he would more or less put thumbs-down on it."[12] Kinney agreed: "We'd give him a quick look at the boards, and that was about it. He wouldn't spend any time."[13] If approved, "you pretty much had full autonomy of the cartoon from the time Walt okayed the story," recalled Hannah.[14]

In terms of producing the work, each director had his own story artist, layout artist, and key animators who would follow them from short to short.

The shorts animators were expected to produce twenty feet a week—around thirteen seconds—whereas feature animators could polish their work, producing between four and ten feet—two and a half to seven seconds per week.

Pictures were rated A, B, C, or D by Walt, influenced by audience reactions, and bonuses were handed out based on this. "If you did a bad picture, you weren't going to get as much money as if you did a picture that he considered A or B," said Kinney. "So you'd try to keep the quality going and still watch the budget."[15]

Though there were many things they shared in common, each of the four directors was quite different in his background and approach.

AUDIENCE RESEARCH INSTITUTE

While Disney had for years used live audiences to confirm his short films were entertaining, he himself had always been the final word on what ended up on-screen. But with his focus now on features, the studio wanted some way to reliably determine how the shorts were playing without drawing on Walt's time.

Following World War II, Disney entered into an agreement with George Gallup's Audience Research Institute (ARI). Story man Leo Salkin recalled that at the point he might normally have had a meeting with Walt, the story was deemed "ready for an ARI." Two groups of employees were recruited to give feedback: the so-called critical group, consisting of "people at high levels in the studio, the directors, the producers, the story men, the layout men, the key animators"; and the noncritical group, "people on lower levels of the studio who were not directly involved in any creative decisions—secretaries, ink and paint girls, maybe inbetweeners."

Salkin would "go into the big projection room and set the storyboards up on easels, and as everybody comes in, they give them two or three pages of stapled-together questions. First, you'd rate the film—whether it was excellent, very good, good, average, fair, poor, not recommended for production. Then there would be a series of questions that were meant to stimulate comments: 'Did you like the title?' 'Did you feel that particular characters were well handled?' 'What did you find funniest about it?' 'What did you find weakest about it?' Usually about two pages of questions. These were never signed; you just turned them in, and then they were averaged out. And both groups would answer the same questions."

Though low ratings would prohibit a story from being made, if Walt happened to like a story even if it didn't get a good rating, after the ARI he'd say, "Okay, I know it didn't get a good score, but I have a good feeling about that thing and I know it'll make a good short."[16]

A second ARI would be held once a film was animated but not yet inked and painted. Screenings were held for an audience of inbetweeners, ink and painters, or anybody who hadn't worked on the picture. Judgment would be passed based on the audible audience reaction as well as written questionnaires. "Walt always was in on those," remembered Hannah. "We'd meet out in the hall with Walt and would immediately go over some maybe very extensive changes, or very little things, or whatever. That's where he would give his final OK. Really basically Walt would only see the picture twice. He would OK the final story to go into production, [and] he would see that pencil test."[17]

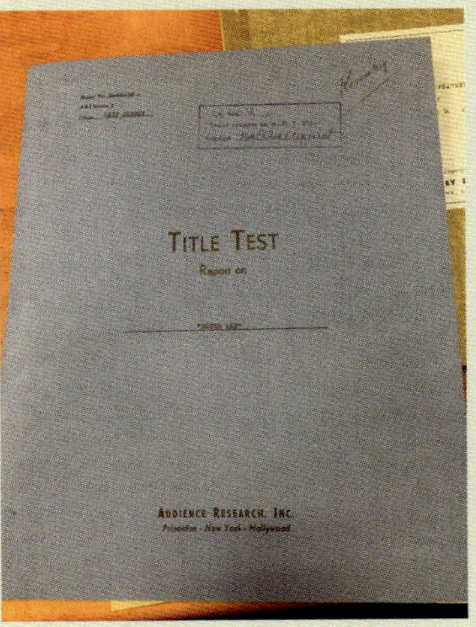

ARI reports were done for the features as well, though not on a consistent basis. This report on *Peter Pan* even tested audience responses to titles for the film, including *Peter Pan and Wendy*, *Peter Pan and Indian Joe*, *Neverland*, and *Straight on 'til Morning*.

JACK KING

Of all the shorts directors, Jack King came with experience. King started his career in 1914, animating for one of the first animation studios, helmed by Raoul Barré. By the time he came to Disney's in 1929, King had worked for Charles Mintz from 1924 to 1927 and Earl Hurd Productions from 1927 to 1929, where he even directed on the Judge Rummy series.

At five foot eight and 192 pounds, the bespectacled King was "a soft, sweet person"[18] with "a very funny high voice, Southern and New Yorkese."[19] Though older than most of the staff, they would nonetheless "rush in to protect Jack because he would stumble into a problem where he would get his head knocked off his shoulders through naïveté."[20]

Born on November 4, 1895, in Birmingham, Alabama, James Patton King served in a field support battalion during World War I, returning to New York to take classes at the Art Students League in 1921 or 1922.

Les Clark remembered King's animation style as tight and stiff, using nickels and dimes to draw Mickey.[21] When Norm Ferguson's rough, loose style became the accepted approach, Kinney remembered that King asked his assistant Roy Williams to "'take this thing and screw it up for me, will you? Put some rough lines around it.' And that's what Roy did. Walt said, 'Jack, you're catching on!' But underneath it was still that hard, stiff drawing."[22]

King left Disney in 1933 citing bad health, and took a job with Leon Schlesinger Productions.

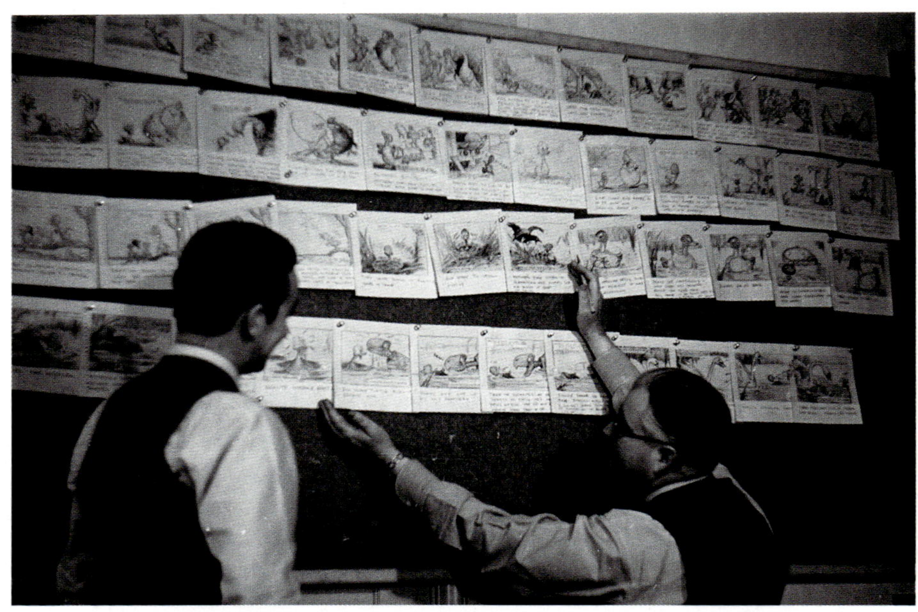

King at work with unknown story artist, around January 1939. According to story man Jack Hannah, who also developed stories in King's unit, "Jack King never got actively involved in the development of the story even though he was directing these cartoons. He'd stop in to say, 'Good morning,' or something like that. He liked everything that Carl [Barks] and I did."[23]

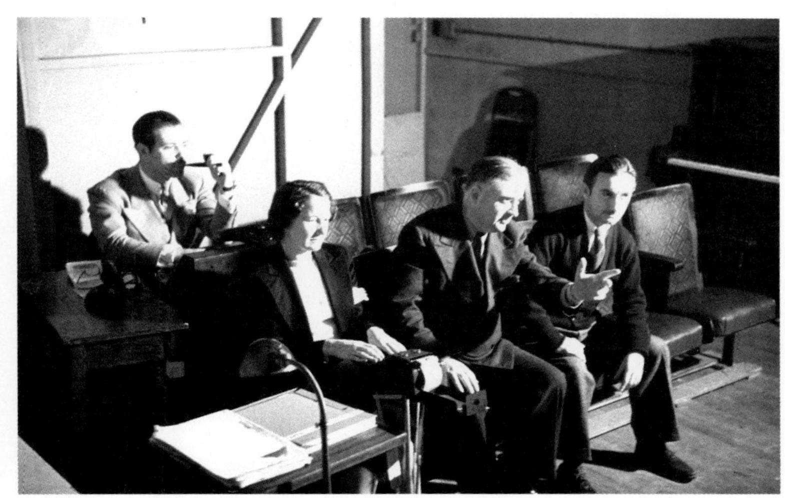

Jack King (CENTER) at work at the Sward Street studio in April or May 1939. Behind King (AT LEFT BEHIND HIS RIGHT SHOULDER) is assistant director Harry Tytle (at that time Harry Tytlebaum).

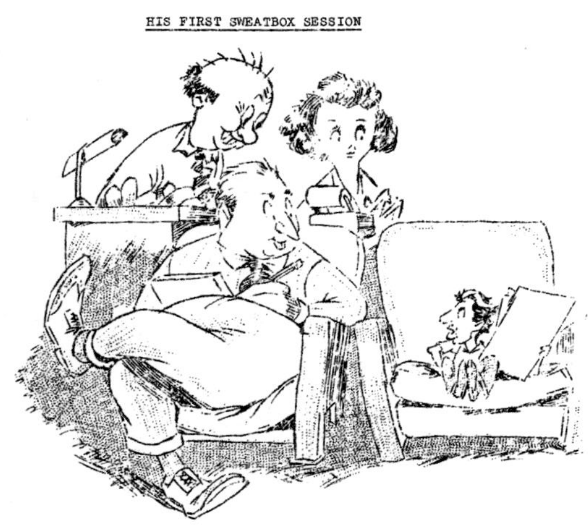

Animator Ted Bonnicksen depicted the feeling of his first director review in this drawing published in *The Bulletin*, an in-house studio magazine, 1940. Director Jack King is seated, while assistant Bob Newman and secretary Marie Dasnoit look on.

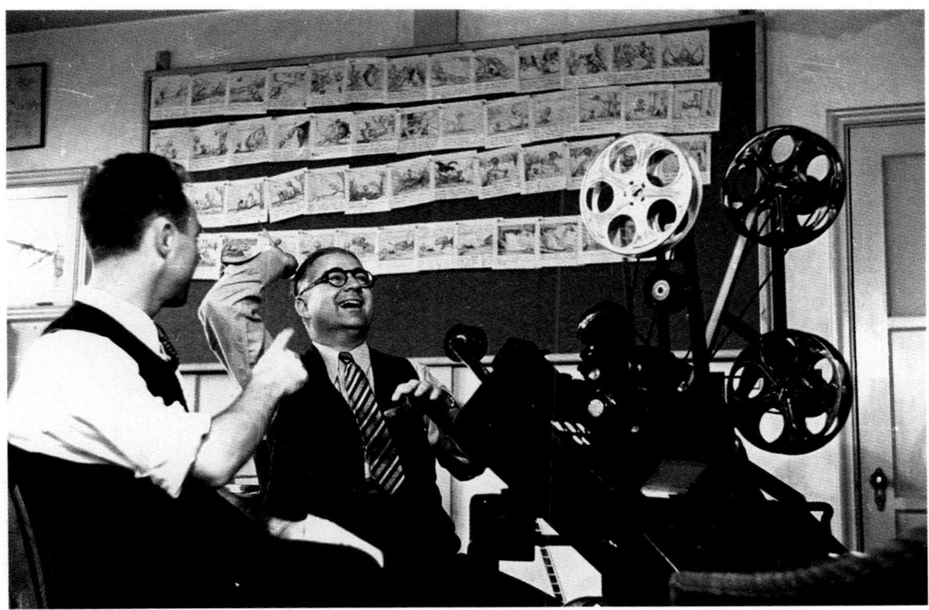

King at the Moviola around January 1939, with an unknown contributor. "He was a guy who was easy to work with," said story man Carl Barks. "His ideas seemed a little old-fashioned sometimes, but he was in on the beginnings of the animated stuff and he knew the limitations. Jack King was a little afraid to experiment on something that was different from what the established and proven trends were. He liked to feel that he was on sure ground."[24]

How working for Schlesinger would have aided King's health is not clear, but while there he returned to directing, working on the Buddy and Beans series. Animator Phil Monroe recalled that King was "a hell of an animator," but "wasn't the director that Friz Freleng was."[25] Strangely, while working at Schlesinger's, King was president of an automobile dealership in Santa Barbara—as he had been in Mamaroneck, New York, while working for Hurd.[26]

King returned to Disney in 1936. "Walt had decided to make Donald Duck a star in his own series of shorts, and Jack King was picked to start directing this series," remembered then-animator Jack Hannah.[27] King would direct forty-seven cartoons starring the ill-tempered duck.[28]

Animator Ed Love worked with King in the late thirties and describes a similar detachment: "He just said, 'Ed, go ahead and do what you want,' and we had a ball."[29] Whereas "the other short directors often called you in for discussion," recalled animator Eric Larson, "you very seldom got to see anything Jack was working on before it was finished."[30] While this level of trust may not apply to all animators, it does paint a picture of King as a rather absentee director.

As the years went on, King's work "just got worse and worse and worse. Roy Williams was his story man and he'd come up with some of the weirdest concepts."[31]

King was laid off in July 1946, his last credit being *The Trial of Donald Duck*, released in 1948.

Though he was only fifty-one, it doesn't seem that King worked in animation after this. Animator Bob McCrea remembered him as "another tragic character. When he left here I don't know what became of him, but the last anybody heard of him, they ran into him serving hamburgers in a hamburger joint in Glendale."[32] King experienced several serious family issues and died of a blood clot, aggravated by acute coronary thrombosis, on October 10, 1958 at age sixty-three.

JACK HANNAH

Serving under King, Jack Hannah determined that if he ever got to direct, he would do things differently. "Jack King wasn't a strong story man, and as director he sometimes missed the personality bits that could really

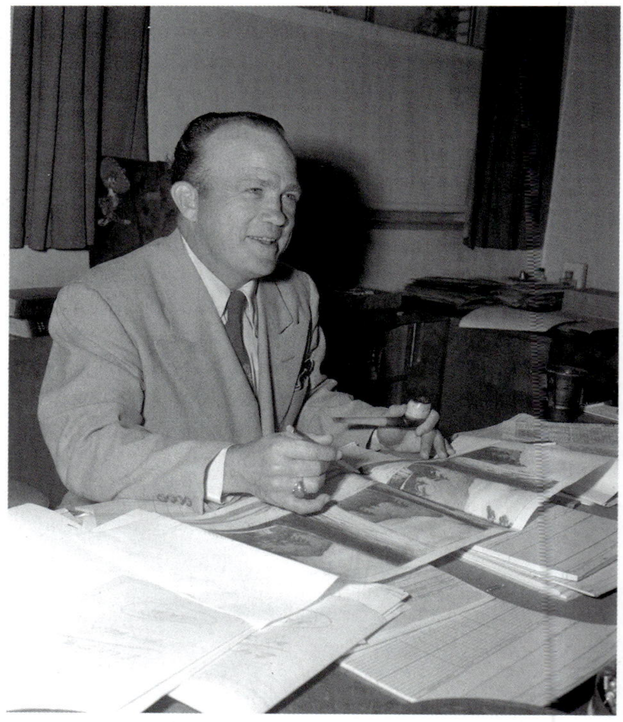

Hannah at his director's desk in March 1954.

add to a story. Carl [Barks] and I were always disturbed that King put one of our stories onto the screen without looking for further development in the personality of the characters. This was very irritating to both Carl and me. We saw a lot of potential in the basic ideas we came up with, but when it was animated, it just fell short a little bit because King never explored the possibilities more fully. It was this type of frustration that made me want to become a director myself. I always felt if I had the chance I could put a little more personality into the stories."[33]

Hannah got that chance, becoming not only a director, but one of the major influences on Donald Duck's animated personality.

John Frederick (Jack) Hannah was born in Nogales, Arizona, on January 5, 1913. Graduating from high school, he hoped to become either a commercial artist or a boxer. The few bucks he made in the ring helped pay his tuition at the Art Guild Academy, and a broken jaw finally cemented his direction.[34]

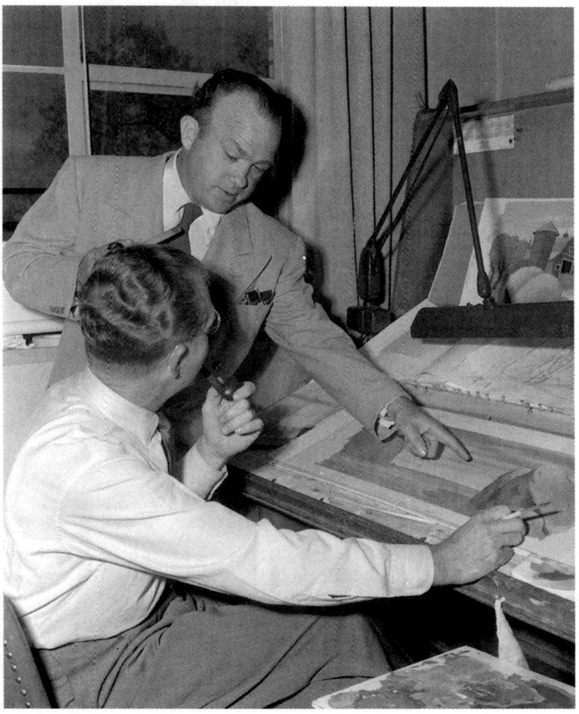

Hannah in the background department.

Jack moved to Los Angeles to take art courses at the Otis and Chouinard art schools in 1931. Working initially as a poster designer, the Great Depression drove him to look for work at Disney's. Driving to the Hyperion Avenue studio "with my portfolio and a little fear in my heart," he was called by Ben Sharpsteen to come in for a two-week tryout, which, he said, laughing, "ended up in thirty years of work at Disney!"[35]

Starting in January 1933 as an inbetweener, Hannah worked his way up to animator for Jack King's unit by 1936. Curious about story, he studied under and alongside story man Carl Barks, and in 1939 moved into story for Jack King's unit. He and Barks built up story ideas, boarded them, road tested it on other story artists, then pitched the story to Jack King and Walt.

Wanting to make some extra cash, Hannah and Barks picked up freelance work drawing and inking comic books for Dell and Whitman/Western Publishing, again featuring Donald Duck. Though Carl Barks would leave the studio to become the best-known Disney comic book artist, Hannah was set on directing.[36]

He finally got his foot in the door with the training film *Out of the Frying Pan Into the Firing Line* (1942), about a housewife saving cooking fats for the war effort. "King wasn't interested in the mechanical part of this picture. You know, showing all these cooking fats and stuff going down a funnel and things like that. So he gave me a little section to direct and I just loved it. That was my first little piece of direction and I started to direct more and more."[37]

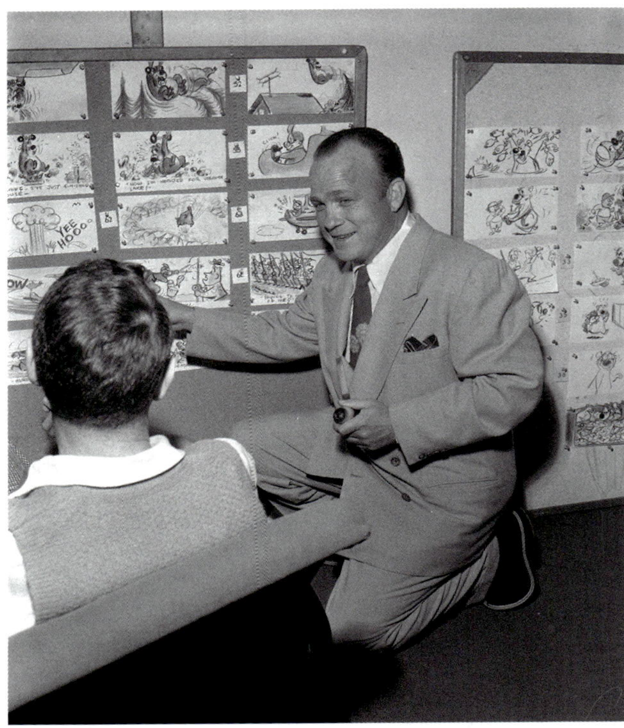

Hannah looks over storyboards for a Humphrey the Bear cartoon.

"When the war was over, they moved me back to being a story man, but I had had a taste of directing and by 1944 I was directing Donald Duck shorts. I spent all my energy trying to be the best director I could,"[38] said Hannah. His first short, *Donald's Off Day* (1944), worked out well enough that Hannah would go on to direct over sixty cartoons at Disney's featuring Chip 'n Dale, Humphrey the Bear, Bootle Beetle, and others—but the large majority would feature Donald.

In contrast to his predecessor Jack King, Hannah's ducks "were much more alive than King's were," felt animator Eric Larson. "Jack King was kind of like this in temperament (draws a smooth curve with hands), where Hannah was like this (steep curve with hands). And it has to come out in what they do, doesn't it?"[39]

Much of this was a result of Hannah's control over his exposure sheets.[40] "A lot of directors gave the animators more say in timing," said Hannah. "I never did that. I timed every foot I directed. I don't care how good the animator was. To me, it was the most important part of the directing—the timing, the pacing, the pauses."[41]

As the production of shorts dwindled, Hannah directed fourteen hour-long Disney television shows, many of which featured Walt Disney interacting with Donald Duck. But this was just a stopgap; Hannah was let go in 1956. He picked up television work for the Walter Lantz Studio, where he directed more than twenty shorts and directed the live-action openings of the *Woody Woodpecker* television show.

In his later years, Jack returned to Disney in the 1960s to work as a story consultant on live-action films, and in 1975 was asked by the Disney Studios to develop a program for character animation at the California Institute of the Arts. There he taught many of the next generation of filmmakers, including Chris Buck, John Musker, Tim Burton, Brad Bird, and John Lasseter. Jack was also a skilled landscape artist, and his paintings were displayed in galleries throughout the West. Jack was given a Winsor McCay Award in 1987 and was made a Disney Legend in 1992. He passed away on June 11, 1994, at the age of eighty-one, at St. Joseph's Hospital in Burbank, California.

NICK NICHOLS

The Pluto expert of the shorts group, Charles August "Nick" Nichols was born on September 15, 1910, in Milford, Utah. He lived in Chicago from 1927 until about late 1934, where he drew several comic book strips, including *The Adventures of Peter Pen* and *Just Supposin'*.

Between 1933 and 1934 he also sold a cartooning course.

He joined Disney in February 1935, probably as an inbetweener, and became an assistant to Woolie Reitherman, cleaning up and inbetweening the magic mirror in *Snow White*. By 1937 Nick was animating the Coachman in *Pinocchio*, as well as on many Pluto shorts.

His expertise with the dog led to his first directing job, *Springtime for Pluto*, and would continue with Pluto into the early fifties. Years later Nick recalled, "Pluto was just a lovable dog and I've gotten letters from many people saying, 'We enjoyed this cartoon and that cartoon because Pluto did exactly the same thing as Old Blue did.' And that always made you feel good. I felt when I did Pluto that I was doing a dog. I remembered my dogs. I remembered dogs that I had been in contact with: how they acted, some of the things they did, And I tried to put that into him, so that he remained as a dog. I think we were quite successful in that respect."[42]

Beyond Pluto, Nichols was known for his action. "When you had a sequence with an element of slapstick to it," recalled animator Eric Larson, "you would call Nichols, and let him have a look."[43]

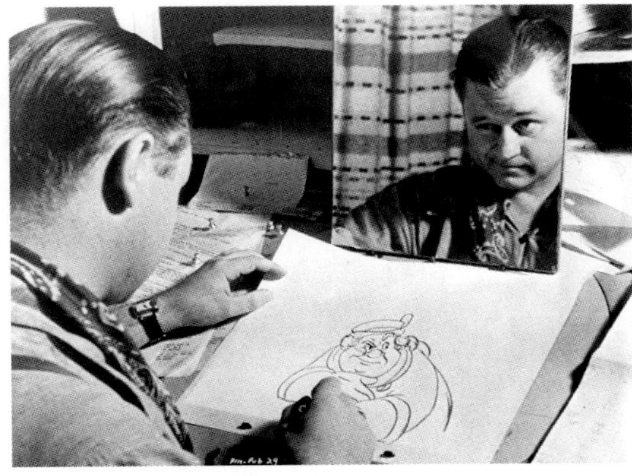

Nichols animating the Coachman on *Pinocchio*.

Paul Carlson, who worked with Nichols for several years, remembered Nick as "a great guy. He was very nice to work with."[44] While animator Victor Haboush also liked Nichols, he described him as "a 'medium' director. He wasn't one of Walt's top guys."[45]

Fellow directors Kinney and Hannah were less than fans of his work. While they all got along well, Kinney felt that some of his Pluto pictures were "the bottom of the barrel," and recalled Hannah complaining: "'Aw, that goddamn Nick, all he does is tink-tink music.' Tink-tink-tink-tink—Pluto going along on his tippy-toes. And everything he did, he had the tink-tink music going." Kinney felt this was due to the fact that "Nick was strictly an animator. He thought as an animator, and his stuff looked like an animator's; his direction was from [an animator's standpoint], that's why you got the tink-tink business. He fell in love with that cute little walk. It was a good little walk, but Jesus, not to do it over and over."[46]

Kinney also noted that Nichols "had an aversion to Scene 13; he never had a Scene 13 in his pictures. I said, '. . . Here are eight or ten of your pictures, and no Scene 13. What the hell's the matter?' He said, 'I'm superstitious, that's all. Shut up.'"[47]

Nick also directed several "one-offs" like *Melody* (1953), *Toot, Whistle, Plunk and Boom* (1953), *Grand Canyonscope* (1954), *How to Have an Accident in the Home* (1956), *How to Have an Accident at Work* (1959), and *The Saga of Windwagon Smith* (1961). While it may seem that *Melody* and *Toot, Whistle* reveal another side to Nichols, for these films he served as codirector with Ward Kimball. "Nichols didn't do anything except fill out the sheets," according to animator Vic Haboush. "Creatively they were Ward's."[48]

As shorts slowed, Nichols reinvented himself as a sequence and commercial director for television. The studio produced hundreds of commercials, including for 7UP (featuring Fresh-Up Freddie), Baker's Instant Chocolate (featuring Jiminy Cricket), Jell-O, Cheerios (featuring Donald Duck), Ipana (featuring Bucky Beaver, voiced by Jimmie Dodd of the *Mickey Mouse Club*), Derby Foods, Inc. (featuring Tinker Bell), and Nash (featuring Mickey Mouse and friends). When the commercials needed live-action footage, Nichols directed that as well. He also directed several of Walt's desk-side introductions for the *Disneyland* television series.

Nichols left Disney's around the end of 1961 and was quickly hired by Hanna-Barbera, where he directed episodes of *The Jetsons*, *The Flintstones*, and *Scooby-Doo*, as well as the feature *Charlotte's Web* (1973). After a stint at Ruby-Spears, Nick Nichols's career ended at Disney, where, in the 1990s, he directed episodes of the animated TV series *Darkwing Duck*, *Goof Troop*, and *Bonkers*. Nichols passed away at the age of eighty-one, on August 23, 1992.

JACK KINNEY

Of all the Disney directors, Jack Kinney was the one you'd most likely enjoy talking with. He told great stories and was a real character himself. A proud member of the "screwball camp" in his personality and taste[49], Jack was an energetic prankster and jazz drummer, and one of the only directors to navigate back and forth between shorts and features. His loud personality is felt in his "How to" Goofy shorts, as well as the sheer volume of work he produced. And his "whatever it takes" approach led to many innovative discoveries along the way. His career was bumpy, hot-and-cold, but never boring, exemplifying the life of a shorts director at Disney: stay flexible, keep the quality up, the budget low, and don't count on anything.

Born March 29, 1909, John Ryan "Jack" Kinney was a born storyteller. Though Kinney wasn't one to let facts get in the way of a good story, the anecdotes, gossip, and practical jokes in his autobiography *Walt Disney and Assorted Other Characters* make for fun reading and reveal Kinney's own high-spirited personality.

Jack came by his rich character genetically. His maternal grandfather was a prospector who struck it rich out West, where Jack's mother met an Irish traveling salesman who became

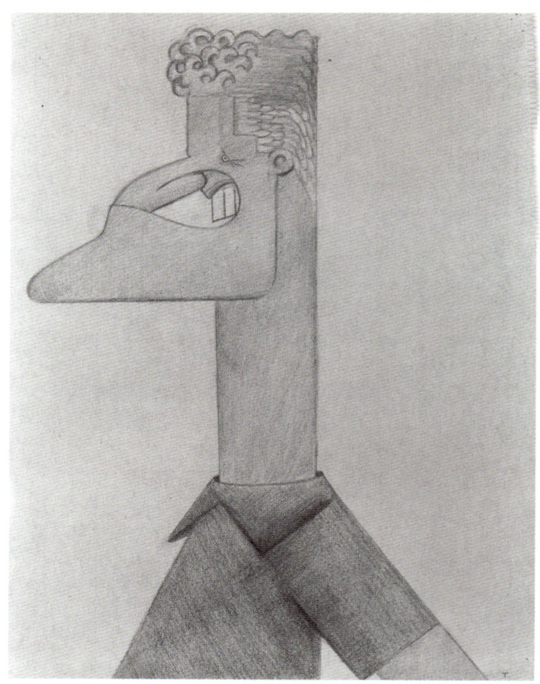

Caricature of Kinney by T. Hee.

Jack's father.[50] Jack was born in Salt Lake City, Utah, and his family moved to California when Jack was about eight. Jack's father's uncle, a tobacco millionaire named Abbott Kinney, had developed a residential district in Santa Monica, and introduced eucalyptus trees to the area. Jack's father owned two dry goods stores in Los Angeles but took his own life during the Great Depression. Jack's mother invested the insurance proceeds but lost all the money, forcing Jack to quit school and go to work, in spite of a football scholarship from USC.[51] "I worked at everything," recalled Jack. "Dug ditches for the Department of Water and Power; Sears, Roebuck; Goodyear Tire & Rubber; Southern California Edison . . . you took anything you could get, because, really, out there people were starving."[52]

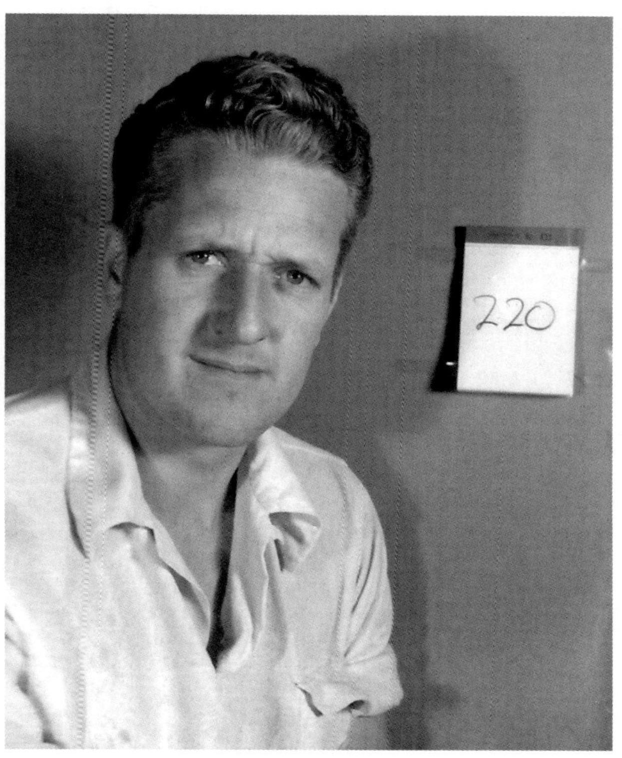

Employee Jack Kinney, taken in 1940.

Jack began at Disney's in 1931 as an inbetweener and worked his way up to animator, but was insecure about his work. "I was just beginning to get the hang of it when Walt shunted me to the story department," he wrote in his autobiography.[53]

As a story artist he worked under Ben Sharpsteen, boarding a sequence on *Moving Day* (1936). "The first one I did, as a story guy all on my own, was *The Brave Little Tailor* (1938). It went through Burt Gillett first, and he blew it like crazy, and then Bill Roberts; that was his first direction."

It was on that film that Kinney came up with the idea of the Leica reel. Developed by Bill Garity, it was a major innovation for Disney story artists and the predecessor to today's story reels, or animatics. Much like "film strips" of the sixties and seventies, Leica reels consisted of a strip of film with a single image on each frame. Projected, the images would be advanced in sync to a live pitch (or, later, a prerecorded soundtrack), allowing an audience to get a sense for what the final film might feel like. Jack and Bill's innovation grew out of the fact that Walt was "a terrible person to tell a storyboard to, because he was always looking down here someplace" instead of where the artist was pointing. "We tried all kinds of tricks." Story man Webb Smith "took long pieces of paper off the layout sheets and laid them across and peeled them back as he went through it. Walt didn't like that. 'Goddammit,' and he goes up and pulls the paper off the board."[54] Kinney knew he couldn't repeat that trick. "I thought, what the hell am I going to do? I took the *Brave Little Tailor* and had them shoot the storyboard on the thing." Kinney pitched the dialogue, doing voices and describing action, while he snapped his fingers to cue Earl Hurd to advance

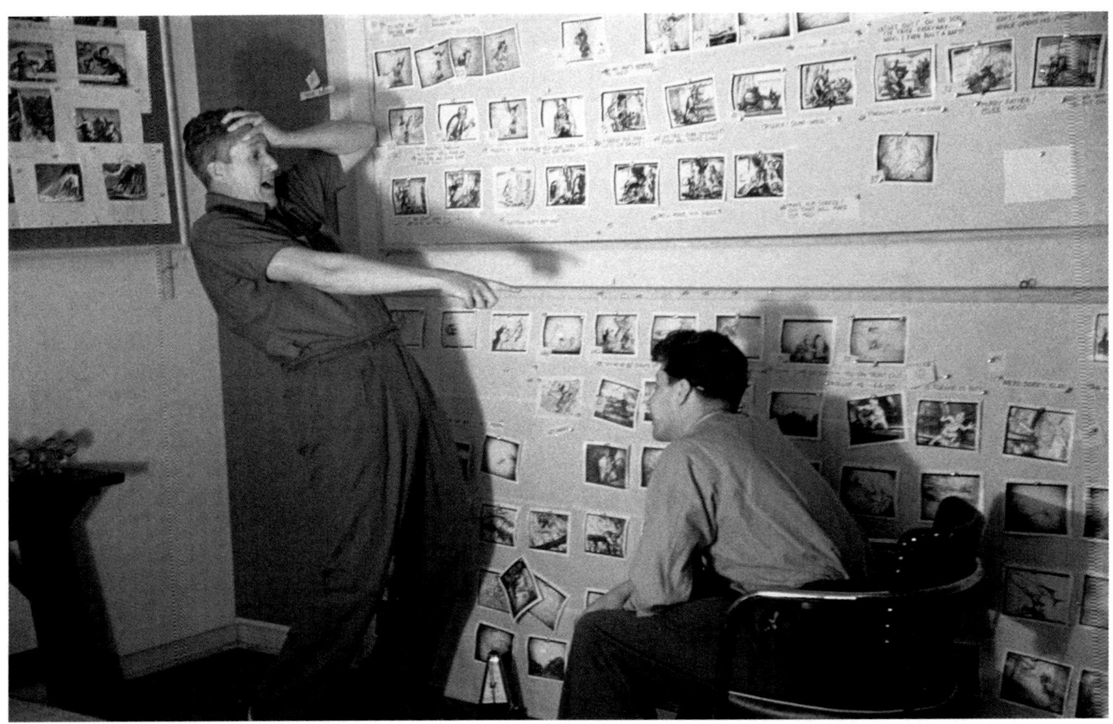

Kinney (LEFT) and someone unknown at work on *Pinocchio*, shot in April/May 1939 in Kinney's office, next to Walt's. Note the metronome on the floor; it was a common tool for the director to determine the pacing and rhythm.

the projector. "It went over like a house afire." Synchronized sound was soon added, along with the ability to advance the images automatically. Leica reels were used extensively on *Snow White*, *Fantasia*, and *Pinocchio*, and continued to be used into the 1950s.

But Kinney's career as a story artist didn't last long. "Walt wanted to make a director out of Jack Kinney on *Pinocchio*," remembered assistant Lou Debney. Kinney and Debney were moved into a music room connected with an adjoining door to Disney's office. (Kinney was disturbed by Walt's habit of walking through his office unannounced, so he rearranged the furniture to block the door, much to Walt's consternation.) Kinney directed five sequences in the movie: "Starving in Belly of Whale," "Geppetto Starts to Fish Tuna," "Reunion in Whale," "Geppetto Fishing for Tuna," and "Coach Ride to Pleasure Island."

Kinney's next assignment was a move into shorts: *Bone Trouble*, a Pluto cartoon released in June 1940. Given the lower status of shorts, it's hard to know what to make of this. Had he failed on *Pinocchio*? Kinney saw himself as the guy they would call when no one else could get the material to work. "I was a garbage can, really. I was a garbage can on 'Bongo' [in *Fun and Fancy Free* (1947)]; they'd bought the story from Sinclair Lewis, and nobody could do anything with it."[55] Kinney returned to features, directing three sequences of *Dumbo*, and would continue to helm both feature sequences and shorts throughout his career, sometimes both concurrently.

As a director, Kinney's favorite material was broad and energetic, informed by his own physicality. "I love sports; I really do," he recalled. "I quit playing football when I was forty-five, because I broke my collarbone playing touch football at Disney's."

Kinney worked with story man Ralph Wright, and the two of them "were a team of real professionals," remembered story artist Carl Barks. "They turned out stuff fast and good."[56] Throughout his directing career, Kinney continued to contribute in story, often in partnership with his brother Dick, who also worked at the studio. "I have always had a hand in the story of any film I directed," he said, "not for ego reasons but to make sure I never got saddled with weak material. I did not get story credit because Walt never credited a man for more than one thing at a time." Kinney later authored several early outlines for *Peter Pan*.

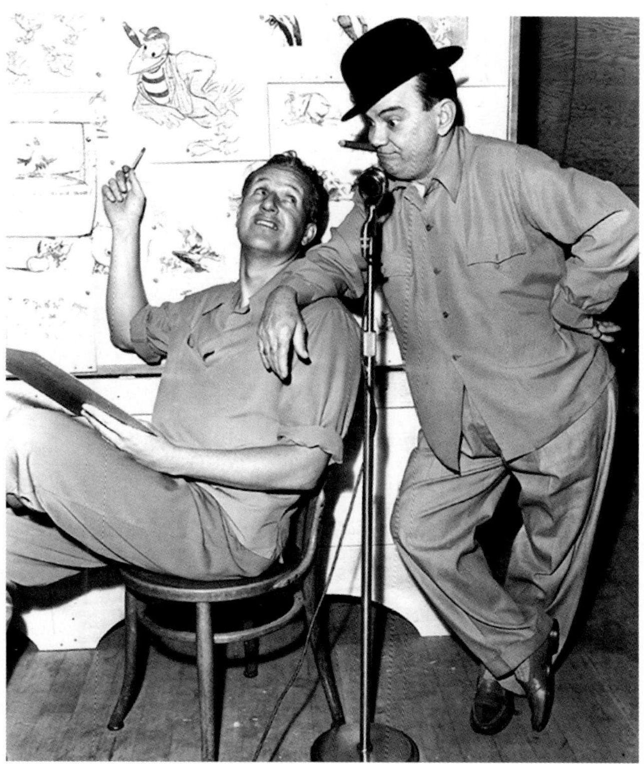

Kinney (LEFT) clowns around with Cliff Edwards on *Dumbo*.

In laying out his films, Kinney felt that the action was where the focus should be. "I always hated when these background guys would get so damned flamboyant with their backgrounds, and fall in love with the background, and the character would turn, and he'd lose a head or a nose or something. I like to see the damned things out there so you can read them. And I don't like anything playing here [holding his arms close to his body], I want their arms out here. They're ham actors, that's what they are, you know; let them be hams. Especially with the Goof; there was nothing subtle about him."[57]

Kinney developed a unique approach that left a lot of freedom to his animators, allowing them to open up the timing and add new ideas. "Jack directed animation like you'd direct live action," said animator Jerry Hathcock. "Where you'd have an 800 foot picture, he'd have maybe 1,600 feet animated, and then cut it, like live action. Particularly on that Goofy stuff."[58] "We did a pose test, from start to finish," Kinney recalled. "We'd see it in continuity and say, okay, it needs tightening here, it needs a better gag here." No other director worked this way, despite the fact that, according to Kinney, "I made a lot of money, on the budget bit [thanks to the bonus system], because we did everything in pose tests, and then [once it was cut down] put the inbetweens in. And it worked."

Kinney's approach as a director is evident in his work. "I think tempo in your picture has to

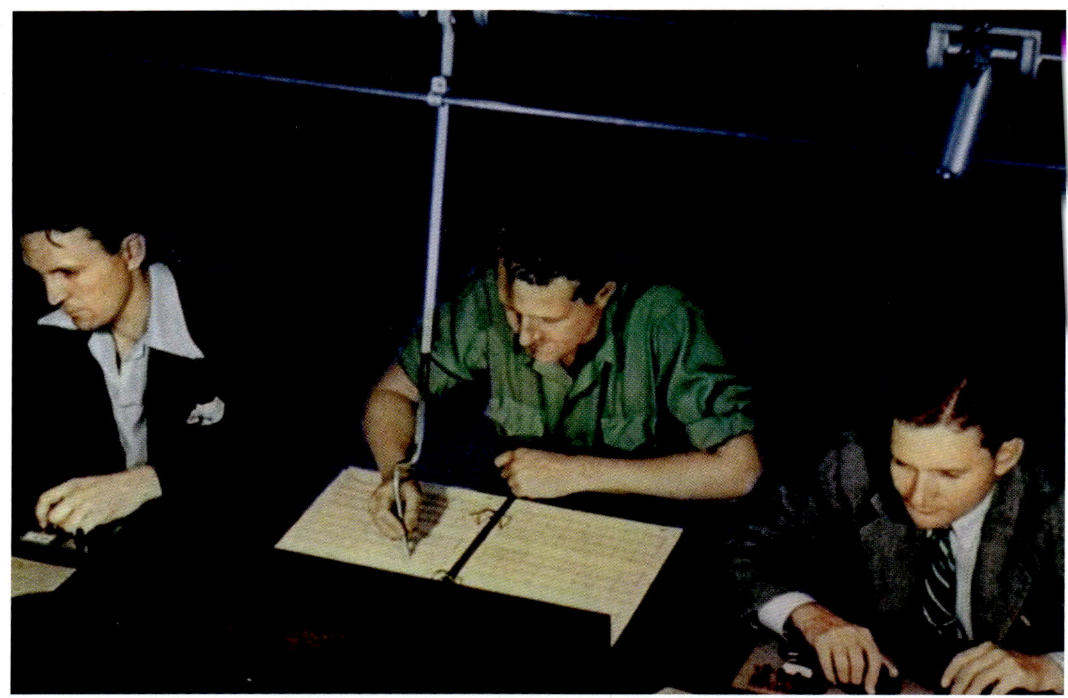

Kinney's background as a musician likely came in handy during final mix, a process referred to at Disney's as "re-re" (as in re-recording—which it actually was, due to the technology at that time). Kinney (CENTER), with sound engineer C. O. "Sam" Slyfield (AT LEFT) and sound effects head Hal Reese (ON RIGHT) watches the image playback and drags a pointer to the correct spot on the bar sheet. The device, nicknamed "The Iron Pencil," in turn shone small overhead spotlights (seen in upper right of photo) down onto the cue sheets in front of up to six engineers, allowing them to follow exactly where they were in the picture. Following instructions indicated on the bar sheets, they manually adjusted the volume of up to twelve tracks of music, sound effects, and dialogue at precise moments; a single error required a redo of the entire short or reel of film.

build. You do it by your cutting of your individual scenes, more than by keeping to a beat. I always try to get a chase someplace, in the last hundred, hundred and fifty feet, going like a bat out of hell. Take a little time to establish it, and then get moving. Let the thing go out, so that even if the gags were dry, they won't be on the scene that long."[59]

Having been assigned to the newly reorganized shorts group, Kinney decided that "the character I'd like to work with would be the Goof. I'd worked with all the other characters at one time or another, but the Goof to me was a nice long, lean character that you could move; you could get poses out of him, crazy poses. I liked his voice, because I thought he was kind of an

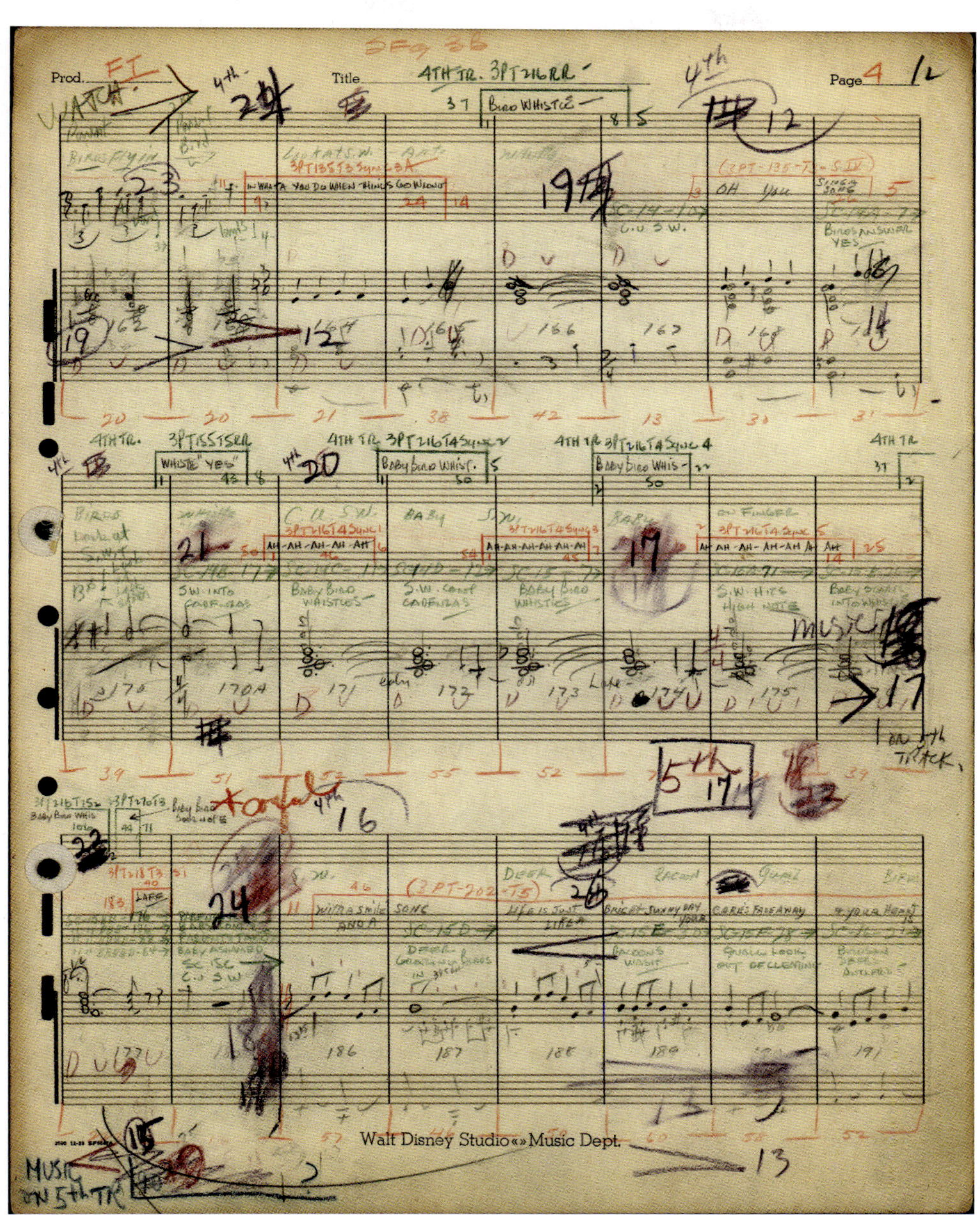

Final bar sheets, like this one from *Snow White*, indicated the relative placement of dialogue, music, and sound effects and would be followed by re-recording mixers using the Iron Pencil method.

easygoing guy that you could associate with, as being dumber than yourself. They always make you feel good, you know." Kinney directed *Goofy's Glider*, released in 1940. But when Pinto Colvig, the voice of Goofy, left the studio. Goofy was left speechless. Kinney had an idea.

> Every Friday, all directors were required to give Walt an interoffice communication report for him to read over the weekend. I submitted my ideas for this new Goofy series. The "how-to" format opened up a vast area. The subject matter could be anything; do-it-yourself repairs, or even the wide world of sports, all open to Goofy's dum-dum exploration. What he would do in any given story would be the hook we'd hang it on. The following Monday, I got a call from Walt, who said, "Jack, this is one hell of an idea! Go ahead on it!" Encouraged by Walt's favorable reaction (this didn't happen every time), I asked, "Which one first?" "Any one of 'em," he said. "Which do you like?" Knowing of Walt's keen interest in polo, I said, "How about How to Ride a Horse?"[60]

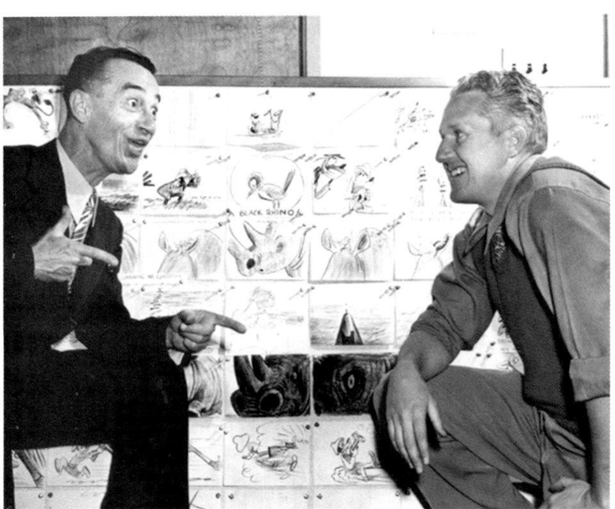

Kinney (RIGHT) clowns with Pinto Colvig on *African Diary*, released in April 1945.

The short was included in *The Reluctant Dragon* and was an immediate hit with audiences. The success of the series hung on wonderfully spirited animation by John Sibley and Woolie Reitherman, as well as distinctive narration by story man John McLeish. The narration, a parody of an existing series of travelogues, was allegedly recorded without McLeish knowing he was doing a spoof. Kinney claimed: "We'll get McLeish for a narrator, and don't tell him that he's not doing it straight. Just let him play it."

"See, that was a fun time at Disney's," reminisced Kinney, "when Walt didn't pay too much attention to the shorts."[61]

Though the "how-to" series was a hit with audiences and continued for years, Disney himself grew to dislike them, particularly the gag-based humor and what he saw as a lack of personality. He also objected to the way Kinney and crew had redesigned Goofy.[62]

Kinney's relationship with Disney was complex. His respect for his boss is often undercut by stories of Disney's own contradictions. "I was in the sweatbox with Walt, all by himself, and we were waiting for other people to show. He leaned back in his chair and saw the ceiling, and he was trying to count [the pushpins in it]; he counted about two hundred pushpins in the ceiling. He turned to me and he says, 'Goddammit, Jack, you know how much these pushpins cost?' I said no. He says, 'You've gotta quit throwing them at that goddamned ceiling. I just can't afford it. They cost a penny and a half apiece.' Then, when the others came in, they were going through a feature picture, he turned around and cut out a $250,000 sequence."[63]

Kinney's "humor wins out over everything" approach was rare at Disney, and animator Lance Nolley felt that Kinney "could take a situation and make it funny, no matter what it was, by his animation and by his drawing and design of the characters."[64] But not everyone was a fan. Frank Thomas and Milt Kahl both complained Kinney didn't know what he wanted. In return Kinney griped about their work on "The Legend of Sleepy Hollow," of which he directed the first half. (Geronimi directed the second.) "I always felt that Crane should have been a loose goose, and instead of that, he came out with the most beautiful walks and stuff—and it wasn't funny, period. He had no character: he was just a guy who moved beautifully. And then when I took some of Frank Thomas's and Milt Kahl's stuff, and cut the hell out of it to make it move, these guys fell in love with every one of their damned drawings. You couldn't let these guys go, because they would pad. Kahl had Brom Bones coming in and leaping over the horse; he did a magnificent job, but I said, 'For Christ's sake, Kahl, you've got thirty-five feet of beautiful animation, and it should be done in ten.'"[65] Kinney felt that too much polish could strangle the spirit and humor. "The value of animation is overrated," Kinney remarked.

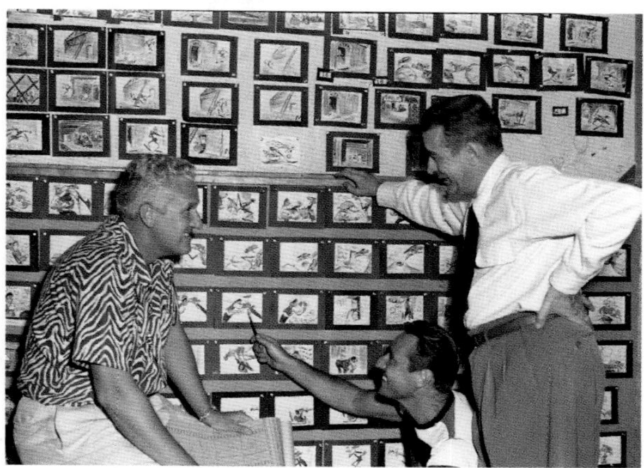

Kinney (LEFT), Joe Rinaldi (KNEELING), and Ed Penner (RIGHT) on "The Legend of Sleepy Hollow," August 1949.

Kinney continued to hop from shorts to features and back. After *Pinocchio* and *Dumbo*, he directed sequences in *The Three Caballeros*, "Bongo" in *Fun and Fancy Free*, and "The Martins and the Coys" and "All the Cats Join In" from *Make Mine Music*. Jack's last feature directing credit was the "Wind in the Willows" segment of *The Adventures of Ichabod and Mr. Toad* (1949).

After this, he continued work on shorts for a time, though begrudgingly. "I had to do pictures I didn't really want to do, like *Fathers Are People* (1951) and all that kind of crap. I said, 'Jesus, Walt, if you're going to do that, make him a human character, take the dog head off of him.' He said, 'Yeah, let's try that.' Then, about an hour later, he called back, 'No, no, the Goof's established, they know him.' But those pictures were disasters, because I didn't fight it hard enough. Afterwards, I thought, this thing is getting to be an awful pain in the ass, to try to do this type of stuff with a character that isn't designed for it. Then I got back to the formula stuff, like *For Whom the Bulls Toil* (1953), back into the old routines again, but by that time the shorts were on their way out." In the end, Kinney directed over fifty shorts at Disney's.

Kinney was one of the first directors to be assigned to Disney's new passion: television. "That wasn't much fun. Then they brought in other people from the outside, and it was a different world, no fun anymore. The spirit had gone out." Kinney was assigned to write the introductions for the show. "Walt said, 'I want you to try and design some things where I'll be master of ceremonies, but one thing,

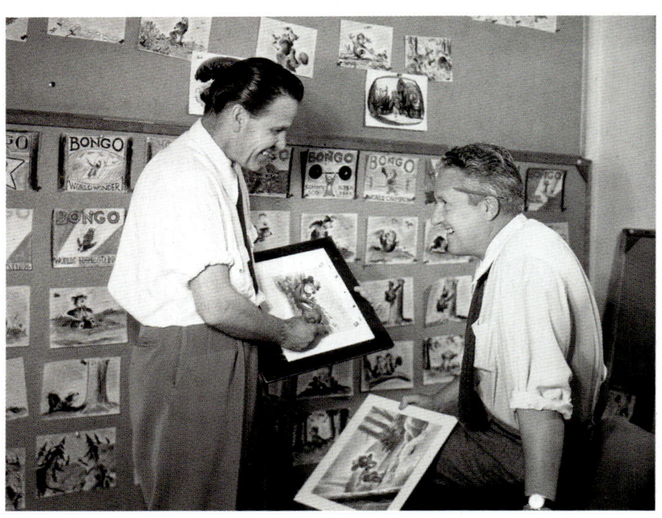

Story artist Lance Nolley (LEFT) and Jack Kinney at work on "Bongo" in late 1946.

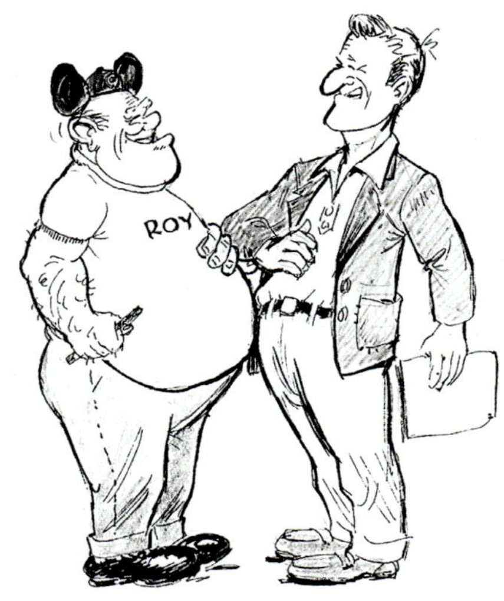

Kinney's self-portrait with story man and Mooseketeer Roy Williams.

goddammit, I don't want, I don't want to be behind a desk. You got that, Jack?' I said, 'Yeah, I got it.' So I tried to come up with all different ways that Walt could be walking around in different departments in the studio, or could be at Disneyland, or on the sound stage, looking over somebody's back, and then going on to a gimmick like that. He ends up behind the desk. He never got out of that library; that was it."[66]

Jack was assigned to create four hours for the Disney TV show on the history of aviation and man in space. He hired Willy Ley and contacted Wernher Von Braun as consultants. But in the end, according to animator Ward Kimball, "Jack was not necessarily interested in the fact that we were going out into space, and I was always a UFO fan anyway. So when I went to Walt with the *Collier's* [article on space exploration] and he said, 'Hey, this is the way we should go,' it was sort of mutual agreement, I think. Jack realized that this was the sort of thing that wasn't his bag."[67]

Kinney also felt that "I was going down the slide at that point."

THE END OF SHORTS

In his book *One of Walt's Boys*, production manager Harry Tytle wrote: "After Walt had pioneered cartoon features with *Snow White and the Seven Dwarfs*, short subjects, the early foundation for the studio's success, began their backward slide in importance." Tytle was in a good position to watch their decline. Though his assignment was to keep shorts alive, that was hard when the bosses weren't on board. As far back as June 19, 1946, Tytle wrote of a conversation with Roy O. Disney:

> He [Roy] threw a bombshell as far as I was concerned. He said after we completed the number of shorts in work, which would be about 2 years, he did not care if we did any more shorts: in fact he preferred we didn't.[68]

Even Walt was losing interest. Tytle's June 20, 1946, journal entry read:

> Walt agreed there was no money in short subjects, and they were not worth the effort, and he said very definitely and openly that he could not put the quality in he wanted to, and consequently had lost interest in them for that reason.

When Jack King's contract was brought up in July 1946, he was let go, "due to the high cost and low quality of his product."[69] With King's exit, just three shorts units remained.

The economics were shifting. Television and changing theatergoing habits meant the market for shorts had diminished, and since theaters had started to show double features to compete with television, shorts and newsreels didn't always have a ready-made spot on the theater bill. Through the early fifties, Disney shorts were no longer being rented as often in theaters. Nick Nichols remembered: "They couldn't get a delivery price. The last price I think they had was between $40,000 to $50,000 per show. When the shows got to costing more, around the $50,000 to $60,000 bracket, Roy said that was okay because they could make the money back in approximately three years. And he didn't mind it, because he figured they were still solvent. But when a picture got to be around $65,000, it was hard to recoup. So they just started to shut them off."[70]

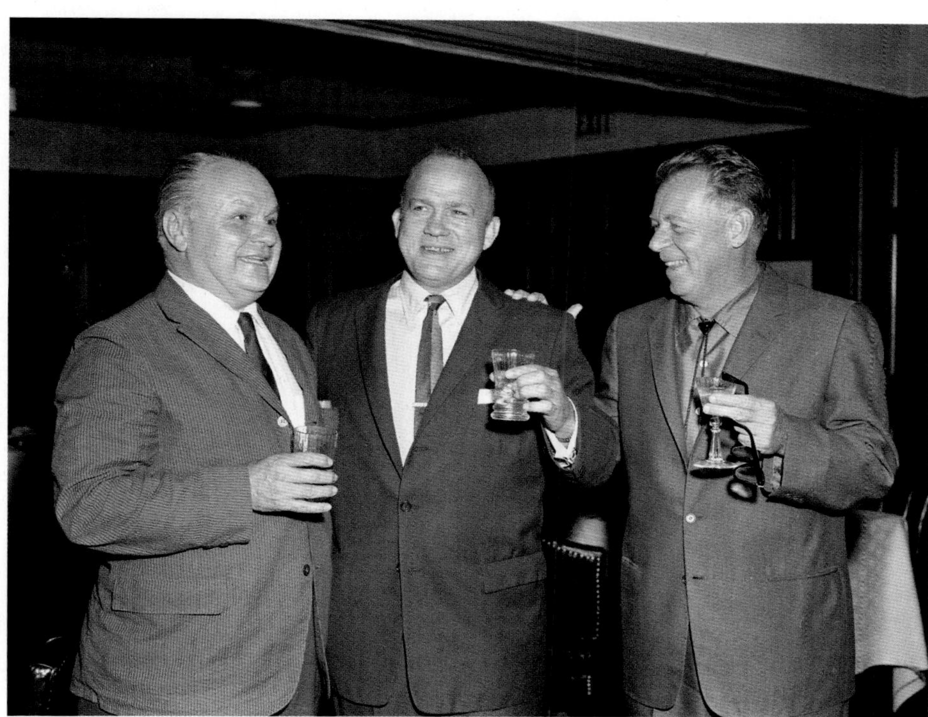

Geronimi (LEFT), Hannah, and Luske at Hannah's goodbye party in May 1959.

By 1956, Harry Tytle noted:

> Hannah was also told that when his contract ran out, there was no job for him at Disney's. He was encouraged to use that time to line up work at other animation studios. Later, returning from vacation on Monday, September 10, 1956, Bill Anderson told me that there were strong indications that Walt was going to release Jack Kinney. He was ultimately correct, though this didn't take place until a year later.

Kinney had run afoul of Walt, both for his gags-forward shorts and for forcing Walt into giving him a raise. Tytle noted on September 4, 1957:

> Kinney had . . . put Walt under pressure. This, I believe, was the time Kinney had an offer from M.G.M. . . . This had upset Walt and he has never forgotten it. In fact, he brought it up this time and said he felt no grief [about letting Kinney go] whatsoever. He felt Kinney had played a dirty trick on the studio and added terrific responsibility to him personally.[71]

After leaving Disney, Kinney directed *1,001 Arabian Nights* starring Mr. Magoo for UPA, and produced and directed more than a hundred Popeye shorts for King Features and dozens of TV shows, documentaries, pilots, training films, and commercials for his own company, Jack Kinney Productions. He was honored with a Winsor McCay Award in 1984, and died at age eighty-two on February 4, 1992, in Los Angeles' Tujunga section of town.

Occasional shorts would continue to be made throughout Disney's life, but only under special circumstances. In some ways, this would result in better work: films like *Noah's Ark* (dir. Bill Justice, 1959), *Goliath II* (dir. Woolie Reitherman, 1960), and *It's Tough to Be a Bird* (dir. Ward Kimball, 1969) are stronger, more distinctive, and interesting. But gone were the days of committed permanent shorts units at Disney's.

From here on, the feature films would carry animation forward. But with live action, television, and theme parks all vying for Walt's attention, for how long would that be?

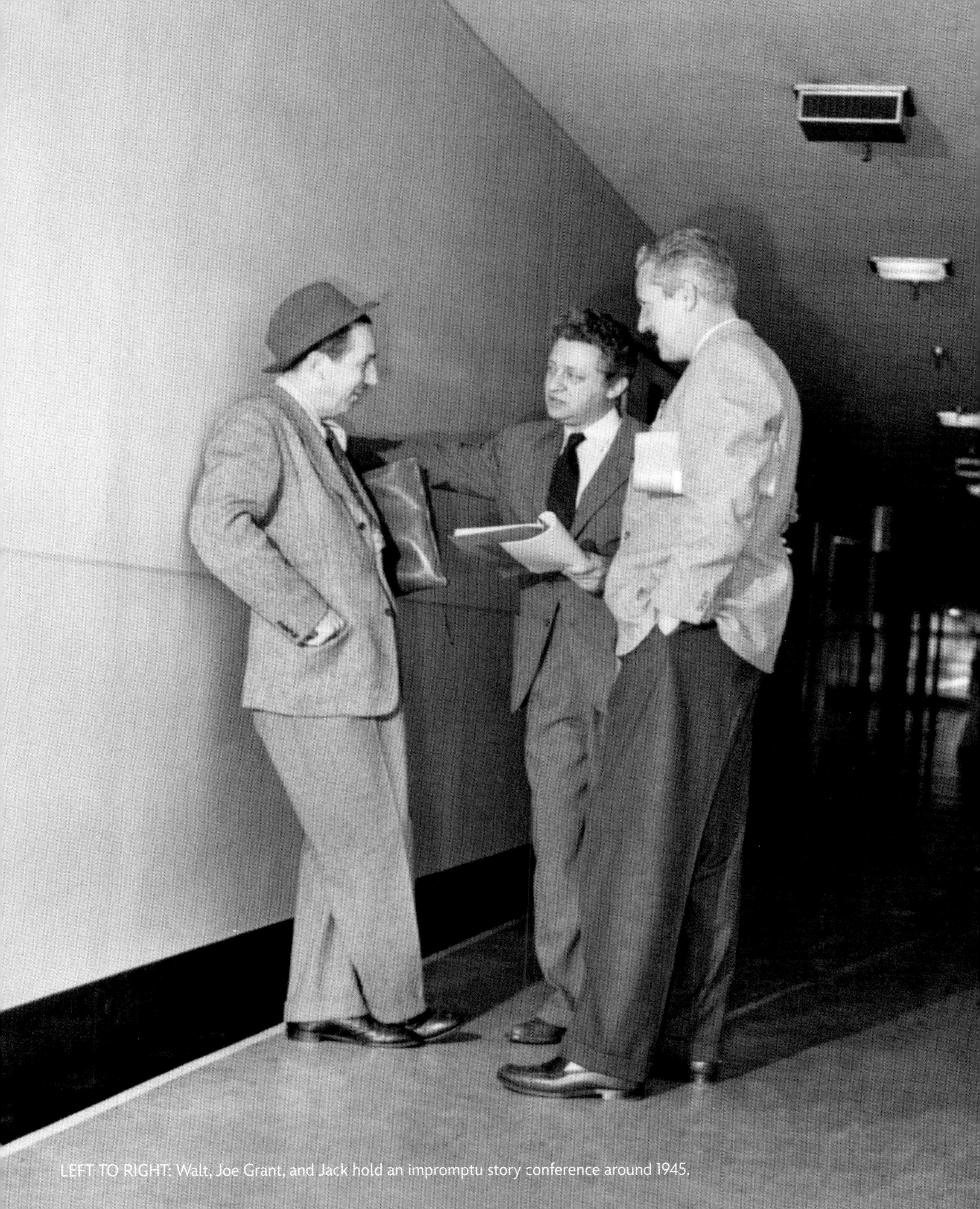

LEFT TO RIGHT: Walt, Joe Grant, and Jack hold an impromptu story conference around 1945.

PART 6

“NO REPLACEMENT FOR WALT”

1962–1973

1962–
1973

DIRECTING FEATURES

with Less Input from Walt

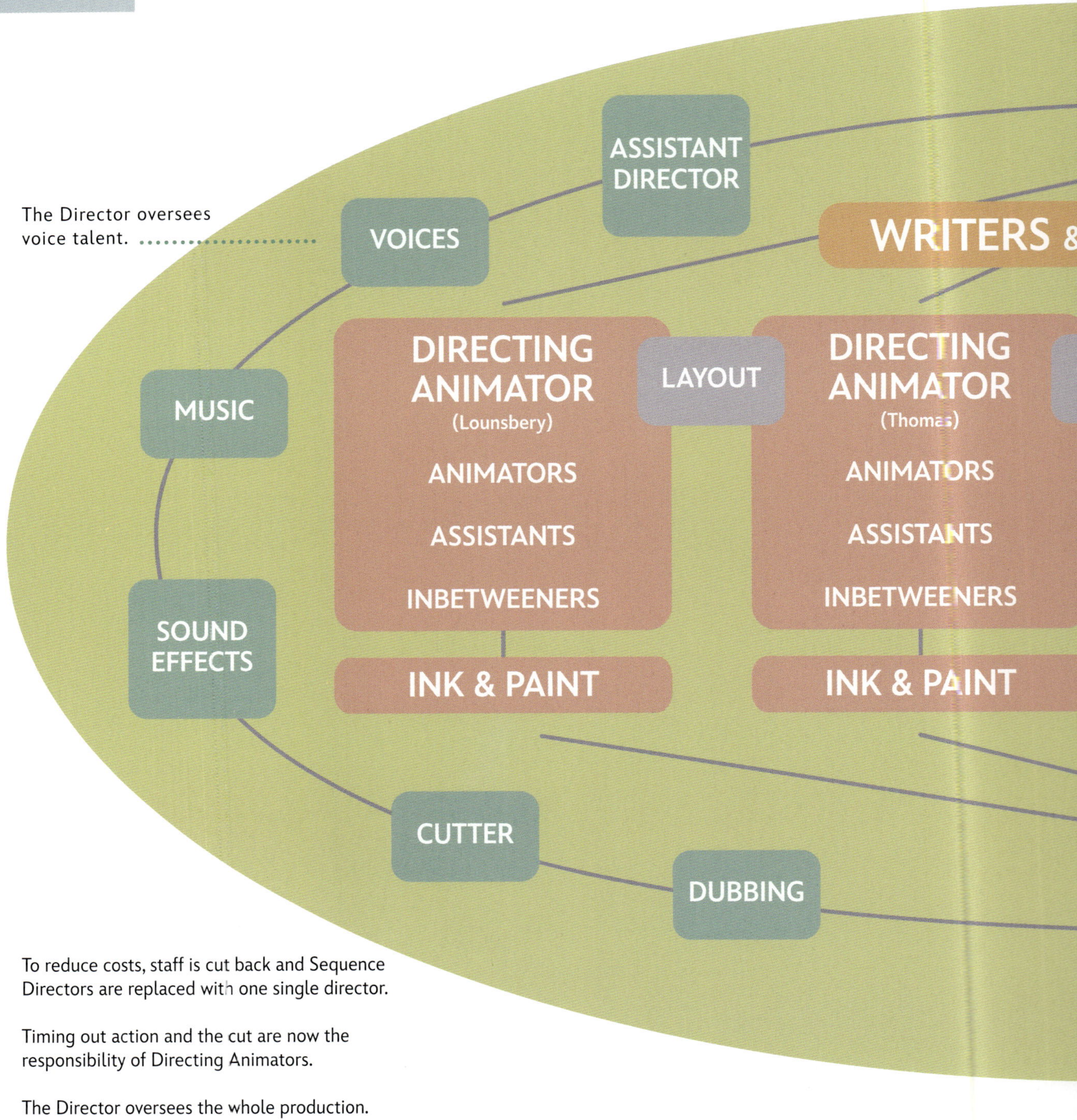

To reduce costs, staff is cut back and Sequence Directors are replaced with one single director.

Timing out action and the cut are now the responsibility of Directing Animators.

The Director oversees the whole production.

Output: one feature approximately every three years

WALT

Now occupied with bicoastal theme park projects, as well as live-action films and television, Walt still selects material and is involved in story development when possible, but the Director largely leads the effort once an idea is selected.

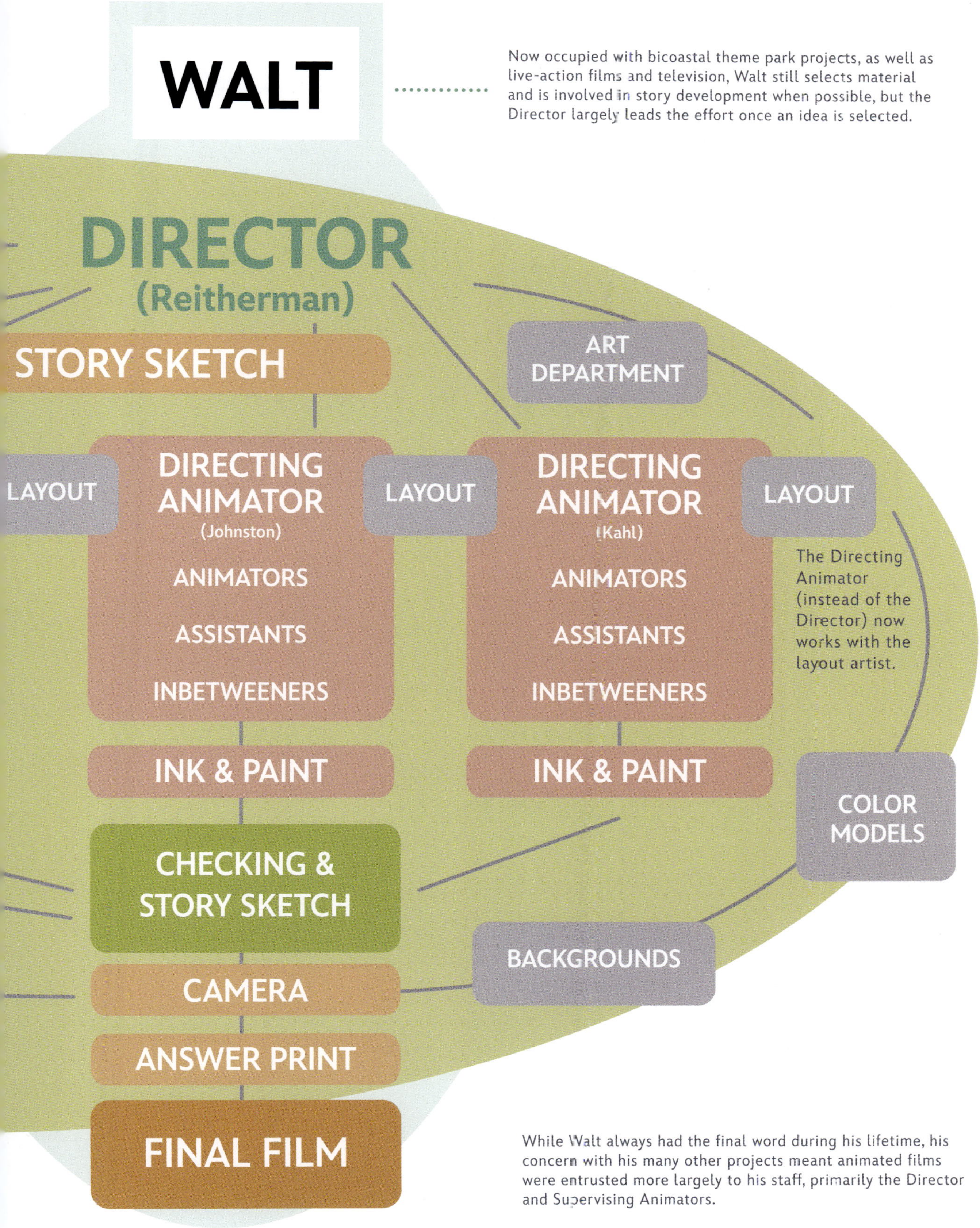

DIRECTOR
(Reitherman)

STORY SKETCH

ART DEPARTMENT

LAYOUT

DIRECTING ANIMATOR
(Johnston)
ANIMATORS
ASSISTANTS
INBETWEENERS

LAYOUT

DIRECTING ANIMATOR
(Kahl)
ANIMATORS
ASSISTANTS
INBETWEENERS

LAYOUT

The Directing Animator (instead of the Director) now works with the layout artist.

INK & PAINT

INK & PAINT

COLOR MODELS

CHECKING & STORY SKETCH

BACKGROUNDS

CAMERA

ANSWER PRINT

FINAL FILM

While Walt always had the final word during his lifetime, his concern with his many other projects meant animated films were entrusted more largely to his staff, primarily the Director and Supervising Animators.

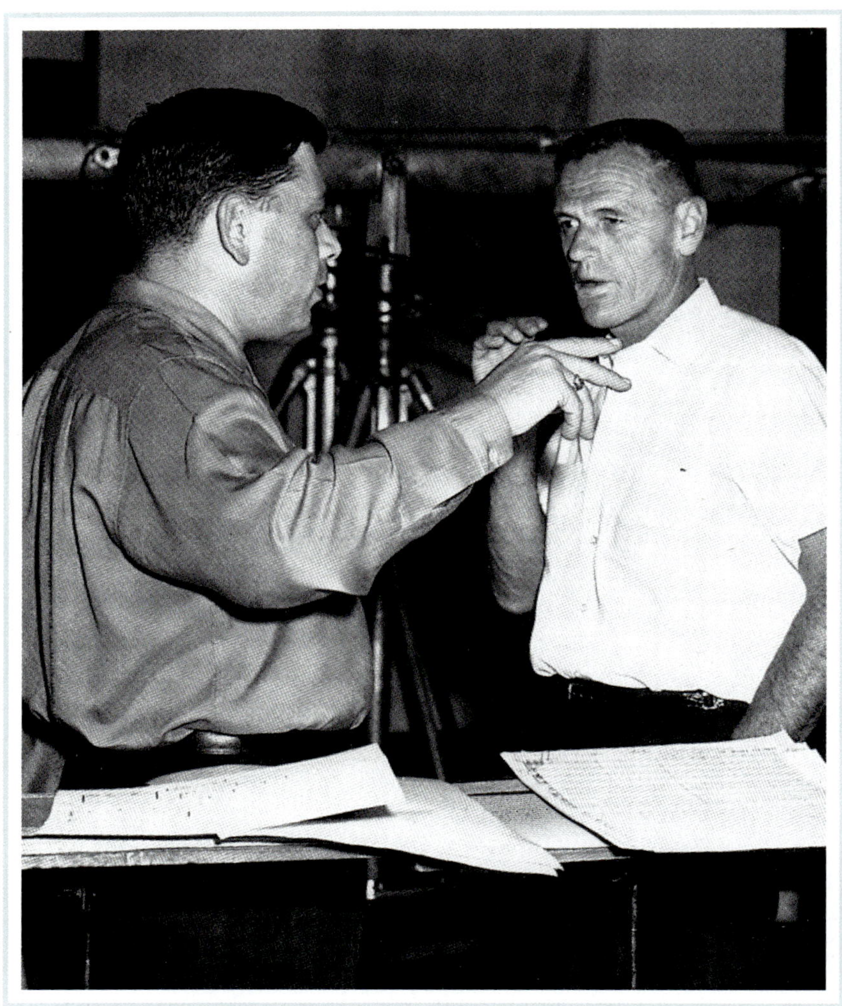

Woolie (right) and Robert Sherman discuss music for *The Jungle Book* (1967).

CHAPTER 9

WOOLIE REITHERMAN—IN THE DIRECTOR'S COCKPIT

"This was so intuitive about Walt: he could put his fingers on the total theme of a picture in a story so quickly. I know it influenced me all the way through *The Jungle Book*, to go for the personalities and not get a complicated story. And then, again this guy left so many roots in all of us; all of the pictures I did since then, I went for personality, strong characterization, strong voices that fit the character. It did make the pictures ever so much simpler to construct."[1]

—Woolie Reitherman

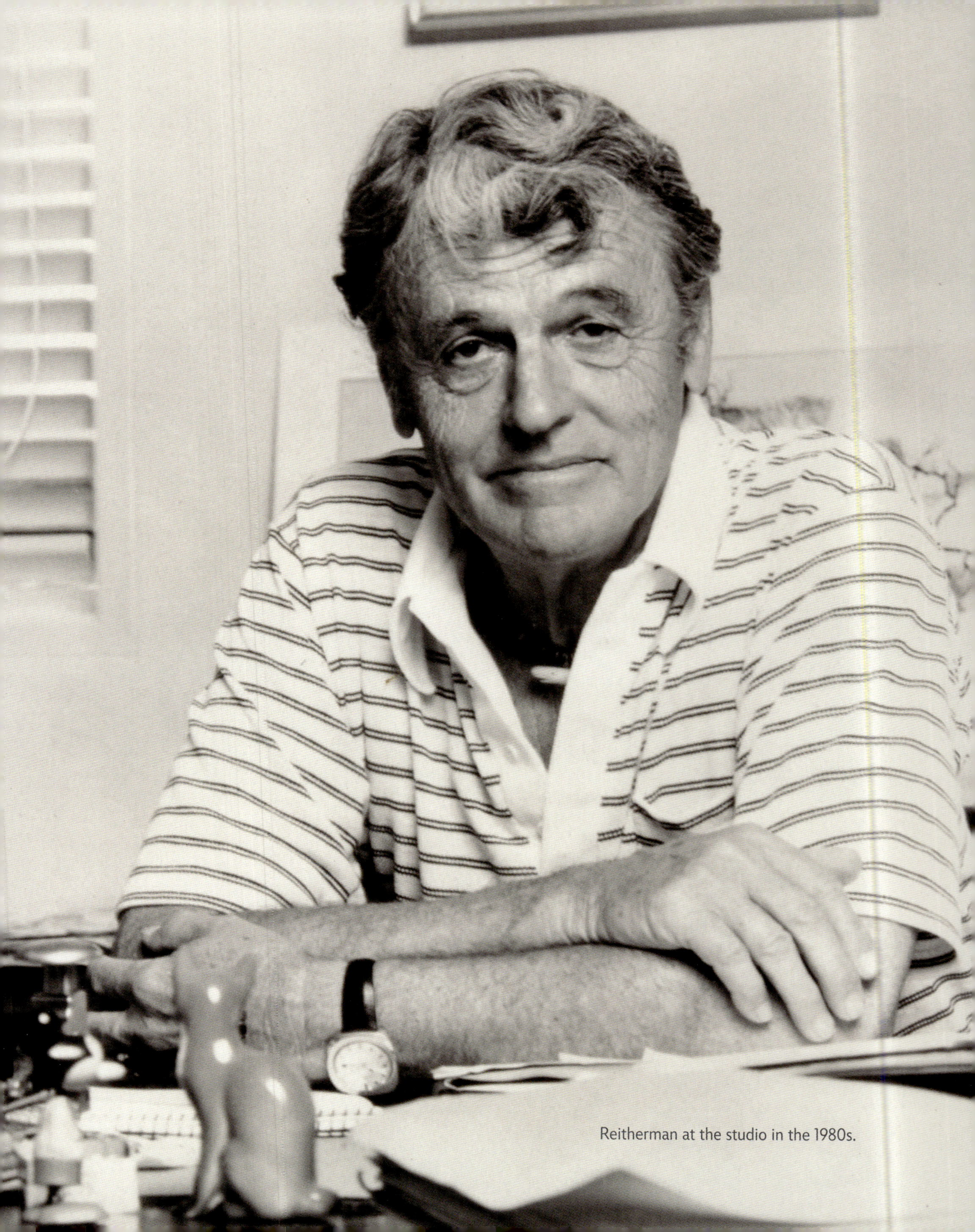

Reitherman at the studio in the 1980s.

ANIMATION ON THE BRINK

The year 1959 was pivotal for the films of Walt Disney. After eight years in production, with multiple directors, a seventy-millimeter format, story rewrites, conflicts over the film's styling, and delays due to the creation of Disneyland—the theme park and the television series—*Sleeping Beauty*, conceived as Walt's animation magnum opus, produced at a record-breaking cost of $6 million, premiered in January. It received mixed reviews on its initial run and would earn only $5.3 million back at the box office, despite reserved-seat pricing.[2] In subsequent releases, the film would fare better with both critics and audiences, but this was its fate in 1959. That same year, Walt released a contemporary live-action comedy, *The Shaggy Dog*, at a production cost of less than $1 million, and it earned back $9 million, exceeding profits for same-year releases *Some Like It Hot* and *North by Northwest*. Only Academy Award–winning Best Picture *Ben-Hur* topped it.[3]

Walt could easily have abandoned animation at this point. He was heavily focused on live-action films, with fifteen live-action films released preceding *The Shaggy Dog* and over forty more to come during the remaining seven years of his life.[4] Indeed, with the success of *Old Yeller* a couple of years earlier, Walt could see the handwriting on the wall. But he kept the animation unit intact, albeit with tighter budgets, to try to placate his financial advisers. As Marc Davis recalled to author Charles Solomon, "The attitude of the business people was, 'it takes too damned long to do these features, they cost too much, we think you shouldn't do any more.' Walt was about ready to dump animation, then he got to thinking, 'I owe these people something'—which he did. So he said, 'Hell, these guys know how to make the films without much input from me,' so Walt convinced the business people that it wasn't fair to do this to the guys."[5]

One Hundred and One Dalmatians kept the three-director structure intact, with the exception that animator Woolie Reitherman replaced the retiring Wilfred Jackson, joining veteran directors Ham Luske and Gerry Geronimi. Cost savings included the widespread use of the Xerox method for transferring animation drawings directly to cells to help with the overwhelming challenge of animating Dalmatians with their multiple spots. Though Walt objected to the graphic, linear look of the film's design, it was very successful and seemed to secure the continuation of Disney animated features.

On the next feature, *The Sword in the Stone*, the cadre of long-term directors had either retired or been moved to television productions. Woolie Reitherman took the reins as the sole director on that film. Speculation runs rampant about why Woolie was singled out—from "he would not cause trouble" to "he had the sensibility of the all-American kid"—but for whatever reason, Walt, busier than ever with television, live-action films, and Disneyland, entrusted this film to Woolie. He always liked Woolie and may have felt that with his everyman sensibility, his military background, and his "never say die" dedication

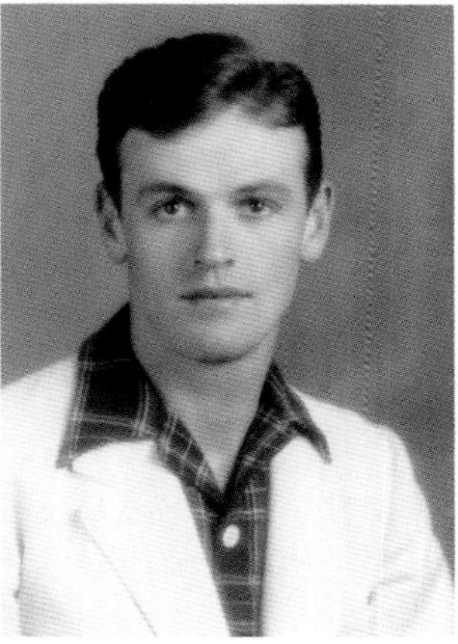

A young Woolie. Reitherman Family Collection.

to animation, he would be a good director. In an ironic turn, Ken Peterson in a 1954 memo to Walt suggested that Woolie "could operate as a Director-Animator for a small TV unit with a small compact unit. Draws well and has a reputation for developing good assistants."[6]

THE MELTING POT

Like Gerry Geronimi, Wolfgang "Woolie" Reitherman was born in Europe, in his case, in Munich, Germany, June 26, 1909, to Philip and Maria Reitherman. The youngest of seven children, Woolie had an adventurous childhood with his older brother, Alfred, as the family migrated to and settled in the Southern California city of Sierra Madre. When Woolie was sixteen, he and Alfred built an airplane in their backyard. Woolie's son Dick said his father's legacy on life and risk-taking can be summed up as: "You learn or intuit what's safe and what can kill you and then stay away from both."[7]

Woolie said he learned by watching, a quality that would serve him well not only in flying an airplane but in learning to animate and, later,

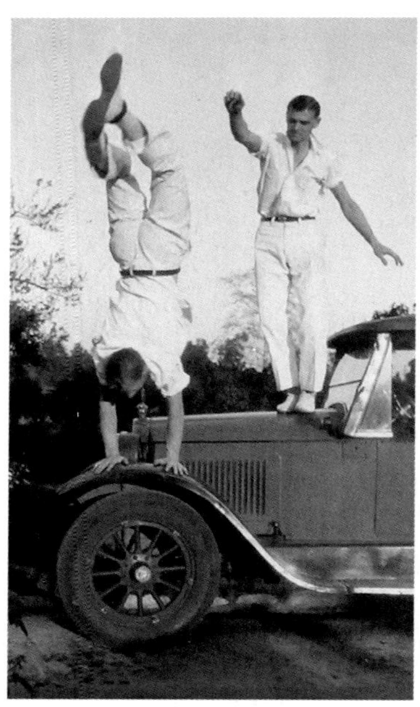

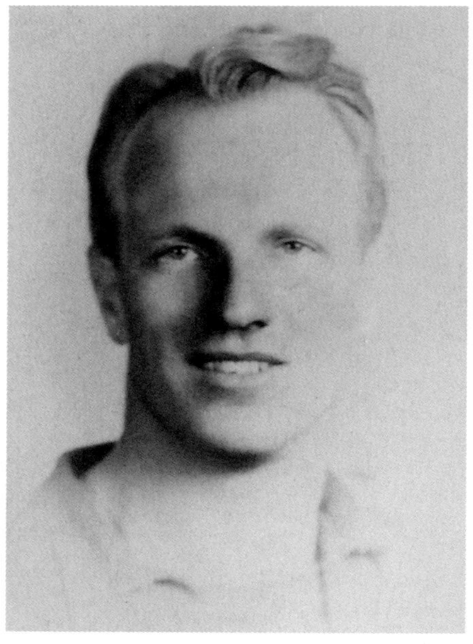

LEFT: Alfred (ON THE LEFT, DOING HANDSTAND) and Woolie in 1930. RIGHT: Brother Alfred. Woolie and Alfred were especially close, and Alfred's death in a test flight during World War II was devastating news to Woolie, who was flying for the military out of China. In a letter to Woolie, Walt said: "Knowing the strong ties that bind your family together, I realize what a blow it is to you. Your sister was, of course, greatly disturbed over Al's passing and, I think, equally disturbed over your reaction to the news. Expressions of regret and sorrow are futile things at a time like this and I know, from my own experience that time alone can heal such scars."[8]

to direct. Flying had become a passion for the Reitherman boys, and for Woolie, so did art. And that began with his teachers. "I was in art school, because somewhere back there in high school, I guess every guy has a teacher somewhere, I've had three or four teachers that have meant a lot to me. They give you a shot in the arm about something, about a talent or whatever. She had told me that I had some kind of a talent. I took freehand drawing on a snap and liked it. . . . The point is that there was a teacher back there. Behind every good man there is either a wife or good woman. There was a teacher back there."[9] Years later, Woolie's wife, Janie, said that Woolie had three great loves: flying, art, and family, and not necessarily in that order![10]

AIRPLANES OR ART?

Woolie zigzagged in career goals. Attending Pasadena Junior College, he planned to be an aircraft engineer. But then in 1931, he changed his mind and enrolled at Chouinard Art Institute. He was having a good deal of success with his watercolor art and was content to follow that path, when Phil Dike, an artist and Chouinard instructor, encouraged Woolie to apply to the Walt Disney Studio. Reluctant at first, Woolie eventually did come over for a one-week trial. Woolie recalled, "I really got turned on. That business of flipping those drawings and making them move and here I was fiddling around with one painting, trying to catch that moment of truth. I just felt I was God, making those damn things move around. Movement captured me, I suppose. . . . In an amateurish way, in an innocent way, I just felt it was the greatest thing that ever happened to art, to be able to move the goddamn stuff. Nobody else had done it. Michelangelo had laid on his back, but he never made it move. All that funny Cubist business didn't make any sense to me. Here it was, moving right in front of my very eyes. I was God back then."[11]

Woolie joined the Disney Studios on May 21, 1933, at age twenty-three. "I was still wet behind the ears. But I was fortunate. I didn't have to go through the inbetweening or the assistant thing. If I had gone that [traditional] route, I don't think I would have lasted long."[12] Woolie began animating on *Funny Little Bunnies* [directed by Jackson]. But early in his career, he came under the wing of Ben Sharpsteen, who remembered the neophyte animator: "I would say another outstanding character who learned in the earlier days before analytical animation was such a dominating factor was Woolie Reitherman. Woolie, from the very start, was a problem to me as I was sort of his teacher and adviser and even a director, because of the abruptness of the way he animated. I criticized him by labeling it

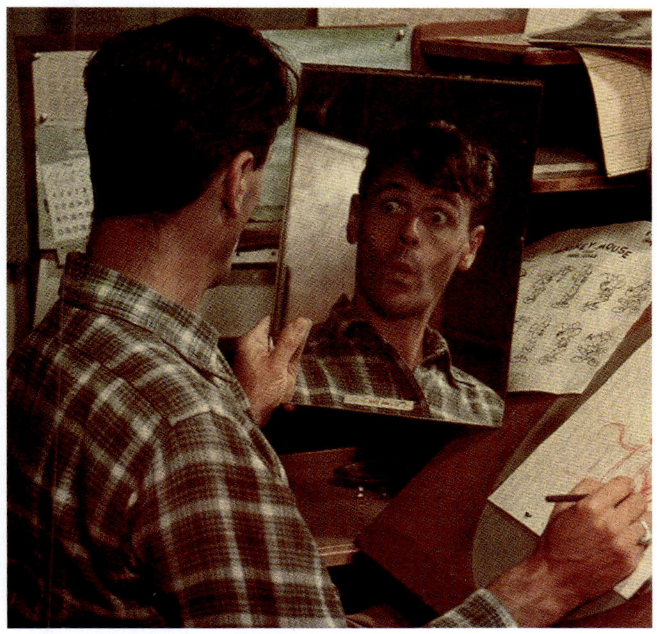

Woolie at his animation table at work on *Fun and Fancy Free*.

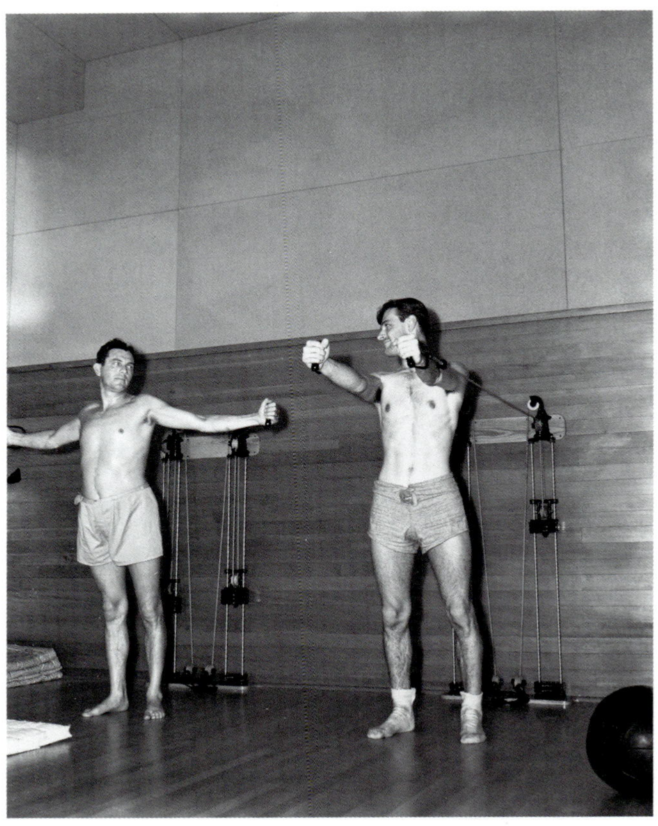

Woolie (LEFT) and Dave Hand keep fit at the new Burbank studio gym, the Penthouse Club, April 1940.

'stop-and-go animation.' There was really nothing too subtle about Woolie's work, but he did have a daring, a certain vitality in his work that gave his characters a certain plus. Walt recognized this in Woolie in early days and he was always a great champion for Woolie."[13]

Woolie animated on over twenty-five shorts before, during, and after the advent of the animated feature films, including such classics as *Two-Gun Mickey*, *The Band Concert*, *Music Land*, *Broken Toys*, *Elmer Elephant*, *Moving Day*, *Clock Cleaners*, *Goofy and Wilbur*, and many more featuring Goofy, a character Woolie excelled at. When Jack Kinney headed up a shorts unit, Woolie played an important role: "For my unit, I drew a Class A team from the studio talent pool: Ralph Wright, a keen story and gag man with a peculiar sense of humor that fit right in with the Goof's oddball antics; Lou Debney as my assistant director; and Woolie Reitherman and John Sibley as my lead animators. All told, we made up a competitive, on-the-ball team that was perfect for turning out shorts of the kind I had planned for Goofy."[14]

Woolie felt that the role of personality was so important to being successful as an animator. At a talk he gave at his alma mater, Chouinard, on April 28, 1937 (Disney-Chouinard Lecture Series), he said: "Try to express your personality in those sketches. . . . I think, especially in the cartoon business, that the thing that makes one person interesting and another dull, the thing that makes you like to talk to one and be bored with another, is personality. If you can get personality into your drawing, you have gone

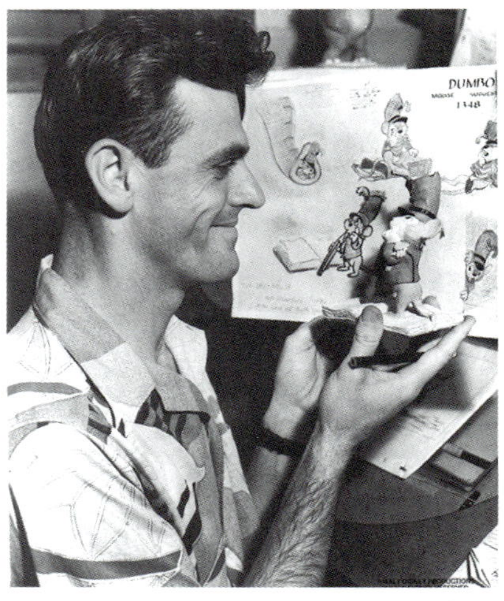

Woolie, along with veteran Fred Moore, animated Timothy Mouse on *Dumbo*.

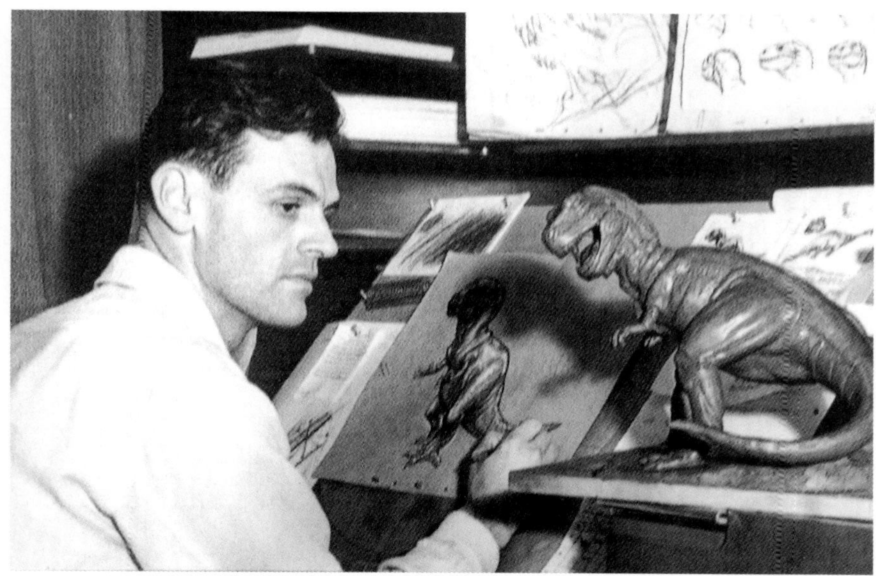

Woolie animating for the "Rite of Spring" segment of *Fantasia.*

a long way toward presenting good entertainment, because that is what people want—they don't want a drab, dull thing." An interesting point coming from an animator best known for broad humor and action scenes.

Ollie Johnston said that "Woolie was always convincing, but it was never through personality, it was just through action—very convincing, solid, believable action, but generally without personality, more with great humor and funny timing."[15] As with his career as a pilot, Woolie seemed most entranced with action and movement.

Woolie was well-known for being tenacious and working and reworking his animation until he achieved what he was seeking. His son Bruce said, "You've heard the stories about his animation. There [are] pieces of animation paper where he's erased right through the paper and had to tape something on. He wouldn't quit. And it seems to me that he, probably compared to some of those other guys, who are Leonardo-esque geniuses when it comes to handling a pencil, may not have had that kind of talent, but he got there in the end."[16]

As an animator, Woolie is best remembered for his action scenes: the escape from Monstro the whale in *Pinocchio*, the battle of the dinosaurs in *Fantasia*, Ichabod Crane's chase by the Headless Horseman in "The Legend of Sleepy Hollow" segment of *The Adventures of Ichabod and Mr. Toad*, and Prince Phillip's battle with

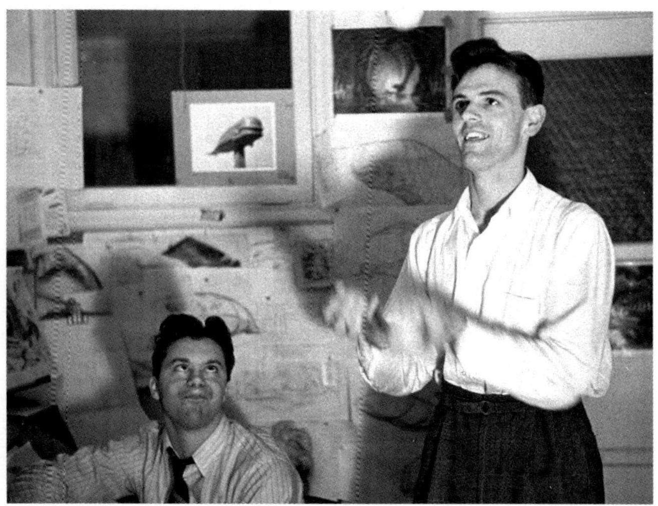

Woolie juggles his duties as an animator on *Pinocchio*.

Maleficent the dragon in *Sleeping Beauty*. These scenes fit an aspect of Woolie's character. He described himself once as "full of life and ginger." He expanded on this: "I am basically action oriented, and I like to get to the extreme of things. I kind of like danger. It's a thrill. I think it's something that everyone should experience once in a while to wake themselves up."[17]

WAR COMES TO AMERICA

When World War II beckoned, Woolie returned to his earlier love of flying and joined the Army Air Forces pilots who flew the treacherous route from India to China known as the Hump. Woolie downplayed the danger he and his crew faced in letters to the studio and friends, but he was on a very perilous mission: "The pilots had no choice but to navigate turbulent weather over the highest mountains in the world—for distances of a thousand miles or more round-trip—in primitive, often overloaded aircraft such as the C-46, nicknamed the "Flying Coffin." Flying over such inhospitable terrain, Hump pilots faced the highest fatality rate of any air mission in World War II. They wore oxygen masks nearly continuously, flying at altitudes of up to twenty-five thousand feet in non-pressurized Depression-era planes."[18]

Due to his preference for action animation and his size and lumbering manner of walking, Woolie projected a kind of John Wayne image at the studio. And later as a director, he often avoided emotionally sensitive story sequences. But he did display a more sensitive side in letters home during World War II when he was seeing action. In a letter begun on June 1 (no year cited) to Wilfred Jackson's wife, Jane, Woolie describes flying and the emotions he feels: "motors droning on and on—your 'insides' free and boundless somehow—master of yourself and all the world—moving, moving, endless on and on." On June 2, he describes a flight: "The clouds heavy and pregnant—lay dark and full just off my wing tip—close—so close and touchable. And a sharp bolt of lightning drove from within it. Golly Jane it was sumpin'!!! Of a sudden a quick bond of understanding—for one fine moment we were brothers—we were scared. Swatting flies within the cockpit—keeping tally of our score—fine thing for us to be doing within this hailstorm—well anyhow it kept us from being scared. Rain driving at us—battering. Over the hill and between the clouds like some great archway—below a rainbow halo following the contour of the hills. The letdown—fine—precisely flown—my own 'super duper'—sure—so sure—grayness parting, drifting by—windshield wiper slapping back and forth—greenness—glimpses now of greenness in the rain—and presto! Whadaya know! Right smack in front of me—Yep you guessed it—The Runway! And all I gotta do is 'chop the power' and we're rolling on the runway!!! Makes a guy feel pretty swell, Jane."

After he described the scenery and the feeling of returning to a welcoming place, he continued: "Walking across the field a great peace came over me—a great peace and a great love. Rain on my upturned face and love in my heart—could anything be richer. Riding along in a jeep, talking with the sergeant driving—talking of his home and children. Talking and watching his face—his character—his feelings. Feeling for him and how he felt. It was like painting a portrait with an exquisite background of purple hills and billowing clouds—only moving, moving—and so very much alive!" He ended this part of the letter contrasting how he felt, full of life and love, with an elderly Chinese woman he saw walking along the road, feet bound and eyes quite dull, with no sign of interest in them. In what may seem typical of

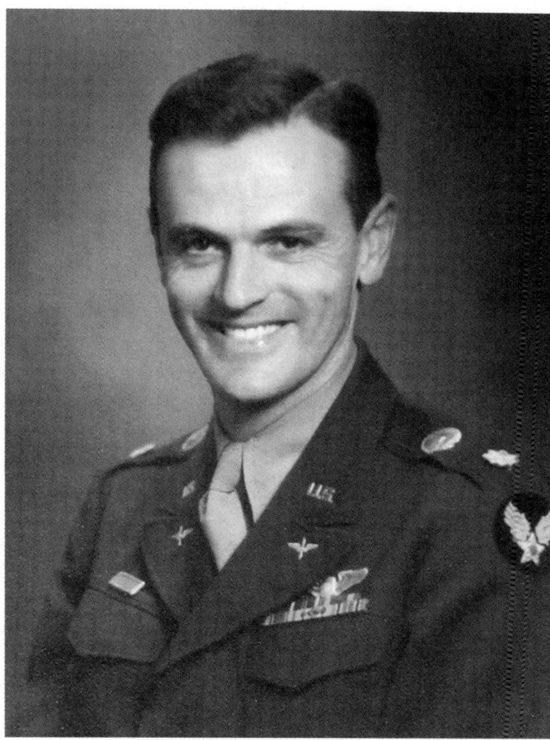

Woolie in the service during World War II.

Woolie to draw back from sharing his feelings, the next section is dated "October 15, '45," and he said he had just found this half-written letter "written long ago, and never finished. On re-reading it it sounds somewhat 'sissy' like but I suppose what's written is written and so I'm sending it on."

In a letter to Walt dated February 20, 1945, Woolie thanked Walt for "a whale of a recommendation" he must have given because Woolie was made deputy wing commander for China. He described in detail a landing without the usual aids, but relying on the "Woolie Vertical System of Letdown" (which one of his sons thinks meant a steep vertical descent rather than a gradual descent). Woolie told Walt, "I feel a tremendous growth taking place within me—being exposed to all the world 'round about me." He talked about seeing a little Chinese child crying, standing by a gutter as people passed by, and he wrote a poem about this scene:

There by the curb in the shadow
There by the curb in the dirt
A child small ragged and crying
Lost from its Mother's long skirt.

Stood by the curb there crying
As all of China went by
Moving, moving, unheeding
Until the day they die.

Rickshaws and harlots and merchants
Shuffling endlessly on
All of China moving and moving
Timeless and ageless and long.

His little bare fanny showing
Barely as high as the curb
The child so small and puny
The seed for a better world

From the child so small and fragile
A sobbing smile at last
Seemed to throw off the weight of China
And the ponderous weight of the past.

Like a rare jewel pure and sparkling
A spirit not yet soiled
A something small and growing
An innocence unspoiled

There by the curb in the sunlight
For one moment so fleeting and fast
A child held the whole weight of China
And the ponderous weight of the past.

Woolie concluded with, "Who would have thought I'd end up writing poetry—beats the hell outa me—Walt! That's what flying an airplane'll do to ya!" He ended the letter with his best regards to his friends at the studio.

Years later, he commented: "Man, what a way to open up your life flying was. I thought, thank goodness I wasn't back at the studio."[19] In fact, Woolie's experience as a pilot would later affect his approach as a director. During World War II, planes didn't have radar, and to find a small island in the middle of the Pacific depended on the skill of the navigator. Woolie was piloting a crew of six in a B-24 bomber, equipped with just enough fuel to get from the mainland to the island. But after thirty to forty-five minutes past when they were due to land, there was still no island in sight. With only an hour's fuel left, Woolie spoke to the navigator, who was bewildered and starting to panic. They were lost in the middle of the Pacific. How would they find land? Woolie knew that when lost, you never fly in circles. As his son Dick recalled, "You commit yourself to one or two trajectories and you GO. If you have enough fuel, you get two

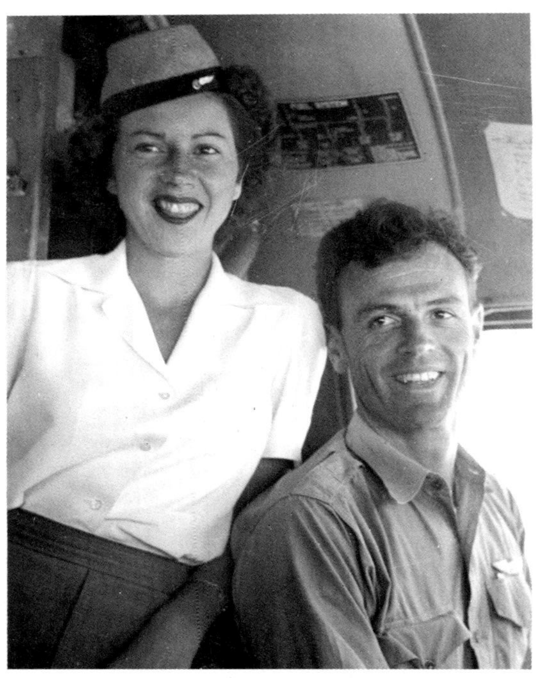

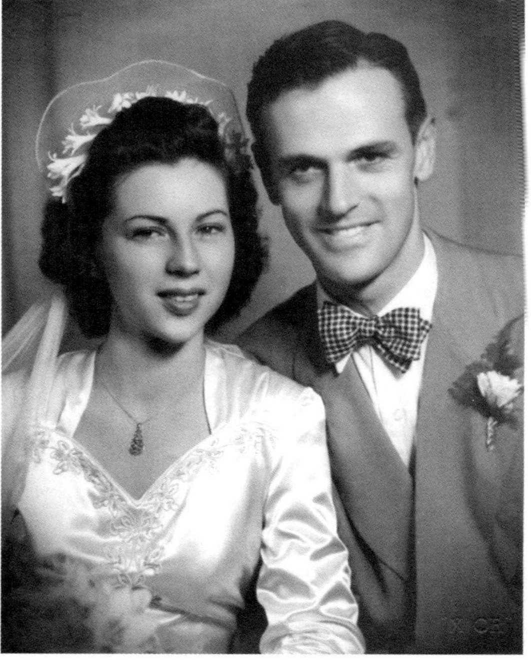

Janie and Woolie in postwar Philippines. Reitherman Family Collection.

shots. If not, you have one. You make your best choice." Woolie assessed the situation the best he could, and made a decision. With the fuel gauge on empty, Woolie made it to the island.[20]

After the war, Woolie flew commercial planes in the Philippines for a while; met his future wife, Janie McMillan; married; and returned to the United States before the birth of Dick, the first of their three sons.

Woolie's love of airplanes would have changed Disney history were it not for Walt's powers of persuasion. After the war, Woolie and Janie had decided to start up an airline company back in the Philippines. As Janie read a book under a tree, Woolie stopped by the studio to say good-bye. After two hours, recounted Woolie's son Bruce, Walt walked out to talk with her. "Woolie and I have had a long talk," Walt told her, "and the only thing preventing Woolie from coming to work back here again is how you might feel about it. So what do you think?"[21] Talk about pressure!

The couple decided to stay. But Woolie always felt that his break from the studio was important so he could remain enthusiastic and committed to his work there.

DIRECTING

Woolie's strong animation performances made him one of Walt Disney's Nine Old Men, Walt's humorous tag for a group of his top animators. As with the others, his responsibilities grew as he and the Disney films matured. He became a directing animator on *Pinocchio*, *Dumbo*, *Fun and Fancy Free*, *The Adventures of Ichabod and Mr. Toad*, *Cinderella*, *Alice in Wonderland*, *Peter Pan*, and *Lady and the Tramp*. (He was a supervising animator on *Fantasia*.) Woolie became a sequence director on *Sleeping Beauty* and

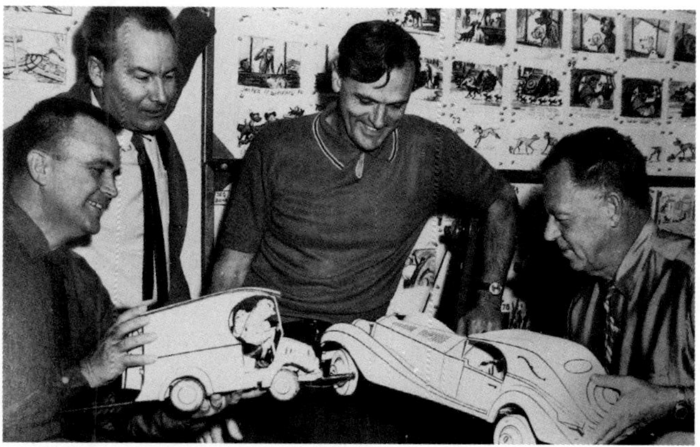

LEFT TO RIGHT: Ken Anderson, Bill Peet, and directors Reitherman and Ham Luske at work on *One Hundred and One Dalmatians*.

continued as a director on *One Hundred and One Dalmatians*. This fit well for Woolie and kept him engaged with his work. "I don't think I would be very happy at the studio there had I not had this respite [military service] and had I not gone on into direction and had a broader scope to what I was doing, than to have animated all of the time."[22] His directing included the memorable "Twilight Bark" sequence in the film.

For *The Sword in the Stone*, Woolie was given the reins as the solo director. Studio publicity ballyhooed this assignment as a first in studio history, which was not accurate; Dave Hand and Ben Sharpsteen had been in that role in earlier animated features. And while those two had sequence directors as well, the position of the directing animator had grown over the years. "By the time we got to *Sword in the Stone*," animator Ollie Johnston said, "as directing animators, we were really directors."[23] They had more control in their sequences over characterization and staging. Even with Woolie at the helm and with a team of top animators, the film was not popular with critics or with audiences. Woolie explained: "I don't think the story was ever right. You didn't feel the right thing for the boy, Wart. . . . We didn't have the sequence where you develop real sympathy for that kid. Surely, they popped up the morale a little bit, but that isn't like when little *Dumbo* goes to see his mother, you know what I mean? You need that warmth in something. Even in the end, when he holds [pulls] out that sword, which I think was a beautiful little sequence, but that wasn't enough to really make you feel something for that kid."[24] Walt was paying less day-to-day attention to the animated films, believing that he could turn more and more over to his artists who had been with him for so many years, and his distractions may have been a factor in the final product.

However, the next film with Woolie as a solo director, *The Jungle Book*, was a major hit for the studio. Even with a generous budget, Walt impressed on Woolie the need to keep down costs, a lesson that Woolie would practice for the rest of his tenure as a director and later as a producer-director on animated feature films. *The Jungle Book* set the stage for Woolie's reign as the director for animated features, especially in the wake of Walt's passing. "Of course, when you talk about *Jungle Book*, you gotta talk about Walt. He checked out about halfway through the picture. He's the one that took us out of—at that time *Jungle Book* was going to be precious, and a lot of Rudyard Kipling dialogue and so on. And he's the one, with his selection of Phil Harris, got us on a track of entertaining personalities which communicate with an audience. And the story came out as the most simple story we've ever done. A little guy that just wants to go back to the man village, and can't make it, everything's against him. This was so intuitive about Walt: he could put his fingers on the total theme of a picture in a story so quickly. I know it influenced me all the way through *Jungle Book*, to go for the personalities and not get a complicated story. And then again this guy left so many roots in all of us; all of the pictures I did since then, I went for personality, strong characterization, strong voices that fit the character. It did make the pictures ever so much simpler to construct."[25]

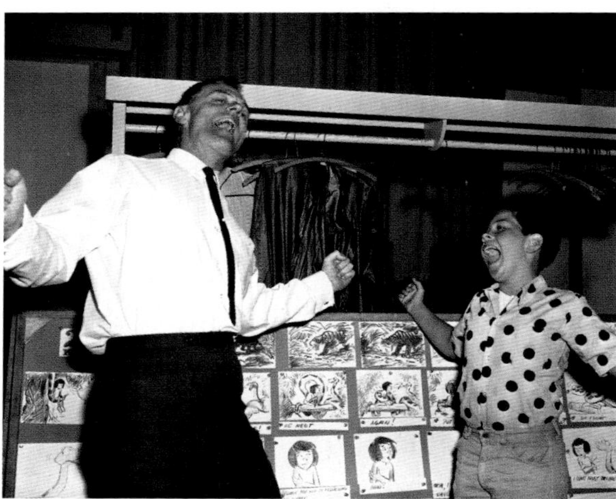

Woolie directing his son Bruce, who was the voice of Mowgli in *The Jungle Book*. Woolie's two older sons, Dick and Bob, provided voices for alternate takes for Rickie Swenson as Wart in *The Sword and the Stone*.

Bill Peet had written and storyboarded a version of *The Jungle Book* that was more faithful to Kipling's book, but was darker than Walt wanted. Before Peet and Walt had a falling out and Peet permanently left the studio, Woolie as the film's director attempted to soothe Peet's ego. In a January 20, 1964, memo, after Woolie met with Walt to discuss the conflicts, Woolie tactfully addressed some of the issues raised:

> Setting all personal feelings and opinions aside and looking objectively towards the common goal of putting good entertainment

on the screen, I feel there are three main problems to resolve:

1. Bagherra's voice and personality. [Peet wanted Howard Morris; Woolie and the animators preferred Sebastian Cabot]
2. Baloo's voice and the handling of the Baloo song.
3. The contribution the animators and the Music Room make to your story and their right to have a voice in these decisions. Remember you are not going to animate the picture. That is our problem and a tough one, too.

After agreeing to provide voice demos for Peet's choices and the choices of Woolie and the animators, Woolie went on to reassure Peet:

> I am sure an early resolution of the above will clear the air and get your story into animation. It might be well to reflect that a cartoon feature represents two years of arduous effort on every one's [sic] part and we'll never put a "fun" picture on the screen if we don't all have "fun" and enthusiasm while we are making it.

The Jungle Book received mostly positive reviews from critics, although at least one saw this and future Reitherman films as a mixed bag: "The Disney features have striven to be amiable and amusing, and little more. In their voices, they are clearly a product of the television age, and they have been consistently successful with a young audience nurtured on TV programs."[26]

WORKING WITHOUT WALT

Walt's passing, sudden and unexpected, not only was a tremendous loss to each individual who knew him and worked with him but also created uncertainty for the future of the company. Roy O. Disney—Walt's brother—took command of the studio and kept it on a steady course, with perhaps his greatest achievement being the development and opening of Walt's last dream, Walt Disney World, just prior to Roy's passing. But according to then vice president Bill Anderson, Roy asked him to shutter the animation unit after the completion of *The Jungle Book*. Anderson did not follow Roy's perhaps hasty and emotion-laden judgment, and the unit stayed on, although with gradually fewer and fewer members. Historian Jay Horan recalled that at the time of Walt's passing, Woolie said, in effect, "that from this day on it will never be like it was, but only as each person remembers it."[27]

WHY WOOLIE?

Woolie was chosen to carry on the Disney legacy as the solo director of Disney animated features. But why Woolie? Some have said that Walt called him to his hospital bed in his last days and "anointed" him to take over the animation unit. But that seems unlikely. Ron Miller doubted that that meeting ever happened, thinking it was more likely that Walt would have called in senior figures like Card Walker or Donn Tatum first, which he apparently did not do.[28] Woolie's son Bruce Reitherman said that even if that meeting had taken place, "what would Woolie have done with that? Get it engraved on a plaque for his desk? Even when Walt was part of the animation process, there were no magic keys or magic wand. The only way to really accomplish what, at times, must have seemed almost impossible was to get down and do the work as a team."[29] Frank Thomas, another of the Nine Old Men, had two versions of why and how Woolie was chosen. First, the ideal version: "When Walt died, we got together and voted, as I recall, [to] leave

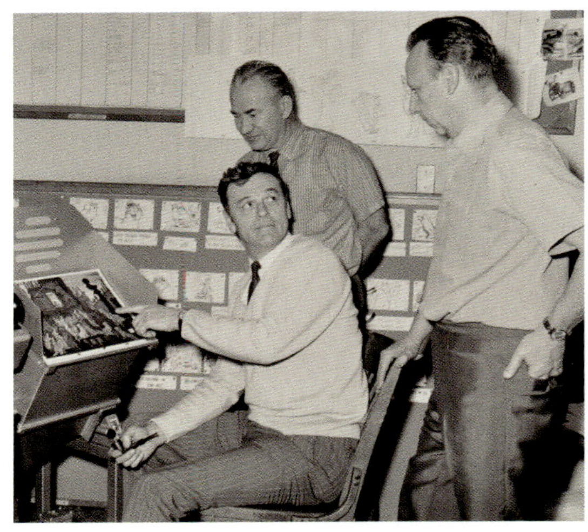

Woolie using the Moviola to make a point, working on *The Aristocats*, circa 1968. Basil Davidovich (LEFT) and Paul Satterfield look on.

things as they are. Woolie is the director, Don Griffith is the layout man, Larry Clemmons is story—that's all we had—and you and you and you and you will be animators, and we'll make the decisions as best we can. Woolie said, 'Golly, guys, I don't know whether I can do it.' We said, 'We'll help you.' He said, 'We're all going to be leaning against each other to stand up. Any one of us by ourselves would fall down. Let's try it and see if it works.'"[30] And then the more practical facts: "Energy and experience. He'd done a lot more different types of scenes." Thomas felt that Walt had already eliminated Ollie Johnston, Milt Kahl, John Lounsbery, and himself from the running as too valuable to animation, and Marc Davis had already moved to Imagineering. "Les [Clark] was off on his commercials. Eric [Larson] was teaching the trainee animators. Kimball was out of the question. So who do you have? I would have picked Woolie."[31]

Regardless of how or why Woolie was chosen, he knew that he was not the new Walt. "There was no replacement for Walt, and in my view the main thing was to keep this team together and keep the same creative juices flowing that they had with Walt."[32] He elaborated: "What you're really missing, of course, is that really, really creative leader. I mean that's what Walt had. You've got all the talent there today, but you don't have the showmanship and *feeling*. God, when old Walt would look at that screen, he was up there. You know what I mean? He expected that thing to bounce back and do something to him. And when it didn't do something to him, he was right every time. And the ordinary person just sits there and it moves alright, and it tells a story—you can't fault it on that—but that's the magic."[33]

Marc Davis once said: "If there is a change in the organization from Walt's time to now, it's this: There is nobody there who could make me feel as good by saying 'I like that' as Walt."[34] Woolie's son Bruce understood this sentiment

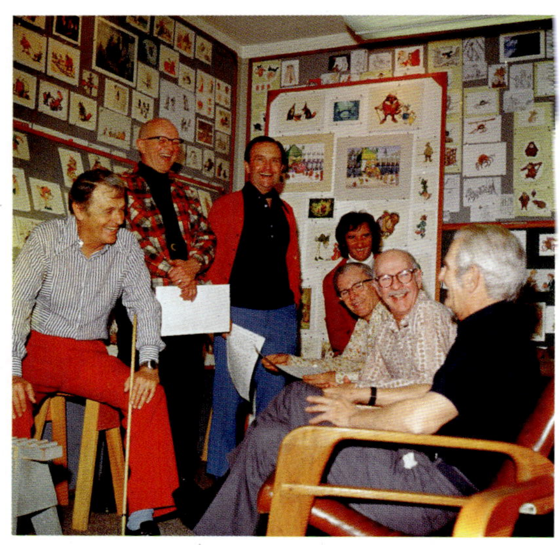

LEFT TO RIGHT: Woolie, Milt Kahl, Ken Anderson, Dave Michener, Frank Thomas, Ollie Johnston, and Larry Clemmons enjoy a lighter moment on *Robin Hood*.

"He was having to fill that vacuum somehow that Walt had left."[35] Other directors have come and gone in the ensuing fifty-plus years since Walt's passing, but Woolie was the first to helm an animated feature without Walt behind him.

DIRECTOR IN CHIEF

In addition to finishing *The Jungle Book*, Woolie faced many challenges, the biggest being to make the films on what seemed to be decreasing budgets in terms of real dollars and to hold the egocentric crew together. And he was elevated from among them, which carried its own burden. Animator Andreas Deja recalled that "Even Frank and Ollie would say, 'He was one of us for so many years, and now we work for him,' and there is a different dynamic all of a sudden, you know, you have to please him. And I think the one who was the most outspoken would be Milt, and tell Woolie that he thinks this is a bunch of crap, you know; he would say that."[36] In fact, Woolie's sons recall that the one event that seemed to upset their father the most from those years involved Milt. Kahl—who ran hot and cold over the years on his assessment of Woolie as a director—made some demands in a memo to Ron Miller that Woolie felt were unacceptable and would have created a rift between Milt and the others. Woolie's son Bruce said, "that was the only time he ever described where it was really hard, where he had to choose between my brother-in-arms and the family."[37] In the end, his demands unmet, Milt retired and, sadly for Woolie, refused to shake his hand at parting.

In the aftermath of Walt's passing, Woolie drew on his experiences in World War II for his leadership philosophy. "Sure sometimes I had to make a decision and stick with it. I guess I got this from the Air Force. Once you make up your mind, fly the flight plan out before you go for a whole bunch of ideas. And that, I think, had a centralizing effect, and a cohesive effect. I remember in World War II when I was flying, the main thing was to keep that airplane up in the air. That was my feeling that this great group of animators—really the best in the world—needed to stay airborne towards a new objective. We had to keep going, going onward and upward."[38]

In John Canemaker's book *Walt Disney's Nine Old Men*, Woolie described his overall approach to directorial leadership. Woolie said he attempted "to open up the communication so that the team was with you. There were maybe ten people who were very, very important to this. There were certain things in the story that you knew were going to happen, but you had to find out whether these animators could feel animation and situation possibilities to create good personalities. They had to get an enthusiasm. You had to respect and listen to everybody because we were all equals. The most important thing was the real cooperation of the four or five animators, and there were some story people that were tremendous, too. I didn't stir conflict, I tried to cool it if I could."

Walt once said that he never made films for children; they were for both adults and children alike. Stories of the frightened children's reactions to scenes in some of his films, beginning with the witch in *Snow White*, the boys turning to donkeys in *Pinocchio*, and Bambi's mother's death, testify to that concept. Woolie's films narrowed the scope. Andreas Deja, in his book *The Nine Old Men*, said: "The tone of the stories being told in Disney films by then were much milder than Walt's earlier achievements. But Woolie wanted to make films for families, and he became increasingly concerned about scaring children with terrifying villains. He stated around this time: 'If we lose the kids we lose everything.'"

THE ARISTOCATS—WOOLIE FLIES THE FLIGHT PLAN

With *The Jungle Book* now in the can, Roy O. was on the fence about continuing the unit. They needed a hit. As Woolie recalled, "This was survival as far as I was concerned and most of the animators were concerned. It was survival to keep this thing going, this thing called Walt Disney animation."[39] But they had an ally: "I think our biggest champion was [production manager] Bill Anderson. And he had worked with Walt a lot and he knew a lot about Walt's philosophy about making pictures, and he knew that you had to leave animators alone to see what they could come up with rather than pushing them around and saying you've got to do it for less money and all those things. Although money was a problem, and we did that picture for a very reasonable negative cost. From then on things went well. At least we were in business."[40] The result was *The Aristocats*, released in December 1970.

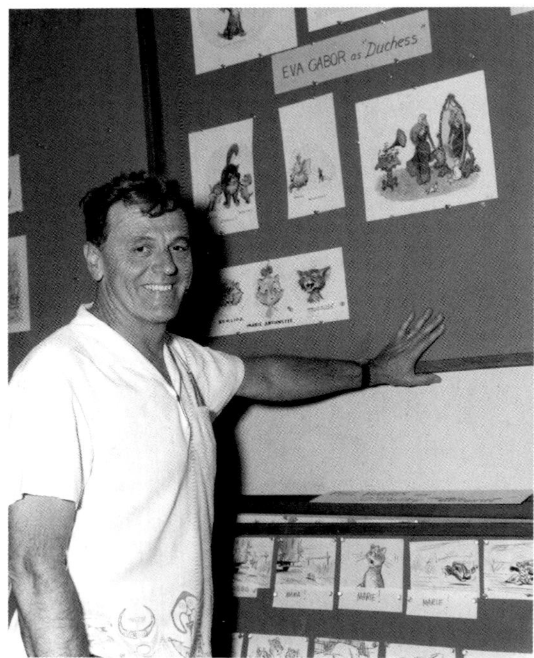

Woolie in position as director of *The Aristocats*, around 1969.

Woolie served as the director *and* producer of *The Aristocats*, *Robin Hood*, the Winnie the Pooh featurettes and feature, and *The Rescuers*, managing to keep feature animation in production and to span the gap between the 1960s and the 1980s, when animation had a resurgence—a huge achievement. Woolie, through good practices and bad, stretched and held the animation unit together, despite the burgeoning egos, tight budgets, reduced staffing, and ever-changing executive management team. His accomplishment cannot be overstated. Walt had focused less of his time and attention on animation in his last years, and with smaller scopes, fewer lavish visuals, and simpler story lines, the films reflected that. Whether Walt would have continued to withdraw his attention had he lived another decade or more is debatable, but his drive was still to produce the best product possible. Woolie, maybe for all the factors just mentioned, took a different tact, and one that Walt might have frowned upon. "When you make a film that is not as good as another, but they make the same money, then you are still in business, so let's not try to make it the most perfect film ever made in our lives, which is sort of what we did with Walt. With the costs going up, the next is going to cost even more than the previous, so you are kind of stuck to clean the costs and balancing it between making it good enough and as good as possible."[41]

In a remarkable overview of how features came together during his time, Woolie discussed the logistics, which were far afield from the departmentalized structure under Walt on the earlier features.

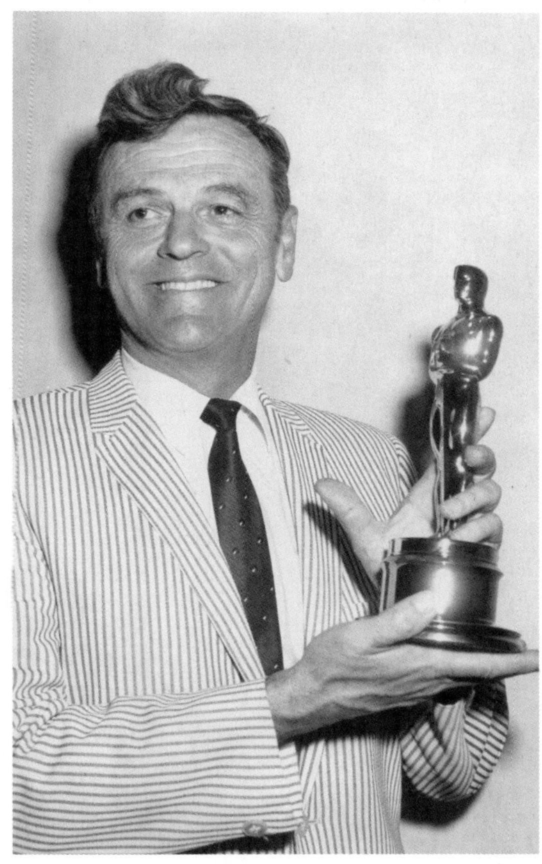

Woolie Reitherman accepting the Academy Award for *Winnie the Pooh and the Blustery Day* as the 1968 Best Short Subject (Cartoon). Woolie directed this featurette as well as *Winnie the Pooh and the Honey Tree*. John Lounsbery directed *Winnie the Pooh and Tigger Too*. Both are credited as directors for *The Many Adventures of Winnie the Pooh*.

> Ken [Anderson] will draw characters and situations that might be in there, and [story man] Larry Clemmons comes along and says, "We've got to have this kind of sequence in here," and he will start writing it. And then, I think that is another thing about the Disney approach: There is a great deal of shuffling and turmoil and flexibility about everything, in an organized way. You say, "For the time being that's pretty good." But you don't say that's great right away. As it develops, you bring in the animators. There are the guys who are going to be the actors, they've got to be with you or you are lost. They begin to have ideas because that's their speciality. And pretty soon you will say, "We took that pilot sequence up to a point, now we better develop something else because we're kind of not right there." You get an intuitive feeling about it when it isn't quite hitting in the ballpark.
>
> Then of course, you've got to go and find the characters. I mean the actual voices. And it isn't until you get the actual voices that things really begin to take hold. Now you can listen to the voice and you say, "That's him." Again, we have quite a few people listening to that. Even before you decide he is it, you take some of those story sketches and you put that together with the voice and pretty soon your eyeballs or your eardrums begin to do something and you say, "That's it."[42]

As animator Glen Keane said, "He was a decision maker from his gut, not an intellectual one at all."[43]

Woolie directed from his music room, with the layout team nearby. He liked to direct voice talent, with Larry Clemmons available to revise dialogue as wanted or needed. He worked through the directing animators primarily. Don Hahn, an assistant director in those days, recalled, "He was pretty deferential to them because I don't think Woolie wanted to get down in the trenches with Eric Cleworth—and with all respect to Eric Cleworth—or Cliff Nordberg or some of those other animators. But he was very willing to listen to or talk to and argue with the Frank and Ollie level of people, the Ward

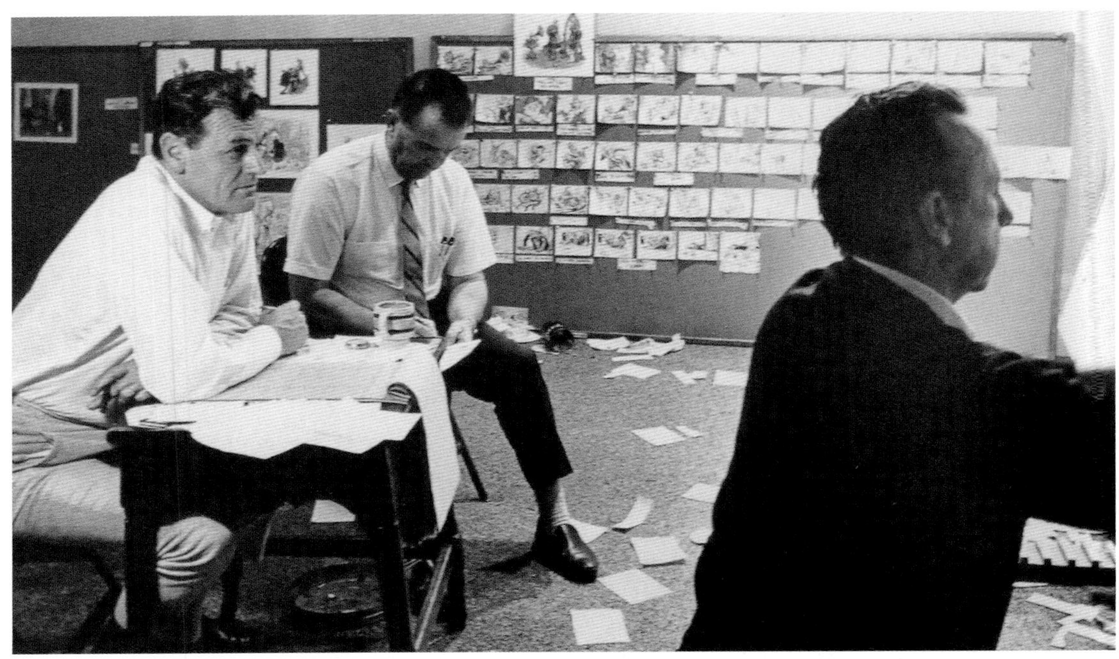

LEFT TO RIGHT: Woolie, Ken Anderson, and Don Griffith.

Kimball level of people, because he saw those as his equals and also he could rely on them to bring back something better than what he might have thought."[44] He felt that his peers respected him, up to a point. "With the large talents there, it wasn't always easy to get respect. I always had little meetings so that those animators who were key to producing any picture were in on the decisions. It wasn't a fearless-leader type of thing by any means. They were part of the creative process, instead of dumping it out there and saying, 'Look, do it!' I think I had the facility to draw people out, to contribute, and keep . . . communication going."[45]

Several characteristics of this new period began emerging. During Woolie's time, next-generation director John Musker saw story and layout atrophy and the animators rise. "They [directing animators] became kings, so they started doing their own layouts and the visual qualities of the film deteriorated, and he didn't really care. I think he felt like, 'You've got to make it for a certain amount of money.'"[46] Frank Thomas felt that the reliance on storyboards diminished. "Woolie never liked story reels because he said they gave you the wrong idea. You can have one concept in your mind and the story reel will seem to support that, and yet the guy who made the story reel has an entirely different concept; you can have three different interpretations of the thing, and a different interpretation of how long a sequence should be, and what the emphasis is. You know, you have a drawing of a deer standing there with wide-open eyes; you can interpret that a lot of different ways. It's tricky, and you can't say this is it, and this is what we're going to do, but I've always been very strong on them, if you view them properly."[47] Still, Woolie was open to new ideas, which was seen as a positive attribute by his colleagues. But perhaps part and parcel with this trait was a tendency to tip over the boat when he didn't understand what was going on, often resulting in cutting a sequence that others thought was promising.

Several animators commented on the fact that Woolie had difficulties visualizing. “The only thing with Woolie is that he wasn’t a great visualizer. In other words, you had to kind of show him the idea; explaining it would only go so far. You had to have pencil and paper and ready to show it to him or even have a board ready to show it to him, and then he could visualize it. So he wasn’t quick on understanding something or visualizing it until you brought it to him, kind of all flushed out.”[48]

Woolie’s treatment of ideas could at times create a great deal of frustration. Frank Thomas felt that Woolie wouldn’t let a tender idea grow but would too often figuratively pound it down. Next-generation director Ron Clements learned that if you were passionate about an idea, Woolie was likely to react negatively. “I did get to go to story meetings, and it was absolutely true, and there are not that many people around that would attest to it, that Woolie, that passion made him uncomfortable, and enthusiasm made him uncomfortable.” Ron had written some story notes in a passionate way, and Woolie got upset about them. Ron said Woolie’s attitude carried over to the storyboard artists, as well. “The storyboard artists had developed this technique, that [your pitch] basically was ‘You could do this or you could do this or you could do this. It doesn’t matter; I don’t care. You could do whatever you want; it doesn’t matter, I don’t care. Here are some thoughts, here are some ideas; you don’t have to use them; you don’t have to like them; it doesn’t matter; I don’t care.’ Because if you did

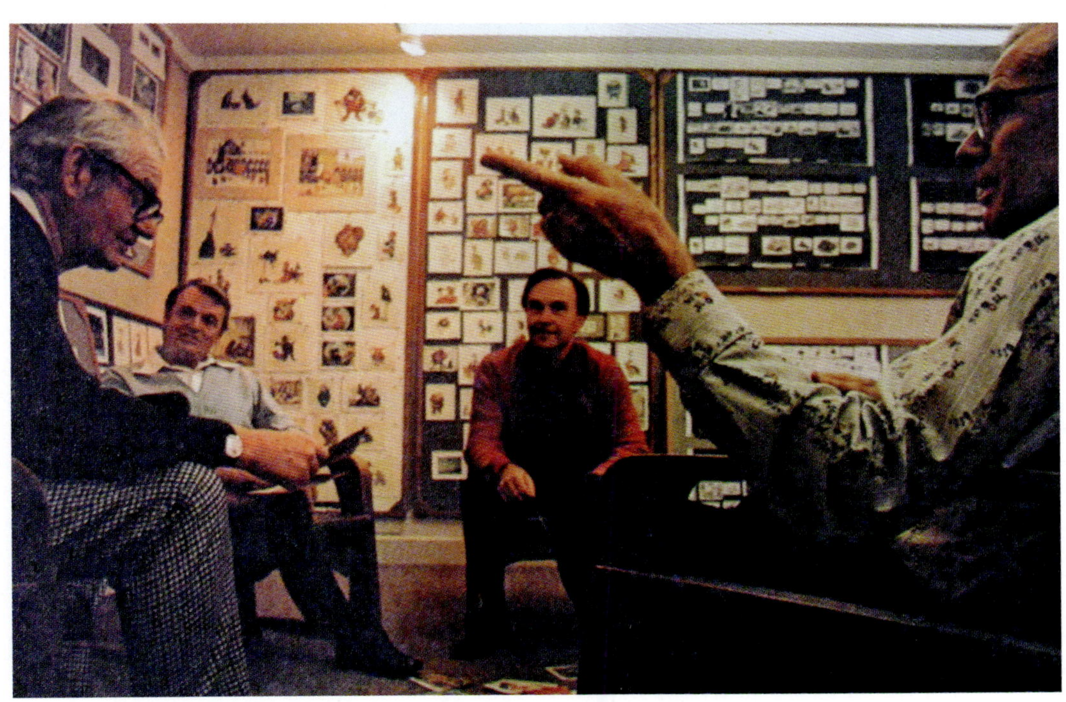

LEFT TO RIGHT: Writer Larry Clemmons, Woolie, designer Ken Anderson, and directing animator Frank Thomas at work on *Robin Hood*.

show any [feeling], like 'I like this idea,' or 'I do care,' Woolie would go out of his way to sort of just destroy it." For most directors, excitement is a measure of the artist's connection to the work and how well it will turn out. Ron is still mystified by Woolie's approach but said, "I think it was just something about his nature that I think he mistrusted that and, I don't know, maybe he felt like, 'You were trying to sell me something.'"[49] John Musker also characterized Woolie as often a contrarian when he thought you were excited about an idea.

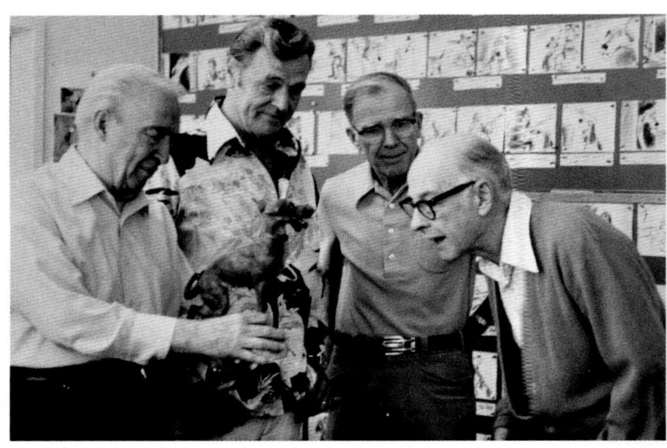

LEFT TO RIGHT: Eric Larson, Woolie, Frank Thomas, and Ollie Johnston inspect a model for the wolf from *The Sword in the Stone*.

In contrast, Dale Baer, also of this younger generation, felt that Woolie was one of the most impressive directors he ever dealt with, and "I have dealt with [Ralph] Bakshi and I've dealt with Richard Williams and Mike Lah and people like that." One of the qualities Dale admired was the empathy that Woolie had for up-and-coming animators. "I think he remembered where he came from. I think he knows; he struggled and I think he could see other people struggle, you know, young people struggle, and he was very fair to it. He mainly wanted to make sure that what you were doing was entertaining, you know. He could care less how well you drew it . . . he just wanted to make sure that you were doing something that was entertaining and doing something that felt right and that fit in the picture." Dale admired his inclusiveness, which may have originated from a lack of confidence. "He wanted everybody's involvement in everything. Like I say, I think that came from when he was animating, because he struggled with everything he did, you know, and he needed reassurance himself on things." And most of all, "he made it fun. Honest to God, he made it fun. In fact, at the end of every film, he says, 'Okay, let's make another one.' You know, he got all excited about it. It wasn't just a job, you know."[50]

One of the criticisms about Woolie was his reuse of animation. Wilfred Jackson even weighed in on this. "He was extremely good at digging up old animation and cleaning up and reusing it. . . . We all kind of had our noses rubbed in it."[51] But as Dale pointed out, "there was a reason for that, because it was a budgetary thing [although it may not have been actually cost-effective], and if he could find something that worked, that fit, just put a different character on top of it and let it go, because all he was mainly trying to do was just make something entertaining, make it fun to watch."[52]

Woolie Reitherman, in his mentoring of Don Bluth as a director, had some strong advice for him: "Being a director will never make you popular. Those people you lead will be jealous of your position, and they'll say mean things and spread ugly rumors. I've heard them all. Ignore them. Develop a thick skin." There was also this from his mentor: "Another lesson Woolie taught me: somebody who's a friend to all won't get a picture made. If you cave in to being friends, the movie will suffer. You have to serve the movie first—not yourself, the powers that be, your own ambition or anyone else's.[53]

John Pomeroy, a contemporary of this younger group, remembered Woolie in a positive light. "I think he was probably one of the best directors I had worked under, because he was extremely encouraging, he was very direct, he wasn't a bully or belligerent at any time. I mean he was always trying to get the very best out of you." He encouraged experimentation until a deadline loomed: "Woolie would give you free reign on just about anything *until* he was about six months away from the finish line on his picture. When the deadline was approaching, you would see him turn up the volume as far as keeping track of where animators were with their scenes, the economy of which they get their footages out. Animators back then were expected to get about five feet a week, I think. It was a low average. That's the pace that they would work, but towards the finish line, there was no more tolerance for any kind of experimentation. You needed to do it as per the direction of the supervisors and the director and no going to the left or the right. Stay right on the path, do what you are told and get it finished."[54]

Burny Mattinson, who had an amazing, record-breaking almost seventy years at the studio, remembered Woolie as a great teacher. "What really helped me more than anything was working with Woolie. He was real quick to bring you into his world and give you his problems [to help solve]."[55] He instilled enough training in Burny that when he came to direct *Mickey's Christmas Carol*, he felt very comfortable. Burny fondly recalled how much Woolie loved the controls on the Moviola; he operated it as though he were flying a plane. The studio abounds with stories about when Walt was in a bad mood, people would say he was wearing his "wounded-bear suit" and those were the days to avoid him. Burny said that on some days, Woolie would be wearing a shark on a gold or silver chain, and that usually meant that someone was going to get fired![56]

Glen Keane remembers Woolie coming in to look at a scene Glen was working on for *The Rescuers*. The story captures Woolie's John Wayne-esque image as seen through the eyes of a trainee: "I had designed a possum, to try to convince him to include a possum in the swamp volunteers for *Rescuers*, and he came down into our little trainee room, and I was so nervous because this had been my, I don't know, ninth week there at the studio and he always had this cigar that he was chewing on; he would never smoke it, he would just suck on it, and it was really disgusting. I don't know how long he had been working on it, but he would get the juice out of it by sucking on it, and he would make this sound when he was looking at your drawings like it was the most painful thing in the world, because he would look at it and go [inhaling, juicy sound]. And it was like 'Oh, gosh, is it that bad?' [sound continues, then smacking sound] 'Aw, well I, you know there's something.' He was kind of like a George Burns kind of thing, and then [smacking, then spit sound] he'd spit and he was spitting right on my other drawings there—but not intentionally. But he was just this bigger-than-life person after World War II, as a bomber pilot, and he'd come walking down the hall, you'd see him from a distance, just this bow-legged, kind of [booming sounds of his walk], and I remember he was just 'Morning, Glen' and that was like 'Wow, he knows my name!' That was so cool!"[57]

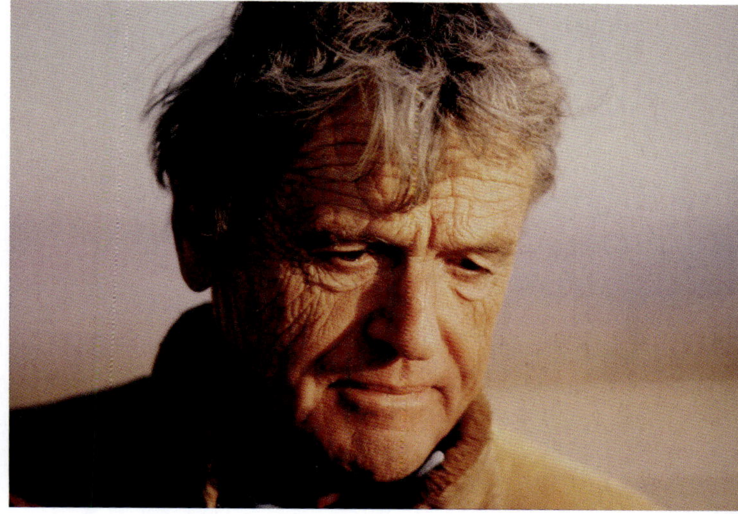

Reitherman in January 1985.

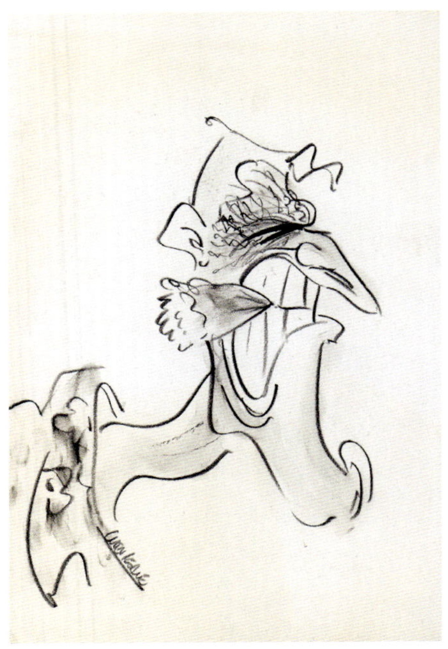

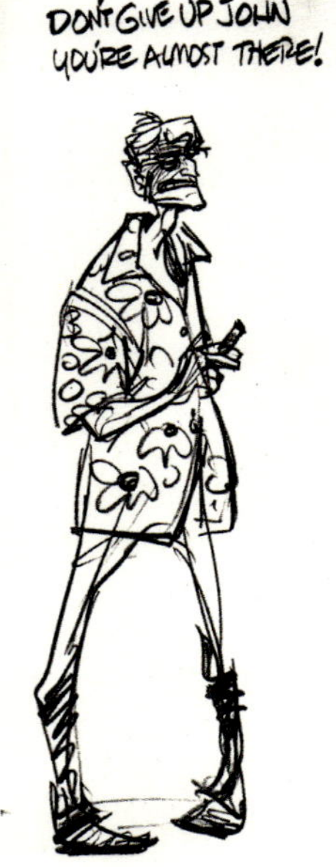

Caricatures of Woolie by Glen Keane (LEFT) and John Musker.

THE FOX AND THE HOUND

As far back as *The Rescuers*, studio chief Ron Miller worried about Woolie's ascendancy. As a result, "John Lounsbery was sort of imposed just to sort of break up Woolie's control of everything," according to Ron Clements. When Lounsbery died of sudden heart failure, Art Stevens was brought in. *The Fox and the Hound* was to represent the changing of the guard: a swan song for the last of Walt Disney's Nine Old Men and the emergence of the rising young animators. But it was not an easy transition—anything but that. Glen remembered:

> So when they retired, when Frank and Ollie and Milt retired, Woolie was the last man standing, and it was really hard on him. Walt was gone, and now all the other Nine Old Men were gone, and there was one of the nine left. And I must have been about twenty-five years old, and Don Bluth had left the studio, and then one day we came down until we only had five animators left at Disney feature animation. I was probably one of the most experienced with zero practical experience and I remember going up to Woolie's office the week after Frank and Ollie retired—they were going to work on their book [*Disney Animation: The Illusion of Life*]—and, it was sort of like—I was honored to be able to stand there with Woolie. Woolie was going through the sequence of Tod and Vixey where they meet and everything, and he's just playing, going through it on the Moviola, and he's looking through different scenes, and I'm standing right next to him, and he says, "Uh, I'm going to have to cut that out of the movie." "Why?" "Because Ollie's the only guy that could animate that." "Oh, I'd—I'd like to try—" "No, no, Ollie was the only guy. Uh, gotta cut this out." "Why?" "Frank was the only guy." "But I—I think I—I think I could do it—" "No, no." I mean he wouldn't even, just not even—because it wasn't really about the fact that I couldn't do it, because I mean,

A DIFFERENT SIDE OF WOOLIE

"Probably one of the most wonderful moments I think I'd ever had with Woolie was him showing me how Penny [*The Rescuers*] would put on the little nightgown, and I was trying to draw it, and he was like, 'No, no, no. It's a little girl that's putting this nightgown on. You know, their arms, they have to kind of get through, it's not easy,' and he's kind of, 'Urr.' And then he grabbed some pen, whatever, something with a point, and he's like 'It's kind of like, you know, she's—' [scribbling with pen and grunting] and he did the most horrible, little ugly drawing, but it was like everything he wanted—it was this awkward little girl, and I was so impressed. It was the most wonderful thing because I thought of Woolie as the guy that did the Tyrannosaurus rex and Ichabod and Monstro and here he was in his scribbly kind of way and he would draw through that. I loved Woolie." Glen Keane re-created Woolie's drawing from memory in November 2021 for this book, with this note: "Now when I see the way it was in my mind I realize how beautifully this 60-something old man (younger than me now!) was so in tune with the charming way a little 5-year-old girl would put on a nightgown. He drew it with a pen (I believe) and held the pen with the tips of his fingers like you would if you were mixing a cocktail."

LOOKS SWELL, GLEN. REAL GOOD.
KEEP UP THE GOOD WORK!
SHOULDN'T HAVE HAD
THAT NINTH MARTINI
AT LUNCH TODAY.
CAN'T FOCUS

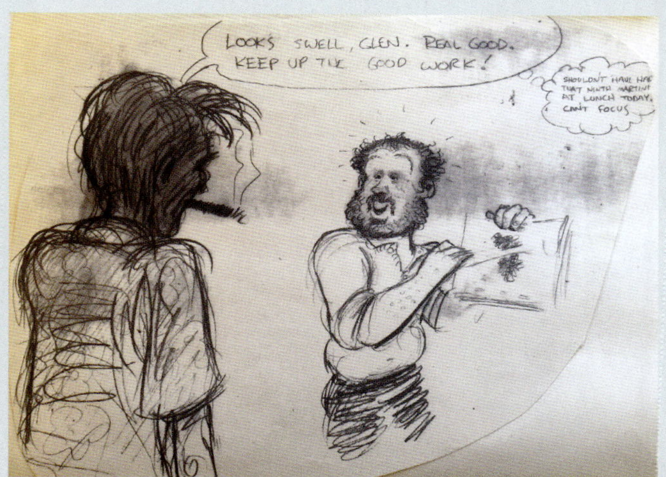

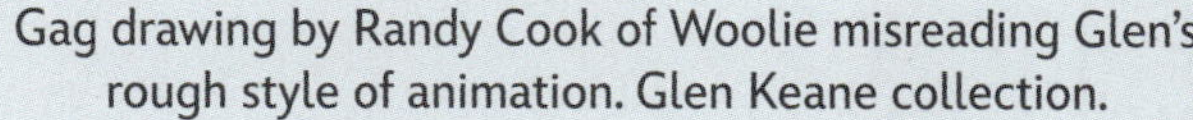
Gag drawing by Randy Cook of Woolie misreading Glen's rough style of animation. Glen Keane collection.

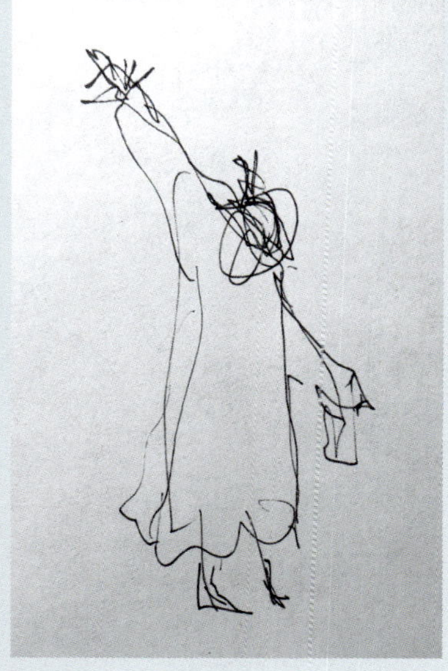

when they were my age, they were doing wonderful things. It was about—"You don't understand, I've had my right and my left arm cut off, what am I supposed to do?" There was such sorrow, I mean real sorrow with Woolie, how much he depended on those three, Frank and Ollie and Milt.[58]

Woolie was codirecting with Art Stevens, who had a long career at Disney, dating back to 1940 and *Fantasia*, and he was more than ready to have an opportunity to direct. But it was difficult for Woolie to let go and share the position. Glen remembered the anguish that Art felt on a sequence they were working on together:

"Art was encouraging, and we collaborated a lot together on that and he was delighted to see me pushing the boundaries of where you could go with animation. It was like—there was this part of him that was really young again and excited. So he and I really got along well, but then he would also come down and feel humiliated because Woolie would shut him down and not give him credit as a director, even though he was now working on this big sequence with me. He was not feeling like Woolie cared at all about him, and Art was extremely emotional. I mean there was a time where he was in tears, and it was a real crisis in his life, you know, 'Okay this is my chance, and its dissolving in my hands.'"[59] Eventually, Art went to Ron Miller to discuss his treatment, resulting in Woolie reluctantly stepping back and focusing on his co-producer responsibilities. This shift created feelings of animosity among some of the team: those who supported Woolie and those who supported Art. Over time, Ted Berman and Rick Rich also joined the directing team on that picture. Woolie worked on some development projects at the studio and some consulting work, but he and they gradually faded from the studio scene. He retired in 1981 and received a Winsor McCay Award in 1983.

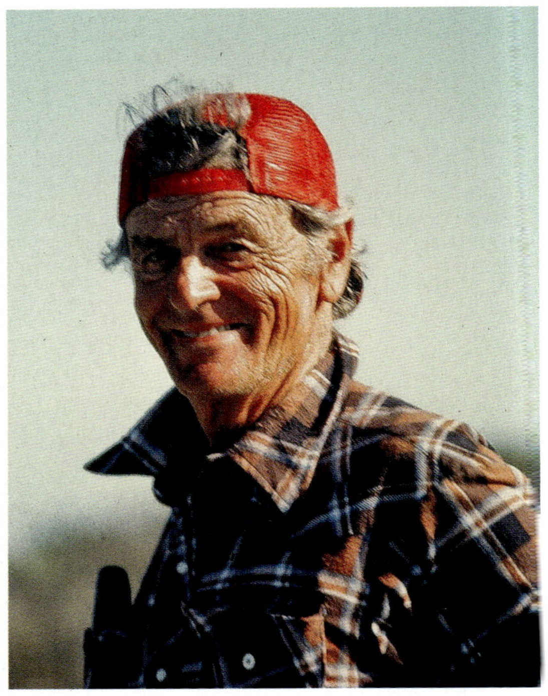

Woolie Reitherman in the winter of 1982, visiting son Bruce at the San Ignacio Lagoon, Baja California Sur, Mexico.

AFTER DISNEY

Woolie had an active homelife involving his growing family, traveling with his travel agent wife, Janie, flying again, and engaging in outdoor sports and activities. Never one to let life pass him by, even on his last day Woolie played tennis in the morning, had lunch with his wife, and stopped at the bank on his way home in preparation for their upcoming trip to Maui. But on his drive home, he had a heart attack and crashed his car. He was conscious when he was transported to the hospital, but died later that day, May 22, 1985, at age seventy-five. He was named a Disney Legend in 1989.

Woolie was the last of the truly legendary figures from the golden age of the studio. Recruited by Walt, stubbornly finding his own path both as an animator and a director, serving his country in a time of war, devoted to his family, Woolie gave his all to everything he undertook, and he helped keep the Disney name magical.

Woolie Reitherman—Disney Director Filmography

Shorts:

- *The Truth About Mother Goose* (1957)
- *Goliath II* (1960)
- *Aquamania* (1961)
- *Winnie the Pooh and the Honey Tree* (1966)
- *Winnie the Pooh and the Blustery Day* (1968)

Features:

- *Pinocchio* (1940) (Directing Animator)
- *Dumbo* (1941) (Directing Animator)
- *Fun and Fancy Free* (1947) (Directing Animator)
- *The Adventures of Ichabod and Mr. Toad* (1949) (Directing Animator)
- *Cinderella* (1950) (Directing Animator)
- *Alice in Wonderland* (1951) (Directing Animator)
- *Peter Pan* (1953) (Directing Animator)
- *Lady and the Tramp* (1955) (Directing Animator)
- *Sleeping Beauty* (1959) (Sequence Director)
- *One Hundred and One Dalmatians* (1961) (Codirector with Ham Luske and Clyde Geronimi)
- *The Sword in the Stone* (1963) (Director)
- *The Jungle Book* (1967) (Director)
- *The Aristocats* (1970) (Producer and Director)
- *Robin Hood* (1973) (Producer and Director)
- *Winnie the Pooh and Tigger Too* (1974) (Producer)
- *The Many Adventures of Winnie the Pooh* (1977) (Producer and Director)
- *The Rescuers* (1977) (Producer and Director)
- *The Fox and the Hound* (1981) (Co-Producer)

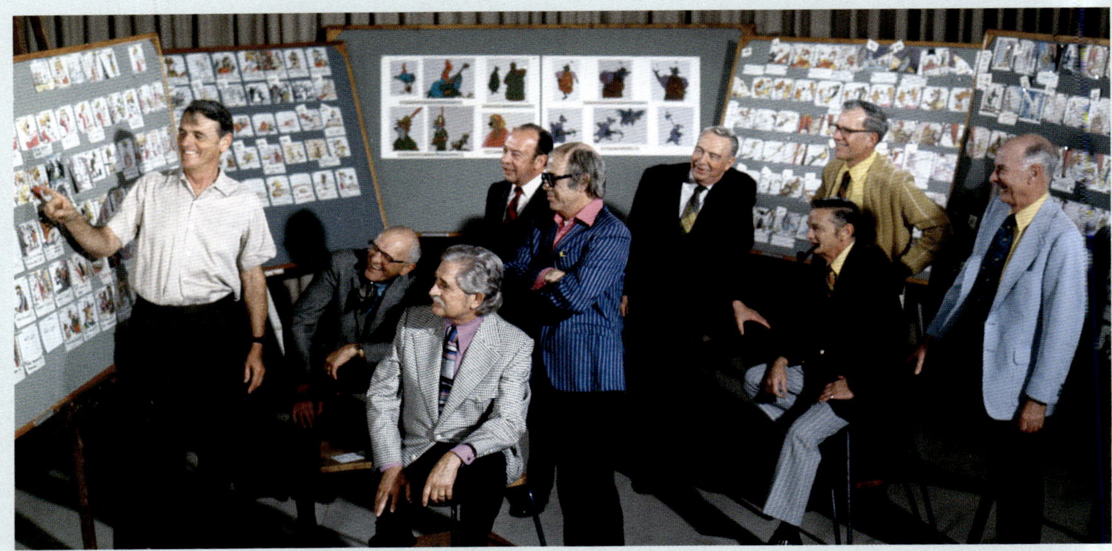

Disney's fabled Nine Old Men were essentially an internal animation review board, pushed forward by the public relations department to give the craft and company a human face after Walt died. FROM LEFT: Woolie Reitherman, Milt Kahl, Les Clark, Marc Davis, Ward Kimball, Eric Larson, John Lounsbery (SEATED), Frank Thomas, and Ollie Johnston.

Did any of the rest of Walt Disney's Nine Old Men harbor an interest in directing? Let's take a look.

Ollie Johnston, Milt Kahl, and Marc Davis are not known to have exhibited any ambition to be the sole director of an animated short or feature. Although as directing animators, they were at times de facto directors, depending on the directorial style of the designated director.

Frank Thomas directed away from the studio, when he enlisted in the Army Air Forces and had an opportunity to direct some training films, including *Camouflage* (1944), as part of the First Motion Picture Unit. Upon returning to Disney, he expressed an interest in directing and he was assigned for a while to the early development of "Johnny Appleseed" with Gerry Geronimi. Over time, Frank returned to his animation desk, where he could probably be most valuable to the studio. (Wilfred Jackson is credited as the director of this short musical segment in *Melody Time*.) Frank would have more opportunities as a supervising animator and a directing animator, especially in the Woolie Reitherman era.

Ward Kimball wanted to direct and had an opportunity with Nick Nichols on two shorts: *Melody* and *Toot, Whistle, Plunk and Boom*, the latter winning the 1954 Academy Award for Best Animated Short Film. Ward said about directing: "I was so relieved to get away from animation. I knew how to do it. I wanted to have a say about the content."[60] Ward also directed three programs for the Tomorrowland segments of the *Disneyland* television series: "Man in Space" (1955), "Man and the Moon" (1955), and "Mars and Beyond" (1957). A directing gig for the live-action *Babes in Toyland* was cut short when Ward was replaced by Jack Donohue. Ward directed the animated shorts *It's Tough to Be a Bird* (1969) and *Dad, Can I Borrow the Car?* (1970), the former winning an Academy Award for Best Animated Short Film. From 1972 to 1973, Ward directed forty-three episodes of television's *The Mouse Factory.*[61]

Eric Larson replaced Wilfred Jackson as the director after he suffered a heart attack during the production of *Sleeping Beauty*. Eric directed a good deal of the film, but due to mounting costs and delays in the production for a variety of reasons, Eric was replaced by Gerry Geronimi. Years later when Eric ran a training program at the studio, he was prepared to direct *The Small One* with his trainees, but Ron Miller assigned it to up-and-coming director Don Bluth, and unbeknownst to Eric, all the art and story work was transferred out of his office over a weekend. Studio colleagues said Eric never really recovered from this loss.

Les Clark was asked by Walt to direct. After he retired, when asked if he preferred animation to direction, Les responded: "It was an advancement. Walt asked me twice to go into direction: first in 1940 and then a few years later. I said I'd rather animate for a while longer because I was enjoying it so. Then when we were preparing for Disneyland, he wanted me to direct a cartoon on the story of oil [*The World Beneath Us*], which the Richfield Oil Company [ARCO today] was financing. From then on, I kept directing. I directed for the *Mickey Mouse Club*'s "Five Senses" with Jiminy Cricket as the narrator. I was a sequence director on *Sleeping Beauty* and then on to educational films [including as a sequence director on *Donald in Mathmagic Land*]."[62] Les directed for his last fifteen years at the studio, including the featurette *Paul Bunyan,* and has over twenty additional directing credits.

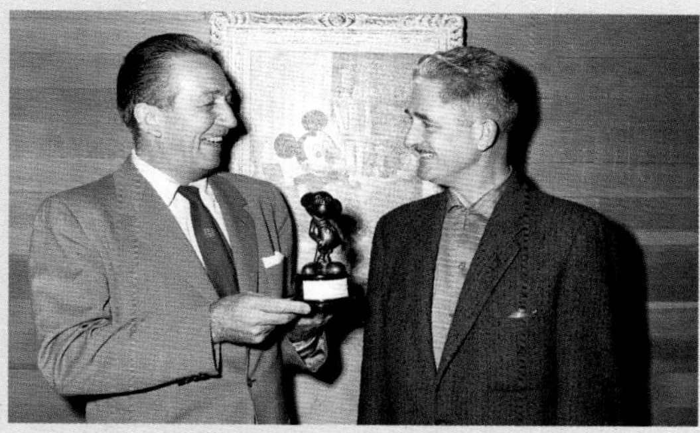

Les Clark gets a lifetime achievement Mousecar, 1957.

John Lounsbery was the other reluctant director who loved his role as an animator. As a directing animator, like his peers, he did have a good deal of directorial clout. But eventually John was "pushed" (his word choice) into directing. Director Richard Williams remembered John saying, "Oh God. If I could just animate! If I could just close the door and have a scene and make it right, I'd get some satisfaction."[63] John directed *Winnie the Pooh and Tigger Too*, and was codirecting *The Many Adventures of Winnie the Pooh* with Woolie and *The Rescuers* at the time of his death. According to Mel Shaw, Ron Miller intended to replace the retiring Woolie Reitherman with John. (Others have suggested that Don Bluth or Dick Sebast were Ron's candidates.)

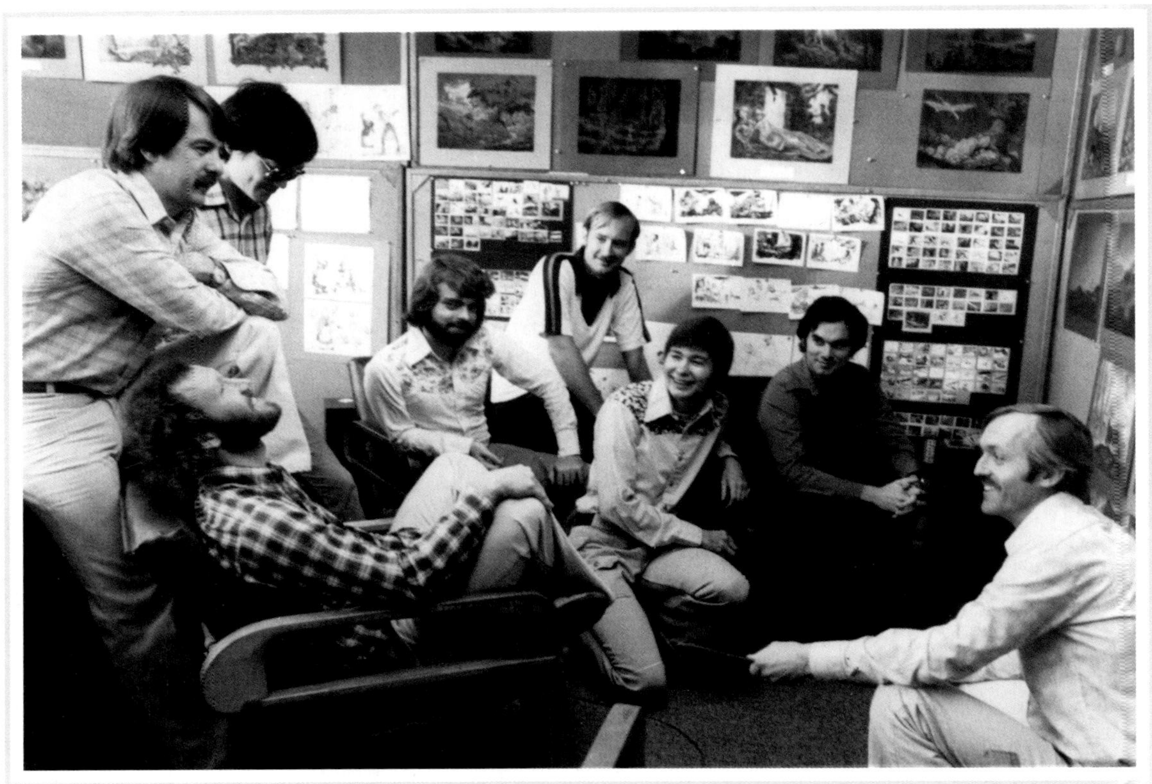

The “second generation” of artists working on *The Fox and the Hound.* LEFT TO RIGHT: Gary Goldman, Glen Keane, Andy Gaskil, Ron Clements, Ed Gombert, Randy Cartwright, John Pomeroy, and Don Bluth.

CHAPTER 10

LEGACY

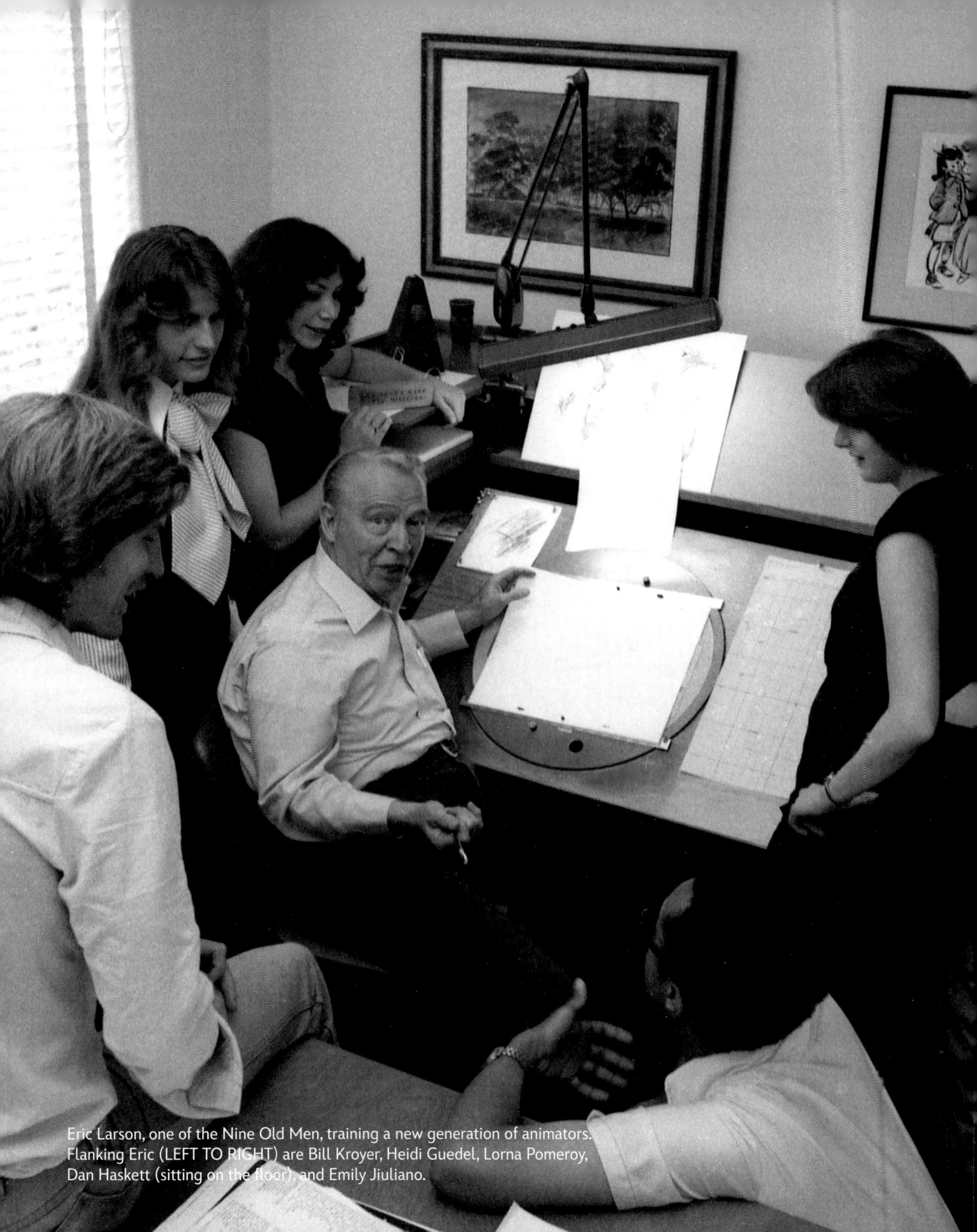

Eric Larson, one of the Nine Old Men, training a new generation of animators. Flanking Eric (LEFT TO RIGHT) are Bill Kroyer, Heidi Guedel, Lorna Pomeroy, Dan Haskett (sitting on the floor), and Emily Jiuliano.

"I DON'T THINK WE CAN CONTINUE"

Walt Disney left no plans for how the studio should be run after he died, nor who should be in charge creatively. Even on his deathbed in St. Joseph's Hospital, rather than strategizing a succession plan, Walt stared at the acoustic tiles of the hospital room ceiling, planning the layout of EPCOT. In fact, there is not much to indicate that he expected the animated films to continue to be made without him. How then did Disney animation not just survive, but, eventually, flourish?

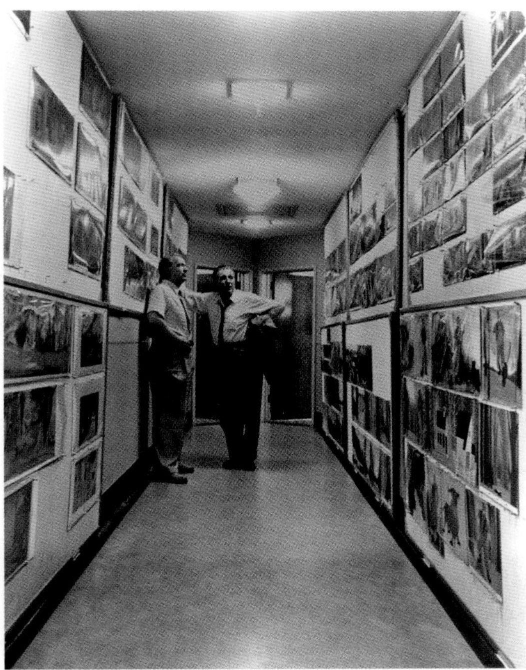

Walt and director Eric Larson, surrounded by beautiful panoramic artwork from *Sleeping Beauty* and *Paul Bunyan*. Eric recalled their conversation in an October 1976 interview with Michael Barrier: "See that picture? That's Walt and me out here in the hall. This was toward the end of *Sleeping Beauty*. Walt's saying, 'I don't think we can continue, it's too expensive.' That was the general conception."

Disney had considered shuttering the department years earlier (Joe Grant recalled that even as early as the mid-1940s, "his interest—you could feel it flagging"[1]), but Walt balked at his brother Roy's suggestion they close the animation department and cash out.[2] By 1960, after *Sleeping Beauty* had absorbed $6 million and six years of Walt's limited attention, Disney seriously considered the suggestion. Instead, perhaps feeling a dedication toward the artists who had devoted their professional lives to developing the art form, Walt kept the department going at greatly reduced staff, and lower cost[3]. Though some associates felt Walt never lost his love for animation, others reported a grouchy, begrudging attitude when he visited the department, as though Walt resented having to leave Imagineering and other interests.[4] "How come Walt lost interest in animation?" pondered director Woolie Reitherman. "I think it was a pain in the ass for him. The personnel problems, the waiting around for animation to come in, and I don't know of any feature that we ever made around here that sailed right through. . . . It's just a tough damn medium the way we do it."[5]

Some speculate that had he lived, Walt would have shut down animation permanently following the retirement of his key artists. So it was no surprise that Walt's death left a gaping hole for animation, and no clarity for how—or even if—it should be filled.

Given the importance of story in Disney's movies, one could argue that someone from the story department would have been a good choice to lead after Walt's death. Bill Peet, the strongest candidate in terms of sheer story ability as well as confidence, was uncompromising and combative, which would have made for difficult relationships. Regardless, Peet had sparred with Walt over *The Jungle Book* and left the studio in January 1964. Woolie Reitherman's charisma did provide organizational leadership, but Woolie had never been asked to provide Walt-level vision for films and the studio for the first thirty-three years of his career. This level of confidence and foresight had taken even Disney years to develop, and Woolie's reluctance or inability to delve deeper into character and story conflict produced *Robin Hood*, *The Aristocats*, and *The Rescuers*—all films more fun to watch in small sections than as a whole.

Directors following Woolie fared even worse. After Don Bluth's departure from the studio in 1979, it seemed new directors got the position by outlasting the Frank Thomases and Bill Peets rather than by merit of their abilities. Ted Berman, Richard Rich, and Art Stevens had been capable in their own fields, but the generation working under them[6] saw no compelling vision. *The Fox and the Hound* and *The Black Cauldron* lacked the joy and fun of earlier films, and even the strong character work of Woolie's efforts. The proven Disney directors, who could have provided guidance and mentorship, were by now long gone, and largely forgotten. "The sad truth," wrote modern director Ron Clements (*The Little Mermaid*, *Aladdin*, *Hercules*, etc.) "is that even when I started at Disney as an animation trainee in the early 1970s, working closely with legendary animators Frank Thomas and Ollie Johnston, the early directors were rarely talked about. I knew that Frank and Ollie loved Wilfred Jackson and hated Gerry Geronimi, and that was about it. While working on *The Rescuers*, we trainees were given tons of lectures on animation, but the director of that film, Woolie Reitherman, never gave one. Everything was about the animation."

Ironically, the director's role had finally come to require creative authorship, yet those now in that role were incapable of providing it.

REBIRTH

And like in a Disney movie, just as the death knell of Disney animation was sounding, it was given another chance.

A lot of things have to go right to make good films. Talent, support from management, and a large audience are all essential for successful big-budget films like those made at Disney's, and the lack of these had nearly strangled the art form. Luckily, a new generation of artists that had grown up on the films of Walt Disney fought passionately to bring forward their own contributions. New management under Roy E. Disney, Michael Eisner, and Jeffery Katzenberg recognized the power animated films still had and committed to bringing it back. The many people and specific efforts are for another book, but a new spirit of energy and enthusiasm slowly took hold. By the late 1980s a rebirth of Disney animation was underway, built on the foundation made by Walt and his directors—but with a new twist.

During this time, the director's job itself would change forever, due to a new focus and new technology.

"When John Musker and I became directors under producer Burny Mattinson on *The Great Mouse Detective*, we worked very much as traditional sequence directors," remembered Ron Clements. "We timed our own story reels" using a stopwatch, noting instructions on X-sheets, which would then be spliced together by a cutter. Clements's and Musker's work on *The Little Mermaid* proceeded the same way.

So when Disney Animation president Peter Schneider suggested they bring on an editor, they were confused. Unlike live action, animation does not have multiple takes of picture options to choose from, and since Clements and Musker selected takes and dictated timing, they suspected Schneider of trying to plant a double agent so Schneider could make changes behind their backs. As it turned out, editor John Carnochan became a shaping force on the film, selecting dialogue takes, rearranging shots, and generally improving the telling of the story—all tasks Musker and Clements had done previously.[7] While they as directors would still supervise and sign off on all these decisions, the editor now owned the massive job of building the story reels. Thanks to the editor, Musker and Clements—and the directors following them—would now be free to focus more extensively on the storytelling.

A second change was technology. Long before computer-generated images appeared on the screen, digital technology was already changing the way films were made, due in large part to the early days of the computer division at Lucasfilm. Nonlinear editing[8] allowed filmmakers to trim, rearrange, and undo edits easily, whereas actual film required it all be pre-timed by a director and hand-spliced together. The benefits seemed clear to John Lasseter and team on *Toy Story*, which was the first Disney animated film to employ digital editing technology—now a standard part of crafting all films.[9] In the past, a director needed the ability to visualize timing and pacing in advance, in their heads. Now they could ask an editor to mock it up quickly, react, and make adjustments. When you look at how early Disney directors used to work, said director Eric Goldberg (*Pocahontas*, *Fantasia 2000*), "the fact that all of it was planned in advance [as opposed to finding the correct path in the editing rooms] is nothing short of miraculous."

The job had shifted hard toward the storytelling, and away from the craft of timing and building reels. Animation directors of the eighties and nineties looked up to Steven Spielberg,

TODAY'S ANIMATION DIRECTOR

While many of the director's tasks have stayed the same since the days of Ub Iwerks and Burt Gillett, the crucial addition of new technology and an editor means the director typically no longer times out the material. A director works with a writer and story artists to craft the characters, plot, and dialogue; directs all the actors (usually scratch actors at first); and often selects music, or at least points to the style they are after. All these pieces go to the editor, who assembles them using their best guesses at timing, pacing, tone, etc. The editor plays their cut for the director, who may have sweeping adjustments or small tweaks, depending on how closely the editor nailed what the director was looking for.

Today's animation directors at Disney and Pixar:

- Come up with concepts for stories
- Work with writer(s) and story department to develop material
- Work with art department to develop character designs, props, and sets
- Approve casting
- Record actors
- Oversee editors who assemble story reels
- Work with story and editor to revise reels until story is working
- Hand cut and approve animation
- Approve simulation, lighting
- Work with musician who creates score
- Oversee final production and sound mix

George Lucas, and Francis Ford Coppola—directors who, while not usually functioning as the screenwriters themselves, did drive the creative direction of their own stories. Spilling over into animation, it was the start of a new era of direction—a new level of creative authorship.

Today, directors at Walt Disney Animation Studios and Pixar Animation Studios are generally asked to generate their own story ideas. They supervise writers and story artists to craft the plan for the film—previously the job of Walt Disney—as well as oversee how that story is executed. The job now consists of both the skills of the directors of years past and, at least to some degree, the storytelling leadership of Walt Disney himself.

"A COMPLICATED LEGACY"

What then have today's directors of animated films inherited from their predecessors? "The directors of Walt Disney's many animated masterpieces left behind a complicated legacy," writes director Brad Bird (*The Iron Giant*, *The Incredibles*, *Ratatouille*). "On one hand, they were subservient to the creative force of Walt Disney, an undeniable genius at developing stories who—strangely—couldn't direct well himself. On the other hand, Disney's overwhelming success and complete dominance in the field of feature animation also led to the mistaken belief that while live-action movies are driven by their directors, animated films are made by corporate entities, a belief widely held to this day."

Most current directors admit to an ignorance of their predecessors' names. Director Don Hall (*Big Hero 6*, *Raya and the Last Dragon*, *Strange World*) remembered being acutely aware of Chuck Jones, Friz Freleng, Bob Clampett, Tex Avery, to the point he "didn't need the credits to tell me who directed the film, because I was so familiar with their unique visual styles," but that Disney films all shared a similar look and sensibility. "Walt's name was so iconic that it cast a shadow over everything that followed."

Still, they were inspired by the work. "I fell in love with animation because of the incredible and timeless art of these great directors," wrote modern-day Disney director Chris Buck (*Tarzan*, *Surf's Up*, *Frozen*). "Subconsciously, my own work is constantly influenced by their genius."[10] Director Brenda Chapman (*The Prince of Egypt*, *Brave*) agreed. "Those films gave me a wonderful sense of stepping into illustrated storybooks—as if I had been bewitched for an hour or so. That feeling became the inspiration for my life's work." John Musker (*The Little Mermaid*, *Aladdin*, *The Princess and the Frog*, and more) remembered being awed by "repeated viewings in a Chicago theatre one summer of *Cinderella*, where the bravura storytelling, animation, and sheer entertainment seemed as alive and engaging as anything I'd ever seen. Who were those filmmakers, and how the heck did they make something that still resonated so powerfully twenty-five years later?" When Musker stepped into the director role, he realized that "the power of the stories and entertainment value those directors put on the screen was both an inspiration, and a gauntlet thrown, daring us as filmmakers to match their mettle."

Director and animator Eric Goldberg admired their varied talents: "story, timing, composition, lighting, use of color, musicality, camerawork, editing, effects animation, and, not the least of them, the acting, performances, and relationships of the characters. Disney animation at its highest point had these varied elements firing on all cylinders, all at once, so that they all contributed to some of the grandest storytelling in cinema." Director Mike Gabriel (*The Rescuers Down Under*, *Pocahontas*) had much to praise, including admiration for their cutting ("They trusted if the character was engaging enough you didn't need to cut away so quickly"—which inspired the scene in *The Rescuers Down Under* where Joanna the iguana tries to steal eggs), their use of music ("They knew to let the action and the music tell their story and carry their emotion, even using music instead of realistic sound effects, which keeps you a part of this whimsically created environment."), and their sincerity ("The key Disney touch was to give them sincerity and appeal. Don't try for anything but being true to the story and its characters with pure sincerity in their performance. Don't waste time trying to be cool or contemporary for its own sake."). But chief among their talents, reflected Gabriel, was that the directors "kept the humor grounded in the characters personalities. The main thing I learned from them as a fellow Disney director was you had to bring to life endearing, entertaining, original personalities first and foremost. The characters' inner drive is going to drive the plot, not vice versa." The combined effort of all this, said Gabriel, was that "their animated films always left me with a glow after I came out of the darkened theater, a weird out-of-body weightless feeling every single time I watched one of their classics."

Don Hall recognized that the early directors contributed "not only to the success of those early films, but to the *process* of making them," a process "built on a relentless drive to tell a great story, driven by visuals, by drawings, and a dedicated commitment to collaboration." Director Byron Howard (*Bolt*, *Tangled*, *Zootopia*) recognized this partnership as well. "Directors frequently directed together, individuals with different strengths focusing together on the single goal of telling a great story. One director was known to be great with music, another had a terrific eye for humor, and others were great with emotion and drama. Teams built these movies," wrote Byron. And while the ultimate vision and creative success or failure still sits at the feet of the director, collaboration is "exactly what we all do now at Disney and Pixar. Generations later, we are still at our best when we bring together diverse people with unique talents, to create great stories that will resonate far beyond our own careers. This group of talented, collaborative directors make it clear to me that teamwork is part of our legacy."

Throughout this book, we've followed Disney's own trajectory throughout his life—from artist, to becoming the first director, to gradually delegating more creative authority to others. But he was unwilling, or perhaps unable, to take the final step: training others to make their own films. While directors working today no longer have Walt's creative genius and vision to guide them, they are given the opportunity to provide this themselves. As such, modern directors are inspired both by Walt Disney himself and the men who worked alongside him.

Director Ron Clements spoke for many working in the field today: "Those early directors, under Walt Disney, starting with shorts and then bringing the knowledge they gained into the making of animated features, figured it all out for us. They created an art form."

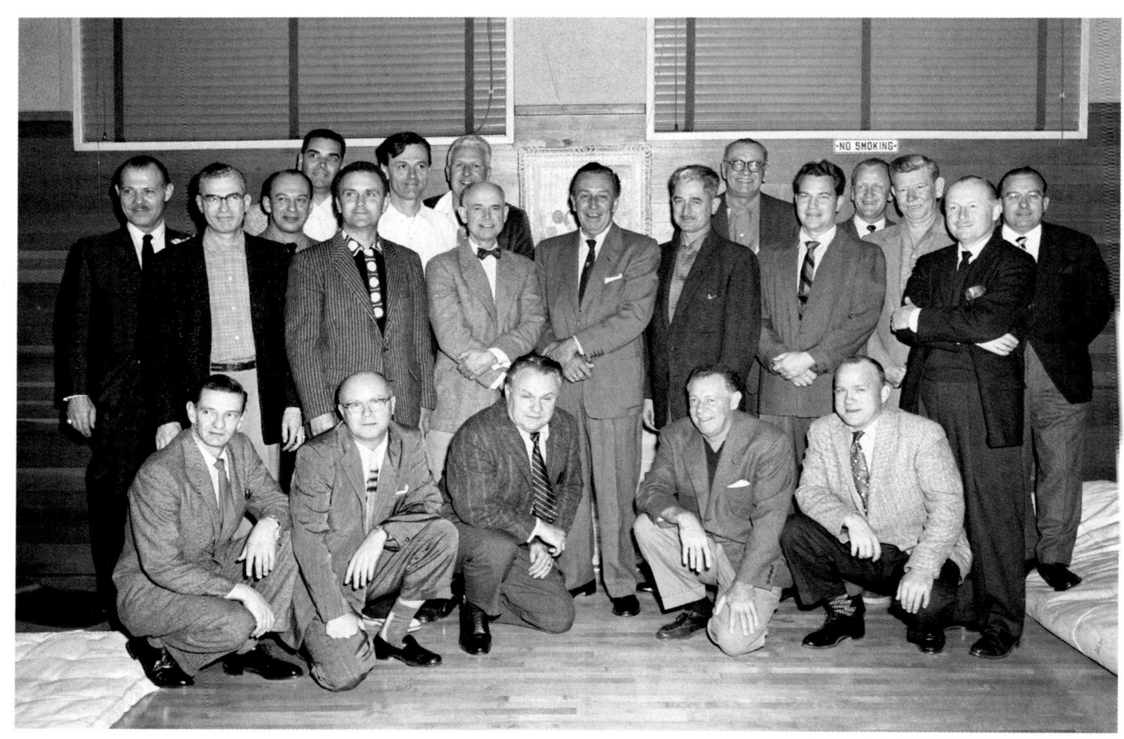

Key directors, animators, and creative leaders at The Walt Disney Studios in 1957: STANDING, LEFT: Harry Tytle, John Sibley, Marc Davis, Claude Coats, Ken Anderson, Woolie Reitherman, Jack Kinney, Ben Sharpsteen, Walt Disney, Les Clark, George Stallings, Bill Justice, Lou Debney, Wilfred Jackson, Jim Algar, Erwin Verity. KNEELING, FROM LEFT: John Lounsbery, McLaren Stewart, Gerry Geronimi, Ham Luske, Jack Hannah.

APPENDIX A

LISTING OF ALL SEQUENCE DIRECTORS AND PRODUCTION SUPERVISORS

Records are often incomplete when it comes to credits, but below is the list of all credited directors we've been able to find at Disney's during Walt's life.

JIM ALGAR

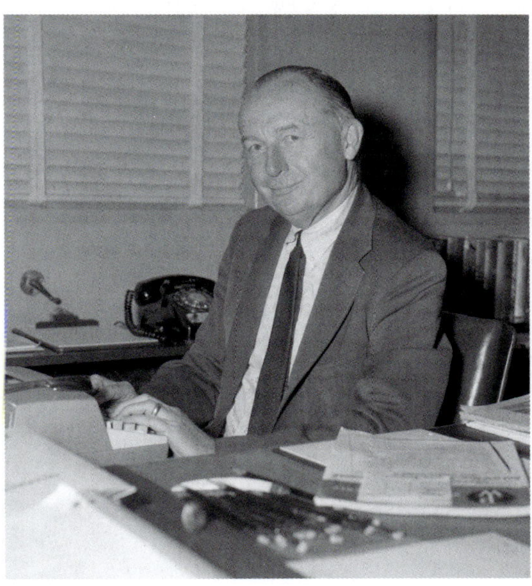

A quiet and thoughtful man, Algar is best remembered for writing and producing many of the True-Life Adventure films. (See Chapter 4.) Recruited by Ben Sharpsteen, Algar started at Disney's as an inbetweener and by 1938 was directing the "The Sorcerer's Apprentice" section of *Fantasia*. He directed ten sequences of *Bambi* (roughly the first half of the film), the "Cyril's Testimony" sequence of *The Adventures of Ichabod and Mr. Toad* (aka "Wind in the Willows"), and sections of *Victory Through Air Power*. He later wrote and produced films for Disneyland and Walt Disney World, as well as produced the theatrical releases *Ten Who Dared* and *The Gnome-Mobile*. He received a Disney Legends Award in 1998.

SAM ARMSTRONG

Armstrong began at Disney in June 1934 and was in charge of backgrounds for the Silly Symphony films. A protégé of director Bill Roberts[1], Armstrong was a sequence director on *Fantasia*, for which he directed the interim orchestra sections as well as the "Nutcracker Suite" sequence. Though "Rite of Spring" segments were directed by Roberts and Satterfield, art director J. Gordon Legg credits Armstrong as "the one who had the mud thing built, with the air hoses to blow the bubbles for the hot lava in 'Rite of Spring.' Now, whether he invented these things, or had the doggedness to pursue them, and work through them—he brought his own 16mm camera to shoot a lot of stuff experimentally and so forth." Armstrong's abilities landed him a stint on *Bambi*, directing the pictorial opening and autumn and winter montages, as well as the "Stork Sequence," "Sad Casey," "Casey Loading," and "Roustabouts" in *Dumbo*. Armstrong's employee file lists him as

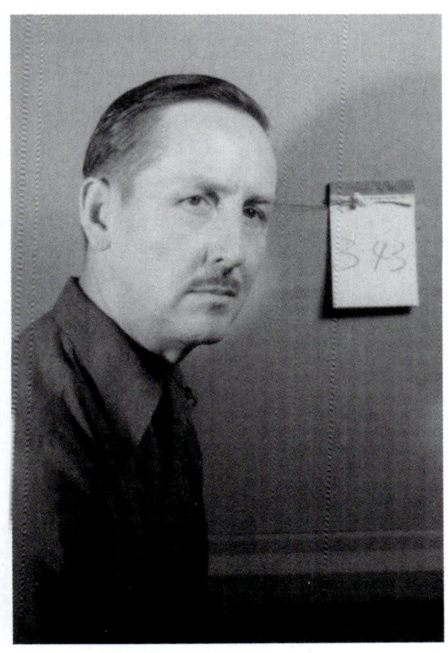

"an excellent color man" with "good knowledge of methods and getting results through the multiplane [camera]"—but also "far too costly" and "bullheaded on points and suspicious of all working with him." Never married, Armstrong brought his mother to the film premieres. She saw herself as the matron of the studio—a move not appreciated by Walt, who, according to Legg, "never missed a chance to get in a nasty dig"[2] at Armstrong. (SEE ALSO SIDEBAR IN CHAPTER 4.)

FORD L. BEEBE JR. (WITH HAM LUSKE)

Son of the famed silent actor, Beebe Jr. was mainly one of several assistant directors for Ham Luske but is credited as codirector (with Luske) on Beethoven's Pastoral Symphony for *Fantasia*, as well as codirecting with Ub Iwerks on several wartime shorts. (SEE ALSO CHAPTER 8.)

ROBERT WILLIAM "BOB" CARLSON

Born November 7, 1906, Bob began as an assistant to Nick Nichols in 1935. Known primarily as an animator, he directed *Crazy with the Heat* (1947), a Donald and Goofy short. Leaving Disney in 1958, he started his own studio for a time, then worked for a number of other studios, including UPA, Filmation, MGM, and Hanna-Barbera.

LES CLARK

The Rest of the Nine Old Men. (SEE SIDEBAR, PAGE 256.)

PINTO COLVIG, ERDMAN "ED" PENNER, WALT PFEIFFER

Directed *Mickey's Amateurs*. (SEE CHAPTERS 2 AND 5.)

ROBERT C. "BOB" CORMACK

Born in Alameda, California, Cormack worked in newspapers in the 1930s until he got a job at Disney's. Primarily a layout artist, he is credited with directing two sequences of *Make Mine Music*: "Without You" and "Two Silhouettes."

WILLIAM "BILL" COTTRELL

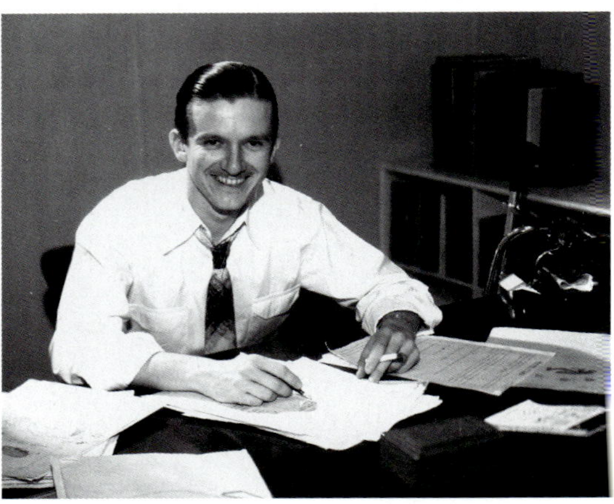

Born in South Bend, Indiana, Cottrell first worked with George Herriman on his famed *Krazy Kat* comic strip. On this strength he was hired at the Disney studio in 1929 as an inker and painter, then in camera, and worked later in the story department, where he teamed with Joe Grant until Disney split up the partnership in the late 1930s. First tapped to be supervising director on *Snow White*, Cottrell ended up directing most of the sequences, including villainous characters, like the Queen, the Magic Mirror, and the Witch, including the frightening transformation sequence. In 1938 he married Lillian Disney's sister Hazel Sewell. As a writer he worked on *Pinocchio* through *Peter Pan*, and in later years he moved over to work at WED, the future Walt Disney Imagineering, as part of the planning and design department for the Disney Parks. Bill was named a Disney Legend in 1994.

JACK CUTTING

See Chapter 8.

JOHN WESLEY "JACK" ELOITTE (WITH BILL ROBERTS)

Born February 6, 1902, Jack directed alongside Roberts in Bill's large unit on *Dumbo*, working on "Fireman Save My Child," "Clowns Celebrate," "Timothy & Dumbo Visit Jail," "Lullaby Sequence," "Clown Sequence," and "Big Town—Dumbo Triumphs." Jack died June 20, 1986.

NORM FERGUSON

See Sidebar in Chapter 4.

GERRY GERONIMI

See Chapter 7.

BURT GILLETT

See Chapter 2.

JOE GRANT

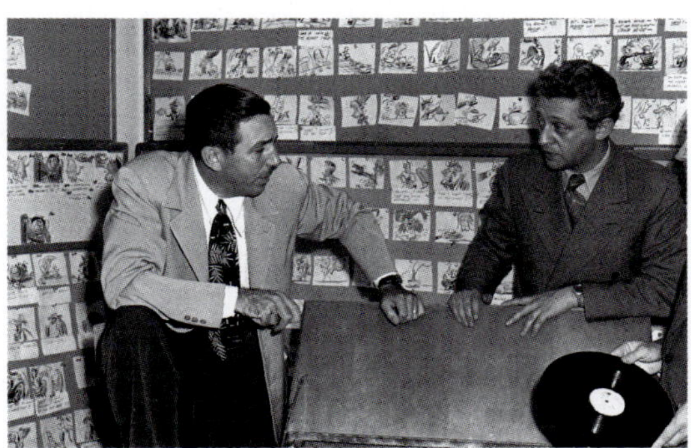

Though not a director, Grant is listed here as production supervisor of *Make Mine Music*. Grant's career as a celebrated newspaper caricature artist landed him a temporary assignment on *Mickey's Gala Premier* (1933), but he stayed at Disney's until the late thirties, returning again to the studio in 1989 and contributing to many films until his death in 2005. Designing characters for *Snow White*, Grant developed clay models to assist the animators, a resource which became the Character Model Department—a small group of amazing artists that developed ideas and characters for new films. As Joe said later, "'Model Department' was the wrong name; Walt called it his think tank."[3] Teamed with Dick Huemer, Grant cowrote *Dumbo*, the "Baby Weems" segment of *The Reluctant Dragon*, and an uncredited early version of *Lady and the Tramp*. Grant said he looked at *Make Mine Music* as a *Fantasia* for the common man.

DAVE HAND

See Chapter 3.

JIM HANDLEY (WITH HAM LUSKE)

Mainly an assistant director for Ham Luske, Handley is credited as codirecting Beethoven's Pastoral Symphony in *Fantasia*. He also assisted Jack King as he directed *Donald's Golf Game*.

JACK HANNAH

See Chapter 8.

T. HEE

Born March 26, 1911, Hee directed "Dance of the Hours" in *Fantasia*. A brilliant designer and caricaturist, he was evidently seen as a somewhat stubborn character by Walt, who fired and rehired Hee several times throughout his career. He later taught at the California Institute of the Arts and died October 30, 1988. He was honored with a Winsor McCay Award in 1981.

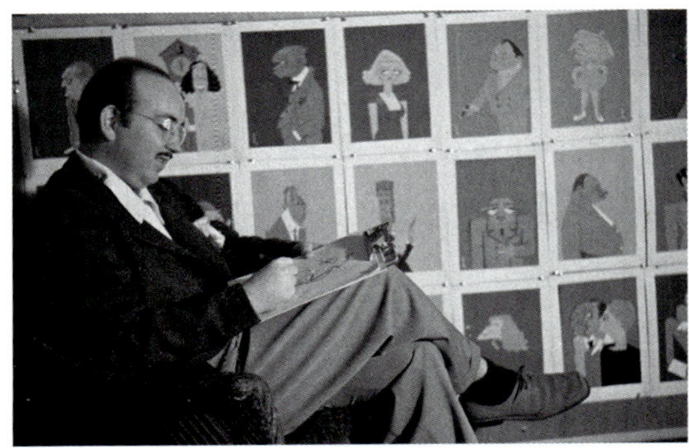

GRAHAM HEID (WITH SAM ARMSTRONG)

Heid described himself as "neither an artist nor a cartoonist, so animation was really not very interesting to me."[4] Nevertheless, Graham Heid is credited as a codirector on *The Old Mill* with Wilfred Jackson. He assisted for Jaxon on *Pinocchio* and Sam Armstrong on the "The Nutcracker Suite" section of *Fantasia*, then codirected the "Raindrop" sequence of *Bambi* with Sam Armstrong. He left the studio to become involved in World War II training films. He wrote and directed for independent producers in Hollywood, produced and directed medical films for the U.S. Public Health Service in Atlanta, and retired in 1971. (See also Chapter 8.)

JOHN HENCH

Later a master designer for the theme parks, Hench served as sequence director for the prologue to *Cinderella*. Hench won a Disney Legends Award in 1990 and a Winsor McCay Award in 2003.

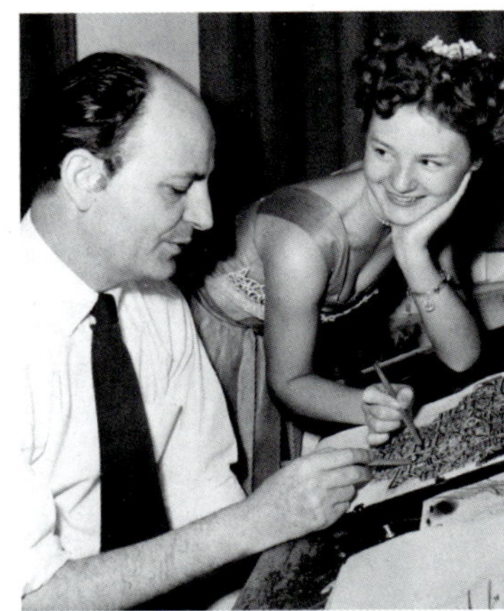

DICK HUEMER

A true animation pioneer, Huemer started his career as an animator in New York in 1916. Once at Disney he branched out as a story artist and idea man, famously partnering with Joe Grant to select music for *Fantasia* and write the story for *Dumbo* until Disney split up the team. Prior to that. Huemer directed *The Whalers* (credited with Dave Hand) and *Goofy and Wilbur*. He described directing as "the most fun of anything I did."[5] He received a Winsor McCay Award in 1978 and a Disney Legends Award posthumously in 2007.

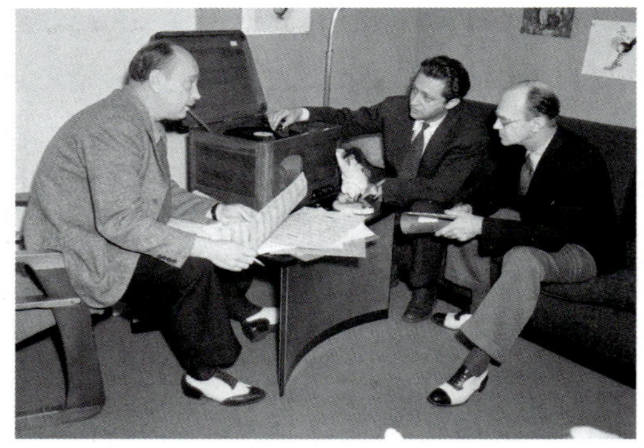

LEFT TO RIGHT: Dick Huemer, Joe Grant, and Deems Taylor discuss musical details for *Fantasia*.

UB IWERKS

See Chapter 1.

WILFRED JACKSON

See Chapter 5.

WARD KIMBALL

The Rest of the Nine Old Men. (See Sidebar Page 256.)

JACK KING

See Chapter 8.

JACK KINNEY

See Chapter 8.

ERIC LARSON

The Rest of the Nine Old Men. (See Sidebar Page 256.)

DICK LUNDY

Primarily a story artist, Lundy directed nine Donald Duck shorts. (See Chapter 8.)

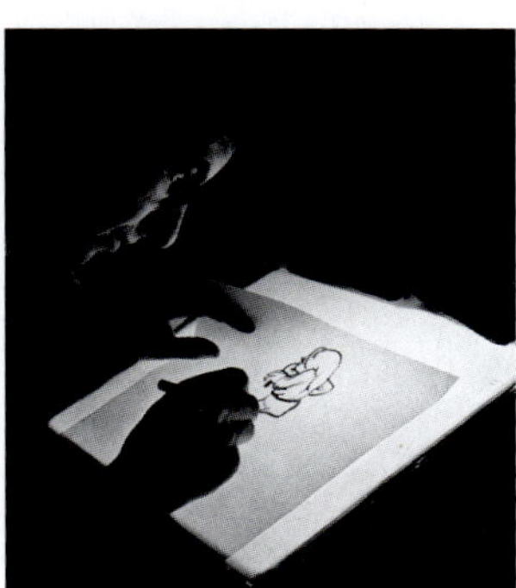

HAM LUSKE

See Chapter 6.

LARRY MOREY

Born in Los Angeles March 26, 1905, Morey worked in vaudeville as an actor and a gag man at Warner Bros. before starting at Disney on November 1, 1933. Working in the story department, Morey wrote a number of lyrics for songs, including "Heigh-Ho" and "Whistle While You Work" from *Snow White*, "You're Nothin' But a Nothin'" from *The Flying Mouse*, "The World Owes Me a Living" from *The Grasshopper and the Ants*, and *Ferdinand the Bull*. Morey became a sequence director on *Snow White*, directing the musical sequences for which he'd written lyrics. Morey next moved into story on *Bambi*, where he wrote "Little April Shower" with Frank Churchill. After writing songs (with Charles Wolcott) for *The Reluctant Dragon*, he left the studio in May 1942. Rehired in April 1947, he wrote lyrics for *So Dear to My Heart* and *The Adventures of Ichabod and Mr. Toad*. Morey left the studio again in September 1947 and died in 1971.

NICK NICHOLS

See Chapter 8.

GAIL PAPINEAU

Papineau was a nephew of Lillian Disney's. Walt wrote in an August 1933 letter, "Everyone seems to like [Gail] and he is working hard. Some day he will probably be a good cameraman." Indeed he was, expanding into the special effects department, where he created mechanical effects for *Fantasia*, and becoming a sequence director on the "Trip through Space" and "Volcanoes" sections of the "Rite of Spring" segment. Later he worked as a technical adviser on *The Three Caballeros*. Despite his relationship, Walt didn't play favorites when salaries or employment was at stake, according to production manager Harry Tytle,[6] and Papineau eventually moved on to Kling Enterprises and then became president of La Brea Productions, both of which produced live-action commercial and industrial films.

PERCE PEARCE

See Sidebar in Chapter 3.

WOOLIE REITHERMAN

See Chapter 9.

RICHARD "DICK" RICKARD

See Chapter 8.

BILL ROBERTS

See Sidebar in Chapter 3.

PAUL MCKINLEY SATTERFIELD

A self-described "mountain hoosier," Satterfield was born March 27, 1896, in Dahlonega, Georgia. Working as a freelance cartoonist, animator, and industrial filmmaker, he was hired at Disney's in 1936 on recommendation from Bill Roberts, with whom he'd worked with at Wallace Carlson's studio in Chicago. At Disney's, Satterfield worked briefly as an effects animator, a character designer in Joe Grant's Model Department (where he designed Cleo for *Pinocchio*), and an assistant director. He directed the "Buck Fight" and "Forest Fire" sequences in *Bambi*, as well as the "Rite of Spring" "Earthquake" sequence of *Fantasia* under Bill Roberts. Layout artist McLaren Stewart remembered Satterfield as working under Bill Roberts. "Bill was the director, but Satterfield was assigned the whole opening section, with all the effects of the creation of the world, and the lava, and all that business."[7] In a 1977 interview with Milt Grey, Satterfield recalled Walt's advice to him as a new director: "You don't have to have 'captain' written across your shirt." After the strike in 1941, Satterfield was one of a group of nonstrikers laid off in an agreement with the new union. He opened a small title and industrial film company in Hollywood, and died on August 14, 1981

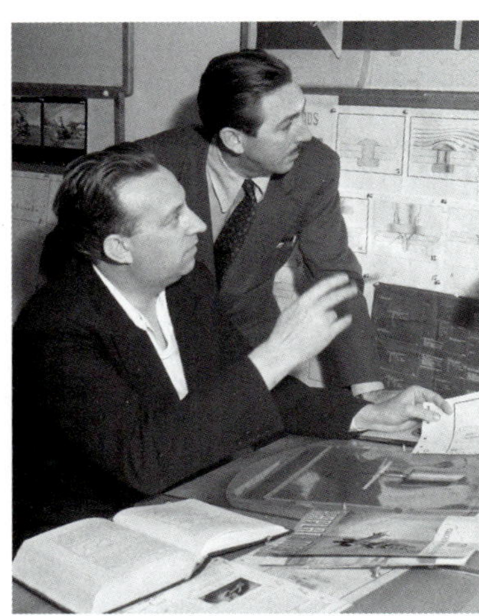

MILTON "MILT" SCHAFFER

Milt started as an assistant animator at Disney's in 1934 and became an animator in 1936 before moving to the story department in 1937. He left the studio to work with Walter Lantz, where he directed Woody Woodpecker (1943), but returned to animate at Disney's in 1947. His one directing credit is *Pluto's Party* (1952). He later did story work at Storyboard, Inc., and De Patie-Freleng and died in March 1993.

BEN SHARPSTEEN

See Chapter 4.

RILEY THOMSON

See Chapter 8.

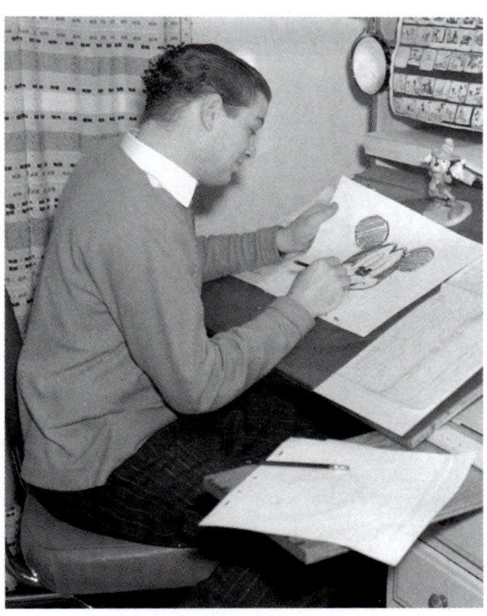

NORMAN WRIGHT

Born in 1910 and educated at USC, Wright started his career at Disney's as an assistant director for a number of Donald shorts in the early forties. After some story development on "The Nutcracker Suite" for *Fantasia*, Wright became a sequence director on *Bambi*, working on both comedic and dramatic sequences: "Owl Tells Kids About Love," "Thumper and Flower Fall in Love," "Bambi and Faline Fall in Love," "Two Winds," "The Drive," "Bambi Rescues Faline from Hounds," and "Introduction to Man." He left Disney's in the late forties or early fifties and produced and directed various documentary shorts, as well as wrote his own children's book, *Chip, Chip*. Wright died in August 2001.

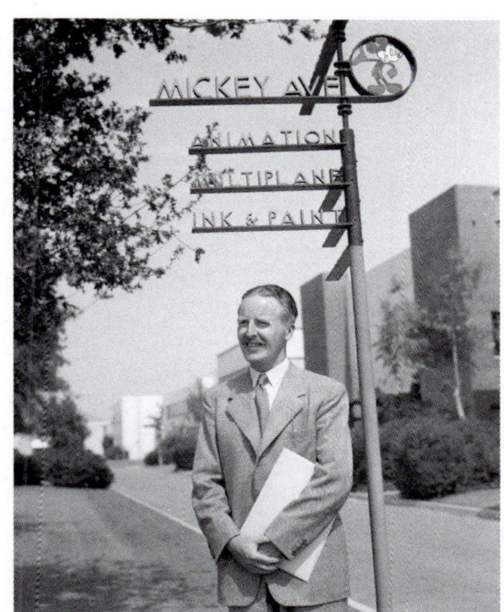

APPENDIX B

DISNEY ANIMATED FILMS BY YEAR AND DIRECTOR

In compiling a list of directors for shorts, featurettes, and feature films, using the lists of different historians and different sources can sometimes lead to disagreements concerning directorial credits. For instance, while studio sources credit Wilfred Jackson with directing *Mickey's Follies* (1929) and *Midnight in the Toy Shop* (1930), he insisted that his directorial debut was on *The Castaway* (1931). Even titles differ by source. In *Walt Disney's Silly Symphonies*, Russell Merritt and J. B. Kaufman prefer the title *The Cat's Nightmare* for *The Cat's Out* (1931). They also credit Dave Hand as a codirector with Wilfred Jackson on *The Country Cousin* (1936), indicating that Hand was originally assigned the short but was replaced by Jackson. The 1930 short *Fiddling Around* has an alternate title of *Just Mickey*. The following list is our best effort at compiling a complete and accurate record.

1928

Steamboat Willie (Short) **Walt Disney**
The Gallopin' Gaucho (Short) **Walt Disney**

1929

The Barn Dance (Short) **Walt Disney**
Plane Crazy (Short) **Walt Disney**
The Opry House (Short) **Walt Disney**
When the Cat's Away (Short) **Walt Disney**
The Barnyard Battle (Short) **Walt Disney**
The Plow Boy (Short) **Walt Disney**
The Karnival Kid (Short) **Walt Disney**
The Skeleton Dance (Short) **Walt Disney**
Mickey's Follies (Short) **Wilfred Jackson**
El Terrible Toreador (Short) **Walt Disney**
Mickey's Choo-Choo (Short) **Walt Disney**
The Jazz Fool (Short) **Walt Disney**
Springtime (Short) **Ub Iwerks**
Hell's Bells (Short) **Ub Iwerks**
Jungle Rhythm (Short) **Walt Disney**
The Haunted House (Short) **Walt Disney**
The Merry Dwarfs (Short) **Walt Disney**
Wild Waves (Short) **Burt Gillett**

1930

Summer (Short) **Ub Iwerks**
Autumn (Short) **Ub Iwerks**
Cannibal Capers (Short) **Burt Gillett**
Fiddling Around (Short) **Walt Disney**
The Barnyard Concert (Short) **Walt Disney**
Night (Short) **Walt Disney**
Frolicking Fish (Short) **Burt Gillett**
The Cactus Kid (Short) **Walt Disney**
Arctic Antics (Short) **Burt Gillett**
The Fire Fighters (Short) **Burt Gillett**
The Shindig (Short) **Burt Gillett**
Midnight in the Toy Shop (Short) **Wilfred Jackson**
The Chain Gang (Short) **Burt Gillett**
Monkey Melodies (Short) **Burt Gillett**
The Gorilla Mystery (Short) **Burt Gillett**
The Picnic (Short) **Burt Gillett**
Winter (Short) **Burt Gillett**
Pioneer Days (Short) **Burt Gillett**
Playful Pan (Short) **Burt Gillett**

1931

The Birthday Party (Short) **Burt Gillett**
Birds of a Feather (Short) **Burt Gillett**
Traffic Troubles (Short) **Burt Gillett**
The Castaway (Short) **Wilfred Jackson**
Mother Goose Melodies (Short) **Burt Gillett**
The Moose Hunt (Short) **Burt Gillett**
The China Plate (Short) **Wilfred Jackson**
The Delivery Boy (Short) **Burt Gillett**
The Busy Beavers (Short) **Burt Gillett**
Mickey Steps Out (Short) **Burt Gillett**

***Associate producer *Cartoon Director *Directing Animator * Director *Producer *Producer; Director *Production Supervisor *Sequence Director *Supervising Director *Story; Director**

Academy Award Winner

The Cat's Out (Short) **Wilfred Jackson**
Blue Rhythm (Short) **Burt Gillett**
Egyptian Melodies (Short) **Wilfred Jackson**
Fishin' Around (Short) **Burt Gillett**
The Clock Store (Short) **Wilfred Jackson**
The Barnyard Broadcast (Short) **Burt Gillett**
The Spider and the Fly (Short) **Wilfred Jackson**
The Beach Party (Short) **Burt Gillett**
The Fox Hunt (Short) **Wilfred Jackson**
Mickey Cuts Up (Short) **Burt Gillett**
Mickey's Orphans (Short) **Burt Gillett**
The Ugly Duckling (Short) **Wilfred Jackson**

1932

The Bird Store (Short) **Wilfred Jackson**
The Duck Hunt (Short) **Burt Gillett**
The Grocery Boy (Short) **Wilfred Jackson**
The Mad Dog (Short) **Burt Gillett**
Barnyard Olympics (Short) **Wilfred Jackson**
Mickey's Revue (Short) **Wilfred Jackson**
Musical Farmer (Short) **Wilfred Jackson**
The Bears and the Bees (Short) **Wilfred Jackson**
Mickey in Arabia (Short) **Wilfred Jackson**
Just Dogs (Short) **Burt Gillett**
Flowers and Trees (Short) **Burt Gillett**
Mickey's Nightmare (Short) **Burt Gillett**
Trader Mickey (Short) **Dave Hand**
King Neptune (Short) **Burt Gillett**
The Whoopee Party (Short) **Wilfred Jackson**
Bugs in Love (Short) **Burt Gillett**
Touchdown Mickey (Short) **Wilfred Jackson**
The Klondike Kid (Short) **Wilfred Jackson**
The Wayward Canary (Short) **Burt Gillett**
Babes in the Woods (Short) **Burt Gillett**
Santa's Workshop (Short) **Wilfred Jackson**
Mickey's Good Deed (Short) **Burt Gillett**

1933

Building a Building (Short) **Dave Hand**
The Mad Doctor (Short) **Dave Hand**
Mickey's Pal Pluto (Short) **Burt Gillett**
Birds in the Spring (Short) **Dave Hand**
Mickey's Mellerdrammer (Short) **Wilfred Jackson**
Ye Olden Days (Short) **Burt Gillett**
Father Noah's Ark (Short) **Wilfred Jackson**
Three Little Pigs (Short) **Burt Gillett**
The Mail Pilot (Short) **Dave Hand**
Mickey's Mechanical Man (Short) **Wilfred Jackson**
Mickey's Gala Premiere (Short) **Burt Gillett**
Old King Cole (Short) **Dave Hand**
Lullaby Land (Short) **Wilfred Jackson**
Puppy Love (Short) **Wilfred Jackson**
The Pied Piper (Short) **Wilfred Jackson**
The Steeplechase (Short) **Burt Gillett**
The Pet Store (Short) **Wilfred Jackson**
Giantland (Short) **Burt Gillett**
The Night Before Christmas (Short) **Wilfred Jackson**

1934

The China Shop (Short) **Wilfred Jackson**
Shanghaied (Short) **Burt Gillett**
The Grasshopper and the Ants (Short) **Wilfred Jackson**
Camping Out (Short) **Dave Hand**
Playful Pluto (Short) **Burt Gillett**
Funny Little Bunnies (Short) **Wilfred Jackson**
The Big Bad Wolf (Short) **Burt Gillett**
Gulliver Mickey (Short) **Burt Gillett**
The Wise Little Hen (Short) **Wilfred Jackson**
Mickey's Steam-Roller (Short) **Dave Hand**
The Flying Mouse (Short) **Dave Hand**
Orphan's Benefit (Short) **Burt Gillett**
Peculiar Penguins (Short) **Wilfred Jackson**
Mickey Plays Papa (Short) **Burt Gillett**
The Goddess of Spring (Short) **Wilfred Jackson**

***Associate producer *Cartoon Director *Directing Animator * Director *Producer *Producer; Director *Production Supervisor *Sequence Director *Supervising Director *Story; Director**

[highlight] Academy Award Winner

The Dognapper (Short) **Dave Hand**
Two-Gun Mickey (Short) **Ben Sharpsteen**

1935

The Tortoise and the Hare (Short) **Wilfred Jackson**
Mickey's Man Friday (Short) **Dave Hand**
The Band Concert (Short) **Wilfred Jackson**
Mickey's Service Station (Short) **Ben Sharpsteen**
The Golden Touch (Short) **Walt Disney**
Mickey's Kangaroo (Short) **Dave Hand**
The Robber Kitten (Short) **Dave Hand**
Water Babies (Short) **Wilfred Jackson**
The Cookie Carnival (Short) **Ben Sharpsteen**
Who Killed Cock Robin? (Short) **Dave Hand**
Mickey's Garden (Short) **Wilfred Jackson**
Mickey's Fire Brigade (Short) **Ben Sharpsteen**
Pluto's Judgement Day (Short) **Dave Hand**
On Ice (Short) **Ben Sharpsteen**
Music Land (Short) **Wilfred Jackson**
Three Orphan Kittens (Short) **Dave Hand**
Cock O' the Walk (Short) **Ben Sharpsteen**
Broken Toys (Short) **Ben Sharpsteen**

1936

Mickey's Polo Team (Short) **Dave Hand**
Orphans' Picnic (Short) **Ben Sharpsteen**
Mickey's Grand Opera (Short) **Wilfred Jackson**
Elmer Elephant (Short) **Wilfred Jackson**
Three Little Wolves (Short) **Dave Hand**
Thru the Mirror (Short) **Dave Hand**
Mickey's Rival (Short) **Wilfred Jackson**
Moving Day (Short) **Ben Sharpsteen**
Alpine Climbers (Short) **Dave Hand**
Mickey's Circus (Short) **Ben Sharpsteen**
Toby Tortoise Returns (Short) **Wilfred Jackson**
Donald and Pluto (Short) **Ben Sharpsteen**
The Three Blind Musketeers (Short) **Dave Hand**
Mickey's Elephant (Short) **Dave Hand**
The Country Cousin (Short) **Wilfred Jackson**
Mother Pluto (Short) **Wilfred Jackson**
More Kittens (Short) **Dave Hand**

1937

The Worm Turns (Short) **Ben Sharpsteen**
Don Donald (Short) **Ben Sharpsteen**
Magician Mickey (Short) **Dave Hand**
Moose Hunters (Short) **Ben Sharpsteen**
Woodland Café (Short) **Wilfred Jackson**
Mickey's Amateurs (Short) **Pinto Colvig**
Mickey's Amateurs (Short) **Erdman "Ed" Penner**
Mickey's Amateurs (Short) **Walt Pfeiffer**
Little Hiawatha (Short) **Dave Hand**
Modern Inventions (Short) Jack King
Hawaiian Holiday (Short) **Ben Sharpsteen**
Clock Cleaners (Short) **Ben Sharpsteen**
The Old Mill (Short) **Wilfred Jackson**
The Old Mill (Short) **Graham Heid**
Pluto's Quin-Puplets (Short) **Ben Sharpsteen**
Donald's Ostrich (Short) **Jack King**
Lonesome Ghosts (Short) **Burt Gillett**
The Moth and the Flame (Short) **Burt Gillett**
Snow White and the Seven Dwarfs (Feature) **Dave Hand**
Snow White and the Seven Dwarfs (Feature) **Bill Cottrell**
Snow White and the Seven Dwarfs (Feature) **Wilfred Jackson**
Snow White and the Seven Dwarfs (Feature) **Larry Morey**
Snow White and the Seven Dwarfs (Feature) **Perce Pearce**
Snow White and the Seven Dwarfs (Feature) **Ben Sharpsteen**

***Associate producer *Cartoon Director *Directing Animator * Director *Producer *Producer; Director *Production Supervisor *Sequence Director *Supervising Director *Story; Director**

Academy Award Winner

1938

Self Control (Short) **Jack King**
Boat Builders (Short) **Ben Sharpsteen**
Donald's Better Self (Short) **Jack King**
Donald's Nephew (Short) **Jack King**
Mickey's Trailer (Short) **Ben Sharpsteen**
Wynken, Blynken, and Nod (Short) **Graham Heid**
Polar Trappers (Short) **Ben Sharpsteen**
Good Scouts (Short) **Jack King**
The Fox Hunt (Short) **Ben Sharpsteen**
The Whalers (Short) **Dick Huemer**
Mickey's Parrot (Short) **Bill Roberts**
Brave Little Tailor (Short) **Bill Roberts**
Farmyard Symphony (Short) **Jack Cutting**
Donald's Golf Game (Short) **Jack King**
Ferdinand the Bull (Short) **Dick Rickard**
Merbabies (Short) **Rudolf Ising**
Mother Goose Goes Hollywood (Short) **Wilfred Jackson**

1939

Donald's Lucky Day (Short) **Jack King**
Society Dog Show (Short) **Bill Roberts**
Mickey's Surprise Party (Short) **Ham Luske**
The Practical Pig (Short) **Dick Rickard**
Goofy and Wilbur (Short) **Dick Huemer**
The Ugly Duckling (Short) **Jack Cutting**
The Ugly Duckling (Short) **Ham Luske**
The Hockey Champ (Short) **Jack King**
Donald's Cousin Gus (Short) **Jack King**
Beach Picnic (Short) **Clyde "Gerry" Geronimi**
Sea Scouts (Short) **Dick Lundy**
The Pointer (Short) **Clyde "Gerry" Geronimi**
Donald's Penguin (Short) **Jack King**
The Autograph Hound (Short) **Jack King**
Officer Duck (Short) **Clyde "Gerry" Geronimi**

1940

The Riveter (Short) **Dick Lundy**
Donald's Dog Laundry (Short) **Jack King**
Tugboat Mickey (Short) **Clyde "Gerry" Geronimi**
Billposters (Short) **Clyde "Gerry" Geronimi**
Mr. Duck Steps Out (Short) **Jack King**
Bone Trouble (Short) **Jack Kinney**
Put-Put Troubles (Short) **Riley Thomson**
Donald's Vacation (Short) **Jack King**
Pluto's Dream House (Short) **Clyde "Gerry" Geronimi**
Window Cleaners (Short) **Jack King**
Mr. Mouse Takes a Trip (Short) **Clyde "Gerry" Geronimi**
Goofy's Glider (Short) Jack Kinney
Fire Chief (Short) Jack King
Pantry Pirate (Short) **Clyde "Gerry" Geronimi**
Pinocchio (Feature) **Ben Sharpsteen**
Pinocchio (Feature) **Ham Luske**
Pinocchio (Feature) **Norm Ferguson**
Pinocchio (Feature) **Thornton "T." Hee**
Pinocchio (Feature) **Wilfred Jackson**
Pinocchio (Feature) **Jack Kinney**
Pinocchio (Feature) **Bill Roberts**
Fantasia (Feature) **Ben Sharpsteen**
Fantasia (Feature) **Jim Algar**
Fantasia (Feature) **Sam Armstrong**
Fantasia (Feature) **Ford Beebe, Jr.**
Fantasia (Feature) **Norm Ferguson**
Fantasia (Feature) **Jim Handley**
Fantasia (Feature) **Thornton "T." Hee**
Fantasia (Feature) **Wilfred Jackson**
Fantasia (Feature) **Ham Luske**
Fantasia (Feature) **Bill Roberts**
Fantasia (Feature) **Paul Satterfield**

1941

Timber (Short) **Jack King**
Pluto's Playmate (Short) **Norm Ferguson**
The Little Whirlwind (Short) **Riley Thomson**

***Associate producer *Cartoon Director *Directing Animator * Director *Producer *Producer; Director *Production Supervisor *Sequence Director *Supervising Director *Story; Director**

Academy Award Winner

Golden Eggs (Short) **Wilfred Jackson**
A Gentlemen's Gentlemen (Short) **Clyde "Gerry" Geronimi**
Baggage Buster (Short) **Jack Kinney**
A Good Time for a Dime (Short) **Dick Lundy**
Canine Caddy (Short) **Clyde "Gerry" Geronimi**
The Nifty Nineties (Short) **Riley Thomson**
Early to Bed (Short) **Jack King**
Truant Officer Donald (Short) **Jack King**
Orphan's Benefit (Short) **Riley Thomson**
Old Mac Donald Duck (Short) **Jack King**
Lend a Paw (Short) **Clyde "Gerry" Geronimi**
Donald's Camera (Short) **Dick Lundy**
The Art of Skiing (Short) **Jack Kinney**
Chef Donald (Short) **Jack King**
The Art of Self Defense (Short) **Jack Kinney**
Dumbo (Feature) **Ben Sharpsteen**
Dumbo (Feature) **Sam Armstrong**
Dumbo (Feature) **Norm Ferguson**
Dumbo (Feature) **Wilfred Jackson**
Dumbo (Feature) **Jack Kinney**
Dumbo (Feature) **Bill Roberts**

1942

The Village Smithy (Short) **Dick Lundy**
The New Spirit (Short) **Wilfred Jackson**
The New Spirit (Short) **Ben Sharpsteen**
Mickey's Birthday Party (Short) **Riley Thomson**
Pluto, Junior (Short) **Clyde "Gerry" Geronimi**
Symphony Hour (Short) **Riley Thomson**
Donald's Snow Fight (Short) **Jack King**
Donald Gets Drafted (Short) **Jack King**
The Army Mascot (Short) **Clyde "Gerry" Geronimi**
Donald's Garden (Short) **Dick Lundy**
The Sleepwalker (Short) **Clyde "Gerry" Geronimi**
Donald's Gold Mine (Short) **Dick Lundy**
T-Bone for Two (Short) **Clyde "Gerry" Geronimi**
How to Play Baseball (Short) **Jack Kinney**
The Vanishing Pirate (Short) **Jack King**
The Olympic Champ (Short) **Jack Kinney**
How to Swim (Short) **Jack Kinney**
Sky Trooper (Short) **Jack King**
Pluto at the Zoo (Short) **Clyde "Gerry" Geronimi**
How to Fish (Short) **Jack Kinney**
Bellboy Donald (Short) **Jack King**
Bambi (Feature) **Dave Hand**
Bambi (Feature) **Jim Algar**
Bambi (Feature) **Sam Armstrong**
Bambi (Feature) **Graham Heid**
Bambi (Feature) **Bill Roberts**
Bambi (Feature) **Paul Satterfield**
Bambi (Feature) **Norman Wright**
Saludos Amigos (Feature) **Norm Ferguson**
Saludos Amigos (Feature) **Jack Kinney**
Saludos Amigos (Feature) **Ham Luske**
Saludos Amigos (Feature) **Wilfred Jackson**
Saludos Amigos (Feature) **Bill Roberts**

1943

Der Fuehrer's Face (Short) **Jack Kinney**
The Spirit of '43 (Short) **Jack King**
Education for Death (Victory) **Clyde "Gerry" Geronimi**
Donald's Tire Trouble (Short) **Dick Lundy**
Pluto and the Armadillo (Short) **Clyde "Gerry" Geronimi**
The Flying Jalopy (Short) **Dick Lundy**
Private Pluto (Short) **Clyde "Gerry" Geronimi**
Fall Out Fall In (Short) **Jack King**
Victory Vehicles (Short) **Jack Kinney**
Reason and Emotion (Short) **Bill Roberts**
Figaro and Cleo (Short) **Jack Kinney**
The Old Army Game (Short) **Jack King**
Home Defense (Short) **Jack King**
Chicken Little (Short) **Clyde "Gerry" Geronimi**

***Associate producer *Cartoon Director *Directing Animator * Director *Producer *Producer; Director *Production Supervisor *Sequence Director *Supervising Director *Story; Director**

Academy Award Winner

Victory Through Air Power (Feature) Jim Algar
Victory Through Air Power (Feature) Clyde "Gerry" Geronimi
Victory Through Air Power (Feature) Jack Kinney

1944

The Pelican and the Snipe (Short) Ham Luske
How to be a Sailor (Short story) Jack Kinney
Trombone Trouble (Short) Jack King
How to Play Golf (Short story) Jack Kinney
Donald Duck and the Gorilla (Short) Jack King
Contrary Condor (Short) Jack King
Commando Donald (Short) Jack King
Springtime for Pluto (Short) Charles "Nick" Nichols
The Plastic Inventor (Short) Jack King
How to Play Football (Short) Jack Kinney
First Aiders (Short) Charles "Nick" Nichols
Donald's Day Off (Short) Jack Hannah
The Three Caballeros (Feature) Norm Ferguson
The Three Caballeros (Feature) Clyde "Gerry" Geronimi
The Three Caballeros (Feature) Jack Kinney
The Three Caballeros (Feature) Bill Roberts

1945

Tiger Trouble (Short) Jack Kinney
The Clock Watcher (Short) Jack King
Dog Watch (Short) Charles "Nick" Nichols
The Eyes Have It (Short) Jack Hannah
African Diary (Short) Jack Kinney
Donald's Crime (Short) Jack King
Californy 'er Bust (Short) Jack Kinney
Canine Casanova (Short) Charles "Nick" Nichols
Duck Pimples (Short) Jack Kinney
The Legend of Coyote Rock (Short) Charles "Nick" Nichols
No Sail (Short) Jack Hannah
Hockey Homicide (Short) Jack Kinney
Cured Duck (Short) Jack King
Canine Patrol (Short) Charles "Nick" Nichols

1946

A Knight for a Day (Short) Jack Hannah
Pluto's Kid Brother (Short) Charles "Nick" Nichols
In Dutch (Short) Charles "Nick" Nichols
Squatter's Rights (Short) Jack Hannah
Donald's Double Trouble (Short) Jack King
The Purloined Pup (Short) Charles "Nick" Nichols
A Feather in his Collar (Commercial) Charles "Nick" Nichols
Wet Paint (Short) Jack King
Dumbbell of the Yukon (Short) Jack King
Lighthouse Keeping (Short) Jack Hannah
Bath Day (Short) Charles "Nick" Nichols
Double Dribble (Short) Jack Hannah
Song of the South (Feature) Wilfred Jackson
Make Mine Music (Feature) Joe Grant
Make Mine Music (Feature) Bob Cormack
Make Mine Music (Feature) Clyde "Gerry" Geronimi
Make Mine Music (Feature) Jack Kinney
Make Mine Music (Feature) Ham Luske
Make Mine Music (Feature) Josh Meador

1947

Pluto's Housewarming (Short) Charles "Nick" Nichols
Rescue Dog (Short) Charles "Nick" Nichols
Straight Shooters (Short) Jack Hannah
Sleepy Time Donald (Short) Jack King
Figaro and Frankie (Short) Charles "Nick" Nichols
Clown of the Jungle (Short) Jack Hannah
Donald's Dilemma (Short) Jack King
Crazy With The Heat (Short) Bob Carlson

*Associate producer *Cartoon Director *Directing Animator * Director *Producer *Producer; Director *Production Supervisor *Sequence Director *Supervising Director *Story; Director

Academy Award Winner

Bootle Beetle (Short) **Jack Hannah**
Wide Open Spaces (Short) **Jack King**
Mickey's Delayed Date (Short) **Charles "Nick" Nichols**
Foul Hunting (Short) **Jack Hannah**
Mail Dog (Short) **Charles "Nick" Nichols**
Chip 'N Dale (Short) **Jack Hannah**
Pluto's Blue Note (Short) **Charles "Nick" Nichols**
Fun and Fancy Free (Feature) **Ben Sharpsteen**
Fun and Fancy Free (Feature) **Jack Kinney**
Fun and Fancy Free (Feature) **Ham Luske**
Fun and Fancy Free (Feature) **Bill Roberts**

1948

They're Off (Short) **Jack Hannah**
The Big Wash (Short) **Clyde "Gerry" Geronimi**
Drip Dippy Donald (Short) **Jack King**
Mickey Down Under (Short) **Charles "Nick" Nichols**
Daddy Duck (Short) **Jack Hannah**
Bone Bandit (Short) **Charles "Nick" Nichols**
Donald's Dream Voice (Short) **Jack King**
Pluto's Purchase (Short) **Charles "Nick" Nichols**
The Trial of Donald Duck (Short) **Jack King**
Cat Nap Pluto (Short) **Charles "Nick" Nichols**
Inferior Decorator (Short) **Jack Hannah**
Pluto's Fledgling (Short) **Charles "Nick" Nichols**
Soup's On (Short) **Jack Hannah**
Three for Breakfast (Short) **Jack Hannah**
Mickey and the Seal (Short) **Charles "Nick" Nichols**
Tea for Two Hundred (Short) **Jack Hannah**
Melody Time (Feature) **Ben Sharpsteen**
Melody Time (Feature) **Clyde "Gerry" Geronimi**
Melody Time (Feature) **Wilfred Jackson**
Melody Time (Feature) **Jack Kinney**
Melody Time (Feature) **Ham Luske**

1949

Pueblo Pluto (Short) **Charles "Nick" Nichols**
Donald's Happy Birthday (Short) **Jack Hannah**
Pluto's Surprise Package (Short) **Charles "Nick" Nichols**
Sea Salts (Short) **Jack Hannah**
Pluto's Sweater (Short) **Charles "Nick" Nichols**
Winter Storage (Short) **Jack Hannah**
Bubble Bee (Short) **Charles "Nick" Nichols**
Honey Harvester (Short) **Jack Hannah**
Tennis Racket (Short) **Jack Kinney**
All in a Nutshell (Short) **Jack Hannah**
Goofy Gymnastics (Short) **Jack Kinney**
The Greener Yard (Short) **Jack Hannah**
Sheep Dog (Short) **Charles "Nick" Nichols**
Slide, Donald, Slide (Short) **Jack Hannah**
Toy Tinkers (Short) **Jack Hannah**
The Adventures of Ichabod and Mr. Toad (Feature) **Ben Sharpsteen**
The Adventures of Ichabod and Mr. Toad (Feature) **Jim Algar**
The Adventures of Ichabod and Mr. Toad (Feature) **Clyde "Gerry" Geronimi**
The Adventures of Ichabod and Mr. Toad (Feature) **Jack Kinney**
So Dear To My Heart (Feature) **Ham Luske**

1950

Pluto's Heart Throb (Short) **Charles "Nick" Nichols**
Lion Around (Short) **Jack Hannah**
Pluto and the Gopher (Short) **Charles "Nick" Nichols**
The Brave Engineer (Short) **Jack Kinney**
Crazy over Daisy (Short) **Jack Hannah**
Wonder Dog (Short) **Charles "Nick" Nichols**
Trailer Horn (Short) **Jack Hannah**
Primitive Pluto (Short) **Charles "Nick" Nichols**
Puss-Café (Short) **Charles "Nick" Nichols**
Motor Mania (Short) **Jack Kinney**

***Associate producer *Cartoon Director *Directing Animator * Director *Producer *Producer; Director *Production Supervisor *Sequence Director *Supervising Director *Story; Director**

Academy Award Winner

Pests of the West (Short) **Charles "Nick" Nichols**
Food for Feudin' (Short) **Charles "Nick" Nichols**
Hook, Lion & Sinker (Short) **Jack Hannah**
Camp Dog (Short) **Charles "Nick" Nichols**
Bee at the Beach (Short) **Jack Hannah**
Hold that Pose (Short) **Jack Kinney**
Morris the Midget Moose (Short) **Jack Hannah**
Out on a Limb (Short) **Jack Hannah**
Cinderella (Feature) **Ben Sharpsteen**
Cinderella (Feature) **Clyde "Gerry" Geronimi**
Cinderella (Feature) **Wilfred Jackson**
Cinderella (Feature) **Ham Luske**

1951

Lion Down (Short) **Jack Kinney**
Chicken in the Rough (Short) **Jack Hannah**
Cold Storage (Short) **Jack Kinney**
Dude Duck (Short) **Jack Hannah**
Home Made Home (Short) **Jack Kinney**
Corn Chips (Short) **Jack Hannah**
Cold War (Short) **Jack Kinney**
Plutopia (Short) **Charles "Nick" Nichols**
Test Pilot Donald (Short) **Jack Hannah**
Tomorrow We Diet (Short) **Jack Kinney**
Lucky Number (Short) **Jack Hannah**
R'Coon Dawg (Short) **Charles "Nick" Nichols**
Get Rich Quick (Short) **Jack Kinney**
Cold Turkey (Short) **Charles "Nick" Nichols**
Fathers Are People (Short) **Jack Kinney**
Out of Scale (Short) **Jack Hannah**
No Smoking (Short) **Jack Kinney**
Bee On Guard (Short) **Jack Hannah**
Alice in Wonderland (Feature) **Ben Sharpsteen**
Alice in Wonderland (Feature) **Clyde "Gerry" Geronimi**
Alice in Wonderland (Feature) **Wilfred Jackson**
Alice in Wonderland (Feature) **Ham Luske**

1952

Father's Lion (Short) **Jack Kinney**
Donald Applecore (Short) **Jack Hannah**
Lambert, The Sheepish Lion (Short) **Jack Hannah**
Hello Aloha (Short) **Jack Kinney**
Two Chips 'N a Miss (Short) **Jack Hannah**
Man's Best Friend (Short) **Jack Kinney**
Let's Stick Together (Short) **Jack Hannah**
Two Gun Goofy (Short) **Jack Kinney**
Susie the Little Blue Coupe (Short) **Clyde "Gerry" Geronimi**
Teachers are People (Short) **Jack Kinney**
Uncle Donald's Ants (Short) **Jack Hannah**
The Little House (Short) **Wilfred Jackson**
Pluto's Party (Short) **Milt Schaffer**
Trick or Treat (Short) **Jack Hannah**
Two Weeks Vacation (Short) **Jack Kinney**
Pluto's Christmas Tree (Short) **Jack Hannah**
How to be a Detective (Short) **Jack Kinney**

1953

Father's Day Off (Short) **Jack Kinney**
The Simple Things (Short) **Charles "Nick" Nichols**
For Whom the Bulls Toil (Short) **Jack Kinney**
Melody (Short) **Ward Kimball**
Melody (Short) **Charles "Nick" Nichols**
Don's Fountain of Youth (Short) **Jack Hannah**
Father's Week End (Short) **Jack Kinney**
How to Dance (Short) **Jack Kinney**
The New Neighbor (Short) **Jack Hannah**
Football Now and Then (Short) **Jack Kinney**
Rugged Bear (Short) **Jack Hannah**
Toot, Whistle, Plunk and Boom (Short) **Ward Kimball**
Toot, Whistle, Plunk and Boom (Short) **Charles "Nick Nichols**
Ben and Me (Featurette) **Ham Luske**

***Associate producer *Cartoon Director *Directing Animator * Director *Producer *Producer; Director *Production Supervisor *Sequence Director *Supervising Director *Story; Director**

Academy Award Winner

Working for Peanuts (Short) **Jack Hannah**
How to Sleep (Short) **Jack Kinney**
Canvas Back Duck (Short) **Jack Hannah**
Peter Pan (Feature) **Clyde "Gerry" Geronimi**
Peter Pan (Feature) **Wilfred Jackson**
Peter Pan (Feature) **Ham Luske**

1954

Spare the Rod (Short) **Jack Hannah**
Donald's Diary (Short) **Jack Kinney**
The Lone Chipmunks (Short) **Jack Kinney**
Pigs is Pigs (Short) **Jack Kinney**
Casey Bats Again (Short) **Jack Kinney**
Dragon Around (Short) **Jack Hannah**
Grin and Bear It (Short) **Jack Hannah**
Social Lion (Short) **Jack Kinney**
The Flying Squirrel (Short) **Jack Hannah**
Grand Canyonscape (Short) **Charles "Nick" Nichols**

1955

No Hunting (Short) **Jack Hannah**
Bearly Asleep (Short) **Jack Hannah**
Beazy Bear (Short) **Jack Hannah**
Up a Tree (Short) **Jack Hannah**
Lady and the Tramp (Feature) **Ed Penner**
Lady and the Tramp (Feature) **Clyde "Gerry" Geronimi**
Lady and the Tramp (Feature) **Wilfred Jackson**
Lady and the Tramp (Feature) **Ham Luske**

1956

Chips Ahoy (Short) **Jack Kinney**
Hooked Bear (Short) **Jack Hannah**
Jack and old Mac (Short) **Bill Justice**
In The Bag (Short) **Jack Hannah**
A Cowboy Needs A Horse (Short) **Bill Justice**
How to Have an Accident in the Home (Short)
Charles "Nick" Nichols

1957

The Story of Anyburg U.S.A. (Short)
Clyde "Gerry" Geronimi
The Truth about Mother Goose (Short)
Woolie Reitherman

1958

Paul Bunyan (Featurette) **Les Clark**

1959

How to Have an Accident at Work (Short)
Charles "Nick" Nichols
Noah's Ark (Featurette) **Bill Justice**
Donald in Mathmagic Land (Featurette)
Ham Luske
Donald in Mathmagic Land (Featurette) **Les Clark**
Donald in Mathmagic Land (Featurette) **Josh Meador**
Donald in Mathmagic Land (Featurette)
Woolie Reitherman
Sleeping Beauty (Feature) **Clyde "Gerry" Geronimi**
Sleeping Beauty (Feature) **Les Clark**
Sleeping Beauty (Feature) **Eric Larson**
Sleeping Beauty (Feature) **Woolie Reitherman**

1960

Goliath II (Short) **Woolie Reitherman**

***Associate producer *Cartoon Director *Directing Animator * Director *Producer *Producer; Director**
***Production Supervisor *Sequence Director *Supervising Director *Story; Director**

Academy Award Winner

1961

Aquamania (Short) **Woolie Reitherman**
The Saga of Windwagon Smith (Short) **Charles "Nick" Nichols**
Donald and the Wheel (Short) **Ham Luske**
The Litterbug (Short) **Hamilton Luske**
101 Dalmatians (Feature) **Clyde "Gerry" Geronimi**
101 Dalmatians (Feature) **Ham Luske**
101 Dalmatians (Feature) **Woolie Reitherman**

1962

A Symposium on Popular Songs (Featurette) **Bill Justice**

1963

The Sword in the Stone (Feature) **Woolie Reitherman**
The Sword in the Stone (Feature) **Milt Kahl**
The Sword in the Stone (Feature) **Ollie Johnston**
The Sword in the Stone (Feature) **John Lounsbery**
The Sword in the Stone (Feature) **Frank Thomas**

1964

Mary Poppins (Feature) **Ham Luske**

1965

Freewayphobia (Featurette) **Les Clark**
Donald's Fire Survival Plan (Short) **Les Clark**
Steel and America (Short) **Les Clark**
Goofy's Freeway Troubles (Short) **Les Clark**

1966

Winnie the Pooh and the Honey Tree (Short) **Woolie Reitherman**

1967

Scrooge McDuck and Money (Short) **Ham Luske**
The Jungle Book (Feature) **Woolie Reitherman**
The Jungle Book (Feature) **Milt Kahl**
The Jungle Book (Feature) **Ollie Johnston**
The Jungle Book (Feature) **John Lounsbery**
The Jungle Book (Feature) **Frank Thomas**

1968

Winnie the Pooh and the Blustery Day (Featurette) **Woolie Reitherman**

1970

The Aristocats (Feature) **Woolie Reitherman**
The Aristocats (Feature) **Milt Kahl**
The Aristocats (Feature) **Ollie Johnston**
The Aristocats (Feature) **John Lounsbery**
The Aristocats (Feature) **Frank Thomas**

1973

Robin Hood (Feature) **Woolie Reitherman**
Robin Hood (Feature) **Milt Kahl**
Robin Hood (Feature) **Ollie Johnston**
Robin Hood (Feature) **John Lounsbery**
Robin Hood (Feature) **Frank Thomas**

1974

Winnie the Pooh and Tigger Too (Featurette) **John Lounsbery**
Winnie the Pooh and Tigger Too (Featurette) **Woolie Reitherman**
Winnie the Pooh and Tigger Too (Featurette) **Milt Kahl**
Winnie the Pooh and Tigger Too (Featurette) **Ollie Johnston**

***Associate producer *Cartoon Director *Directing Animator * Director *Producer *Producer; Director *Production Supervisor *Sequence Director *Supervising Director *Story; Director**

Academy Award Winner

Winnie the Pooh and Tigger Too (Featurette)
Eric Larson
Winnie the Pooh and Tigger Too (Featurette)
Frank Thomas

1977

The Many Adventures of Winnie the Pooh (Feature)
Woolie Reitherman
The Many Adventures of Winnie the Pooh (Feature)
John Lounsbery
The Rescuers (Feature) **Woolie Reitherman**
The Rescuers (Feature) **Don Bluth**
The Rescuers (Feature) **Milt Kahl**
The Rescuers (Feature) **Ollie Johnston**
The Rescuers (Feature) **Frank Thomas**

1981

The Fox and the Hound (Feature) **Art Stevens**
The Fox and the Hound (Feature) **Woolie Reitherman**
The Fox and the Hound (Feature) **Ron Miller**
The Fox and the Hound (Feature) **Ted Berman**
The Fox and the Hound (Feature) **Rick Rich**

***Associate producer *Cartoon Director *Directing Animator * Director *Producer *Producer; Director *Production Supervisor *Sequence Director *Supervising Director *Story; Director**

APPENDIX C

SEQUENCES BY DIRECTOR

FEATURES: SELECTED DIRECTORS AND SEQUENCES DIRECTED

JIM ALGAR		
BAMBI	Seq. 1.1	Approach to Thicket
BAMBI	Seq. 1.2	Animals at Thicket
BAMBI	Seq. 2.1	Learning to Walk
BAMBI	Seq. 2.2	Learning to Walk (aka Learning to Talk)
BAMBI	Seq. 4.1	Dawn on the Meadow
BAMBI	Seq. 4.3	Bambi Meets Faline
BAMBI	Seq. 4.8	Bucks on the Meadow
BAMBI	Seq. 8	Fun In the Snow
BAMBI	Seq. 9.2	Death of the Mother
BAMBI	Seq. 15	Birth of Twins and Finale
FANTASIA	Seq. 7	Sorcerer's Apprentice
THE ADVENTURES OF ICHABOD AND MR. TOAD	Seq. 10.1, Draft Sec. 9	Cyril's Testimony

SAM ARMSTRONG		
FANTASIA	Seq. 10	Interim Orchestra
FANTASIA	Seq. 11a	Interim Orchestra
FANTASIA	Seq. 2.1 & 2.2	Interim Orchestra: Intermission
FANTASIA	Seq. 3.1	Toccata
FANTASIA	Seq. 3.2	Fugue
FANTASIA	Seq. 4	Interim Orchestra
FANTASIA	Seq. 5	Interim Orchestra
FANTASIA	Seq. 5.1	Nutcracker Suite: Sugar Plum Fairy
FANTASIA	Seq. 5.2	Nutcracker Suite: Chinese Dance
FANTASIA	Seq. 5.3	Nutcracker Suite: Dance of the Reed Flutes
FANTASIA	Seq. 5.4	Nutcracker Suite: Arabian Dance
FANTASIA	Seq. 5.5	Nutcracker Suite: Trepak—Russian Dance
FANTASIA	Seq. 5.6	Nutcracker Suite: Waltz of the Flowers
FANTASIA	Seq. 7a	Interim Orchestra
FANTASIA	Seq. 8	Interim Orchestra
DUMBO	Seq. 1	Stork Sequence
DUMBO	Seq. 11.3	Sad Casey
DUMBO	Seq. 3	Casey Loading
DUMBO	Seq. 4	Roustabouts

BAMBI	Seq. 2.4	Raindrop Sequence
BAMBI	Seq. 1	Pictorial Opening
BAMBI	Seq. 7	Autumn Montage
BAMBI	Seq. 9.1	Winter Montage
LES CLARK		
SLEEPING BEAUTY	Seq. 01.0	Opening—To Entrance of Maleficent
BOB CORMACK		
MAKE MINE MUSIC	Seq. 4	Without You
MAKE MINE MUSIC	Seq. 6	Two Silhouettes
BILL COTTRELL		
SNOW WHITE AND THE SEVEN DWARFS	Seq. 1B	First Queen & Mirror Sequence
SNOW WHITE AND THE SEVEN DWARFS	Seq. 2B	Queen Orders Snow White's Death
SNOW WHITE AND THE SEVEN DWARFS	Seq. 7A	Queen Leaves Mirror—Prepares Disguise
SNOW WHITE AND THE SEVEN DWARFS	Seq. 9A	Witch at Cauldron—Prepares Apple, aka Witch at Cauldron
SNOW WHITE AND THE SEVEN DWARFS	Seq. 13A	Snow White Making Pies—Witch Enters House (aka Snow White Making Pies Witch Enters House)
SNOW WHITE AND THE SEVEN DWARFS	Seq. 14C	Witch Urges S.W. to Make Wish
SNOW WHITE AND THE SEVEN DWARFS	Seq. 14F	Snow White Starts Wish
SNOW WHITE AND THE SEVEN DWARFS	Seq. 14H	Snow White Dies
NORM FERGUSON		
SALUDOS AMIGOS	Seq. 3	Chile—Reel 3-A
SALUDOS AMIGOS	Seq. 1	Titles—Reel 1-A
SALUDOS AMIGOS	Seq. 5	Argentine—Reel 3-A
THE THREE CABALLEROS—LA PINATA	Seq. 4	Solamente una Vez
THE THREE CABALLEROS—LA PINATA	Seq. 5	Montage
THE THREE CABALLEROS—LA PINATA	Seq. 6	Zandunga
THE THREE CABALLEROS—LA PINATA	Seq. 7	Jesusita (The Cactus March)
THE THREE CABALLEROS	n/a	The Flying Gauchito
DUMBO	Seq. 11	Pyramid Act
DUMBO	Seq. 17	Hiccups and Cure
DUMBO	Seq. 18	Pink Elephants
DUMBO	Seq. 5	Circus Parade

CLYDE "GERRY" GERONIMI		
THE THREE CABALLEROS—LA PINATA	Seq. 2	Las Posadas & Breaking Pinata
THE THREE CABALLEROS—LA PINATA	Seq. 3	Folio
THE THREE CABALLEROS—LA PINATA	Seq. 8	Finale
THE THREE CABALLEROS—LA PINATA	Seq. 1	Intro to Charro
MAKE MINE MUSIC	Seq. 10	The Whale Who Wanted To Sing at The Met
MELODY TIME: BLAME IT ON THE SAMBA	Seq. 6	Blame It on the Samba
MELODY TIME: LITTLE TOOT	Seq. 1	Little Toot
MELODY TIME: PECOS BILL	Seq. 7, 7.1	Pecos Bill
ICHABOD CRANE	Seq. 7	The Dance
ICHABOD CRANE	Seq. 8	Story Telling
ICHABOD CRANE	Seq. 9	The Ride and The Chase
ICHABOD CRANE	Seq. 10	Epilogue
CINDERELLA	Seq. 04.2	Duke Awakens the King
CINDERELLA	Seq. 05.0	Cinderella Locked Up
CINDERELLA	Seq. 05.1	Slipper Fitting
ALICE IN WONDERLAND	Seq. 5	Walrus and the Carpenter
ALICE IN WONDERLAND	Seq. 7.1	Bird in the Tree
ALICE IN WONDERLAND	Seq. 7.5	Cheshire Cat
ALICE IN WONDERLAND	Seq. 8	Mad Tea Party
ALICE IN WONDERLAND	Seq. 9	Tulgey Wood
PETER PAN	Seq. 11	Hook Tricks Tinker Bell
PETER PAN	Seq. 13	Captured by the Pirates
PETER PAN	Seq. 14	The Fight with the Pirates
PETER PAN	Seq. 4	Introduction to Hook & Smee
PETER PAN	Seq. 9	Hook Has a Cold
LADY AND THE TRAMP	Seq. 01.1	Introduction of Tramp
LADY AND THE TRAMP	Seq. 05.0	Lady Escapes
LADY AND THE TRAMP	Seq. 06.0	At the Zoo
LADY AND THE TRAMP	Seq. 07.0	Dinner at Tony's
LADY AND THE TRAMP	Seq. 07.1	Bella Notte
LADY AND THE TRAMP	Seq. 10.0	Lady at Dog Pound
SLEEPING BEAUTY	Seq. 13.0	Kings at King Stefan's Castle
SLEEPING BEAUTY	Seq. 15.0	Fairies Put Castle to Sleep

SLEEPING BEAUTY	Seq. 17.0	Prince Captured, Fairies Discover His Capture
SLEEPING BEAUTY	Seq. 18.0	Maleficent and Prince in Dungeon—Escape
SLEEPING BEAUTY	Seq. 21.0	Girl Awakens—Ending
ONE HUNDRED AND ONE DALMATIANS	Seq. 1	Opening
ONE HUNDRED AND ONE DALMATIANS	Seq. 3	Puppies Arrive
ONE HUNDRED AND ONE DALMATIANS	Seq. 12	Cruella at Hell Hall
THORNTON T. HEE		
PINOCCHIO	Seq. 3	Fox & Cat Meet Pino for First Time / On to the Theatre
PINOCCHIO	Seq. 7.0	Fox, Cat & Coachman Plot in Inn
PINOCCHIO	Seq. 7.1	Fox & Cat Sell Pino on Pleasure Island
FANTASIA	Seq. 10.1	Dance of the Hours: Ostrich Ballet
FANTASIA	Seq. 10.2	Dance of the Hours: Hippo Ballet
FANTASIA	Seq. 10.3	Dance of the Hours: Elephant Ballet
FANTASIA	Seq. 10.4	Dance of the Hours: Alligators—Finale
JOHN HENCH		
CINDERELLA	Seq. 01.1	Prologue
WILFRED JACKSON		
SNOW WHITE AND THE SEVEN DWARFS	Seq. 8A	Entertainment
SNOW WHITE AND THE SEVEN DWARFS	Seq. 8B	Story Telling
SNOW WHITE AND THE SEVEN DWARFS	Seq. 8C	Going to Bed
SNOW WHITE AND THE SEVEN DWARFS	Seq. 15A	Snow White Dead
SNOW WHITE AND THE SEVEN DWARFS	Seq. 15B	Titles
SNOW WHITE AND THE SEVEN DWARFS	Seq. 16A	S.W. In Coffin—Back to Life—Away with Prince (aka S.W. In Coffin Back to Life Away with Prince)
PINOCCHIO	Seq. 1.1	Geppetto Carves Marionette
PINOCCHIO	Seq. 2	Going to School
PINOCCHIO	Seq. 3.1	Geppetto Awaiting Pino's Return
PINOCCHIO	Seq. 4.2	Marionette Show
PINOCCHIO	Seq. 4.4	Stromboli Imprisons Pinocchio
PINOCCHIO	Seq. 4.7	Geppetto Continues Search for Pino
FANTASIA	Seq. 11	Night on Bald Mountain
FANTASIA	Seq. 12	Ave Maria
DUMBO	Seq. 10	Ringmaster's Idea for Pyramid Act

DUMBO	Seq. 12	Gossips Disown Dumbo
DUMBO	Seq. 3.1	Stork Chases Circus Train
DUMBO	Seq. 3.2	Stork Delivers Dumbo—Dumbo Named
DUMBO	Seq. 6	Menagerie—Mrs. Jumbo Goes Berserk
DUMBO	Seq. 7	Elephants Gossip
DUMBO	Seq. 9	Timothy Befriends Dumbo
SALUDOS AMIGOS		Aquarela Do Brasil
SONG OF THE SOUTH	n/a	Laughing Place
SONG OF THE SOUTH	n/a	Tar Baby Section 1
SONG OF THE SOUTH	n/a	Tar Baby Section 2
SONG OF THE SOUTH	n/a	Tar Baby Section 3
SONG OF THE SOUTH	n/a	Tar Baby Combination
SONG OF THE SOUTH		Ending
MELODY TIME	Seq. 10, 40	Titles & Inserts
MELODY TIME: JOHNNY APPLESEED	Seq. 2, 2.2	Johnny Appleseed
CINDERELLA	Seq. 01.2	Introduction
CINDERELLA	Seq. 01.4	Mice Decoy Cat
CINDERELLA	Seq. 01.5	Shell Game
CINDERELLA	Seq. 01.6	Serving Breakfast
CINDERELLA	Seq. 02.4	Dress Building
CINDERELLA	Seq. 2.3	Work Fantasy (Mice Sing Work Song)
ALICE IN WONDERLAND	Seq. 1	Opening—River Bank
ALICE IN WONDERLAND	Seq. 10	Croquet Game
ALICE IN WONDERLAND	Seq. 11	Trial
ALICE IN WONDERLAND	Seq. 12	Ending—Chase
ALICE IN WONDERLAND	Seq. 2	Down the Rabbit Hole
PETER PAN	Seq. 1	Opening—Introduction to Family
PETER PAN	Seq. 15	Voyage Home—Ending
PETER PAN	Seq. 2	Wendy Meets Peter
PETER PAN	Seq. 2.1	Learning to Fly
PETER PAN	Seq. 3	Flight to Neverland
LADY AND THE TRAMP	Seq. 02.0	Dogs Discuss Baby—Enter Tramp
LADY AND THE TRAMP	Seq. 03.0	Calendar

JACK KINNEY		
PINOCCHIO	Seq. 10.1	Starving in Belly of Whale
PINOCCHIO	Seq. 10.3	Geppetto Starts to Fish Tuna
PINOCCHIO	Seq. 10.5	Reunion in Whale
PINOCCHIO	Seq. 10.8	Geppetto Fishing for Tuna
PINOCCHIO	Seq. 7.2	Coach Ride to Pleasure Island
DUMBO	Seq. 19	Up in the Tree
DUMBO	Seq. 19.1	I've Seen Everything Song
DUMBO	Seq. 19.2	Dumbo Learns to Fly
SALUDOS AMIGOS	n/a	El Gaucho Goofy
SALUDOS AMIGOS	Seq. 6	Brazil Reels 3-B and 4-A
THE THREE CABALLEROS	Seq. 1	Intro—Into Penguin Picture
THE THREE CABALLEROS	Seq. 2	Birds—Insert from Penguin to Gauchito
THE THREE CABALLEROS	Seq. 3	Lead Into Baia
MAKE MINE MUSIC	Seq. 1	The Martins and the Coys
MAKE MINE MUSIC	Seq. 3	All the Cats Join In
MAKE MINE MUSIC	Seq. 8	After You've Gone
MAKE MINE MUSIC	Seq. 9	Johnny Fedora and Alice Blue Bonnet
FUN AND FANCY FREE: BONGO	Seq. 1	Circus
FUN AND FANCY FREE: BONGO	Seq. 2	Lazy Countryside
FUN AND FANCY FREE: BONGO	Seq. 3	Night
FUN AND FANCY FREE: BONGO	Seq. 4	Bongo Meets Lulubelle
FUN AND FANCY FREE: BONGO	Seq. 5	Too Good To Be True (Fantasy)
FUN AND FANCY FREE: BONGO	Seq. 6	Lumpjaw Entrance
FUN AND FANCY FREE: BONGO	Seq. 7	Say It with a Slap
FUN AND FANCY FREE: BONGO	Seq. 8	Flight and Finale
MELODY TIME: BUMBLE BOOGIE	Seq. 3, 3.1	Bumble Boogie
ICHABOD CRANE	Seq. 2	Intro Ichabod Song
ICHABOD CRANE	Seq. 3	School Room
ICHABOD CRANE	Seq. 3.1	Eating
ICHABOD CRANE	Seq. 3.2	Social Calendar
ICHABOD CRANE	Seq. 3.3	Choral Society (aka Singing Lesson)
ICHABOD CRANE	Seq. 4	Picnic—Katrina Song (aka Picnic)

ICHABOD CRANE	Seq. 4.1	Dream
ICHABOD CRANE	Seq. 4.2	Shopping—Ichabod Meets Katrina (aka Shopping Tour)
ICHABOD CRANE	Seq. 5	Rivalry with Brom
ICHABOD CRANE	Seq. 6	Dressing for Party
ERIC LARSON		
SLEEPING BEAUTY	Seq. 02.0	Entrance of Maleficent
SLEEPING BEAUTY	Seq. 06.0	Fairies Start Dress and Cake
SLEEPING BEAUTY	Seq. 07.0	Fairies Plan
SLEEPING BEAUTY	Seq. 08.0	Boy Meets Girl
SLEEPING BEAUTY	Seq. 09.0	Fairies Finish Dress and Cake
SLEEPING BEAUTY	Seq. 12.0	Girl Returns
SLEEPING BEAUTY	Seq. 14.0	Girl Pricks Finger
HAM LUSKE		
PINOCCHIO	Seq. 8.5	Lampwick Changes—Pino Escapes
PINOCCHIO	Seq. 1	Introduction of the Cricket
PINOCCHIO	Seq. 1.5	Blue Fairy Gives Pinocchio Life
PINOCCHIO	Seq. 1.6	Cricket Sings for Pinocchio
PINOCCHIO	Seq. 1.7	Pino Meets Geppetto, Figaro & Clio
PINOCCHIO	Seq. 12	Pino Becomes Real Boy, Cricket Gets Badge
PINOCCHIO	Seq. 4.8	Cricket Finds Pinocchio in Cage
PINOCCHIO	Seq. 4.9	Blue Fairy Frees Pinocchio from Cage
PINOCCHIO	Seq. 8.3	Poolroom Sequence
FANTASIA	Seq. 4.1	Beethoven—First Movement
FANTASIA	Seq. 4.2	Beethoven—Second Movement
FANTASIA	Seq. 4.5	Beethoven—Fifth Movement: Sunset
FANTASIA	Seq. 4.3	Beethoven—Third Movement
FANTASIA	Seq. 4.4	Beethoven—Fourth Movement: Storm
SALUDOS AMIGOS	n/a	Pedro
MAKE MINE MUSIC		Titles
FUN AND FANCY FREE	Seq. 1	Inserts
FUN AND FANCY FREE	Seq. 2	Inserts
FUN AND FANCY FREE	Seq. 3	Inserts

FUN AND FANCY FREE	Seq. 4	Inserts
FUN AND FANCY FREE	Seq. 5	Inserts
MELODY TIME: ONCE UPON A WINTERTIME	Seq. 4	Once Upon a Wintertime
MELODY TIME: TREES	Seq. 5	Trees
CINDERELLA	Seq. 02.0	Introduction of King & Duke
CINDERELLA	Seq. 03.0	Fairy Godmother
CINDERELLA	Seq. 04.0	King & Duke at Ball
CINDERELLA	Seq. 06.0	Epilogue
CINDERELLA	Seq. 2.1	Bubble Sequence & Music Lesson
CINDERELLA	Seq. 2.5	Sisters Bedroom
CINDERELLA	Seq. 4.1	Clock Strikes
ALICE IN WONDERLAND	Seq. 3	Alice and the Doorknob
ALICE IN WONDERLAND	Seq. 4	Caucus Race
ALICE IN WONDERLAND	Seq. 6	The Rabbit's House
ALICE IN WONDERLAND	Seq. 6.5	Garden of Live Flowers
ALICE IN WONDERLAND	Seq. 7	Caterpillar
ALICE IN WONDERLAND	Seq. 9.5	Painting the Roses Red
PETER PAN	Seq. 10	Indian Dance
PETER PAN	Seq. 12	Underground Home
PETER PAN	Seq. 13.1	Underground Explosion
PETER PAN	Seq. 5	Arrival in Neverland
PETER PAN	Seq. 6	Captured by Indians
PETER PAN	Seq. 7	Mermaid Lagoon
PETER PAN	Seq. 7.1	Boys Tied To Stake
PETER PAN	Seq. 8	Skull Rock
LADY AND THE TRAMP	Seq. 01.0	Introduction Lady, Family & Friends
LADY AND THE TRAMP	Seq. 03.2	What Is a Baby?
LADY AND THE TRAMP	Seq. 04.1	Siamese Cats & Pet Store
LADY AND THE TRAMP	Seq. 08.0	Morning After
LADY AND THE TRAMP	Seq. 09.0	Lady in the Chicken Yard
LADY AND THE TRAMP	Seq. 11.0	Jock and Trosty Propose
LADY AND THE TRAMP	Seq. 12.0	Tramp Kills Rat
LADY AND THE TRAMP	Seq. 12.1	Christmas Party—End
ONE HUNDRED AND ONE DALMATIANS	Seq. 12	Cruella at Hell Hall

ONE HUNDRED AND ONE DALMATIANS	Seq. 15	The Dairy Barn
ONE HUNDRED AND ONE DALMATIANS	Seq. 17	The Happy Ending
ONE HUNDRED AND ONE DALMATIANS	Seq. 2	Introduction of Cruella
ONE HUNDRED AND ONE DALMATIANS	Seq. 4	Introduction of Puppies (TV Sequence)
ONE HUNDRED AND ONE DALMATIANS	Seq. 6	Dogs Make Decision
ONE HUNDRED AND ONE DALMATIANS	Seq. 7	Pongo Sends Message
GAIL PAPINEAU		
FANTASIA	Seq. 8.1	Rite of Spring: Trip Through Space
FANTASIA	Seq. 8.2	Rite of Spring: Volcanoes
PERCE PEARCE		
SNOW WHITE AND THE SEVEN DWARFS	Seq. 2A	S.W. & the Prince in the Garden
SNOW WHITE AND THE SEVEN DWARFS	Seq. 4A	Dwarfs at Mine
SNOW WHITE AND THE SEVEN DWARFS	Seq. 4D	Spooks
SNOW WHITE AND THE SEVEN DWARFS	Seq. 5A	Bedroom
SNOW WHITE AND THE SEVEN DWARFS	Seq. 5B	Snow White Tells Dwarfs to Wash
SNOW WHITE AND THE SEVEN DWARFS	Seq. 6A	Dwarfs at Washing Tub
SNOW WHITE AND THE SEVEN DWARFS	Seq. 6B	Soup
SNOW WHITE AND THE SEVEN DWARFS	Seq. 10A	Dwarfs Leave for Mine
SNOW WHITE AND THE SEVEN DWARFS	Seq. 3A	Snow White and Huntsman (aka S.W. & Huntsman, aka S.W. & Huntsman—S.W. Into Woods—Montage)
SNOW WHITE AND THE SEVEN DWARFS	Seq. 3B	Snow White Meets Animals
SNOW WHITE AND THE SEVEN DWARFS	Seq. 3C	S.W. Discovers Dwarfs' House
SNOW WHITE AND THE SEVEN DWARFS	Seq. 3D	S.W. and Animals Clean House
SNOW WHITE AND THE SEVEN DWARFS	Seq. 4C	Snow White Discovers Bedroom
WOOLIE REITHERMAN		
SLEEPING BEAUTY	Seq. 07.1	Maleficent Kicks Goons Around
SLEEPING BEAUTY	Seq. 19.0	The Fight
ONE HUNDRED AND ONE DALMATIANS	Seq. 13	Escape from Hell Hall
ONE HUNDRED AND ONE DALMATIANS	Seq. 14	Family Reunion
ONE HUNDRED AND ONE DALMATIANS	Seq. 16	Final Escape
ONE HUNDRED AND ONE DALMATIANS	Seq. 5	Puppies Stolen
ONE HUNDRED AND ONE DALMATIANS	Seq. 7.1	Twilight Bark

ONE HUNDRED AND ONE DALMATIANS	Seq. 8	Puppies Discovered
ONE HUNDRED AND ONE DALMATIANS	Seq. 9	Pongo Gets the News
SWORD IN THE STONE	Seq. 001	Prologue
SWORD IN THE STONE	Seq. 002	Wart Meets Merlin
SWORD IN THE STONE	Seq. 003	Castle of the Forest Sauvage
SWORD IN THE STONE	Seq. 004	Tilting Practice
SWORD IN THE STONE	Seq. 005	Wart Becomes a Fish
SWORD IN THE STONE	Seq. 006	Wart Becomes a Squirrel
SWORD IN THE STONE	Seq. 007	Kitchen Battle
SWORD IN THE STONE	Seq. 008	Educational Sequence
SWORD IN THE STONE	Seq. 009	Madam Mim
SWORD IN THE STONE	Seq. 01.1	Introduction of Merlin, Owl, Wart & Klay
SWORD IN THE STONE	Seq. 03.1	Pelinore Visits Castle
SWORD IN THE STONE	Seq. 08.1	The Flying Lesson
SWORD IN THE STONE	Seq. 10	Wizards' Duel
SWORD IN THE STONE	Seq. 12.0	Ending
SWORD IN THE STONE	Seq. 14.0	Wart Becomes Kay's Squire, Off to London
SWORD IN THE STONE	Seq. 5.1	Wart Tells Fish a Story
BILL ROBERTS		
PINOCCHIO	Seq. 10	Pinocchio & Cricket Undersea
PINOCCHIO	Seq. 10.2	Whale Awakens—Sees Tuna
PINOCCHIO	Seq. 10.4	Pinocchio Meets Monstro & Screams
PINOCCHIO	Seq. 10.6	Ext: Whale on Fire
PINOCCHIO	Seq. 10.7	Int: Pino and Geppetto Launch Raft
PINOCCHIO	Seq. 10.9	Pinocchio Swallowed by Whale
PINOCCHIO	Seq. 11	Pinocchio & Geppetto Escape Whale
PINOCCHIO	Seq. 8.1	Pleasure Island
PINOCCHIO	Seq. 9.1	Pino & Jiminy Escape from Boobyland, Return Home, Get Message, Go to Find Geppetto
PINOCCHIO	Seq. 9.4	Jiminy Discovers Coachman Crating Donkeys
FANTASIA	Seq. 8.3	Rite of Spring: Undersea Live
FANTASIA	Seq. 8.4	Rite of Spring: Pterodactyls
FANTASIA	Seq. 8.5	Rite of Spring: Family Life
FANTASIA	Seq. 8.6	Rite of Spring: Fight

FANTASIA	Seq. 8.7	Rite of Spring: Trek
DUMBO	Seq. 14	Fireman Save My Child
DUMBO	Seq. 14.1	Clowns Celebrate
DUMBO	Seq. 14.2	Timothy & Dumbo Visit Jail
DUMBO	Seq. 15.1	Lullaby Sequence
DUMBO	Seq. 16	Clown Sequence
DUMBO	Seq. 20	Big Town—Dumbo Triumphs
SALUDOS AMIGOS	Seq. 2	Lake Titicaca
THE THREE CABALLEROS	n/a	Cold Blooded Penguin
FUN AND FANCY FREE: MICKEY AND THE BEANSTALK	Seq. 1	Opening—Happy Valley
FUN AND FANCY FREE: MICKEY AND THE BEANSTALK	Seq. 3	Starvation
FUN AND FANCY FREE: MICKEY AND THE BEANSTALK	Seq. 1	Opening—Happy Valley
FUN AND FANCY FREE: MICKEY AND THE BEANSTALK	Seq. 5	Opera
FUN AND FANCY FREE: MICKEY AND THE BEANSTALK	Seq. 7	Beanero
FUN AND FANCY FREE: MICKEY AND THE BEANSTALK	Seq. 8	Early Morning
FUN AND FANCY FREE: MICKEY AND THE BEANSTALK	Seq. 10	Dragonfly
FUN AND FANCY FREE: MICKEY AND THE BEANSTALK	Seq. 13	Discover Harp
FUN AND FANCY FREE: MICKEY AND THE BEANSTALK	Seq. 14	Introduction of the Giant (aka Introduction to Giant)
FUN AND FANCY FREE: MICKEY AND THE BEANSTALK	Seq. 17.5	Pink Bunny
FUN AND FANCY FREE: MICKEY AND THE BEANSTALK	Seq. 15	Lullaby
FUN AND FANCY FREE: MICKEY AND THE BEANSTALK	Seq. 16	Key Stealing
FUN AND FANCY FREE: MICKEY AND THE BEANSTALK	Seq. 18	Ending (Chase Down Beanstalk)
PAUL SATTERFIELD		
FANTASIA	Seq. 8.8	Rite of Spring: Earthquake
BAMBI	Seq. 10.4	Buck Fight
BEN SHARPSTEEN		
SNOW WHITE AND THE SEVEN DWARFS	Seq. 4B	Dwarfs March Home from the Mine
SNOW WHITE AND THE SEVEN DWARFS	Seq. 10B	Queen on Way To Dwarfs' House
SNOW WHITE AND THE SEVEN DWARFS	Seq. 11A	The Lodge Meeting
SNOW WHITE AND THE SEVEN DWARFS	Seq. 11B	Bed Building
SNOW WHITE AND THE SEVEN DWARFS	Seq. 14B	Dwarfs at Mine—Animals Warn Them
SNOW WHITE AND THE SEVEN DWARFS	Seq. 14E	Dwarfs Start for House to Rescue S.W.—Meet Turtle

SNOW WHITE AND THE SEVEN DWARFS	Seq. 14G	Dwarfs on Way to House
SNOW WHITE AND THE SEVEN DWARFS	Seq. 14J	Dwarfs Chase the Queen
DUMBO	Seq. 23	Success Montage
NORMAN WRIGHT		
BAMBI	Seq. 4.9	Introduction to Man
BAMBI	Seq. 10.1	Owl Tells Kids About Love
BAMBI	Seq. 10.2	Thumper and Flower Fall in Love
BAMBI	Seq. 10.3	Bambi and Faline Fall in Love
BAMBI	Seq. 11	Two Winds
BAMBI	Seq. 12.1	The Drive (aka The Driver)
BAMBI	Seq. 12.2	Bambi Rescues Faline from Hounds

APPENDIX D

ANIMATION DIRECTORS TIME LINE

List of films, directors, production supervisors, and animators from 1928 to 1966.

	1928	1929	1930	1931	1932	1933
NATURE & PEOPLE/ PLACES						
LIVE-ACTION CARTOON MIX						
ANIMATED FEATURE						
SHORTS (AA WINNERS LISTED)	STEAMBOAT	SHORTS	SHORTS	SHORTS	FLOWERS/TREES	3 LITTLE PIGS
LIVE ACTION FILMS						
TELEVISION						
THEME PARKS						

	1928	1929	1930	1931	1932	1933
WALT DISNEY	DIRECTOR	DIRECTOR	DIRECTOR	VISIONARY	VISIONARY	VISIONARY
UB IWERKS (1924)	ANIMATOR/DIR	DIRECTOR	DEPARTS JAN.			
WILFRED JACKSON	ANIMATOR	ANIMATOR	ANIMATOR	DIRECTOR	DIRECTOR	DIRECTOR
BEN SHARPSTEEN		ANIMATOR	ANIMATOR	ANIMATOR	ANIMATOR	ANIMATOR
BURT GILLETT		ANIMATOR/DIR	DIRECTOR	DIRECTOR	DIRECTOR	DIRECTOR
DAVE HAND			ANIMATOR	ANIMATOR	ANIMATOR	DIRECTOR
HAM LUSKE				ANIMATOR	ANIMATOR	ANIMATOR
GERRY GERONIMI				ANIMATOR	ANIMATOR	ANIMATOR
JACK KINNEY				ANIMATOR	ANIMATOR	ANIMATOR
JACK KING		ANIMATOR	ANIMATOR	ANIMATOR	RESIGNS	
JACK HANNAH						ANIMATOR
NICK NICHOLS						
WOOLIE REITHERMAN						ANIMATOR

1934	1935	1936	1937	1938	1939	1940
				SNOW WHITE		PIN/FANTASIA
TORTOISE	3 ORPH. KIT.	COUNTRY C.	OLD MILL	FERDINAND	UGLY DUCK.	SHORTS

1934	1935	1936	1937	1938	1939	1940
VISIONARY	VISIONARY	VISIONARY	VISIONARY	VISIONARY	VISIONARY	VISIONARY
						RETURNS
DIRECTOR	DIRECTOR	DIRECTOR	DIRECTOR	DIRECTOR	DIRECTOR	DIRECTOR
DIRECTOR	DIRECTOR	DIRECTOR	DIRECTOR	DIRECTOR	DIRECTOR	DIRECTOR
RESIGNS		RETURNS	RESIGNS			
DIRECTOR	DIRECTOR	DIRECTOR	DIRECTOR	DIRECTOR	DIRECTOR	DIRECTOR
ANIMATOR	ANIMATOR	ANIMATOR	ANIMATOR	ANIMATOR	ANIMATOR	DIRECTOR
ANIMATOR	ANIMATOR	ANIMATOR	ANIMATOR	ANIMATOR	DIRECTOR	DIRECTOR
ANIMATOR	ANIMATOR	ANIMATOR	ANIMATOR	ANIMATOR	ANIMATOR	DIRECTOR
		RETURNS	DIRECTOR	DIRECTOR	DIRECTOR	DIRECTOR
ANIMATOR	ANIMATOR	ANIMATOR	ANIMATOR	ANIMATOR	ANIMATOR	ANIMATOR
	ANIMATOR	ANIMATOR	ANIMATOR	ANIMATOR	ANIMATOR	ANIMATOR
ANIMATOR	ANIMATOR	ANIMATOR	ANIMATOR	ANIMATOR	ANIMATOR	DIRECTOR

	1941	1942	1943	1944	1945	1946
NATURE & PEOPLE/ PLACES						
LIVE-ACTION CARTOON MIX	RELUCT. DRAGON		SALUDOS	THREE CABS		SOTS
ANIMATED FEATURE	DUMBO	BAMBI				MAKE MINE
SHORTS (AA WINNERS LISTED)	LEND A PAW	DER FUEHRER	SHORTS	SHORTS	SHORTS	SHORTS
LIVE ACTION FILMS						
TELEVISION						
THEME PARKS						

	1941	1942	1943	1944	1945	1946
WALT DISNEY	VISIONARY	VISIONARY	VISIONARY	VISIONARY	VISIONARY	VISIONARY
UB IWERKS (1924)	CAMERA/EFX	CAMERA/EFX	CAMERA/EFX	CAMERA/EFX	CAMERA/EFX	CAMERA/EFX
WILFRED JACKSON	DIRECTOR	DIRECTOR	DIRECTOR	DIRECTOR	DIRECTOR	DIRECTOR
BEN SHARPSTEEN	DIRECTOR	PROD. SUP	PROD. SUP	PROD. SUP	PROD. SUP	PROD. SUP
BURT GILLETT						
DAVE HAND	DIRECTOR	DIRECTOR	DIRECTOR	RESIGNS		
HAM LUSKE	DIRECTOR	DIRECTOR	DIRECTOR	DIRECTOR	DIRECTOR	DIRECTOR
GERRY GERONIMI	DIRECTOR	DIRECTOR	DIRECTOR	DIRECTOR	DIRECTOR	DIRECTOR
JACK KINNEY	DIRECTOR	DIRECTOR	DIRECTOR	DIRECTOR	DIRECTOR	DIRECTOR
JACK KING	DIRECTOR	DIRECTOR	DIRECTOR	DIRECTOR	DIRECTOR	DIRECTOR
JACK HANNAH	ANIMATOR	ANIMATOR	ANIMATOR	DIRECTOR	DIRECTOR	DIRECTOR
NICK NICHOLS	ANIMATOR	ANIMATOR	ANIMATOR	DIRECTOR	DIRECTOR	DIRECTOR
WOOLIE REITHERMAN	DIRECTOR	WWII	WWII	WWII	WWII	DIRECTOR

1947	1948	1949	1950	1951	1952	1953
		SEAL ISLAND	NATURE	NATURE	NATURE	NATURE
		SO DEAR				
FUN & FANCY	MAKE MM	ICHABOD/TOAD	CINDERELLA	ALICE		PETER PAN
SHORTS	SHORTS	SHORTS	SHORTS	SHORTS	SHORTS	TOOT, WHISTLE
			TREASURE ISL.		ROBIN HOOD	SWORD/ROSE

1947	1948	1949	1950	1951	1952	1953
VISIONARY	VISIONARY	VISIONARY	VISIONARY	VISIONARY	VISIONARY	VISIONARY
CAMERA/EFX	CAMERA/EFX	CAMERA/EFX	CAMERA/EFX	CAMERA/EFX	CAMERA/EFX	CAMERA/EFX
DIRECTOR	DIRECTOR	DIRECTOR	DIRECTOR	DIRECTOR	DIRECTOR	DIRECTOR
PROD. SUP	PROD. SUP	PROD. T-L	PROD. T-L	PROD. T-L	PROD. T-L	PROD. T-L
DIRECTOR	DIRECTOR	DIRECTOR	DIRECTOR	DIRECTOR	DIRECTOR	DIRECTOR
DIRECTOR	DIRECTOR	DIRECTOR	DIRECTOR	DIRECTOR	DIRECTOR	DIRECTOR
DIRECTOR	DIRECTOR	DIRECTOR	DIRECTOR	DIRECTOR	DIRECTOR	DIRECTOR
DIRECTOR	RETIRES					
DIRECTOR	DIRECTOR	DIRECTOR	DIRECTOR	DIRECTOR	DIRECTOR	DIRECTOR
DIRECTOR	DIRECTOR	DIRECTOR	DIRECTOR	DIRECTOR	DIRECTOR	DIRECTOR
DIRECTOR	DIRECTOR	DIRECTOR	DIRECTOR	DIRECTOR	DIRECTOR	DIRECTOR

	1954	1955	1956	1957	1958	1959
NATURE & PEOPLE/ PLACES	NATURE	NATURE/PP	NATURE/PP	NATURE/PP	NATURE/PP	NATURE/PP
LIVE-ACTION CARTOON MIX						
ANIMATED FEATURE		LADY/TRAMP				SL. BEAUTY
SHORTS (AA WINNERS LISTED)	SHORTS	SHORTS	SHORTS			
LIVE ACTION FILMS	20,000 + 1	LADY/TRAMP	3 FILMS	J TREMAIN	2 FILMS	SL. BEAUTY
TELEVISION	TV	TV	TV	TV	TV	TV
THEME PARKS		DISNEYLAND	DISNEYLAND	DISNEYLAND	DISNEYLAND	DISNEYLAND

	1954	1955	1956	1957	1958	1959
WALT DISNEY	VISIONARY	VISIONARY	VISIONARY	VISIONARY	VISIONARY	VISIONARY
UB IWERKS (1924)	CAMERA/EFX	CAMERA/EFX	CAMERA/EFX	CAMERA/EFX	CAMERA/EFX	CAMERA/EFX
WILFRED JACKSON	TV	TV	TV	TV	TV	TV
BEN SHARPSTEEN	PROD. T-L	PROD. T-L	PROD. T-L	PROD. T-L	PROD. T-L	RETIRES
BURT GILLETT						
DAVE HAND						
HAM LUSKE	DIRECTOR	DIRECTOR	DIRECTOR	DIRECTOR	DIRECTOR	DIRECTOR
GERRY GERONIMI	DIRECTOR	DIRECTOR	DIRECTOR	DIRECTOR	DIRECTOR	RESIGNS
JACK KINNEY	DIRECTOR	DIRECTOR	DIRECTOR	LAID OFF		
JACK KING						
JACK HANNAH	DIRECTOR	DIRECTOR	LAID OFF			
NICK NICHOLS	DIRECTOR	DIRECTOR	DIRECTOR	DIRECTOR	DIRECTOR	DIRECTOR
WOOLIE REITHERMAN	DIRECTOR	DIRECTOR	DIRECTOR	DIRECTOR	DIRECTOR	DIRECTOR

1960	1961	1962	1963	1964	1965	1966
PP						
				M. POPPINS		
	101 DAL.		SWORD			JUNGLE BOOK
6 FILMS	5 FILMS	6 FILMS	5 FILMS	PLUS 5 FILMS	3 FILMS	4 FILMS
TV	TV	TV	TV	TV	TV	TV
DISNEYLAND	DISNEYLAND	DISNEYLAND	DISNEYLAND	DISNEYLAND	DISNEYLAND WDW PLANS	DISNEYLAND WDW PLANS

1960	1961	1962	1963	1964	1965	1966
VISIONARY	VISIONARY	VISIONARY	VISIONARY	VISIONARY	VISIONARY	DIES
CAMERA/EFX	CAMERA/EFX	CAMERA/EFX	CAMERA/EFX	CAMERA/EFX	CAMERA/EFX	CAMERA/EFX
TV	RETIRES					
DIRECTOR	DIRECTOR	DIRECTOR	DIRECTOR	DIRECTOR	DIRECTOR	DIRECTOR
DIRECTOR	DIRECTOR	RESIGNS				
DIRECTOR	DIRECTOR	DIRECTOR	DIRECTOR	DIRECTOR	DIRECTOR	DIRECTOR

APPENDIX E

DAVE HAND'S 1938 ORGANIZATION DIAGRAM

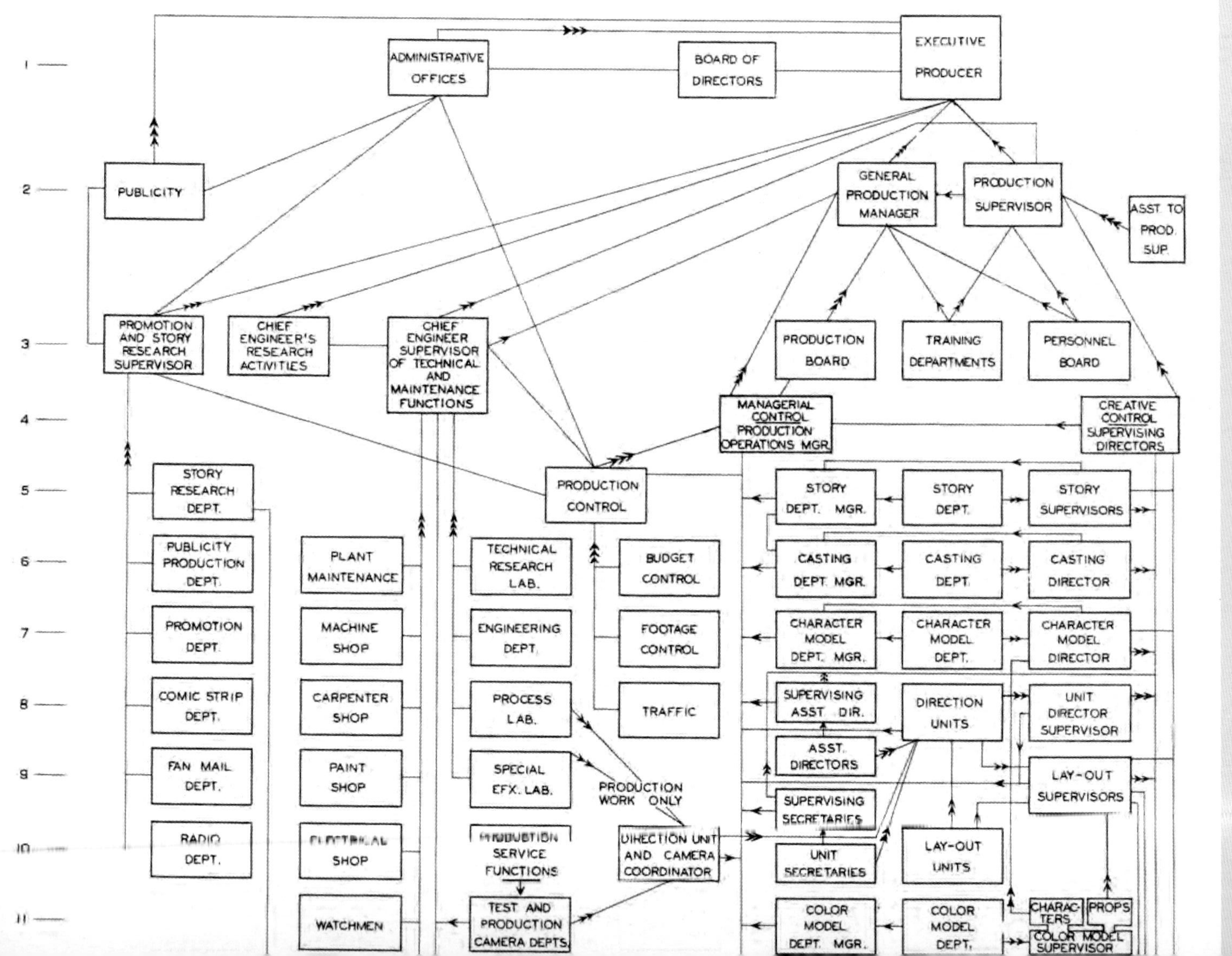

Just months after *Snow White*'s release on May 16, 1938, Dave Hand published a 58-page handbook titled *The Organization*, proposing elaborate instructions and structure "to facilitate the movement of work and to avoid wastes through the proper distribution of help where the need is the greatest." Included were job descriptions for each role, along with the objectives, responsibilities, and functions of each department.

To make clear the chain of command, this not-so-easy to follow chart was also included. The Supervising Director ("in complete creative supervision of their assigned productions")

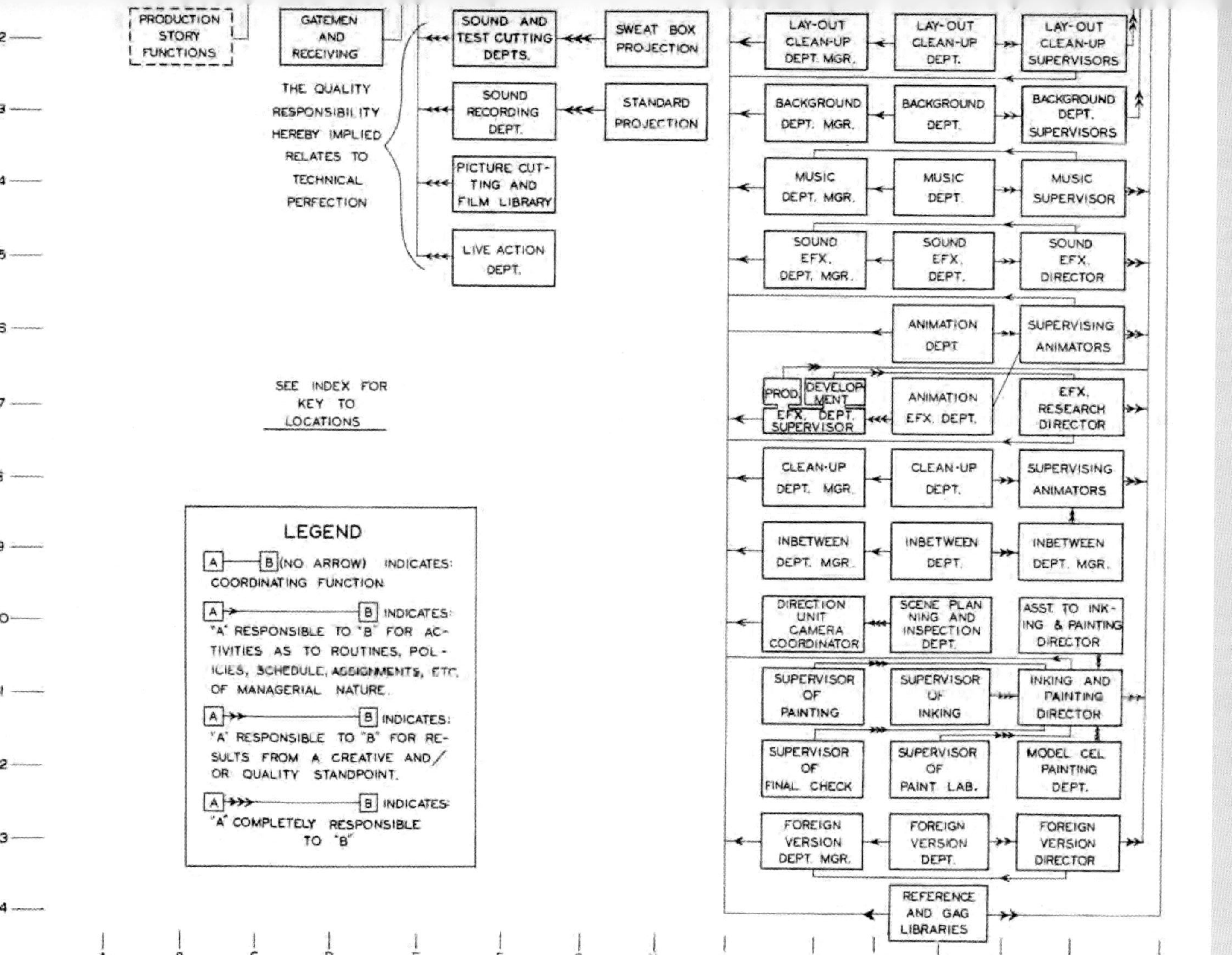

is shown at position N-4, and Unit or Sequence Directors (directly responsible for all creative results of production, from completion of story to the final screen results) are shown at position L-8.

Hand served as both General Production Manager (authority over direction units in a secondary capacity to Walt, working under Walt's direction at all times, supervising the directorial functions of the units) and Production Supervisor (the balancing factor between the creative and managerial aspects of the Producing Organization), shown at K-2 and M-2 respectively.

See also pages 67 and 68 for additional information.

ACKNOWLEDGMENTS

Creating this book has been like making a film: so many people play a role in the creation, and it could not have succeeded without the help of so many. This book has been a labor of love for us, and we hope those who helped us will be pleased with our final product.

First we would like to thank all those generous people who we had the privilege of interviewing personally: Laurie Adams; Dale Baer; Michael Barrier; Brad Bird; Mike Bonifer; Sybil Byrnes; John Canemaker; Ron Clements; Rolly Crump; Andreas Deja; Peg Finefrock; Nancy Fadis; Gary Geronimi; Lynn Geronimi; Andrea Lounsbery Gessell-Severe; Don Hahn; Joe Hale; David Hale Hand; Natha Horbach; Ben Harris; J. B. Kaufman; Glen Keane; Margaret Kerry; John Kinney, Jr.; Judy LaPrade; Kathryn Beaumont Levine; John Lounsbery (son); Ken Lounsbery; Carol Luske; James Luske; Burny Mattinson; Ron Miller; John Musker; Floyd Norman; Cathy Nourafshan; John Pomeroy; Sylvia Roemer; Dick Sherman; Ted Thomas; Gail Sharpsteen; Bob, Bruce, and Dick Reitherman; and Mary Weible.

A note: We interviewed family members of many of the directors in this book, and they were all very gracious with sharing family photos and stories. But they may or may not concur with our assessments of their relatives at work. These men would be well known at home as fathers and grandfathers, but it would be uncommon for a family member to know what they were like to work with in a high-pressure studio setting. We doubt that our own families could accurately assess our working relationships. We have attempted to portray each director as fairly as possible based on their film output, their comments about directing, and what others said about them as directors. In a 1989 note to Michael Barrier, Frank Thomas touched on this dilemma:

> "As you no doubt have learned, there are very few absolutes in this world, and especially at the animation studios. One guy was a hero to some, a sometimes friend to others, and a real heel to the rest. Should we appraise his value on the contribution to a specific film without regard to the damage he caused to others and to the production? Or should we judge him only as a fallible human being like the rest of us? Or as an influence on his coworkers? Or as a talented artist whatever he did? Or just in animation?"

We would like to thank our team of transcribers who made the interviews accessible for us, including Sue, Julie, and Emily Peri; Elie Docter; Corky Mau; Mary Horton; Vic Manley; Chris Meyers; and Xotchil Sarabia.

Thanks to these contemporary animation directors who provided quotes for us: Brad Bird, Chris Buck, Brenda Chapman, Mike Gabriel, Eric Goldberg, Don Hall, Byron Howard, and Jennifer Lee.

Thanks to George Lucas for writing our introduction and Lynne Hale and Connie Wethington for making that happen.

Thank you, Howard Green, the patron saint of retired animators (and researchers), for your many connections and boundless passion and enthusiasm.

This book would not have happened without the support of Wendy Lefkon, who likely didn't realize how many years she'd be dealing with us when she said yes to this project. Wendy has been a joy to work with. She has guided and been there with us through good and stressful times, including Covid and a myriad of other factors affecting our progress to creating this book. We are grateful for our brief but productive work with Jennifer Eastwood and for the talent Winnie Ho has brought to the design of the book.

The Walt Disney Archives is ground zero for research on Disney history, and we are most grateful for the professionalism and the hours of assistance we received from Becky Cline, Kevin Kern, Nicole Carroll, Ed Ovalle, and Justin R. Arthur.

At the photo library of the archives, Michael Buckoff, Holly Brobst, and Maggie Evenson helped us navigate the literally millions of images there. Ann Hansen and Fox Carney of the Animation Research Library guided us through the paper trails of early cartoons.

Thanks also to the wonderful folks at the Disney Music Library—Lisa Janacua and Leslie Smith Buttars—and to Gena Cadiente, Vice-President of Music Research and Administration.

The Walt Disney Family Museum was a valuable source of research material for us, and we appreciate the support and assistance of Diane and Ron Miller, Kirsten Komoroske, Michael Labrie, Bri Bertolaccini, and Nicole Meldahl.

Sophie Glidden-Lyon at the Fales Library and Special Collections at New York University's Elmer Bobst Library graciously accommodated our visit to peruse the papers and collection of eminent historian John Canemaker, housed there.

Thanks to Kristen Ray, Med de Waal, and Warren Sherk of the Herrick Research Library at the Academy of Motion Pictures Arts and Sciences.

Thanks to the University Press of Mississippi for permission to quote from Don Peri's books *Working with Walt* and *Working with Disney.*

We are indebted to these folks who kindly provided never-before-published photos for the book: David Hale Hand and Judy LaPrade, Gail Sharpsteen, Natha Horbach, the Luske family, the Geronimi family, the Reitherman family, Jennifer Castrup, Dave Bossert, Jake Friedman, Ted Thomas, and Hans Perk.

But the majority of information came from people who worked directly with Walt, captured by historians, friends, and admirers before anyone else realized what they were about to lose.

J. B. Kaufman, Didier Ghez, and Ted Thomas were particularly helpful as deep sources of knowledge and passion as we engaged in what felt at times to be never-ending research.

Special thanks to Joe Campana, who can find anything about anybody (so watch out!).

Deep thanks to Hans Perk for his knowledge, passion, and extensive collection of animation history—all of which he graciously shared with us. As a director of animation himself, Hans understands X-sheets and bar sheets like no one else. We're indebted to Hans's detective-worthy discoveries of both Hyperion and Burbank studios, as well as locations and dates of photographs. We want to thank readers of all or part of our manuscript, whose suggestion made this a much better book: Jonas Rivera, Pete Sohn, Chris Buck, John Canemaker, Mike Barrier, and, of course, Hans Perk.

One of the unexpected delights of our years of research was our visit to the Little Rock, Arkansas, home of Michael Barrier, one of the preeminent Disney historians, to talk with him and to spend time researching in what he calls the Vast Barrier Archives. We spent two days discovering for ourselves so much material that really helped define this book. Anyone who cares about the history of animation owes an enormous debt of gratitude to Mike, who did extensive, careful, and thorough research at a time when seemingly few others seemed to care. Thanks also to his partner in crime Milton Gray. The two collected hours of interviews, as well as (literally) file cabinets full of letters and other material that we drew from liberally. Michael has been a friend and mentor of Don's for almost fifty years.

DON I want to thank Walt Disney for being such an inspirational figure in my life. From the first movie I saw in a theater—*Peter Pan* in its initial run—to the thrill of the mid-1950s when Walt came to us through his movies, his television programs—*Disneyland* and my beloved *Mickey Mouse Club*—and Disneyland, the theme park, Walt Disney has been a big part of my life and has had an inordinate influence on me. We know from the research for this book that he could be a hard taskmaster, but the lives of all these directors would have been diminished had they not worked for him. They were in awe of him, and I remain so.

I also want to acknowledge the debt of gratitude I have to all the Disney artists I had the privilege of interviewing over the years, and especially for this book: Ben Sharpsteen, Dick Huemer, Wilfred Jackson, Dave Hand (by correspondence), Les Clark, and Ward Kimball. They were very generous to a neophyte interviewer who learned on the job. My life is richer for having known them.

I want to thank Pete Docter for agreeing to coauthor this book. We did our first interview in 2013, so the book has been in the works for more than a decade. Pete has been wonderful to work with, and it has been his stature in the animation field that opened a lot of doors for us. I think we each brought different skills and perspectives to this project, but we complemented each other and our affection and appreciation of Walt Disney and what he accomplished was the same. Our travels naturally took us to Southern California, but also to New York City and to Maplewood, Minnesota; Wichita, Kansas; and Little Rock, Arkansas. Through it all and countless emails and conversations about our band of directors, Pete has always been upbeat, considerate, curious, and the best writing partner I could have hoped for. I have a friend in him, and he has a friend in me.

PETE Thank you, Don, for being such a great writing partner, for your patience as I attempted to write a book while directing a film AND running a studio, and for catching my many errors and omissions.

Thanks to John Musker and Ron Clements for their patient and thorough answers to my many harassing emails, as well as these Pixar folks who listened patiently as I enthusiastically bored them with my many discoveries: Jonas Rivera, Peter Sohn, Lee Unkrich, Dan Scanlon, and Jamie Datz. Thank you, Charles Solomon, Jenny Lerew, Ross Care, Don Iwerks, Leslie Iwerks, Jennifer Castrup, Børge Ring, Fox Carney, Theo Gluck, Jeff Miller, and Robert Tieman. And thanks to Victoria Manley for her help, organization, enthusiasm, and support.

Writing this book has allowed me to see myself in the future by looking into the past. Seeing how

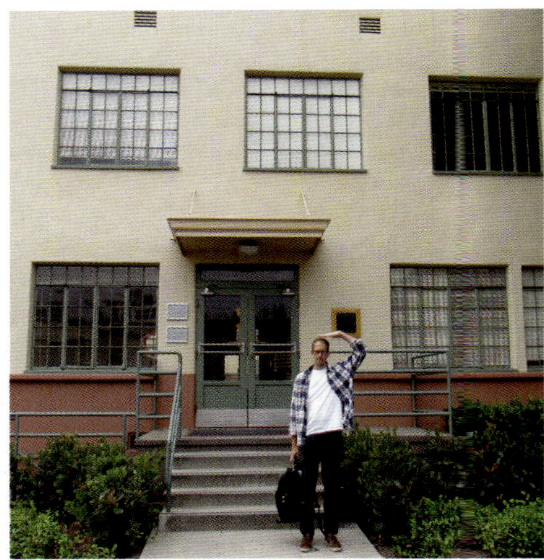

The “world’s tallest animator” in front of the Shorts Building on the Disney Studios lot.

other directors looked back on their careers has given me an almost daily recognition of how truly lucky I am to do what I love, while being surrounded by people I love.

Speaking of which, we want to thank our families.

PETE Thanks to my wife, Amanda, who at this point knows much more about Disney directors than she ever wanted to. I used to quiz my kids, Nick and Elie, on which animators did which scenes (no, Nicholas, the answer is not ALWAYS Milt Kahl)—but now they have a whole other category of knowledge, and I'm thankful to them and my daughter-in-law, Michelle, for putting up with me having my nose in the computer (as if that doesn't happen enough while directing movies).

DON My wife, Sue, and my daughters, Julie and Emily, have graciously listened to *hours and hours* of my stories about these directors and have even spent hours themselves transcribing some of the interviews. I so appreciate their support of these projects that I have undertaken over the years. All our lives are touched by the Disney magic, whether it is by seeing the films or by visiting the parks or by hearing the music, and I hope that knowing more of the history behind the magic enhances their lives as it does mine. I am forever grateful for their encouragement and love.

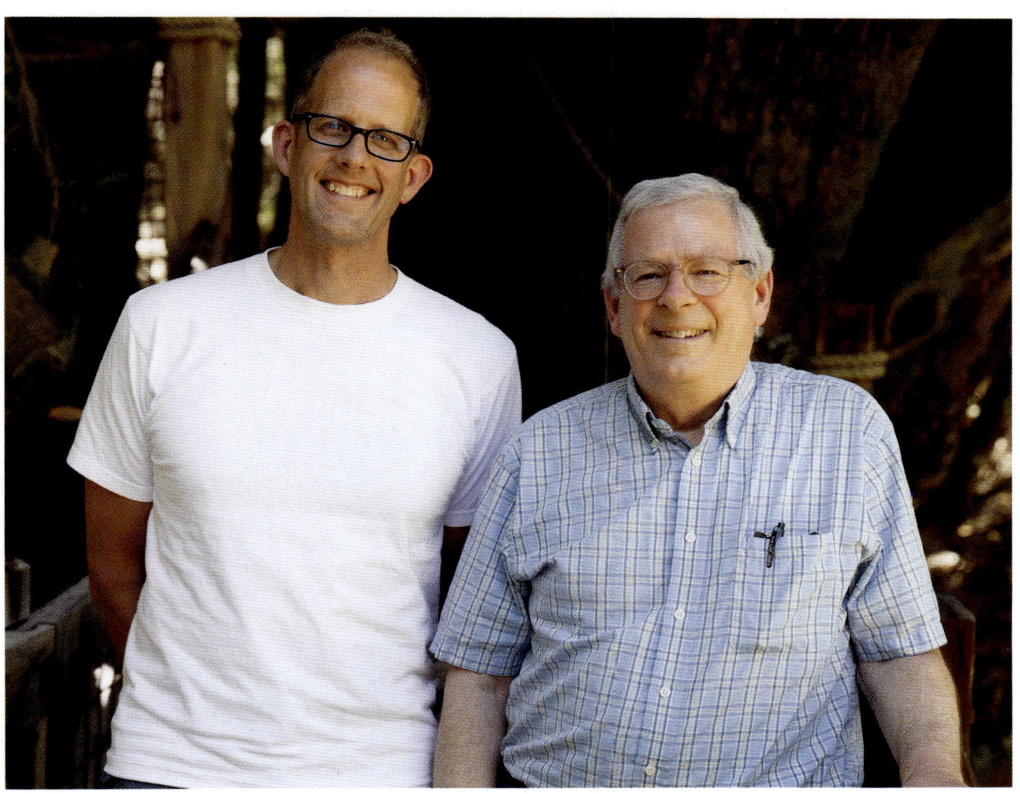

THIS BOOK'S PRODUCERS WOULD LIKE TO SPECIALLY THANK

Jennifer Black, Ann Day, Monique Diman, Tony Fejeran, Michael Freeman, Susan Gerber, Daneen Goodwin, Maureen Graham, Tyra Harris, Winnie Ho, Denise Horn, Dianne Hosmer, David Jefferson, Kim Knueppel, Vicki Korlishin, Kaitie Leary, Meredith Lisbin, Taryn Maister, Warren Meislin, Stacy Mendoza, Estella Morero, Anne Peters, Scott Piehl, Paula Potter, Holly Rice, Zan Schneider, Alexandra Serrano, Fanny Sheffield, Dina Sherman, Marina Shults, Megan Speer, Marybeth Tregarthen, Pat Van Note, Monica Vasquez, Lynn Waggoner, Jessie Ward, Meredith Wilcox, and Rudy Zamora.

ENDNOTES

Introduction

1. Michael Barrier, *The Animated Man*, University of California Press, Berkeley, 2007, page 6. As Barrier points out, Disney's speech exists in three versions. The version delivered on February 10, 1941, in manuscript and on discs at WDA, includes remarks directed specifically to the animators. The version of February 11, which is Lessing exhibit 29, NLRB/Bab-bitt, was delivered to lower-ranking employees at the studio, particularly the women who inked and painted the cels. An abbreviated version of the February to speech, with Disney's profanity removed, is part of CSUN/SCG. Memos listing the departments summoned to each of the two speeches are also part of that collection.

Chapter 1

1. Dick Huemer, interview with Michael Barrier, November 27, 1973.
2. Clyde "Gerry" Geronimi, interview with Michael Barrier, Newport Beach, California, November 5, 1976.
3. Leonard Maltin, *Of Mice and Magic: A History of American Animated Cartoons*.
4. *The Official Walt Disney Quote Book*, compiled by the staff of the Walt Disney Archives, Disney Editions, Los Angeles, 2023.
5. Ub Iwerks, interview with George Sherman, July 30, 1970, WDA.
6. Leslie Iwerks and John Kenworthy, *The Hand Behind the Mouse*, Disney Editions, New York, 2001.
7. The *Silly Symphony* series was suggested by composer Carl Stalling and Walt liked the idea, in no small part because it freed him from gag-oriented stories and reliance on the cartoon "stars."
8. Letter from Wilfred Jackson to Michael Barrier. November 13, 1975. Michael Barrier Collection.
9. Ben Sharpsteen, interview with Don Peri, November 4, 1976. First appeared in *Working with Walt*. Don Peri would like to thank the University Press of Mississippi for permission to quote from his two books, *Working with Walt* and *Working with Disney*, here and throughout this book.
10. Dick Huemer, "Huemeresque," *Funnyworld* Number 18, Summer 1978.
11. The Walt Disney Archives credits Ub with also directing *Arctic Antics*, but J. B. Kaufman and Russell Merritt, in their book *Walt Disney's Silly Symphonies*, credit Burt Gillett with this short. Hans Perk, in correspondence with the authors, pointed out that Ub was no longer at the studio when the short was animated.
12. Dave Hand, interview with Frank Thomas and Ollie Johnston, June 22, 1978. Ted Thomas Collection.
13. January 25, 1930, letter from Roy O. Disney to Walt Disney, Walt Disney Archives.
14. Bob Broughton, interview with Don Peri, October 12, 2002. Walt Disney Family Foundation.
15. January 25, 1930, letter, Walt Disney Archives.
16. Ben Sharpsteen, interview with Don Peri, February 6, 1974.
17. Interoffice communication to Walt Disney from Ben Sharpsteen. August 12, 1940. Walt Disney Archives.
18. Dick Huemer, acceptance speech, October 19, 1978. Don Peri Collection.

Chapter 2

1. Eric Larson, interview with Michael Barrier, October 27, 1976.
2. Shamus Culhane, *Talking Animals and Other People: the Autobiography of One of Animation's Legendary Figures*, St. Martin's Press, March 1, 1986.
3. Disney Family collection.
4. Michael Barrier, *The Animated Man: A Life of Walt Disney*, Berkeley, University of California Press, 2007.
5. Michael Barrier, interview with Ben Sharpsteen, October 23, 1976.
6. Jack Kinney, *Walt Disney and Assorted Other Characters*, Harmony Books, New York, 1988.
7. Wilfred Jackson, "Third Installment of June 3, 1975" letter to Michael Barrier.
8. Wilfred Jackson, "Second Installment of June 3, 1975" letter to Michael Barrier.
9. Wilfred Jackson, "Third Installment of June 3, 1975" letter to Michael Barrier.
10. Wilfred Jackson, "Third Installment of June 3, 1975" letter to Michael Barrier.

11. Eric Larson, *Fifty Years in the Mouse House*, Theme Park Press, 2015.
12. Wilfred Jackson, "Third Installment of June 3, 1975" letter to Michael Barrier.
13. Third Installment of June 3, 1975 letter to Michael Barrier.
14. Wilfred Jackson, "Third Installment of June 3, 1975" letter to Michael Barrier.
15. Dick Huemer, notes on a telephone call with Michael Barrier, October 27, 1976.
16. Fredric M. Gillett, letter to Dave Smith, May 10, 1982, WDA.
17. Ben Sharpsteen, interview with Don Peri, April 24, 1974.
18. Joe Barbera, *My Life in 'toons: From Flatbush to Bedrock in Under a Century*, Turner Publishing, Inc., Atlanta, 1994.
19. Frank Thomas and Ollie Johnston interview with Mary Tebb, May 15, 1979.
20. Ben Sharpsteen, interview with Don Peri, April 24, 1974.
21. Ben Sharpsteen, interview with Don Peri, November 20, 1976.
22. Memo in the Gillett file at the Walt Disney Archives.
23. Devon Baxter, "Animator Profiles: Burt Gillett," https://cartoonresearch.com/index.php/animator-profiles-burt-gillett/, October 3, 2018.
24. With the exception of credit for *Arctic Antics*, which comes from *Walt Disney's Silly Symphonies* (Merritt and Kaufman), the credit list comes from the Walt Disney Archives.

Chapter 3

1. Dave Hand, studio lecture *The Director's Relationship to the Picture and to the Animator*, February 27, 1936.
2. Dick Lundy, interview with Michael Barrier, Sunland, California, November 26, 1973.
3. Joe Grant, interview with Michael Barrier, December 14, 1986.
4. Jack Cutting, interview with Frank Thomas and Ollie Johnston, May 25, 1978.
5. Dick Lundy, interview with Michael Barrier, Sunland, California, November 26, 1973.
6. Dave Hand, interview with Michael Barrier, November 21, 1973.
7. We've noted that people who worked with Walt Disney (the man) tend to refer to the studio as "Disney's." Those who worked there after his death label it "Disney," as in "Disney Studios."
8. Dave Hand, interview with Frank Thomas and Ollie Johnston, June 22, 1978.
9. Ben Sharpsteen, interview with Don Peri, April 24, 1974.
10. Dick Huemer, interview with Michael Barrier, North Hollywood, November 27, 1973.
11. Dick Huemer Oral History, interviewed by Joe Adamson. Huemer's opinion was shared by instructor Don Graham, who praised the "spirit" of the film in a 1936 analysis class.
12. https://www.intanibase.com/iad_entries/entry.aspx?shortID=179
13. In his biography "One of Walt's Boys," Harry Tytle describes Walt's methods for promoting personnel as "curious, but certainly consistent. He was quite severe when he gave [Gerry] Geronimi the job of associate producer on the live-action productions from Vienna . . . but Walt had given me the same treatment when he included the live-action portion of the evening television show as my responsibility. Walt once (at least once!) gave Ub Iwerks hell before moving him to a more important position . . ."
14. Dave Hand, interview with Frank Thomas and Ollie Johnston, June 22, 1978.
15. Dave Hand, interview with Frank Thomas and Ollie Johnston, June 22, 1978.
16. Barrier lists *The Flying Mouse* (1934), *Who Killed Cock Robin?* (1935), *Pluto's Judgment Day* (1935), and *Alpine Climbers* (1936).
17. Eric Larson, interview with Michael Barrier, Burbank, California, October 27, 1976.
18. Dick Huemer Oral History, interview by Joe Adamson, 1968.
19. Chuck Couch, interview with Milt Grey, Santa Monica, California, March 22, 1977.
20. Jack Cutting, interview with Don Peri, April 24, 1979. First appeared in *Working with Walt*.
21. Jack Cutting, interview with Don Peri, April 24, 1979. First appeared in *Working with Walt*.
22. Jack Cutting, interview with Frank Thomas and Ollie Johnston, May 25, 1978.

ENDNOTES

23. Frank Thomas, letter to Michael Barrier, August 22, 1991.
24. Judy La Prade, interview with the authors, Benicia, California, October 6, 2015.
25. Judy La Prade, interview with the authors, Benicia, California, October 6, 2015.
26. David Hale Hand, interview with the authors, personal communication, August 10, 2015.
27. Judy La Prade, interview with the authors, Benicia, California, October 6, 2015.
28. Judy La Prade, interview with the authors, Benicia, California, October 6, 2015.
29. Joe Grant, interview with Michael Barrier, December 14, 1986.
30. Dick Huemer, interview with Michael Barrier, North Hollywood, California, November 27, 1973.
31. Dick Lundy, interview with Michael Barrier, Sunland, California, November 26, 1973.
32. Bill Cottrell, interview with Frank Thomas and Ollie Johnston, November 3, 1976.
33. Dick Huemer, interview with Michael Barrier, North Hollywood, California, November 27, 1973.
34. Jack Brunner, interview with Milt Gray, March 31, 1977.
35. Don Duckwall, interview with Don Peri, July 16, 1980. First appeared in *Working with Walt.*
36. Dick Huemer Oral History, July 1968.
37. Ben Sharpsteen, interview with Don Peri, March 26, 1975.
38. For example, Bill Cottrell was assigned to direct most sequences containing the Queen; Perce Pearce many of the personality scenes with the Dwarfs, etc.
39. Ben Sharpsteen, interview with Don Peri, April 24, 1974.
40. Dave Hand, interview with Michael Barrier, 1973.
41. Dave Hand, interview with Michael Barrier, November 1973.
42. Ollie Johnston, interviewer unknown.
43. Frank Tashlin, interview with Michael Barrier, Beverly Hills, California, May 29, 1971.
44. Jack Kinney autobiography, *Walt Disney and Assorted Other Characters*.
45. Jack Cutting, interview with Frank Thomas and Ollie Johnston, May 25, 1978.
46. Dave Hand, interview with Michael Barrier, 1973.
47. Jack Cutting, interview with Frank Thomas and Ollie Johnston, May 25, 1978.
48. Frank Thomas and Ollie Johnston, interviewer unknown, 1993.
49. *Snow White* production notes.
50. Dave Hand, interview with Michael Barrier, November 21, 1973.
51. Leo Salkin, interview with Milt Gray, November 27, 1976.
52. Wilfred Jackson, interview with Michael Barrier, 1973.
53. *Snow White* premiered at the Carthay Circle Theatre on December 21, 1937, but began its general release on January 13, 1938, with an engagement at the Radio City Music Hall.
54. Frank Thomas, letter to Michael Barrier, May 22, 1988.
55. Dick Huemer, interview with Michael Barrier, North Hollywood, California, November 27, 1973.
56. Ben Sharpsteen, interview with Don Peri, May 2, 1974. First appeared in *Working with Walt.*
57. Michael Barrier, interview with Frank Thomas "on dead batteries," likely late 1978 or 1979.
58. Internal studio memo: "Discussion of New Studio Unit Set-up, October 24, 1938–Sweatbox 4."
59. Walt made this decision as early as December 1937, more or less concurrent with the release of *Snow White.*
60. Chuck Couch, interview with Milt Gray, Santa Monica, California, March 22, 1977.
61. Chuck Couch, interview with Milt Gray, Santa Monica, California, March 22, 1977.
62. Dave Hand, telephone conversation with Michael Barrier, August 17, 1975.
63. Chuck Couch, interview with Milt Gray, Santa Monica, California, March 22, 1977.
64. Zach Schwartz, interview with Leonard Maltin, August 18, 1977. *Walt's People*, Volume 14
65. David Dodd Hand, *Memoirs*, Lighthouse Litho, January 1991.
66. Dave Hand, interview with Frank Thomas and Ollie Johnston, June 22, 1978.
67. Meeting notes following a private screening on March 4, 1941.
68. Ben Sharpsteen, interview with Michael Barrier, October 23, 1976.

69. Frank Thomas, interviewer unknown, 1993.
70. Joe Grant, interview with Michael Barrier, Glendale, California, October 14, 1988.
71. David Dodd Hand, *Memoirs*, Lighthouse Litho, January 1991.
72. Jim Algar, letter to Frank Thomas, approximately 1975.
73. David Dodd Hand, *Memoirs*, Lighthouse Litho, January 1991.
74. David Hale Hand, interview with the authors, personal communication, August 10, 2015.
75. Jim Algar, letter to Frank Thomas, approximately 1975.
76. Excerpt from 1993 interviews with Frank Thomas and Ollie Johnston, interviewer unknown.
77. Dave Hand, interview with Michael Barrier, November 21, 1973.
78. Dave Hand, interview with Frank Thomas and Ollie Johnston, June 22, 1978.
79. David Lewin, *The Daily Express*. https://c3z3.com/www.animatormag.com/1987/issue-19/issue-19-page-27/
80. Though credited to Hand, Gillett notes that he directed it, and the timing sheets look to be in Gillett's hand.
81. Roy Williams was a story artist who was legendary for practical jokes and funny personal incidents. Best known to the *Mickey Mouse Club* audience as the Big Mooseketeer.
82. Jack Kinney, "Bambi and the Goof," *Funnyworld*, Number 21.
83. Interview with Don Peri, October 4, 1975.
84. Interview with Don Peri, October 4, 1975.
85. J. B. Kaufman, *The Fairest One of All*, San Francisco, The Walt Disney Family Foundation Press, 2012.
86. Michael Barrier, *Hollywood Cartoons*, Oxford University Press, 1999.
87. *Disney's Bambi: The Story and the Film* by Ollie Johnston and Frank Thomas, Stewart, Tabori & Chang Inc. 1990.
88. For an extensive examination of Perce's career, see "Piercing the Perce Pearce Mystery," by Didier Ghez and George Grant, in *Walt's People*, Volume 12.
89. Interview with Don Peri, October 4, 1975.
90. Interview with the authors, September 17, 2015.
91. According to the California Death Index, Bill was born on August 14. Bill himself wrote his birth was on August 2, 1899, in Jordan Station, Kentucky. According to Wikipedia: "Jordan is an unincorporated hamlet in Fulton County, Kentucky, United States. Jordan Station was a station on the Memphis and Ohio Railroad. It currently consists of a few houses and a liquor store."
92. Shamus Culhane, *Talking Animals and Other People*, St. Martin's Press, 1986.
93. Interview with Milt Gray, March 31, 1977.
94. Correspondence with Michael Barrier.
95. Correspondence with Michael Barrier.
96. Interview with Michael Barrier and Milt Gray, November 4, 1976.
97. John Canemaker, *Walt Disney's Nine Old Men*, Disney Editions, New York, 2001.
98. Interview with Milt Gray, March 31, 1977.
99. None of the Disney directors we are highlighting in this book, considered to be part of management, went out on strike.
100. Interview with Michael Barrier, August 15, 1978.
101. Interview with Michael Barrier, July 13, 1987.
102. Jack Kinney, *Walt Disney and Assorted Other Characters*, Harmony Press, New York, 1988.

Chapter 4

1. Interview with Don Peri, August 14, 1974. First appeared in *Working with Walt*.
2. Interview with Lorin Sorenson, September 25, 1973. Gail Sharpsteen collection.
3. David Bennett, "Ben Sharpsteen," *Ford Life*, Volume 4, Number 3.
4. According to Gail Sharpsteen, the spelling of the last name has alternated from "Sharpstein" to "Sharpsteen" from

ENDNOTES

generation to generation. Ben's grandfather preferred Sharpstein; Ben's father, Sharpsteen. Ben was Sharpstein during his college years and in the Marine Corps, but he changed it to Sharpsteen sometime in the 1920s.

5. Phyllis Schaumberg, "About the Cover Painting . . . ," *Horseless Carriage Gazette*, March–April 1966.
6. Interview by W. S. Fullerton, Sharpsteen Museum Association newsletter, August 1989, reprinted in *About Ben Sharpsteen: Second Impressions*, Sharpsteen Museum Reprints, July 1990.
7. Interview with Lorin Sorenson, September 25, 1973. Gail Sharpsteen collection.
8. Interview with Don Peri, August 14, 1974.
9. Interview with Don Peri, August 14, 1974.
10. Interview with Lorin Sorenson, September 25, 1973. Gail Sharpsteen collection.
11. Interview with Don Peri, February 6, 1974. First appeared in *Working with Walt*.
12. Interview with Michael Barrier, October 23, 1976.
13. Dave Smith, "Ben Sharpsteen: 33 years with Disney," *Millimeter Magazine*, April 1975.
14. Interview with Don Peri, February 6, 1974. First appeared in *Working with Walt*.
15. Interview with Lorin Sorenson, September 25, 1973. Gail Sharpsteen collection.
16. Interview with Lorin Sorenson, September 25, 1973. Gail Sharpsteen collection.
17. Interview with Don Peri, no date.
18. Interview with Don Peri, February 6, 1974. First appeared in *Working with Walt*.
19. Interview with Don Peri, February 6, 1974. First appeared in *Working with Walt*.
20. Interview with Don Peri, February 6, 1974. First appeared in *Working with Walt*.
21. Copy of page 18 of a ledger sheet in, I believe, Roy Disney's handwriting. No date. Don Peri collection.
22. Interview with Don Peri, February 6, 1974. First appeared in *Working with Walt*.
23. Interview with Don Peri, February 6, 1974. First appeared in *Working with Walt*.
24. Interview with Don Peri, March 5, 1975.
25. Correspondence with Michael Barrier, November 15, 2017.
26. Interview with Don Peri. February 6, 1974. First appeared in *Working with Walt*.
27. Interview with Don Peri, January 19, 1975. First appeared in *Working with Walt*.
28. Interview with Don Peri, February 7, 1975. First appeared in *Working with Walt*.
29. Interview with Don Peri, March 26, 1975.
30. Interview with Don Peri, February 6, 1974. First appeared in *Working with Walt*.
31. Interview with Don Peri, February 7, 1975. First appeared in *Working with Walt*.
32. Jack Kinney, *Walt Disney and Assorted Other Characters*, 1988.
33. Interview with Don Peri, October 4, 1975.
34. Interview with Michael Barrier, October 23, 1976.
35. Interview with Michael Barrier and Milton Gray, November 4, 1976.
36. Interview with Ron Merk, *Walt's People*: Volume 18.
37. Steven Watts, *The Magic Kingdom: Walt Disney and the American Way of Life*, 1997.
38. Interview with Milton Gray, March 22, 1977.
39. Interview with Michael Barrier, October 27, 1976.
40. Interview with George Sherman, *Walt's People*, Volume 1.
41. Interview with Frank Thomas and Ollie Johnston, 1993, interviewer unknown.
42. Interview with Ron Merk, *Walt's People*: Volume 18.
43. Interview with Don Peri, February 6, 1974. First appeared in *Working with Walt*.
44. Interview with Don Peri, August 14, 1974.
45. Interview with Don Peri, August 14, 1974.
46. Interview with Don Peri, February 1, 1975. First appeared in *Working with Walt*.
47. Interview with Michael Barrier, October 23, 1976.
48. Interview with Don Peri, August 14, 1974.

49. Interview with Don Peri, February 6, 1974. First appeared in *Working with Walt*.
50. Interview with Don Peri, March 20, 1976. See Chapter 1.
51. Interview with Don Peri, March 26, 1975.
52. Interview with Don Peri, August 14, 1974.
53. Interview with Don Peri, February 6, 1974.
54. Correspondence with Michael Barrier, November 24, 2017.
55. Interview with Don Peri, February 7, 1975.
56. Interview with Don Peri, January 11, 1976.
57. In a 1940 radio interview for *Hollywood Whispers* with George Fisher (KHJ-Mutual), Ben gave a different version of how the story of *Pinocchio* was chosen. "There are two main reasons why we settled on *Pinocchio*. The first is people have been writing into us over a period of years suggesting this story. There were probably thousands of letters on the subject, but it was especially significant we thought that a great many of them came from schoolteachers and librarians. In addition, our own people around the studio thought it would make a swell picture. Finally, in the face of all this, Walt broke down and read the book. He liked it and well you know what happened. *Pinocchio* won because it was a good story and because it lent itself to cartooning." This was recorded on January 31, 1940, and is on a record in a private collection.
58. Interview with Don Peri, February 6, 1974.
59. Interview with Don Peri, February 6, 1974.
60. George Fisher: Well I should think Walt feels pretty good about it, having done a job like that. Ben: No. On the contrary, Walt is the worrying kind. The thing is never so good but what it could be better. He's already found a thousand faults, little things that could be improved. He's never satisfied. Now that he has heard how the preview crowd has received it, naturally he's pleased.
61. Michael Barrier, *The Animated Man: A Life of Walt Disney*, 2007.
62. The Animated Man: A Life of Walt Disney, Barrier, page 152.
63. Ken Peterson, interview with Frank Thomas and Ollie Johnston, May 21, 1979.
64. Ken Anderson, interview with Frank Thomas and Ollie Johnston, April 8, 1978.
65. Created by Helen Aberson and her husband, Harold Pearl, *Dumbo* was published as a Roll-a-Book, with illustrations by Helen Durney. Walt Disney Productions bought the rights to develop it in 1939.
66. Interview with Don Peri, August 14, 1974.
67. Interview with Don Peri, March 26, 1975.
68. Michael Barrier, *The Animated Man: A Life of Walt Disney*, 2007.
69. Interview with Don Peri, November 20, 1976.
70. Interview with Don Peri, November 20, 1976.
71. Ben Sharpsteen, interview with Don Peri, April 26, 1974. First appeared In *Working with Walt*.
72. Interview with Don Peri, November 20, 1976.
73. Bob Thomas, *Walt Disney: An American Original*, 1994.
74. Dave Smith, *Millimeter Magazine*, April 1975.
75. Interview with Richard Hubler, *Walt's People*, Volume 5.
76. Interview with Don Peri, February 6, 1974. First appeared in *Working with Walt*.
77. Interview with Don Peri, February 6, 1974. First appeared in *Working with Walt*.
78. Interoffice communication between Ben and Walt Disney, October 2, 1956.
79. Interoffice communication between Ben and Walt Disney, October 2, 1956.
80. Correspondence from Walt Disney to Ben, March 22, 1956 from Ben's personal collection.
81. Interview with Don Peri, February 6, 1974.
82. Interview with Richard Hubler, October 19, 1968.
83. Interview with Don Peri, February 6, 1974.
84. Interview with Don Peri, August 30, 1974.
85. Interview with Don Peri, February 22, 2003, for the Walt Disney Family Foundation.

ENDNOTES

86. Interview with Don Peri, February 6, 1974. First appeared in *Working with Walt.*
87. Ben left the studio in 1959, but his retirement became effective on January 31, 1962.
88. Letter from Walt Disney to Emil Mrak, July 29, 1966.
89. Filmography from the Walt Disney Archives.
90. Frank Thomas and Ollie Johnston, *Disney Animation: The Illusion of Life*, Abbeville Publishers, New York, 1981.
91. Frank Thomas and Ollie Johnston, *Disney Animation: The Illusion of Life*, Abbeville Publishers, New York, 1981.
92. Interview with Don Peri, November 20, 1976.
93. J. B. Kaufman, *South of the Border with Disney*, Disney Editions, New York, 2009.
94. Interview with Don Peri, November 20, 1976.
95. Interview with Richard Huemer by Joe Adamson, UCLA Department of Theater Arts. October 8, 1968.
96. Interview with Don Peri, November 20, 1976.
97. Interview with Don Peri, January 19, 1975.
98. Interview with Robin Allan and Dr. William Moritz, June 9, 1985, appearing in *Walt's People*, Volume 1.
99. Jack Kinney, *Walt Disney and Assorted Other Characters*, Harmony Press, New York, 1988.
100. Compiled from various sources.

Chapter 5

1. Interview with Don Peri, January 12, 1977. First appeared in *Working with Walt.*
2. Interview with Michael Barrier, 1986.
3. Correspondence with Michael Barrier, 1973.
4. Correspondence with Michael Barrier, 1977.
5. Correspondence with Michael Barrier, 1973.
6. Interview with Don Peri, January 12, 1977. First appeared in *Working with Walt.*
7. Interview with Don Peri, January 12, 1977. First appeared in *Working with Walt.*
8. Copy of letter to Harry and Marian Tytle, April 7, 1979.
9. Interview with Michael Barrier, Milt Gray, and Bob Clampett, 1973.
10. Interview with Michael Barrier, Milt Gray, and Bob Clampett, 1973.
11. Letter to Jane Jackson, no date. Natha Horbach collection.
12. Interview with Don Peri, January 12, 1977. First appeared in *Working with Walt.*
13. Interview with Don Peri, January 12, 1977. First appeared in *Working with Walt.*
14. Correspondence with Michael Barrier, 1977.
15. Interview with Don Peri, January 12, 1977. First appeared in *Working with Walt.*
16. Interview with Don Peri, January 12, 1977. First appeared in *Working with Walt.*
17. Interview with Don Peri, January 12, 1977. First appeared in *Working with Walt.*
18. Interview with Don Peri, January 12, 1977. First appeared in *Working with Walt.*
19. Correspondence with Michael Barrier, 1975.
20. Interview with Don Peri, January 12, 1977. First appeared in *Working with Walt.*
21. Correspondence with Michael Barrier, 1975.
22. Interview with Michael Barrier, Milt Gray, and Bob Clampett, 1973.
23. Interview with Michael Barrier, Milt Gray, and Bob Clampett, 1973.
24. The term "sweatbox" first referred to a small closet at the Hyperion Avenue studio where the animators and Walt crowded in to view footage. The closeness of the space caused people to sweat. Even later in spacious rooms at the Burbank studio location, the term stuck, because people were likely to sweat when their work was reviewed, especially by Walt.
25. Interview with Michael Barrier, Milt Gray, and Bob Clampett, 1973.
26. Interview with Michael Barrier, 1986.
27. Interview with Don Peri, January 12, 1977. First appeared in *Working with Walt.*

28. Correspondence with Michael Barrier, 1975.
29. Wilfred Jackson, lecture on "Musical Stories," January 12, 1939, Walt Disney Studios.
30. Correspondence with Michael Barrier, 1975.
31. Interview with Michael Barrier, Milt Gray, and Bob Clampett, 1973.
32. Correspondence with Michael Barrier, 1975.
33. Jaxon's lecture on "Musical Stories," January 12, 1939, Walt Disney Studios.
34. Interview with Michael Barrier, Milton Gray, and Bob Clampett, 1973.
35. Interview with Dave Johnson, *Snow White's People*, Volume 1.
36. Interview with Michael Barrier, Milton Gray, and Bob Clampett, 1973.
37. Correspondence with Michael Barrier, 1975.
38. Interview with Steve Hulett, *Mouse in Transition*.
39. Interview with Michael Barrier, Milton Gray, and Bob Clampett, 1973.
40. Frank Thomas and Ollie Johnston, *The Disney Villain*, 1993.
41. Jackson notes from WDA, undated.
42. Neal Gabler, *Walt Disney: The Triumph of the American Imagination*, 2006.
43. Diary of Wilfred Jackson (1943–1959). Natha Horbach collection.
44. Diary of Wilfred Jackson, March 15, 1944. Natha Horbach collection.
45. Interview with Don Peri, January 12, 1977. First appeared in *Working with Walt*.
46. Interview with Michael Barrier and Milton Gray, 1976.
47. Interview with Michael Barrier, Milt Gray, and Bob Clampett, 1973.
48. Interview with Michael Barrier and Milt Gray, 1976.
49. Correspondence with Michael Barrier, 1975.
50. Correspondence with Michael Barrier, 1991.
51. Interview with Michael Barrier and Milton Gray, 1976.
52. Interview with Michael Barrier and Milton Gray, 1976.
53. Interview with Michael Barrier and Milton Gray, 1976.
54. Interview with Michael Barrier and Milton Gray, 1976.
55. Interview with Michael Barrier and Milton Gray, 1976.
56. Interview with Christopher Finch and Linda Rosenkrantz, 1972, in *Walt's People*, Volume 11.
57. Bob Thomas notes from a 1956 interview, WDA.
58. Interview with Don Peri, April 24, 1974.
59. Correspondence with Michael Barrier, 1978.
60. Michael Barrier, *The Animated Man*, 2007.
61. Interview with Don Peri, January 12, 1977. First appeared in *Working with Walt*.
62. Interoffice communication, April 23, 1954, to Walt Disney.
63. Jackson notes from WDA, undated.
64. Jackson notes from WDA, undated.
65. Interview with Dave Smith, May 5, 1976—Volume 17 of *Walt's People*.
66. Interoffice communication, handwritten copy, Natha Horbach collection.
67. Handwritten note, October 6, 1961, Natha Horbach collection.
68. Handwritten note, October 6, 1961, Natha Horbach collection.
69. Interview with Michael Barrier and Milton Gray, 1976.
70. *Midnight in the Toy Shop* (1930) is credited to Jackson in *Walt Disney's Silly Symphonies*.

Chapter 6

1. Eric Larson, *50 Years in the Mouse House*, Theme Park Press, 2015.
2. Eric Larson, *50 Years in the Mouse House*, Theme Park Press, 2015.

ENDNOTES

3. Correspondence with Peggy Finefrock, August 6, 2018.
4. Correspondence with Peggy Finefrock, August 6, 2018.
5. Walt Disney Studio internal newsletter, *Bulletin*, March 3, 1939.
6. *The Blue and Gold: A Complete Record of the College Year 1925–1926*, University of California at Berkeley.
7. Walt Disney Studio internal newsletter, *Bulletin*, March 3, 1939.
8. Walt Disney Studio internal newsletter, *Bulletin*, March 3, 1939.
9. Walt Disney Studio internal newsletter, *Bulletin*, March 3, 1939.
10. Correspondence with Michael Barrier, February 27, 1968.
11. Interview with Don Peri, November 20, 1976.
12. Eric Larson, *50 Years in the Mouse House*, Theme Park Press, 2015.
13. Interview with Don Peri, November 24, 2002, for the Walt Disney Family Foundation.
14. Frank Thomas and Ollie Johnston, *Disney Animation: The Illusion of Life*, Abbeville Press, New York, 1981.
15. Interview with Michael Barrier and Bill Spicer, 1969.
16. Correspondence with Michael Barrier, November 27, 1973.
17. Woolie Reitherman interview with Christopher Finch and Linda Rosenkrantz, May 9, 1972, Didier Ghez, *Walt's People*, Volume 23, Theme Park Press, 2019.
18. J. B. Kaufman, *The Fairest One of All*, The Walt Disney Family Foundation Press, San Francisco, 2012.
19. Interoffice communication from Walt to Paul Hopkins, November 25, 1935, quoted in Neal Gabler, *Walt Disney: The Triumph of the American Imagination*, Alfred A Knopf, 2006.
20. Michael Barrier, *The Animated Man: A Life of Walt Disney*, University of California Press, Berkeley, 2007.
21. Frank Thomas and Ollie Johnston, *Disney Animation: The Illusion of Life*, Abbeville Press, New York, 1981.
22. Interview with Don Peri, November 20, 1976.
23. Michael Barrier, *Hollywood Cartoons: American Animation in Its Golden Age*, Oxford University Press, New York, 1999.
24. Interview with Jim Korkis, March 2012, Didier Ghez, *Walt's People*, Volume 15, Theme Park Press, 2014.
25. Interview with Aline Mosby, UPI, quoted in Leonard Maltin, *The Disney Films*, Disney Editions, New York, 2000.
26. Wilfred Jackson, "Third Installment of June 3, 1975" letter to Michael Barrier.
27. Wilfred Jackson, "Third Installment of June 3, 1975" letter to Michael Barrier.
28. Interview with Michael Barrier and Milton Gray, November 4, 1976.
29. Interview with Michael Barrier and Milton Gray, October 1976.
30. Interview with John Culhane, February 7, 1978.
31. Interview with Pete Docter and Don Peri, September 2016.
32. Ralph Wright, interview with Michael Barrier, February 1, 1977.
33. Wilfred Jackson, "Third Installment of June 3, 1975" letter to Michael Barrier.
34. Interview with Pete Docter and Don Peri, October 14, 2015.
35. Interview with Don Peri, June 1977, first appeared in *Working with Walt*.
36. Otto Englander letter to Izzy Klein, September 16, 1965, in Didier Ghez, *Walt's People*, Volume 24, Theme Park Press, 2020.
37. Filmography from the Walt Disney Archives.

Chapter 7

1. Gerry Geronimi, interview with Michael Barrier and Milt Gray, November 5, 1976.
2. Quotes from animator Rudy Larriva, animator Ed Love, and layout artist Thor Putnam; interviews by Mike Barrier.
3. Letter to authors from Geronimi's granddaughter Megan Hills, February 2, 2018.
4. https://theworld.org/stories/2015-11-26/brief-history-america-s-hostility-previous-generation-mediterranean-migrants
5. Letter to authors from Geronimi's granddaughter Megan Hills, February 2, 2018.
6. Geronimi, interview with Michael Barrier, 1976.

7. Gerry Geronimi, interview with Michael Barrier and Milt Gray, Newport Beach, California, November 5, 1976.
8. Gerry Geronimi, interview with Michael Barrier and Milt Gray, Newport Beach, California, November 5, 1976.
9. https://www.mouseplanet.com/10821/The_History_of_Oswald_the_Lucky_Rabbit_Part_Two.
10. Gerry Geronimi, interview with Michael Barrier and Milt Gray, Newport Beach, California, November 5, 1976. Disney's records indicate Geronimi was hired on August 28, 1931, but records of exact employment dates from this time are often unreliable.
11. Hans Perk, http://afilmla.blogspot.com/2009/06/prod-rm7-boat-builders_26.html.
12. Thor Putnam, interview with Michael Barrier, December 1, 1990.
13. Gerry Geronimi, interview with Michael Barrier and Milt Gray, Newport Beach, California, November 5, 1976.
14. Jack Cutting, interview with Michael Barrier, December 11, 1986.
15. Gerry Geronimi, interview with Michael Barrier and Milt Gray, Newport Beach, California, November 5, 1976.
16. Don Duckwall, interview with Don Peri, July 16, 1980. First appeared in *Working with Walt*.
17. Donald Duckwall, interview with Dave Smith, January 30, 1980. Duckwall's reference to bonuses was an economic incentive set by the studio: budgets kept below a certain amount meant the production team took home the difference.
18. Gerry Geronimi, interview with Michael Barrier and Milt Gray, Newport Beach, California, November 5, 1976.
19. Charles August "Nick" Nichols (1910–1992) from *Walt's People,* Volume 16.
20. Don Duckwall, interview with Don Peri, July 16, 1980. First appeared in *Working with Walt*.
21. Lance Nolley, interview by Don Peri, August 11, 1978. First appeared in *Working with Walt*.
22. Gerry Geronimi, interview with Michael Barrier and Milt Gray, Newport Beach, California, November 5, 1976.
23. Donald Duckwall, interview with Dave Smith, January 30, 1980.
24. Donald Duckwall, interview with Dave Smith, January 30, 1980.
25. Gerry Geronimi, interview with Michael Barrier and Milt Gray, Newport Beach, California, November 5, 1976.
26. Gerry Geronimi, interview with Michael Barrier and Milt Gray, Newport Beach, California, November 5, 1976.
27. John Sibley and Woolie Reitherman also animated a substantial part of this section, according to the records.
28. Typically music would be written in advance of the animation being drawn, called prescoring. This music would be written once animation was completed, a process that became more common after *Cinderella*.
29. Gerry Geronimi, interview with Michael Barrier and Milt Gray, Newport Beach, California, November 5, 1976.
30. Frank Thomas, recorded memo to self, 1978.
31. See Wilfred Jackson chapter for more info on this.
32. Jack Brunner, interview with Milt Gray, March 31, 1977.
33. Don Jurwich, interview with Milt Gray, December 20, 1976.
34. Jack Cutting, interview with Michael Barrier, December 11, 1986. Geronimi's New York accent can be heard as he works with animator Woolie Reitherman on the *Wonderful World of Disney* "The Story of Dogs."
35. Ed Love, interview with Michael Barrier, September 25, 1990.
36. Lance Nolley, interview with Don Peri, August 11, 1978. First appeared in *Working with Walt*.
37. Les Clark, interview with Michael Barrier, December 1, 1973.
38. Frank Thomas, letter to Michael Barrier, October 11, 1989.
39. Gerry Geronimi, interview with Michael Barrier and Milt Gray, Newport Beach, California, November 5, 1976.
40. Eleanor Audley, interview with Charles Solomon, February 1986.
41. Gerry Geronimi, interview with Michael Barrier and Milt Gray, Newport Beach, California, November 5, 1976.
42. Jack Brunner, interview with Milt Gray, March 31, 1977.
43. Floyd Norman, interview with the authors, August 1, 2011.
44. Jerry Hathcock, interview with Michael Barrier, November 29, 1986, pp. 30, 31.
45. Gerry Geronimi, interview with Michael Barrier and Milt Gray, Newport Beach, California, November 5, 1976.
46. Gerry Geronimi, interview with Michael Barrier and Milt Gray, Newport Beach, California, November 5, 1976.
47. Ward Kimball, interview with Steve Hulett, spring 1978 (*Walt's People,* Volume 6, p. 74).
48. Harry Tytle, *One of Walt's Boys*, ASAP Publishing, January 1, 1997.

ENDNOTES

49. Megan Hills (Gerry's granddaughter), letter to authors, February 2, 2018; Lyn Geronimi (Gerry's son), letter to authors, July 2017.
50. The ten being the famed Nine Old Men plus Norm Ferguson. The only exceptions to this were Hal King on *Lady and the Tramp* and Don Bluth on *The Rescuers*.
51. Gerry Geronimi, interview with Michael Barrier and Milt Gray, Newport Beach, California, November 5, 1976.
52. Dick Huemer, interview with Michael Barrier, North Hollywood, California, October 27, 1976.
53. Wilfred Jackson, interview with Michael Barrier.
54. While many attribute storyboards to story artist Webb Smith, animation pioneer Dick Huemer wrote in his "Huemeresque" column in Funnyworld #18, Summer 1978: "Would you like to know the name of the genius who invented the concept of the storyboard? Most think that it was Walt Disney's idea and there are those who claim the honor for Webb Smith. But take it from me, an unimpeachable source, it was Ted Sears who first thought of it and submitted it to the Fleischers back in New York when he was working for them in the late 20's. According to how I heard it, they didn't go for it. So later when Ted made the switch to Disney and again unveiled the idea to that perfectionist, his nibs, being in the concept still another way to improve the product, promptly ordered it done. The rest, to uncoin a phrase, is no mystery." See also Dick Huemer, interview with Michael Barrier, North Hollywood, California, October 27, 1976, as well as Jack Kinney interviews with Michael Barrier.
55. Wilfred Jackson, interview with Michael Barrier.
56. Dick Huemer, interview with Michael Barrier, North Hollywood, California, October 27, 1976. See also Jack Kinney interviews with Michael Barrier.
57. Jack Kinney, interview with Michael Barrier; Wilfred Jackson diary, January 6, 1944.
58. Gerry Geronimi, interview with Michael Barrier and Milt Gray, Newport Beach, California, November 5, 1976; Burny Mattinson and Ellen Sirola, interview with the authors, October 29, 2018; Wilfred Jackson diary.
59. Ron Clements, interview with Pete Docter, June 9, 2021.
60. Ron Clements, interview with Pete Docter, June 9, 2021; June 11, 2021, email with John Musker; June 19 email with Mike Gabriel.

Chapter 8

1. Don Duckwall, interview by Don Peri, July 16, 1980. First appeared in *Working with Walt.*
2. Jackson would direct only three more shorts in his career: *Golden Eggs* in 1941, *The New Spirit* in 1942, and *The Little House* in 1952.
3. According to *One of Walt's Boys* by Harry Tytle.
4. Graham Heid, letter to Michael Barrier, May 24, 1975. Heid left Disney in 1945 and worked with independent producers and the U.S. Public Health Service producing medical teaching films until his retirement in 1971.
5. Having started directing with a commercial short for Standard Oil, Thompson went into comics in the 1950s, leaving the studio with Jack Hannah in 1959. For more, see *The Life and Times of Riley Thomson* (1912–1960) by Alberto Becattini, *Walt's People*, Volume 15.
6. Ben Sharpsteen, interview with Michael Barrier, October 23, 1976.
7. Ben Sharpsteen, interview with Michael Barrier, October 23, 1976.
8. Don Duckwall, interview with Dave Smith. *Walt's People*, Volume 13.
9. Ben Sharpsteen, interview with Michael Barrier, October 23, 1976.
10. Interviewed in February 1985, interviewer unknown, *Walt's People*, Volume 16.
11. Jack Kinney, interview with Michael Barrier, 1973.
12. Nick Nichols, interviewer unknown, February 1985, *Walt's People*, Volume 16.
13. Jack Kinney, interview with Michael Barrier.
14. Jack Hannah, interview with Dave Smith, date unknown.
15. Jack Kinney, interview with Michael Barrier and Milt Gray, November 28, 1973.
16. Leo Salkin, interview with Milt Gray, November 27, 1976.

17. Jack Hannah, interview with Dave Smith, date unknown.
18. Donald Duckwall, interview with Dave Smith, January 30, 1980.
19. Jack Kinney, interview with Michael Barrier and Milt Gray, 1976.
20. Donald Duckwall, interview with Dave Smith, January 30, 1980.
21. Les Clark, interview with Frank Thomas and Ollie Johnston, September 14, 1976.
22. Jack Kinney, interview with Michael Barrier and Milt Gray, 1976.
23. Jack Hannah, interview with Jim Korkis, *Mindrot* #11, July 24, 1978.
24. Carl Barks, interview with Michael Barrier, October 5–6, 1974.
25. Phil Monroe, interview with Michael Barrier and Milt Gray, 1976.
26. Disney Archives 3/97, "A note for the Jack King file."
27. Jack Hannah, interview with Jim Korkis, *Mindrot* #11, July 24, 1978.
28. Historian David Gerstein indicates King directed *A Haunted House*, a black-and-white Mickey Mouse short from 1929, which is often credited to Disney.
29. Notes from an interview with Ed Love, September 25, 1990.
30. Eric Larson, interview with Thorkil B. Rasmussen, February 22, 1978.
31. Bob McCrea, interview with Dave Smith.
32. Bob McCrea, interview with Dave Smith.
33. Jack Hannah, interview with Jim Korkis.
34. 1987 Annie Awards mini-biography.
35. Jack Hannah, interview with Jim Korkis.
36. "An Animated Life: The Story of Jack Hannah" by Jim Korkis, published in *Persistence of Vision* #8, June 1996.
37. "An Animated Life: The Story of Jack Hannah" by Jim Korkis, published in *Persistence of Vision* #8, June 1996.
38. "An Animated Life: The Story of Jack Hannah" by Jim Korkis, published in *Persistence of Vision* #8, June 1996.
39. Eric Larson, interview with Thorkil B. Rasmussen, February 22, 1978.
40. See sidebar in Chapter 2 for more on exposure sheets.
41. Interviews with Jim Korkis in July 1978 and May 1981, plus additional conversations until 1994, *Walt's People*, Volume 1.
42. Interviewed in February 1985, interviewer unknown, *Walt's People*, Volume 16.
43. Eric Larson, interview with Thorkil B. Rasmussen on February 22, 1978, *Walt's People*, Volume 2.
44. Paul Carlson, interview with Didier Gehz, *Walt's People*, Volume 9.
45. Victor Haboush, interview with Didier Gehz on July 3, 2007, *Walt's People*, Volume 9.
46. Jack Kinney, interview with Michael Barrier and Milt Grey, 1973.
47. Jack Kinney, interview with Michael Barrier, 1973.
48. Victor Haboush, interview with Didier Gehz on July 3, 2007, *Walt's People*, Volume 9.
49. Bob McCrea, interview with Dave Smith, May 5, 1976. McCrea also mentions Ward Kimball and Roy Williams as part of this group.
50. Jack Kinney, interview with Michael Barrier, December 14, 1986.
51. Kinney and Roy Williams had played football together at Fremont High School.
52. Jack Kinney, interview with Michael Barrier, December 14, 1986.
53. *Walt Disney and Assorted Other Characters* by Jack Kinney.
54. Jack Kinney, notes from interviews with Michael Barrier, December 1986.
55. Jack Kinney, interview with Michael Barrier, 1973.
56. Carl Barks, interview with Michael Barrier, October 5–6, 1974.
57. Jack Kinney, interview with Michael Barrier and Milt Gray, November 28, 1973.
58. Jerry Hathcock, interview with Michael Barrier, November 29, 1986.
59. Jack Kinney, interview with Michael Barrier and Milt Gray, November 28, 1973.
60. *Walt Disney and Assorted Other Characters* by Jack Kinney.
61. Jack Kinney, interview with Michael Barrier and Milt Gray, 1973.

ENDNOTES

62. Harry Tytle, One Of "Walt's Boys," page 26: "The new Goofy also received adverse comment from Walt; he just was not a fan of the revised Goofs. Walt wanted the dangly, dog-like ears back on Goofy. He felt the character did not aid in the studio's merchandising effort.
63. Jack Kinney Interview by Michael Barrier, December 8, 1986. Kinney was likely exaggerating the actual dollar amount for humor.
64. Lance Nolley, interview with Don Peri, August 11, 1978. First appeared in *Working with Walt.*
65. Jack and Jane Kinney, interview with Michael Barrier and Milt Gray, November 3, 1976.
66. Jack Kinney, interview with Michael Barrier, 1973.
67. Ward Kimball, interview with Michael Barrier, http://www.michaelbarrier.com/Interviews/Kimball/interview_ward_kimball.htm.
68. *One of Walt's Boys*, Harry Tytle.
69. *One of Walt's Boys*, Harry Tytle.
70. Interviewed in February 1985, interviewer unknown, *Walt's People*, Volume 16.
71. *One of Walt's Boys*, Harry Tytle.

Chapter 9

1. Mica Productions, footage and transcripts for "Disney Family Album" television program featuring Woolie Reitherman
2. Leonard Maltin, *The Disney Films*, Disney Editions, New York, 2000.
3. Reel History, "The Shaggy Dog," March 10, 2021, https://norlinreelhistory.blogspot.com/2021/03/the-shaggy-dog.html
4. https://d23.com/list-of-disney-films/
5. Interview with Marc Davis by Charles Solomon, August 19, 1986; appeared in Daniel Kotheenschulte (ed.), *The Walt Disney Film Archives: The Animated Movies 1921–1968*, Taschen, Hohenzollernring, 2016.
6. Interoffice communication, April 5, 1954.
7. Interview with the authors, May 5, 2016.
8. March 27, 1945, letter from Walt Disney to Woolie Reitherman.
9. Cecilia _____ (last name unknown), *Family Circle* magazine, date unknown, appears in *Walt's People*, Volume 23, Didier Ghez, editor; Theme Park Press, 2019.
10. Janie Reitherman, interview with John Canemaker, July 9, 1998.
11. Cecilia _____ (last name unknown), *Family Circle* magazine, date unknown, appears in *Walt's People*, Volume 23, Didier Ghez, editor; Theme Park Press, 2019.
12. Chuck Champlin, Jr., "The Disney Days of Reitherman," *Los Angeles Times*, August 10, 1981.
13. Interview with Don Peri, November 20, 1976.
14. Jack Kinney, *Walt Disney and Assorted Other Characters*, Harmony Press, New York, 1988.
15. Michael Barrier, interview with Frank Thomas and Ollie Johnston, July 13, 1987.
16. Authors, interview with Bruce Reitherman, May 5, 2016.
17. Mica Productions, footage and transcripts for "Disney Family Album" television program featuring Woolie Reitherman.
18. Becky Hughes, "How 'Hump Pilots' Defied Death Flying Over the Himalayas During World War II," *Parade*, December 6, 2017.
19. Chuck Champlin, Jr., "The Disney Days of Reitherman," *Los Angeles Times*, August 10, 1981.
20. Dick Reitherman, interview with authors, May 5, 2016.
21. Bruce Reitherman, interview with authors, May 5, 2016.
22. Mica Productions, footage and transcripts for *Disney Family Album* television program featuring Woolie Reitherman.
23. Michael Barrier, *Hollywood Cartoons*, Oxford University Press, New York, 1999.
24. Interview with Thorkil B. Rasmussen, February 24, 1978, in *Walt's People*, Volume 2, Didier Ghez (ed.), Theme Park Press, 2006.
25. Mica Productions, footage and transcripts for *Disney Family Album* television program featuring Woolie Reitherman.

26. Michael Barrier review, *The Jungle Book*, reprinted from *Funnyworld* Number 19, http://www.michaelbarrier.com/Funnyworld/JungleBook/JungleBook.html
27. Jay Horan, interview with Claude Coats, *Walt's People*, Volume 16, Didier Ghez (ed.), Theme Park Press, 2015.
28. Authors interview with Ron Miller, May 8, 2018.
29. Walt Disney Family Museum blog, "More from Mowgli: Outtakes with Bruce Reitherman," Lucas Seastrom, posted 2/10/2023.
30. Michael Barrier, interview with Frank Thomas and Ollie Johnston, July 13, 1987.
31. John Canemaker, *Walt Disney's Nine Old Men*, Disney Editions, New York, 2001.
32. Mica Productions, footage and transcripts for *Disney Family Album* television program featuring Woolie Reitherman.
33. Interviewer unknown, 1984, *Walt's People*, Volume 17, Didier Ghez (ed.), Theme Park Press, 2015.
34. Interview with Don Peri, October 14, 1978, in *Working with Disney*, University Press of Mississippi, Jackson, 2011.
35. Interview with the authors, May 5, 2016.
36. Andreas Deja, interview with the authors, October 24, 2015.
37. Interview with the authors, May 5, 2016.
38. Mica Productions, footage and transcripts for *Disney Family Album* television program featuring Woolie Reitherman.
39. Mica Productions, footage and transcripts for *Disney Family Album* television program featuring Woolie Reitherman.
40. Mica Productions, footage and transcripts for *Disney Family Album* television program featuring Woolie Reitherman.
41. Interview with Thorkil B. Rasmussen, February 24, 1978, in *Walt's People*, Volume 2, Didier Ghez (ed.), Theme Park Press, 2006.
42. Interview with Christopher Finch and Linda Rosenkrantz, May 9, 1972, in *Walt's People*, Volume 23, Didier Ghez (ed.), Theme Park Press, 2019.
43. John Canemaker, *Walt Disney's Nine Old Men*, Disney Editions, New York, 2001.
44. Interview with the authors, October 15, 2015.
45. John Canemaker, *Walt Disney's* Nine *Old Men*, Disney Editions, New York, 2001.
46. Interview with the authors, November 23, 2013.
47. Michael Barrier, interview with Frank Thomas and Ollie Johnston, July 13, 1987.
48. Authors' interview with John Pomeroy, August 22, 2018.
49. Interview with the authors, August 17, 2015.
50. Interview with the authors, October 25, 2018.
51. Michael Barrier correspondence December 3, 1986.
52. Interview with the authors, October 25, 2018.
53. Bluth, Don, *Somewhere Out There: My Animated Life*, Smart Pop Books, Dallas, 2022.
54. Interview with the authors, August 22, 2018.
55. Interview with Clay Kaytis, 2006, in *Walt's People*, Volume 9, Didier Ghez (ed.), Theme Park Press, 2010.
56. Interview with the authors, October 14, 2015.
57. Interview with the authors, March 21, 2016.
58. Interview with the authors, March 21, 2016.
59. Interview with the authors, March 21, 2016.
60. John Canemaker, *Walt Disney's Nine Old Men*, Disney Editions, New York, 2001.
61. Wikipedia, https://en.wikipedia.org/wiki/Ward_Kimball.
62. Interview with Don Peri, August 13, 1978. First appeared in *Working with Walt*.
63. John Canemaker, *Walt Disney's Nine Old Men*, Disney Editions, New York, 2001.

Chapter 10

1. Joe Grant, interview with Michael Barrier, October 14, 1988.
2. Roy's suggestion, around 1947, allegedly led to a fight between the brothers that lasted for months. But Walt's

ENDNOTES

selection of *Cinderella* was telling; as Frank Thomas put it, "the only thing the audience seems to like is a young girl in trouble, and people trying to help her out. So let's do *Cinderella* and try not to make it like *Snow White*."

3. Story teams on earlier films numbered in the dozens, while *One Hundred and One Dalamtians* consisted of Bill Peet and a couple of associates. The ink and paint department was replaced by the xerox process. Lavish multiplane camera moves were phased out in favor of simpler, flat staging
4. Bill Peet book; Dick Huemer interview.
5. Woolie Reitherman, interview with Frank Thomas and Ollie Johnston.
6. Ron Musker, John Lasseter, Brad Bird, etc.
7. Ron Clements interview with Pete Docter, June 9, 2021; John Musker correspondence with Pete Docter, June 11, 2021.
8. Computer programs like Final Cut, Pro Tools and Avid.
9. When Lasseter and team told Disney of their plans to use nonlinear editing, they were told initially that Jeffery Katzenberg refused to watch movies on video, preferring the look of film. Whether this was true or a misunderstanding, the benefits quickly outshined the downsides.
10. This and all quotes from modern-day directors from correspondence with Pete Docter, September 3, 2021, through October 4, 2021.

Appendix A

1. Dan MacManus, interview with Milt Gray, March 22, 1977.
2. Gordon Legg, interview with Milt Gray, March 13, 1976.
3. Joe Grant, interview with Michael Barrier, October 14, 1988.
4. Heid letter to Michael Barrier, May 24, 1975.
5. Dick Huemer Oral History, July 1968–June 1969.
6. Harry Tytle, "One of Walt's Boys."
7. McLaren Stewart, interview with Milt Gray: March 31, 1977.

INDEX

A

The Adventures of Ichabod and Mr. Toad (feature) 110, 173, 182, 221, 237, 271, 275, 286, 294
Algar, Jim 73, **96**, **106**, **266**, 271, **271**
  directing credits by year 283, 284, 286
  feature film sequences directed by 294
  True-Life Adventure films 104, 271
Alice in Wonderland (feature) 103, 142, 157, 158, 180, 183, 241
  in director filmographies 110, 114, 147, 163, 192, 255
  live-action reference **159**, 180, 185
  in production **159**, **188**
  selected directors and sequences directed 196, 298, 301
  year and directors 287
Ama Girls (short) 98, 107, 110
Anderson, Bill **106**, 224, 243, 246
Anderson, Ken 94, 100, **241**, **244**, **247**, **248**, **249**, **266**
Animation directors, modern 263–265
Animation directors time line 308–313
Animation process: explained by Mickey Mouse **40–41**
Animators, lead
  credits on features 193
  role of 21, 44
"The Animator's Prayer" ix
Arctic Antics (short) **27**, 39, 280, 319, 324
The Aristocats (feature) 244, 246, 255, 262, 289
Armstrong, Sam 102, 204, **271**, 271–272, 274, 283, 284, 294
Audience Research Institute (ARI) 207
Audley, Eleanor 185, **188**

B

Babbitt, Art 62–63, 115, 121, 131, 187
Bambi (feature) 49, 58, 69–71, 82, 102, 189, 271, 276, 277
  as box-office disappointment 183, 205
  "Death of the Mother" sequence 245
  in director filmographies 75, 83
  involvement of Walt Disney 71, 102
  Leica reel 194
  music 128, 276
  "Raindrop" sequence 204, 295
  selected directors and sequences directed 292, 293, 304, 305
  story development 69–70, 77–78, 156
  Supervising Animators (credit) 193
  year and directors 284
The Band Concert (short) 132, 133, 147, 175, 236, 282
Bar sheets 27–31, **29–31**, 60, 126, **127**, 218, **219**
Barks, Carl 208, 209, 211, 217
Barrier, Michael 33, 52, 59, 79, 82, 92, 99, 101, 131, 140, 145, 155, 160, 261
Baskett, James 139
Beaumont, Kathryn **158**, **159**, 180
Beebe, Ford L., Jr. 204, 272, 283
Belcher, Marjorie **134**, 155
Blair, Mary 139–140, **140**
Blue Rhythm (short) **37**, 39, 281
Bluth, Don 250, 252, 257, **258**, 262, 289, 290
Bone Trouble (short) **28**, 216, 283
The Brave Little Tailor (short) 38, 81, 83, 194, 215–216, 283
Bray Productions 25, 170, 174
Brodie, Don L. **99**
Building a Building (short) 52, 75, 281

C

Cannon, Johnny 11, **11**, **13**, **22**, **26**, **48**, **50**, 52, 126
Carlson, Robert William "Bob" 272
The Castaway (short) 128–129, 147, 280
Cels (celluloid sheets) 3, 4, 20, 33, **34**, 126
Churchill, Frank **13**, **26**, **34**, **36**, **130**, **135**
  as composer and songwriter 36, 124, 128, 275
  one-sentence description of 115
Cinderella (feature) 103, 113, 140, 142–143, 158, 183, 195, 241, 274
  in director filmographies 110, 114, 147, 163, 192, 255
  legacy 264
  live-action reference **144**, **159**, 185, **185**
  role of Walt Disney 142, 143, 183
  selected directors and sequences directed 296, 297, 298, 301
  strength of Geronimi's work 173, 187
  year and directors 287
Clark, Les 11, **11**, **13**, 16, **16**, **48**, **51**, 52, 153, 155, 257
  directing credits by year 288, 289
  in group photos **xvii**, **22**, **26**, **48**, **256**, **266**
  honored with Mousecar **xvii**, **257**
  as one of Nine Old Men **256**, 257
  one-sentence description of 115
  recollections of 184, 208, 257
  on *Sleeping Beauty* 257, 295
  X-sheet assigned to **32**
Clements, Ron 249, 252, **258**, 262–263, 265
Clemmons, Larry 105, 115, 156, 180, 244, **244**, 247, **249**
Coats, Claude **266**
Colonna, Gerry **188**
Colvig, Pinto 220, **220**, 272, 282
Conried, Hans **188**
Cook, Randy: gag drawing by **253**
Cormack, Robert C. "Bob" 272, 28[illegible], 295
Cottrell, William "Bill" 59, 61, 94, 100, **272**, 272, 282, 295
Couch, Chuck 53, 69–70, 71, 94
Crosby, Bing 182–183
Culhane, Shamus 25, 79, 94
Cutting, Jack **11**, **13**, **26**, 184, 204, **204**
  bar sheet prepared by **29**
  on Dave Hand 53, 58, 62
  supervision of foreign dubbing 95, 204
  The Ugly Duckling and 156, 176, 204, 283

D

Davidovich, Basil **244**
Davis, Marc 140, **188**, 233, 244, 256, **256**, **266**
De Trémaudan, Gilles "Frenchy" **26**, 52, 80
  caricature by **137**
Disney, Lillian **66**, 78, **105**, 273
Disney, Roy E. 262
Disney, Roy O. 35, 73, 91, **107**, 108, 129, 243, 246
  and end of shorts 203, 222
  and Iwerks 9, 15–16
Disney, Walter Elias
  as animator 9
  caricature of **13**
  death 109, 195, 243, 261
  directing credits by year 280, 281
  diversification 78, 118–119, 142, 158, 189, 229
  efforts to organize studio 38, 61, 66–67, 68, 99
  experimentation with directors 204–205
  with film crews **28**, **51**, **81**, **84**, **130**, **133**, **189**, **261**
  in group photos **22**, **26**, **48**, **266**
  and Iwerks **6**, 9, 12, 14–17, **16**
  loss of interest in animation 261
  memos from **37**, 155
  presenting Mousecars **xvi**, **107**, **257**
  relationships with directors 49, 65, 68, 72, 102–105, 109, 140, 220
  role in film production process: flowcharts 4, 5, 21, 44–45, 118–119, 199, 228–229
  "shaping crew" 100
  Snow White, involvement with 11, 61, [illegible], 133–134
  time line 308 - 313
Disneyland (television series) 104, **104**, [illegible], 214, 233, 256
Disneyland, Anaheim, California 189, 233, 271
Donald Duck (character) 82, 96, 113, 175, 210, 211, 212, 214
Duckwall, Donald 60, 176–178, 203, 204, 205
Dumbo (feature) 82, 101–102, 112, 137, 20[illegible], 216, **217**, 241, 271–273

Boldface indicates illustrations.

Animation Directors (credit) 193
in director filmographies 83, 110, 114, 147, 255
music 128
selected directors and sequences directed 294, 295, 298, 299, 304, 305
story development 204, 273, 274
Timothy Mouse 101, **236**
train model **15**
year and directors 284

E

Edwards, Cliff **79, 217**
Eisner, Michael 262
Elmer Elephant (short) 147, **154**, 154–155, 236, 282
Eloitte, John Wesley "Jack" 273

F

Fantasia (feature) 69, 71, 80–81, 101, 135–137, 205, 241
Animation Supervision (credit) 193
"Ave Maria" sequence 137, 271, 298
"Dance of the Hours" sequence 112, 274, 295
in director filmographies 83, 110, 114, 147, 163
as disappointment in initial release 101, 183
Leica reels 194, **194**, 216
music 137, 274, 275
"Night on Bald Mountain" sequence 135, 136, 297
"Nutcracker Suite" sequence 271, 274, 277, 294
"Pastoral Symphony" sequence 157, 204, 272, 274
in production **82, 237, 275**
"Rite of Spring" sequence 81–82, 237, 271, 276, 302-304
selected directors and sequences directed 292, 295, 296, 298, 302-304
"Sorcerer's Apprentice" sequence 77, 271, 294
story development 77, 78, 204, 277
year and directors 283
Feature directors: flowcharts
under Walt's creative leadership (1936–1948) 44–45
as Walt diversified (1949–1961) 118–119
with less input from Walt (1963–1966) 228–229
Ferdinand the Bull (short) 204, 276, 283
Ferguson, Norman "Fergy" **13**, 38, **91**, 111–114, **111–114**
animation experience 25, 91, 111, 129
directing credits by year 283–285
Disney director filmography 114
feature film sequences directed by 295
in group photos **22, 26, 48, 99**
rough animation style 111, 208
and *The Three Little Pigs* 36, 112
as top animator 38, 111, 114, 151
Ferrer, Pilar **113**
Flowers and Trees (short) 33, 39, 175, 281, 306
The Fox and the Hound (feature) 252–254, 255, 262, 290
Freleng, Friz 210, 264
Fun and Fancy Free (feature)
"Bongo" sequence 216, 221, 222, 299
Directing Animators (credit) 193
in director filmographies 83, 110, 163, 255
"Mickey and the Beanstalk" sequence 82, 304
as "package" film 103, 157
in production **222, 235**
selected directors and sequences directed 297, 298, 304
year and directors 285

G

Garity, Bill **13, 130**, 194, 215
Geronimi, Clyde "Gerry" 113, 142, 156, **170**, 171–191, **172–191**, 256, 257
and *Alice in Wonderland* 142, 158, 183, **188**
as animator 52, 173–176
caricatures of **178, 179**
criticism of 173, 183–185, 189, 191, 262
directing credits by year 283–288
as director 142, 158, 176–190, 233
Disney director filmography 192
feature film sequences directed by 294–295
in group photos **xvi, 106, 223, 266**
New York animation experience 9, **170**, 173–174, **174**
praise for 173, 176, 184, 187
role as sequence director: flowchart 119
as shorts director 176–178, 205
and *Sleeping Beauty* 185, 189, **189**
time line 306–310
Ghez, Didier 123
Gillett, Burton Fred "Burt" 12, **13**, 17, 23–38, **24–26, 34**
as animator 26, 91, **91**, 129
approach to directing 33, 35, 81
and *The Brave Little Tailor* 38, 194, 215
directing credits by year 280–281
Disney director filmography 39
and Frank Churchill **25**, 36, **36**
in group photos **22, 26, 34, 48**
New York studio experience 25, 33, 35, 90–91, 111
time line 308-309
Gillett, Fredric 36
Gilson, Merle **22, 91**, 92
Goldberg, Eric 263, 264–265
The Golden Touch (short) 38, 59, 112, 281
Goofy (character) 96, 175, 205, 206, 217, 236
"how-to" series 214, 220
redesigned 220, 331n62
Goofy and Wilbur (short) 131, 204, 236, 274, 283
Gottfredson, Floyd 35, **48**
Gramatke, Hardie 59, 94
Grant, Joe 65, 67, **81**, 100, **220, 225**, 272, 273, **273, 275**
caricatures by **65**
and Dick Huemer 82, 101, 204, 273, 274
Make Mine Music production supervisor 273, 285
recollections of 49, 59, 68, 72, 108, 261
Gray, Milt 140
Griffith, Don 244, **248**
Guinle, Jorge **113**
Gurney, Eric: caricature by **179**

H

Hand, David Dodd **46**, 47–75, **64–67, 73, 74, 236**
as animator 49, **50**, 52
and *Bambi* **69**, 69–71, **70**, 78
caricatures of **51, 65**
directing credits by year 281, 282, 284
as director 52–53, 58–59, 94–95, 203, 241
Disney director filmography 75
in group photos **26, 48**
New York studio experience 33, 49, 111
one-sentence description of 115
passion for organization 67, 71, 141
as production supervisor 66–68
relationship with Walt Disney 49, 72–73, 75
and *Snow White* 59, 61–66, **62**, 76, 156, 157, 175, 203
as supervising director 61–66, 134
time line 308-311
Hand, David Hale 58, **58**, 73
Handley, Jim 273–274, 283
Hanna-Barbera 214, 272
Hannah, John Frederick "Jack" 130, 206–208, **210–212**, 210–213
bar sheets **30–31**
directing credits by year 285–288
goodbye party (1959) **223**
in group photos **xvii, 266**
laid off (1956) 212, 224, 310
one-sentence description of 115
time line 308-313

Boldface indicates illustrations.

INDEX

Harline, Leigh 124, **129**
Hathcock, Jerry 189, 217
Hee, Thornton "T." 112, 274, **274**, 283
 caricatures by **94**, **141**, **214**
Heid, Graham 147, 204, 274, 282, 284, 329n4
Hench, John **131**, 274, **274**, 297
Hennesy, Hugh **24**, **34**, 115, **129**, **182**
Hibler, Winston 103, 104, **106**, 168, 180
Hopkins, Paul 115, 155
Huemer, Dick 7, 9, 17, 25, 131–132, 204, 274–275, **275**
 directing credits by year 282, 283
 and Joe Grant 82, 101, 204, 273
 recollections of 9, 14, 36, 52–53, 59, 61, 66, 113, 153, 154
 self-caricature **17**
Humphrey the Bear cartoons 212, **212**
Hurd, Earl 90, 97, 210, 215–216
Hyperion Avenue Studio, Los Angeles, California
 dialogue recording session **79**
 Dictaphone system 61
 map **35**
 music rooms 26, **26**, **53**, **122**
 parking lot **67**
 soundstage **99**
 "sweatbox" 325n24

I

"Iron Pencil" **218**, 219
Iwerks, Ub **6**, 9, **11**, **12**, 14–17, **22**, 142
 departure from Disney (1930) 16, 308
 directing credits by year 280
 Disney director filmography 17
 personality 11, 15, 25
 proto-storyboard drawings by **8**
 return to Disney (1940) 16–17, 97, 308
 and *Steamboat Willie* 11
 time line 306–311
 wartime shorts 17, 272
 weekly salary 91

J

Jackson, Jane Ames 125, **125**, 126, **135**, 144, 146, 238
Jackson, Wilfred Emmons "Jaxon" 12–13, 33, 80–81, **84**, 121–146, **122–124**, **129**, **138**, 203, 250
 Academy Award–winning shorts 133, 203
 and *Alice in Wonderland* **131**, 142
 as animator **11**, 126–128
 bar sheets 28, 126, **127**
 caricatures of **128**, **137**, **141**, **142**
 and *Cinderella* 142–143, **144**
 directing credits by year 280–288
 as director 65, 95, 118, 121, 123, 128–144, 158, 183, 184, 189, 233
 Disney director filmography 147
 feature film sequences directed by 297-298
 flowchart: role as sequence director 118
 in group photos **xvii**, **22**, **26**, **48**, **96**, **130**, **266**
 on Ham Luske 160, 161
 heart attack 142, 144, 256
 innovations 126–128, 194
 as live-action reference model 135, **136**, 155
 military training films 102, 137
 one-sentence description of 115
 and *Peter Pan* 142, **143**, **144**
 and *Pinocchio* 134–135, **135**
 retirement 107, 145, **146**, 233, 312
 and *Saludos Amigos* 112–113, **113**
 and *Sleeping Beauty* 142, 189, 256
 and *Snow White* 61, 76, 133–134, **134**, **135**
 and *Song of the South* **120**, 138–139, **139**
 and *Steamboat Willie* 11, 126, 127
 time line 308-312
Jindrak, Elska "Alice" 174, 175
Johnston, Ollie 61, 95, 100, **182**, 204, 237, 244, 252
 books 2, 76, 93, 140, 153, 252
 as directing animator 241, 256
 directing credits by year 288, 289
 and Gerry Geronimi **179**, 262
 and Ham Luske 153, 160
 as one of Nine Old Men 141, **256**
 and Robin Hood **244**, 289
 and *The Sword in the Stone* 241, **250**, 288
 and Wilfred Jackson 140, 141, 262
The Jungle Book (feature) 230, 231, 242–243, 262, 289
Justice, Bill 224, **266**, 288
 caricatures by **76**, **142**, **179**

K

Kahl, Milt 81, 141, **144**, 152, 221, 244, **244**, 245
 directing credits by year 289
 as one of Nine Old Men 141, 256, **256**
 recollections of 81, 94, 113, 160
Katzenberg, Jeffrey 262
Keane, Glen 141, 247, 251, 253, **253**, **258**
 caricature by **252**
Kerry, Margaret **143**
Kimball, Ward 52, 59, **106**, 108, 154, 222, **256**
 caricature by **157**
 as director 213–214, 224, 256, 287
 and Gerry Geronimi 182, 183, 187, 189, 191
 and Wilfred Jackson 141–142
King, James Patton "Jack" 25, 91, **91**, 111, 129, 206, 208–212, **209**
 caricatures of Disney staff **13**, **51**, **128**
 directing credits by year 282–28[illegible]
 in group photos **22**, **26**, **48**
 time line 306–309
Kinney, John Ryan "Jack" 112–113, 205–206, 213–224, **215–218**, **220–223**, **225**
 Bone Trouble **28**, 216
 caricature of **214**
 directing credits by year 283–288
 feature film sequences directed by 297–298
 in group photos **xvi**, **266**
 invention of concept of Leica reels 194, 215–216
 laid off (1957) 224, 310
 recollections of 33, 76, 82, 93, 194, 206, 213
 time line 308-311

L

Lady and the Tramp (feature) 142, 158, 183, 241, 273
 in director filmographies 147, 163, 1[illegible]2, 255
 live-action model for Lady 157
 selected directors and sequences directed 296, 298, 301
 spaghetti scene 173, 184
 year and directors 288
Laemmle, Carl 175
Lantz, Walter 38, 49, 90, 173–175, **174**, [illegible]1, 277
Larson, Eric 35, 113, 161, **182**, **250**, **256**, 256–257
 as assistant to Ham Luske 35, 151, 154
 on Burt Gillett 23, 35
 directing credits by year 288
 feature film sequences directed by 2[illegible]6
 as one of Nine Old Men **256**, 256–257
 recollections of 52, 81, 94, 142, 153, 21[illegible], 212, 213
 and *Sleeping Beauty* 142, 189, 256–25[illegible], **261**
 training animators 244, 257, **260**
 on Wilfred Jackson 140, 142
Legg, J. Gordon 271, 272
Leica reels 69, 194, **194**, 215–216
Leon Schlesinger Productions 208, 210
Lewis, Bert **26**, **48**
Lewis, Sinclair 216
Lounsbery, John 189, 244, 247, 252, 257, **256**
 directing credits by year 288, 289
 as one of Nine Old Men **256**, 257
 role as directing animator 228–229
Lundy, Dick **13**, 49, 52, 59, **91**, 205, 275, **275**
 directing credits by year 283, 284
 in group photos **22**, **26**, **48**

Boldface indicates illustrations.

Luske, Hamilton Somers "Ham" **62**, **148**, 149–162, **150–151**, **157**, **161**, 205, **223**
and *Alice in Wonderland* 142, 158, **159**, 183
as animator 153–155, 161–162
assistants 35, 151, 204, 272, 273
and *Cinderella* **140**, 142, 158, **159**, 183
directing credits by year 283, 284, 286–289
Disney director filmography 163
and *Fantasia* 157, 205, 272
feature film sequences directed by 300-302
flowchart: role as sequence director (1949–1961) 119
in group photos **xvii**, **106**, **241**, **266**
and *Mary Poppins* 158, **162**
one-sentence description of 115
and *Peter Pan* 142, 157, 158, **158**, 183
and *Pinocchio* 100, 156, **156**, 205
and *The Reluctant Dragon* 157, **157**
and *Snow White* 155–156
time line 308-313
Luske, Tom 157, **158**

M

Make Mine Music (feature) 157, 182, 221, 272, 273
"Casey at the Bat" sequence 179, 182
in director filmographies 163, 192
selected directors and sequences directed 295, 296, 298, 299
year and directors 285
The Many Adventures of Winnie the Pooh (feature) 247, 255, 257, 289
Mary Poppins (feature) 158, 162, 163, 289
Mattinson, Burny 161, 251, 262
McCrea, Bob 145, 210
McLeish, John 220
Melody Time (feature) 103, 182, 183
in director filmographies 110, 147, 163, 192
"Johnny Appleseed" segment 139–140, 256, 298
selected directors and sequences directed 296, 298-301
year and directors 286
Mickey Mouse (character) 11, 28, 33, **40–41**, 206, 208
Mickey Mouse series
artistic and technical innovations 203
early cartoons 11, 14, 33, 133, 194
fast-paced schedule 92
Mickey Steps Out (short) **27**, 39, 280
Mickey's Amateurs (short) 38, 204–205, 272, 282
Mickey's Circus (short) 94, 101, 110, 282
Mickey's Grand Opera (short) **32**, 147, 282
Mickey's Nightmare (short) **10**, 39, 281
Miller, Ron 243, 245, 252, 254, 257
Milotte, Alfred and Elma 104
Mintz, Charles 125, 153, 175, 208
Moore, Fred 33, 36, 38, 94, 101, 112, 151, 236
Morey, Larry 76, 81, 275–276, 282
Mousecars **xvi–xvii**, **107**, **110**, **257**
Moviola 37, **111**, **148**, 160, 178, 182, **244**, 251
Musker, John 195, 212, 248, 250, 262–264
caricatures by **xv**, **252**

N

Natwick, Grim 155, 156
Nelson, Mique 155
The New Spirit (short) 102, 110, 137, 147, 284
New York, New York
animation studios 3, 9, 11, 17, 25, 33, 49, 90–91
flowchart: animator's job (1920s) 3
Steamboat Willie premiere (1928) 12
Nichols, Charles "Nick" 130, 176, 206, 212–214, **213**, 223, 256, 272
directing credits by year 285–288
pose testing 176, 183
time line 308-313
Nine Old Men 35, 112, 141, 184, 241, 252, **256**, 256–257
Nolley, Lance 140, 176, 184, 221, **222**

O

O'Connor, Ken 94, 95, 108, 109, 140, 162
The Old Mill (short) 133, 147, 203, 282
On Ice (short) 96–97, 101, 110, 282
One Hundred and One Dalmatians (feature) 158, 189, 195, 233, 241
in director filmographies 163, 192, 255
selected directors and sequences directed 297, 301-302
year and directors 288
Oswald the Lucky Rabbit (character) 11, 91, 125, 175, 194

P

"Package" films 44, 103, 157, 182–183
Palmer, Tom **13**, **26**, **48**, **51**, 52, 91, 111
Papineau, Gail 276, 302
Paul Bunyan (featurette) 257, 261, 288
Pearce, Percival C. "Perce" 61, 69, **69**, **76**, 76–78, **77**, 194, 282, 300
Peet, Bill 38, 82, **83**, 140–141, 195, **241**, 242–243, 261–262
Penner, Erdman "Ed" **187**, **189**, **221**, 272, 288
Perk, Hans 164, 175
Persephone (character) 153, **153**
Personality animation, development of 111, 112, 154
Peter Pan (feature) 142, 158, 183, 195, 217, 241, 273
ARI title test report 207, **207**
in director filmographies 114, 147, 163, 192, 255
live-action reference **143**, **144**, 157, **158**, 180, 185
selected directors and sequences directed 296, 298, 301
year and directors 287
Peterson, Ken 100, 189, 234
Pfeiffer, Walt 272
Philippi, Charlie **24**, **34**
Pinocchio (feature) 69, 100, 112, 134–135, 156, 205, 241, 245, 273, 274
Animation Direction (credit) 193
as box-office disappointment 100, 183
the Coachman 213, **213**
in director filmographies 83, 110, 114, 147, 163, 255
involvement of Walt Disney 71, 134, 142
Leica reels 194, 216
Monstro the whale 237, 253
in production **81**, **83**, **135**, **148**, **156**, **213**, **216**, **237**
selected directors and sequences directed 297, 299, 300, 302
year and directors 283
Pixar Animation Studios 263, 264, 265
Plane Crazy (short) **8**, 11, 12, 280
Plumb, Ed **70**, 137
Pluto (character) 80, 96–97, 111, **112**, 176, 205–206, 212–213. *see also* Bone Trouble
The Pointer (short) **29**, 176, 192, 283
Pomeroy, John 250–251, **258**

Q

Quimby, Fred 38

R

Reeves, Harry 94, 115
Reitherman, Alfred 234, **234**
Reitherman, Bruce 237, 241, **242**, 243, 244–245, 254
Reitherman, Dick 234, 240–241
Reitherman, Janie 144, 235, **240**, 241, 254
Reitherman, Wolfgang "Woolie" **230**, 231–255, **232–237**, **240–242**, **247**

Boldface indicates illustrations.

INDEX

after Walt Disney's death 243–245, 261–262
as animator 81–82, 130, 154–155, 220, **235**, 235–238, **236**, **237**
and *The Aristocats* **244**, 246, **246**, 262
caricatures of **252**
directing credits by year 288-290
as director 180, 241–254
Disney director filmography 255
feature film sequences directed by 302-303
flowchart: directing with less input from Walt (1963–1966) 228–229
gag drawing of **253**
and *The Jungle Book* **230**, 231, **242**, 242–243
and *One Hundred and One Dalmatians* 158, 189, 241
as one of Nine Old Men 241, **256**, 257
time line 308-312
during World War II 234, 238–241, **239**, 245

The Reluctant Dragon (feature) 15, 157, 220, 273, 276
The Rescuers (feature) **40–41**, 193, 246, 251, 257, 262, 290
Rickard, Richard "Dick" 204, 283, 284
Rinaldi, Joe **183**, **187**, **189**, **221**
Roberts, Bill 79–83, **79–83**, **96**, 112–113, 129–130, 205
and *The Brave Little Tailor* 81, 83, 194, 205, 215, 283
directing credits by year 282–285
Disney director filmography 83
and *Dumbo* 82, 205, 273
and *Fantasia* 205, 271, 276
feature film sequences directed by 303-304
Robin Hood (feature) 244, 246, 249, 255, 262, 289, 311
Robinson, Edward G. **181**
Running reels, development of 126, 128, 194

S

Salkin, Leo 63, 207
Saludos Amigos (feature) 82, 112–113, 139–140, 157
in director filmographies 83, 114, 147, 163
selected directors and sequences directed 293, 296–298, 304
year and directors 284
Satterfield, Paul McKinley **96**, **244**, **276**, 276–277, 283, 284, 288, 304
Schaffer, Milton "Milt" 115, 277, 287
Sears, Ted **13**, 26, **26**, 27, **34**, **63**, 100, 115
invention of storyboard 14–15, 194
Sewell, Hazel **13**, 115, 273
The Shaggy Dog (feature) 233
Sharpsteen, Benjamin Luther "Ben" **84**, 85–110, **86**, **96**, **105**, **107**, **109–110**, 193, 203, 241
as animator 52, 90–95, **91**
caricature of **94**
directing credits by year 281–284, 286, 287
Disney director filmography 110
Disneyland television show 104, **104**
and Don Peri **97**, 97–98, **98**
feature film sequences directed by 304-305
friendship with Burt Gillett 25, 38
in group photos **xvi**, **22**, **26**, **48**, **51**, **266**
on Ham Luske 153, 156, 204
in the Marine Corps 88–89, **89**
memos from 16–17, **103**, 105
and *The New Spirit* 137
New York studio experience 13, 25, 33, 49, 52, 90
one-sentence description of 115
and *Pinocchio* 100–101, **101**, 134, 156
recollections of 27, 36–38, 61, 66–67, 72, 76, 79, 111, 142, 153, 205, 235–236
recruitment of talent 92, 211, 271
retirement party **93**, **106**, 107, **107**, 109
and *Snow White* 61, 76, **99**, 99–100
time line 306-313
True-Life Adventures 104, **104**, 134
Sharpsteen, Bernice 59, 89, 90, **97**, 98, **105**, 108, 109
Sherman, Robert **230**
Shorts, culture of 205–206
Shorts, end of 222–224
Shorts directors: flowcharts
New York studios (1920s) 3
early days at Disney Studios (1926–1928) 4
proto-directors (1929–1931) 5
evolution of director (1932–1936) 21
short film directors (1936–1957) 199
Sibley, John 220, 236, **266**
Silly Symphony series 12, 14, 26, 33, 36, 49, 52, 92, 271
Academy Award winners 33, 133
artistic and technical innovations 203
see also Three Little Pigs
Sleeping Beauty (feature) 142, 144, 185, 189, 233, 237–238, 241, 256–257, 261
in director filmographies 192, 255
involvement of Walt Disney 142, 189, **189**, 261, **261**
selected directors and sequences directed 295, 297, 300, 302
year and directors 288
Smith, Dave 36, 102
Smith, Webb 14, **26**, 215
Snow White and the Seven Dwarfs (feature) 59–66, 72, 76–77, 99–100, 133–134, 155–156, 272–273
bar sheet **219**
in director filmographies 75, 78, 110, 147
involvement of Walt Disney 11, 61, 71, 133–134
Leica reels 194, 216
live-action reference footage 99, **134**, 156
music 128, 275
premiere 98, 134, **135**, 205, 321n5[illegible]
selected directors and sequences directed 295, 297, 302, 304, 305
soundstage **99**
Supervising Animators (credit) 195
the Witch 99, 112, 245, 273
year and directors 282
Song of the South (feature) 78, **120**, 138–139, **139**, 146, 147, 193, 285, 298
Stalling, Carl 16, **22**, 27, 319n7
Stallings, George 59, 174, **266**
Stanley, Helene **144**, **159**, **186**
Steamboat Willie (short) 11–12, 126, **127**, 280
Stevens, Art 252–254, 262, 289
Stewart, McLaren 80, 81, **266**, 276
Stokowski, Leopold 71, 137
Story artists 44, 119, 180, 194, 206, 215, 263, 264
Story men (proto-directors) 5, 12–14, 27, 38
Storyboard, invention of 14–15, 194, 329n54
Storytelling tools: time line 194–195
Stravinsky, Igor **82**
The Sword in the Stone (feature) 233, 241–242, 250, 255, 288, 302-303

T

Terry, Paul 37, 111
Thomas, Frank 38, 82, 160, 183, 184, 20[illegible], 221, 252, 256, 262
and Ben Sharpsteen 93, 95
books 2, 76, 93, 140, 153, 252
and Dave Hand 58, 62, 66, 67, 70–73, 141
directing credits by year 288, 289
and Gerry Geronimi 184, 256, 262
and *Ichabod Crane* 182, 221
as one of Nine Old Men 243, 256, **256**
one-sentence description of 115
and *The Rescuers* 195, 262, 289
and *Robin Hood* **244**, **249**, 289
and *The Sword in the Stone* **250**, 288
and Wilfred Jackson 141, 160, 262
and Woolie Reitherman 243–244, 248, 249
Thomson, Riley 204, **277**, 283, 284
The Three Caballeros (feature) 82, 113, 18[illegible], 221, 276

Boldface indicates illustrations.

in director filmographies 83, 114, 192
selected directors and sequences directed 295, 296, 299, 304
year and directors 285
Three Little Pigs (short) 33, 36–37, 39, 105, 112, 128, 281
Timothy Mouse (character) 101, **236**
Toot, Whistle, Plunk and Boom (short) 213, 256, 287
The Tortoise and the Hare (short) 130, 132, 133, 153–154, **154**, 281
Touchdown Mickey (short) **10**, 147, 281
Treasure Island (feature) 77, 78, 143, 183
True-Life Adventure series 103, 104, **104**, 134, 271
Tugboat Mickey (short) **178**, 192, 283
Tytla, Vladimir "Bill" 94–95, 112, **135**, 135–137, 151
Tytle, Harry 190, **209**, 222–224, **266**, 276, 320

U

The Ugly Duckling (1931 short) 147, 280
The Ugly Duckling (1939 short) 156, 176, 204, 283, 309
Uncle Remus (character) 139

V

Victory Through Air Power (feature) 71, 75, 78, 182, 192, 271, 284

W

Walker, Card **106**, 243
Wallace, Ollie 124, 143, 182
The Walt Disney Studios, Burbank, California
animation process **40–41**
animation staff (1929) **11**
buildings **72**, **164**, **200**, **316**
floor plans (1950) **165–167**
flowcharts: feature film directors 44–45, 118–119, 228–229
flow charts: short film directors 4–5, 21, 199
in-house magazine 151, **178**, 209, **209**
internal memo 54–57
job descriptions 20
key personnel (1957) **266**
maps **168**, **202**
new employees' pamphlet (mid-1940s) **168**, **169**
organizational charts **70–71**, **169**
organizational manual (1938) 67–68, **68**
recruitment brochure (1977) **40–41**
shorts department 200–224
staff caricatures **13**
success with synchronized sound 11–12, 49, 128
Who Killed Cock Robin? (short) 75, 80, 154, **154**, 175, 282
"Who's Afraid of the Big Bad Wolf?" (song) 36
Williams, Richard 250, 257
Williams, Roy 76, 92, 93, **93**, 208, 210, **222**, 322n81
Winnie the Pooh featurettes 246, 247, 255, 257, 289
World War II: military training films 17, 102, 137, 157
Wright, Norman 277, **277**, 284, 305
Wright, Ralph 217, 236
Wynn, Ed **188**

X

X-sheets (exposure sheets) 20, 27, 32, **32**, 60, 212, 262
Xerox 20, 233, 333

Z

Zamora, Rudy **13**, **26**, **51**

Boldface indicates illustrations.

SELECTED BIBLIOGRAPHY

In addition to the books listed below, the references in the chapter footnotes, and our own personal archives, we were so fortunate not only to have access to the Walt Disney Archives but to have access to the John Canemaker Animation Collection at the Elmer Holmes Bobst Library at New York University and the personal archives of Disney historian Michael Barrier.

Adamson, Joe, *The Walter Lantz Story, with Woody Woodpecker and Friends*, G. P. Putnam's Sons, New York, 1985.

Anderson, Paul F., *Jack of All Trades: Conversations with Disney Legend Ken Anderson*, Theme Park Press, 2017.

Barbera, Joe, *My Life in 'Toons: From Flatbush to Bedrock in Under a Century*, Turner Publishing, Atlanta, 1994

Barrier, Michael, *The Animated Man: A Life of Walt Disney*, University of California Press, Berkeley, 2007.

Barrier, Michael, *Hollywood Cartoons: American Animation in Its Golden Age*, Oxford University Press, New York, 1999.

Cabarga, Leslie, *The Fleischer Story in the Golden Age of Animation*, Nostalgia Press, New York, 1976.

Canemaker, John, *Paper Dreams: The Art and Artists of Disney Storyboards*, Hyperion, New York, 1999.

Canemaker, John, *Walt Disney's Nine Old Men and the Art of Animation*, Disney Editions, New York, 2001.

Care, Ross, *Disney Legend Wilfred Jackson: A Life in Animation*, Theme Park Press, 2016.

Clark, Miriam Leslie, *Glimpses into the Golden Age of Disney Animation*, Theme Park Press, 2019.

Clark, Steven and Rebecca Cline, *The Walt Disney Studios: A Lot to Remember*, Disney Editions, Glendale, 2019.

Culhane, Shamus, *Talking Animals and Other People*, St. Martin's Press, New York, 1986.

Deja, Andreas, *The Nine Old Men: Lessons, Techniques, and Inspiration from Disney's Greatest Animators*, CRC Press, Boca Raton, 2016.

Field, Robert D., *The Art of Walt Disney*, Collins, London and Glasgow, 1944.

Finch, Christopher, *The Art of Walt Disney: From Mickey Mouse to the Magic Kingdoms*, Harry N. Abrams, Inc., New York, 1973.

Gabler, Neal, *Walt Disney: The Triumph of the American Imagination*, Alfred A. Knopf, New York, 2006.

Ghez, Didier, *Walt's People*, volumes 1–24, Xlibrus Corp and Theme Park Press, 2005–2020.

Hahn, Don and Tracey Miller-Zarneke, *Before Ever After: The Lost Lectures of Walt Disney's Animation Studio*, Disney Editions, Los Angeles, 2015.

Hand, David, *Memoirs: David Dodd Hand*, Lighthouse Litho, Cambria, California, no date.

Hannah, Jack, *From Donald Duck's Daddy to Disney Legend*, Theme Park Press, 2016.

Horowitz, James, *They Went Thataway: A Front-Row Kid's Search for His Boyhood Heroes—The Old-Time Hollywood Cowboys*, Ballantine Books, New York, 1976.

Hulett, Steve, *Mouse in Transition: An Insider's Look at Disney Feature Animation*, Theme Park Press, 2014.

Iwerks, Leslie and John Kenworthy, *The Hand Behind the Mouse*, Disney Editions, New York, 2001.

Johnson, David, *Snow White's People: An Oral History of the Disney Film "Snow White and the Seven Dwarfs,"* Volumes I and II, Theme Park Press, 2017, 2018.

Jones, Chuck, *Chuck Amuck: The Life and Times of an Animated Cartoonist*, Farrar Straus Giroux, New York, 1989.

Justice, Bill, *Justice for Disney*, Tomart Publications, Dayton, 1992.

Kaufman, J. B., *The Fairest One of All: The Making of Walt Disney's "Snow White and the Seven Dwarfs,"* The Walt Disney Family Foundation Press, San Francisco, 2012.

Kaufman, J. B., *The Making of Walt Disney's "Fun and Fancy Free,"* Hyperion Historical Alliance Press, 2019.

Kaufman, J. B., *"Pinocchio": The Making of the Disney Epic*, The Walt Disney Family Foundation Press, San Francisco, 2015.

Kaufman, J. B., *"Snow White and the Seven Dwarfs": The Art and Creation of Walt Disney's Classic Animated Film*, The Walt Disney Family Foundation Press, San Francisco, 2012.

Kaufman. J. B., *South of the Border with Disney: Walt Disney and the Good Neighbor Program 1941–1948*, Disney Editions, New York, 2009.

Kaufman, J. B. and David Gerstein, *Walt Disney's Mickey Mouse: The Ultimate History*, Taschen GmbH, 2018.

Kaufman, J. B. and Russell Merritt, *Walt Disney's Silly Symphonies: A Companion to the Classic Cartoon Series*, Disney Editions, Glendale, 2016.

Kinney, Jack, *Walt Disney and Assorted Other Characters: An Uncuthorized Account of Early Years at Disney's*, Harmony Books, New York, 1988.

Kothenschulte, Daniel, *The Walt Disney Film Archives: The Animated Movies 1921–1968*, Taschen GmbH, 2016.

Lanpher, Dorse A., *Flyin' Chunks and Other Things to Duck: Memoirs of a Life Spent Doodling for Dollars*, IUniverse, New York, 2010.

Larson, Eric, *50 Years in the Mouse House: The Lost Memoir of One of Disney's Nine Old Men*, Theme Park Press, 2015.

Maltin, Leonard, *The Disney Films*, Fourth Edition, Disney Editions, New York, 2000.

Maltin, Leonard, *Of Mice and Magic: A History of American Animated Cartoons*, Plume, New York, 1987.

Merritt, Russell and J. B. Kaufman, *Walt in Wonderland: The Silent Films of Walt Disney*, Le Giornate del Cinema Muto, 1992.

Miller, Diane Disney, *The Story of Walt Disney*, Dell Publishing, New York, 1957.

Peri, Don, *Working with Disney: Interviews with Animators, Producers, and Artists*, University cf Press, Jackson, 2011.

Peri, Don, *Working with Walt: Interviews with Disney Artists*, University Press of Mississippi, Jackson, 2008.

Schatz, Thomas, *The Genius of the System*, MacMillan, New York, 1996.

Sito, Tom, *Drawing the Line: The Untold Story of the Animation Unions from Bosko to Bart Simpson*, University Press of Kentucky, 2006.

Smith, Dave, *Disney A to Z: The Official Encyclopedia*, Disney Editions, New York, 2006.

Takamoto, Iwao, *My Life with a Thousand Characters*, University Press of Mississippi, Jackson, 2009.

Thomas, Bob, *The Art of Animation*, Simon and Schuster, New York, 1958.

Thomas, Bob, *Walt Disney: An American Original*, Simon and Schuster, New York, 1976.

Thomas, Frank and Ollie Johnston, *Disney Animation: The Illusion of Life*, Abbeville Press, New York, 1981.

Thomas, Frank and Ollie Johnston, *Too Funny for Words: Disney's Greatest Sight Gags*, Abbeville Press, New York, 1987.

Tytla, Adrienne, *Disney's Giant and the Artist's Model*, Valley Press and New Era Printing Company, Deep River, 2004.

Tytle, Harry, *One of Walt's Boys*, A.S.A.P. Publishing, 1997.

Watkin, Larry, *Larry Watkin: A Memoir of an American Man of Letters*, Pulp Hero Press, 2018.

Watkin, Larry, *Walt Disney*, unpublished biography in the Walt Disney Archives.

Watts, Steven, *The Magic Kingdom: Walt Disney and the. American Way of Life*, Houghton Mifflin Company, Boston, 1997.

IMAGE CREDITS

Cover	Courtesy of the Walt Disney Archives
p. ix	Courtesy of the Walt Disney Archives
p. x	Courtesy of George Lucas
p. xv	Courtesy of John Musker
p. xvi–xvii	Courtesy of the Walt Disney Archives
p. 6	Courtesy of the Walt Disney Archives
p. 8	Courtesy of the Walt Disney Archives
p. 10	Courtesy of Hans Perk
p. 11	Courtesy of the Walt Disney Archives
p. 12	Courtesy of the Walt Disney Archives
p. 13	Courtesy of the Walt Disney Archives
p. 15	Courtesy of the Walt Disney Archives
p. 16	Courtesy of the Walt Disney Archives
p. 17	Courtesy of Don Peri
p. 22	Courtesy of the Walt Disney Archives
p. 24	Courtesy of the Walt Disney Archives
p. 25	Courtesy of the Walt Disney Archives
p. 26	(top and bottom) Courtesy of the Walt Disney Archives
p. 27	Courtesy of Hans Perk
p. 28–29	Courtesy of the Walt Disney Animation Research Library
p. 30–31	Courtesy of the Walt Disney Animation Research Library
p. 32	Courtesy of the Walt Disney Animation Reserach Library
p. 34	(top) Courtesy of the Walt Disney Animation Research Library (bottom) Courtesy of the Walt Disney Archives
p. 35	Courtesy of Hans Perk
p. 36	Courtesy of the Walt Disney Archives
p. 37	Courtesy of Hans Perk
p. 40–41	(top) Courtesy of the Walt Disney Archives
p. 40–41	(bottom) Courtesy of National Geographic Library
p. 46	Courtesy of the Walt Disney Archives
p. 48	Courtesy of the Walt Disney Archives
p. 50	Courtesy of the Walt Disney Archives
p. 51	Courtesy of the Walt Disney Archives
p. 53	Courtesy of the Walt Disney Archives
p. 54–57	Courtesy of the Walt Disney Archives
p. 58	Courtesy of Judy LaPrade
p. 62	Courtesy of the Walt Disney Archives
p. 64	Courtesy of the Walt Disney Archives
p. 65	Courtesy of Jennifer Grant Castrup
p. 65	Courtesy of Judy LaPrade
p. 66	Courtesy of the Walt Disney Archives
p. 67	Courtesy of Ward Kimball collection
p. 68	Courtesy of Ward Kimball collection
p. 69	(top and bottom) Courtesy of the Walt Disney Archives
p. 70–71	(top and bottom) Courtesy of the Walt Disney Archives
p. 72	Courtesy of the Walt Disney Archives
p. 73	Courtesy of Judy LaPrade
p. 74	(top) Courtesy of Ted Thomas
p. 74	(bottom) Courtesy of Michael Barrier
p. 76	Courtesy of the Walt Disney Archives
p. 77	(top and bottom) Courtesy of the Walt Disney Archives
p. 79	(top and bottom) Courtesy of the Walt Disney Archives
p. 80	Courtesy of Gilles "Frenchy" de Trémaudan collection
p. 81	Courtesy of the Walt Disney Archives
p. 82	Courtesy of the Walt Disney Archives
p. 83	Courtesy of the Walt Disney Archives
p. 84	Courtesy of the Walt Disney Archives
p. 86	Courtesy of the Walt Disney Archives
p. 88	Courtesy of Ben Sharpsteen collection
p. 89	Courtesy of Ben Sharpsteen collection
p. 91	Courtesy of the Walt Disney Archives
p. 93	Courtesy of the Walt Disney Archives
p. 94	Courtesy of the Walt Disney Archives
p. 96	Courtesy of the Walt Disney Archives
p. 97	Courtesy of Don Peri
p. 98	Photo by Mary Horton, courtesy of Don Peri
p. 99	Courtesy of Ben Sharpsteen collection
p. 101	Courtesy of the Walt Disney Archives
p. 103	Courtesy of the Walt Disney Archives
p. 104	(top and bottom) Courtesy of the Walt Disney Archives
p. 105	(left) Courtesy of Ben Sharpsteen collection
p. 105	(right) Courtesy of the Walt Disney Archives
p. 106	(top and bottom) Courtesy of the Walt Disney Archives
p. 107	Courtesy of the Walt Disney Archives
p. 108	(left and right) Courtesy of Ben Sharpsteen collection
p. 109	Courtesy of Don Peri
p. 110	Courtesy of Don Peri
p. 111	Courtesy of the Walt Disney Archives
p. 112	(left and right) Courtesy of the Walt Disney Archives
p. 113	Courtesy of Dave Bossert
p. 114	Courtesy of Jennifer Grant Castrup
p. 115	Courtesy of the Walt Disney Archives
p. 120	Courtesy of the Walt Disney Archives
p. 122	Courtesy of the Walt Disney Archives
p. 123	Courtesy of Natha Horbach
p. 124	Courtesy of Natha Horbach
p. 125	(left) Courtesy of Natha Horbach
p. 125	(right) Courtesy of Natha Horbach
p. 127	Courtesy of the Walt Disney Archives
p. 128	Courtesy of the Walt Disney Archives
p. 129	Courtesy of the Walt Disney Archives
p. 130	Courtesy of the Walt Disney Archives
p. 131	Courtesy of the Walt Disney Archives
p. 134	Courtsy of Michael Barrier
p. 135	(top) Courtesy of Natha Horbach
p. 135	(bottom) Courtesy of the Walt Disney Archives

p. 136 (left) Courtesy of Don Peri
p. 136 (top and right) Courtesy of the Walt Disney Archives and Don Peri
p. 137 Courtesy of Gilles "Frenchy" de Trémaudan collection
p. 138 Courtesy of the Walt Disney Archives
p. 139 Courtesy of the Walt Disney Archives
p. 140 Courtesy of the Walt Disney Archives
p. 141 Courtesy of the Walt Disney Archives
p. 142 Courtesy of the Walt Disney Archives
p. 143 Courtesy of the Walt Disney Archives
p. 144 (top and bottom) Courtesy of the Walt Disney Archives
p. 145 Courtesy of Don Peri
p. 146 Courtesy of Natha Horbach
p. 148 Courtesy of the Walt Disney Archives
p. 150 Courtesy of the Walt Disney Archives
p. 151 Courtesy of Ham Luske collection
p. 152 Courtesy of Ham Luske collection
p. 153 Courtesy of the Walt Disney Animation Research Library
p. 154 (all) Courtesy of Walt Disney Studios Media Library
p. 156 Courtesy of the Walt Disney Archives
p. 157 (top and bottom) Courtesy of the Walt Disney Archives
p. 158 Courtesy of the Walt Disney Archives
p. 159 (all) Courtesy of the Walt Disney Archives
p. 161 Courtesy of the Walt Disney Archives
p. 162 Courtesy of the Walt Disney Archives
p. 164 Courtesy of the Walt Disney Archives
p. 165 Courtesy of Hans Perk
p. 166–167 (left and right) Courtesy of Hans Perk
p. 168–169 Courtesy of the Walt Disney Archives
p. 170 Courtesy the Geronimi Family Collection
p. 172 Courtesy the Geronimi Family Collection
p. 174 Courtesy the Geronimi Family Collection
p. 175 (left and right) Courtesy the Geronimi Family Collection
p. 176 Courtesy the Geronimi Family Collection
p. 177 (all) Courtesy the Geronimi Family Collection
p. 178 (top) Courtesy of the Walt Disney Archives
p. 178 (bottom) Courtesy of the Walt Disney Archives
p. 179 (top left) Courtesy the Geronimi Family Collection
p. 179 (top right) Courtesy of the Walt Disney Archives
p. 179 (left and right) Courtesy of the Walt Disney Archives
p. 181 Courtesy the Geronimi Family Collection
p. 182 Courtesy the Geronimi Family Collection
p. 183 Courtesy of the Walt Disney Archives
p. 185 (all) Courtesy of the Walt Disney Archives
p. 186 (all) Courtesy of the Walt Disney Animation Research Library
p. 187–189 (all) Courtesy of the Walt Disney Archives
p. 190 Courtesy of the Walt Disney Archives
p. 191 Courtesy the Geronimi Family Collection
p. 194 Courtesy of the Walt Disney Archives
p. 200 Courtesy of Don Peri
p. 201 Courtesy of the Walt Disney Archives
p. 204 Courtesy of the Walt Disney Archives
p. 207 Courtesy of Pete Docter
p. 208–209 (all) Courtesy of the Walt Disney Archives
p. 210–212 (all) Courtesy of the Walt Disney Archives
p. 213 Courtesy of the Walt Disney Archives
p. 214–217 (all) Courtesy of the Walt Disney Archives
p. 218 Courtesy of the Walt Disney Archives
p. 219 Courtesy of Walt Disney Studios Music Department
p. 220–221 (all) Courtesy of the Walt Disney Archives
p. 222 (left) Courtesy of the Walt Disney Archives
p. 222 (right) Courtesy of Jack Kinney Family Collection
p. 223 Courtesy of the Walt Disney Archives
p. 225 Courtesy of the Walt Disney Archives
p. 230 Courtesy of the Walt Disney Archives
p. 232 Courtesy of the Walt Disney Archives
p. 233 Courtesy of Woolie Reitherman collection
p. 234 (left and right) Courtesy of Woolie Reitherman collection
p. 235 Courtesy of the Walt Disney Archives
p. 236–237 (all) Courtesy of the Walt Disney Archives
p. 239 Courtesy of Woolie Reitherman collection
p. 240 (left and right) Courtesy of Woolie Reitherman collection
p. 241 Courtesy of the Walt Disney Archives
p. 242 Courtesy of the Walt Disney Archives
p. 244 (top and botom) Courtesy of the Walt Disney Archives
p. 246 Courtesy of the Walt Disney Archives
p. 247 Courtesy of the Walt Disney Archives
p. 248–250 (all) Courtesy of the Walt Disney Archives
p. 251 Courtesy of Woolie Reitherman collection
p. 252 (left) Courtesy of Glen Keane collection
p. 252 (right) Courtesy of John Musker collection
p. 253 (top and bottom) Courtesy of Glen Keane collection
p. 254 Courtesy of Woolie Reitherman collection
p. 256–261 (all) Courtesy of the Walt Disney Archives
p. 266 Courtesy of the Walt Disney Archives
p. 271 (top and bottom) Courtesy of the Walt Disney Archives
p. 272–273 (both) Courtesy of the Walt Disney Archives
p. 274 (left and right) Courtesy of the Walt Disney Archives
p. 275 (top and botom) Courtesy of the Walt Disney Archives
p. 276 Courtesy of the Walt Disney Archives
p. 277 (left and right) Courtesy of the Walt Disney Archives
p. 320 Courtesy of Don Peri
p. 321 Photo by Sue Peri, courtesy of Don Peri
p. 350 Courtesy of the Walt Disney Archives

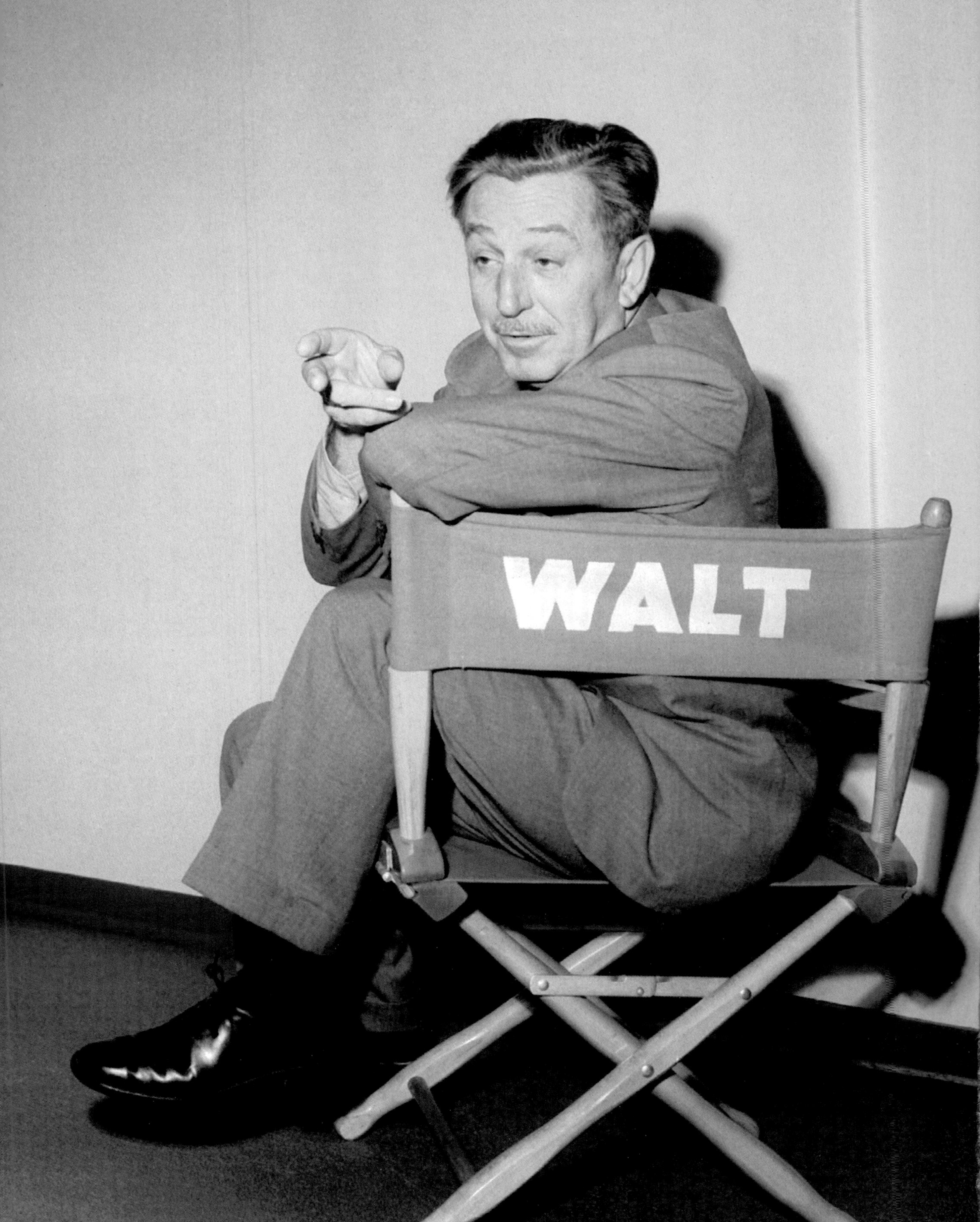
WALT